Thyroid Eye Disease: Understanding Graves' Ophthalmopathy

Thyroid Eye Disease: Understanding Graves' Ophthalmopathy

Editor: Edgar Harrison

FOSTER ACADEMICS

www.fosteracademics.com

www.fosteracademics.com

FOSTER ACADEMICS

Cataloging-in-Publication Data

Thyroid eye disease : understanding graves' ophthalmopathy / edited by Edgar Harrison.
p. cm.
Includes bibliographical references and index.
ISBN 978-1-64646-549-1
1. Thyroid eye disease. 2. Graves' disease. 3. Eye--Diseases.
4. Thyroid gland--Diseases. I. Harrison, Edgar.
RE715.T48 T49 2023
617.7--dc23

Foster Academics,
118-35 Queens Blvd., Suite 400,
Forest Hills, NY 11375, USA

ISBN 978-1-64646-549-1 (Hardback)

Contents

Preface

Graves' disease refers to a disorder affecting the immune system which leads to the over production of thyroid hormones. Graves' ophthalmopathy, also called Graves' orbitopathy, is an autoimmune disease affecting the retro-ocular tissues in patients having Graves' disease. It is primarily the disease of the orbit and can have severe implications, such as loss of sight. It causes swelling in the area around the eyes, which causes bulging of the eyes. The symptoms of Graves' ophthalmopathy include double vision, bulging eyes, swelling in the eyelids, vision loss, sensitivity to light, redness or inflammation, and difficulty in moving eyes. This disease results in increased extraocular muscle volume and orbital fat in the orbital space. The targets of autoimmune attack within Graves' ophthalmopathy are the fibroblasts residing in the orbital tissues. Radiation, immunosuppression and surgical procedures, like orbital decompression surgery, eye muscle surgery and eyelid surgery are utilized to treat severe forms of this disease. This book contains some path-breaking studies on Graves' Ophthalmopathy. It is a valuable compilation of topics, ranging from the basic to the most complex advancements in the study of this disease. The book will serve as a reference to a broad spectrum of readers.

This book has been the outcome of endless efforts put in by authors and researchers on various issues and topics within the field. The book is a comprehensive collection of significant researches that are addressed in a variety of chapters. It will surely enhance the knowledge of the field among readers across the globe.

It gives us an immense pleasure to thank our researchers and authors for their efforts to submit their piece of writing before the deadlines. Finally in the end, I would like to thank my family and colleagues who have been a great source of inspiration and support.

Editor

1

Teprotumumab as a Novel Therapy for Thyroid-Associated Ophthalmopathy

Terry J. Smith[1,2*]

[1] *Department of Ophthalmology and Visual Sciences, Kellogg Eye Center, Ann Arbor, MI, United States,* [2] *Division of Metabolism, Endocrinology, and Diabetes, Department of Internal Medicine, University of Michigan Medical School, Ann Arbor, MI, United States*

***Correspondence:**
Terry J. Smith
terrysmi@med.umich.edu

Thyroid-associated ophthalmopathy (TAO) has remained a vexing and poorly managed autoimmune component of Graves' disease where the tissues surrounding the eye and in the upper face become inflamed and undergo remodeling. This leads to substantial facial disfigurement while in its most severe forms, TAO can threaten eye sight. In this brief paper, I review some of the background investigation that has led to development of teprotumumab as the first and only US FDA approved medical therapy for TAO. This novel treatment was predicated on recognition that the insulin-like growth factor I receptor plays an important role in the pathogenesis of TAO. It is possible that a similar involvement of that receptor in other autoimmune disease may lead to additional indications for this and alternative insulin-like growth factor I receptor-inhibiting strategies.

Keywords: autoimmune, insulin-like growth factor I receptor, monoclonal antibody, Graves' disease, thyroid-associated ophthalmopathy, connective tissue

INTRODUCTION

Thyroid-associated ophthalmopathy (TAO), also known as thyroid eye disease or Graves' orbitopathy, remains a vexing disease process most frequently occurring in individuals with Graves' disease (GD) (1). Less commonly, TAO can occur in patients with Hashimoto's thyroiditis. Autoimmunity similar to that found in the thyroid is presumed to underlie TAO, although responses to the specific autoantigen(s) in the two tissues may not be identical. The medical treatment of TAO has been woefully inadequate, in large part as a consequence of our poor understanding of its pathogenesis. Thus, until very recently, no drug had been approved by the U.S. Food and Drug Administration (FDA) for TAO. TAO can present with a variety of physical signs and symptoms, many of which are shared with other more common diseases of the tissues surrounding the eye. In this brief review, I attempt to provide the historical background underpinning efforts to identify an effective and safe medical therapy for TAO. That direction of study has yielded substantial evidence for meaningful involvement of the insulin-like growth factor-I receptor (IGF-IR) in the development of TAO (2). At the heart of this evidence is the over-expression of IGF-IR by orbital fibroblasts, T and B cells (3–5), the generation of autoantibodies targeting the receptor in patients with GD (3, 6), and the apparent physical and functional collaboration between IGF-IR and the thyrotropin receptor (TSHR) (7). Based nearly entirely on a series of studies conducted *in vitro*, a β arrestin-biased agonist that acts as an IGF-IR inhibitor, teprotumumab, now marketed as Tepezza, was repurposed from its initially intended clinical use as an anti-neoplastic agent, to its consideration as a medical therapy for TAO (8). On the strength of two successful clinical trials involving patients with active, moderate to severe disease, teprotumumab has recently been approved by the FDA for use in TAO (9). This approval has therefore ushered in to clinical practice a new era for medically managing this serious and historically underserved manifestation of thyroid autoimmunity.

CURRENT UNDERSTANDING OF TAO PATHOGENESIS

A number of key insights have been generated in the recent past by several laboratory groups across North America and abroad. At the heart of TAO is the growing and sometimes reluctant recognition that orbital fibroblasts from diseased orbits (GD-OF) comprise a heterogeneous cell population and are involved in pathogenesis as a consequence of the unique presence of $CD34^+$ cells where CD34 indicates a cell phenotype with specific characteristics (10–14). These cells have been proposed as the dominant mediators of TAO development by virtue of their extraordinary responsiveness to inflammatory mediators such as cytokines and growth factors (15–19) (**Figure 1**). They express key promoters of inflammation including both prostaglandin endoperoxide H synthase 1 and 2, the latter of which is highly inducible (15, 16, 20, 21) and 15-lipoxygenase (22). We contend that the identification of $CD34^+CXCR4^+Col\ I^+$ fibroblasts in the TAO orbit as a discrete subset of GD-OF and their putative derivation from circulating fibrocytes represents a plausible explanation for the markedly heterogeneous behavior found among these disease-derived fibroblasts (14). The aggregate of these markers identifies fibrocytes and distinguishes them from fibroblasts and other cell types (23). These cells can undergo adipogenic differentiation (24). The Thy-1^- subset of GD-OF is particularly susceptible to pro-adipogenic factors while those of the Thy-1^+ phenotype can undergo differentiation into myofibroblasts through the actions of TGF-β and the activation of the Smad pathway (25, 26). $CD34^+$ OF exhibit unique phenotypic attributes which can be attributed, at least in part, to their promiscuous expression of the autoimmune regulator protein (27). They synthesize several proteins, the expressions of which were previously thought to be restricted to the thyroid, including TSHR, thyroglobulin, thyroperoxidase, and sodium iodide symporter (28, 29). But the expression of tissue-specific proteins that behave as autoantigens is not limited to those relevant to the thyroid. Fibrocytes have also been found to express those protein antigens implicated in type 1 diabetes mellitus (29). Fibrocytes cross-talk with T cells, and especially with those polarized to the Th17 paradigm, the cytokines from which appear to play important roles in driving orbital inflammation in TAO (30). IL-17A promotes the expression of regulated on activation, normal T cell expressed and secreted (RANTES, CCL5) by orbital fibroblasts, effects mediated through the CD40/CD154 (CD40 ligand) bridge (31).

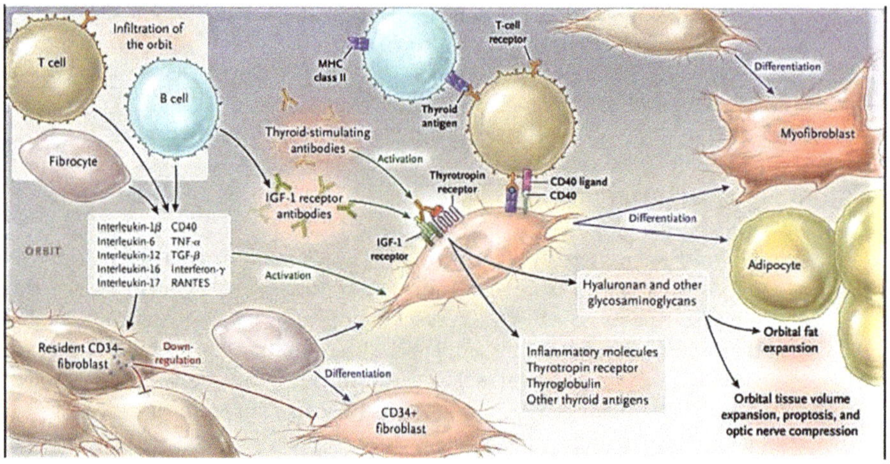

FIGURE 1 | Cartoon proposed model of thyroid-associated ophthalmopathy (TAO) pathogenesis. At the center of the disease are orbital fibroblasts which exhibit particularly robust responses to inflammatory mediators. Among them are $CD34^+$ cells which we propose derive from fibrocytes, monocyte-derived progenitor cells trafficked from bone marrow. Fibrocytes circulate in Graves' disease at higher frequency than that found in healthy individuals. When cultivated from the peripheral circulation, fibrocytes express several thyroid-specific proteins, including thyrotropin receptor (TSHR), thyroglobulin, thyroperoxidase, and sodium-iodide symporter. They also express Class II major histocompatibility complex (MHC) when unstimulated by interferon γ and can present antigens. When exposed to the appropriate culture conditions, they undergo differentiation into myofibroblasts (through Smad pathway activation by TGF-β) and adipocytes (through the activation of PPAR-γ). Many of the genes expressed by fibrocytes are detected at considerably lower levels in $CD34^+$ orbital fibroblasts. We have found that these lower levels of expression result from the actions of Slit2. When activated, $CD34^+$ fibrocytes and $CD34^+$ fibroblasts generate several pro-inflammatory or anti-inflammatory cytokines, including interleukins 1β, 6, 8, 10, 12, 16, tumor necrosis factor α, and regulated on activation, normal T expressed and secreted (RANTES), CXCL-12 and CD40-CD154. Both $CD34^+$ and $CD34^-$ orbital fibroblasts cell-surface display insulin-like growth factor-I receptor (IGF-IR). Orbital fibroblasts express three mammalian hyaluronan synthase isoenzymes and UDP glucose dehydrogenase and synthesize hyaluronan, the glycosaminoglycan associated with expanding orbital tissue in TAO. The vast majority of hyaluronan synthesis occurs in $CD34^-$ orbital fibroblasts. From N. Engl. J. Med, Smith T.J. and Hegedus L., Graves' Disease, 375; 1552-1565.

GD-OF and fibrocytes have been found to express TSHR (14, 32). This receptor was subsequently found to be functional and could mediate effects of both TSH and thyroid-stimulating autoantibodies (7, 14). Activation of several genes, including those encoding cytokines implicated in the pathogenesis of TAO, has been reported (19, 33–35). Fibrocytes are trafficked to sites of tissue injury through several chemokine networks, most notably the CXCL-12/CXCR4 pathway (36) which is under the control of TSHR signaling. A potentially important molecular conduit, the activation of which can influence gene expression in GD-OF, is the CD40–CD154 bridge (21, 37). Ligation of CD40 displayed on the surface of these cells results in substantial upregulation of hyaluronan synthesis and the generation of prostaglandin E_2 through the induction of prostaglandin endoperoxide H synthase 2.

TAO HAS LONG BEEN A DISEASE THE TREATMENT FOR WHICH EXEMPLIFIES INADEQUACY

Despite its initial published descriptions, dating to the 19th century (38), precious little progress had been made in identifying safe and effective medical therapy for TAO (39, 40). Of the available medications, glucocorticoids have been the most widely used. Standardization of their use, including indications, exclusions, treatment duration, and dosages has yet to be established with placebo-controlled, prospective, and adequately powered clinical trials. Some clinicians taking care of patients with TAO extoll them as the "gold standard", but the basis for this often strongly expressed opinion appears to rest on dubious grounds rather than on firm scientific evidence. Both oral and intravenous routes of steroid administration have been advocated. More recent reports suggest that IV pulse may be more effective and associated with fewer side effects than those delivered by the oral route (41). But even staunch advocates of steroid use in TAO typically concede that these agents fail to consistently provide benefit to patients and that only 50% respond meaningfully (42). Further, many experts acknowledge that responses to steroids are essentially limited to amelioration of inflammatory signs and symptoms. Among the most informative reports of steroid use in active, moderate to severe TAO, was that of Bartalena and colleagues (43). They examined three different cumulative dosages (2.25, 4.98, and 7.47 g) administered as 12 weekly infusions. Their study demonstrated that short-term response, as measured by improvement in the clinical activity score (CAS), was greatest in those receiving the highest dosage. Patients receiving 7.47 g also showed a 0.6 mm proptosis reduction at 12 weeks compared to baseline, a result widely considered to be lacking clinical importance. Evidence suggests that glucocorticoids in combination with external beam radiation may be somewhat superior to steroids alone (44–47). Other agents have been proposed for combination with steroids, including rituximab, mycophenolate and azathioprine (48–50). In my view, whether used as a single agent or in combination with radiotherapy, systemic steroids should play a progressively less frequent role in the treatment of TAO. In distinction, locally administered steroids, such as those delivered in eye drops or intraorbital injections, may have some utility, especially in mild but symptomatic disease. Steroid therapy in TAO poses substantial risk. Given their limited efficacy, these agents are deemed unsafe since they are associated with several potentially serious side-effects, including hypertension, bone loss, psychiatric illness, and peptic ulcer disease. Moreover, high-dosage intravenous steroids can deleteriously affect liver function and in rare cases, result in fatal hepatic failure (48, 51, 52). Having articulated these objections to steroid use, several biological agents are currently under development or already have been repurposed for potential use in severe TAO. Among them tocilizumab, an IL-6 receptor antagonist, has been subjected to a placebo controlled trial of 32 patients with steroid-resistant TAO at 10 performance sites in Spain (53). Drug or placebo was administered at weeks 0, 4, 8, and 12. Of those receiving active drug, 93.3% met the primary response of a ≥2 point reduction in CAS at week 16 while 58.8% of those treated with placebo met the response ($p = 0.04$). Notably, a 1.5 mm reduction in proptosis was detected in those receiving the active drug *versus* 0.0 mm in the placebo group at week 16. Observations made later in the study revealed that the small change in proptosis seen with tocilizumab was not durable. A clinical trial of belimumab is currently underway for TAO (54). In addition, preliminary studies examined the potential for immune retolerizing of TSHR in GD and TAO (55).

IGF-IR AND ITS SIGNALING PATHWAY AS THERAPEUTICALLY EXPLOITABLE TARGETS

The IGF-I pathway is complex, comprising several molecules that either enhance signaling initiated by IGF-I or play inhibitory/modulatory roles. IGF-I influences regulation of both normal and abnormal development, metabolism/energy expenditure and immune surveillance (56, 57). It is generated either by the liver or in peripheral tissues. In the latter, it can act locally. IGF binding proteins (IGF-IBP), of which six have been identified, can enhance the half-life of IGF-I within the circulation (58) and can modulate the interactions between IGF-I and IGF-IR (59). The actions of IGF-I and IGF-II are mediated through their interactions with the two cell surface receptors, IGF-IR and IGF-IIR/mannose-6-phosphate receptor (60). IGF-IR is a member of the insulin receptor (IR) family of cell surface-displayed tyrosine kinases. We had suggested some time ago that this pathway might be exploitable for the therapeutic targeting of autoimmune diseases, including GD and TAO (61). The first clue that the IGF-IR pathway might be involved in TAO emanated from the laboratory of Kendall–Taylor nearly three decades ago (62). They reported that IgGs found in sera of patients with TAO could compete for binding of radiolabeled IGF-I to the surface of orbital fibroblasts collected from patients with the disease. While the identity of the binding site was surmised to be IGF-IR by that group, results in a later study conducted by those in another laboratory definitively demonstrated that IGF-IR harbored the binding site and therefore the epitope for autoantibodies circulating in TAO (3). These later studies indicated that IgGs from patients with GD (GD-IgG) could initiate signaling and that the PI3 kinase/FRAP/mTor/p70^{S6k} and Erk p42/44 pathways become activated in GD-OF (3, 6) and thyroid epithelial cells (63). Those studies failed to examine whether GD-IgGs could initiate autophosphorylation of tyrosine residues intrinsic to IGF-IR. Their findings did however raise the possibility that GD-IgG was initiating signaling directly through interactions with IGF-IR. Subsequently, several laboratory groups reexamined this question that GD-IgGs activate IGF-IR autophosphorylation. One group reported that GD-IgGs from a subset of patients could activate receptor kinase activity above levels seen with control (healthy) IgGs (64). In contrast, other investigators have failed to detect GD-IgG-stimulation of IGF-IR kinase activity (65, 66). The concept of anti-IGF-IR antibodies playing a role in TAO has been vigorously argued against by some investigators [summarized in ref (2)]. Their viewpoints have relied heavily on selective reviews of the literature rather than on comprehensive consideration and reconciliation of opposing opinions. The discrepancy between the findings generated by several laboratory groups has yet to be explained satisfactorily. It should be noted that the methods used for detecting IGF-IR activity have varied widely, experimental conditions have not been standardized, and cell treatment protocols have generally relied on single time points, potentially inappropriate target cells, and the uniform absence of assessing endogenous IGF-I concentrations in the culture media. GD-IgG was found to induce the synthesis of hyaluronan in orbital fibroblasts from patients with TAO but not in orbital fibroblasts from healthy individuals (67). Those effects could be mimicked by recombinant IGF-I but not by recombinant human TSH. Subsequent to the detection of anti-IGF-IR autoantibodies in GD and TAO, Tsui et al. reported that IGF-IR and TSHR co-localize in thyroid epithelial cells, orbital fibroblasts and *in situ* in orbital fat (7). Further, in pull-down studies, these investigators found that monoclonal antibodies directed against either receptor protein could precipitate both. They also found that the IGF-IR inhibitory monoclonal antibody, 1H7, could attenuate the activation of Erk 42/44 MAPK initiated by rhTSH, GD-IgG and IGF-I. Those results suggested that signaling emanating from either receptor depended on the activation of IGF-IR. Another report demonstrated that the cellular distribution of IGF-IR was altered in fibroblasts derived from TSHR-null mice (68). A similar pattern of response to disease-derived IgGs was subsequently observed in synovial fibroblasts from patients with rheumatoid arthritis (69). Based on the aggregate of findings implicating IGF-IR in the pathogenesis of TAO, the receptor became a plausible therapeutic target. Further it was suggested that multiple autoimmune diseases, besides GD and rheumatoid arthritis, might share IGF-IR-dependent disease mechanisms and that therapeutic development could be successfully focused on that receptor (61).

TWO CLINICAL TRIALS OF TEPROTUMUMAB REVEAL AN EFFECTIVE AND SAFE THERAPY FOR MODERATE TO SEVERE, ACTIVE TAO

Phase 2 Trial

Based on the preclinical studies outlined above, which demonstrated the plausibility of IGF-IR inhibition as a potential treatment strategy for GD and TAO, an initial trial was organized by River Vision Development Company beginning in 2010. The phase 2 study of teprotumumab (RV001, R1507), a fully human monoclonal β-arrestin biased agonist IGF-IR inhibitor, involved the repurposing of that drug from its initially intended use in cancer where it had proven ineffective in treating several disease types (70, 71). This trial was a double-masked, randomized, placebo-controlled and multi-centered study with 15 performance sites in North America and Europe (72). Enrolment commenced on 2 July, 2013 and was completed 23 September, 2015. Exclusionary factors included uncontrolled hyper- and hypothyroidism, a history of receiving >1 g of steroids for the treatment of TAO, prior rehabilitative ocular surgeries for TAO and prior treatment with either rituximab or tocilizumab. A total of 88 patients, age range from 18 to 75 years, with moderate to severe, active [clinical activity scores (CAS) ≥4 on a 7-point scale] TAO were randomized to receive either teprotumumab or placebo in a 1:1 ratio. Participants were uniformly within 9 months of the onset of TAO, included both cigarette smokers and non-smokers, and were clinically euthyroid. Once randomized, patients were included in the intention-to-treat (ITT) cohort. Participants in both treatment groups received dosing every 3 weeks for a total of eight infusions over a 24-week intervention phase. The primary response was defined as improvement in the study (worse) eye of both, improvement in CAS of ≥2 points, AND reduction in proptosis of ≥2 mm. This improvement must have occurred in the absence of a similar degree of worsening in the fellow eye. Secondary endpoints, measured as independent variables, included improvement from baseline of CAS of ≥2 points, reduction in proptosis of ≥2 mm, improvement in subjective diplopia, and improved results from a fully validated quality of life questionnaire (GO-QoL). The occurrence and severity of adverse events were also assessed. Any subjects failing to complete the 24-week treatment phase or the assessment at week 24 for any reason were considered treatment failures.

The responses used to judge drug efficacy included reduction in CAS, proptosis, improvement in diplopia, and GO-QoL. These parameters were comparable at the baseline assessment in the two treatment arms. Despite attempts to stratify participants with regard to cigarette smoking, an imbalance in group assignment was detected, with a great number who used tobacco randomized to the placebo group. Analysis of the results demonstrated that of those in the ITT group receiving teprotumumab, 29 of 42 (69%) exhibited a response at 24 weeks. In contrast, nine of 45 (20%) patients receiving placebo responded ($p < 0.001$). Similar numbers of participants in the two treatment arms completed the intervention phase (87% in the placebo and 88% in the teprotumumab cohorts). The time to response was considerably shorter in the teprotumumab cohort than in those receiving placebo. The onset of response was very rapid. Nearly one-half of those receiving teprotumumab achieved the primary response at week 6, *i.e.* those who had received the half-dose and a single full-dose. The proportion of patients achieving a response was greater in the teprotumumab group and continued to increase throughout the duration of the treatment phase with striking differences compared to placebo which continued to be significant at every time point (all $p < 0.001$). When the responses were graded, considerably more patients exhibited a high response at week 24 (≥3 point improvement in CAS and ≥3 mm proptosis reduction in the study eye). With regard to the secondary outcomes, those patients receiving teprotumumab responded with a change in proptosis from baseline and CAS from baseline when compared to those receiving placebo. Both responses were significantly different when compared to controls at the 6-week time point ($p < 0.001$ for both), and the differences continued to increase throughout the treatment phase which ended at week 24 (both $p < 0.001$). On the basis of this trial, the FDA designated teprotumumab a "breakthrough" therapy for TAO.

Phase 3 Trial

A pivotal phase 3 study was initiated shortly after the results of the phase 2 trial had been reported (73). The study was organized and funded by Horizon Pharmaceutical (now Horizon Therapeutics) and included many of the same investigators and institutions participating in the preceding phase 2 trial. It was conducted between October 24, 2017 and August 31, 2018, when 107 patients were screened and 83 underwent randomization (**Figure 2A**). The trial followed an experimental

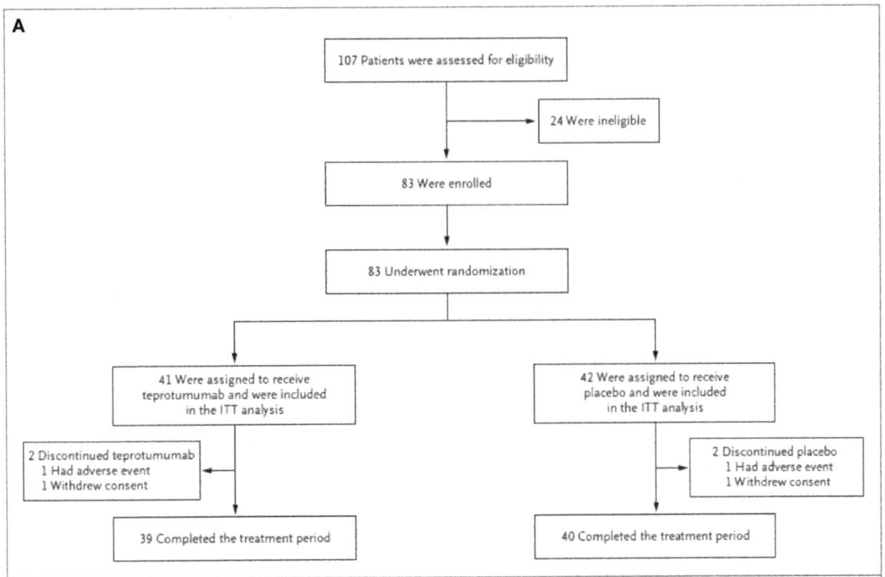

B

Efficacy Outcomes	Teprotumumab	Placebo	Difference (95% CI)	P Value
Primary outcome of proptosis response at wk 24				
In the ITT population — % of patients (no./total no.)	83 (34/41)	10 (4/42)	73 (59 to 88)	<0.001
In the per-protocol population — % of patients (no./total no.)	88 (29/33)	12 (4/34)	76 (61 to 92)	<0.001
Secondary outcomes in the ITT population				
Overall response at wk 24 — % of patients (no./total no.)	78 (32/41)	7 (3/42)	71 (56 to 86)	<0.001
Clinical Activity Score of 0 or 1 at wk 24 — % of patients (no./total no.)	59 (24/41)	21 (9/42)	36 (17 to 55)	<0.001
Mean change in proptosis from baseline through wk 24 — mm	−2.82±0.19	−0.54±0.19	−2.28 (−2.77 to −1.80)	<0.001
Diplopia response at wk 24 — % of patients (no./total no. with diplopia at baseline)	68 (19/28)	29 (8/28)	39 (16 to 63)	0.001
Mean change in GO-QOL score from baseline through wk 24	13.79±2.07	4.43±2.10	9.36 (4.08 to 14.64)	<0.001

FIGURE 2 | (A) Trial profile. **(B)** Efficacy endpoints. * CMH weighting was used to estimate the common risk difference and the 95% Confidence Interval (95% CI) of the common risk difference for the primary and secondary endpoints of overall responder, percent with CAS 0 or 1, and diplopia responder; least squares mean difference was calculated for secondary endpoints of change in proptosis from baseline and change in Graves' Orbitopathy quality of life (GO-QOL) questionnaire from baseline using the Mixed-Model Repeated-Measures (MMRM) analysis of covariance (ANCOVA) model described below. ¥ 28 patients in each treatment group had diplopia at baseline ‡ GO-QOL score was calculated and transformed to a 0 to 100 scale. Transformed score = [(sum of each score − number of completed items)/(2 * number of completed items)] * 100 § Change from baseline in proptosis or GO-QOL as a continuous variable is based on MMRM ANCOVA model with an unstructured covariance matrix including the following terms: baseline score, tobacco use status (non-user, user), treatment group, visit, and visit-by-treatment and visit-by-baseline-score interactions; data presented as least squares mean ± standard error. All analyses were controlled for multiplicity. From N. Engl. J. Med, Douglas R.S, Kahaly G.J., Patel A., Sile E.H.Z., Thompson R et al. Teprotumumab for the treatment of active thyroid eye disease. 382; 341-352.

protocol that was very similar to that of the earlier study. It allowed a widened patient age limit (18 years to 80 years) and the inclusion of a study extension, which enabled treatment cross-over for patients failing to respond during the 24-week treatment period and those who had responded initially and then relapsed. Individuals with a history of inflammatory bowel disease were excluded since at least one participating patient in the earlier trial with that diagnosis experienced worsening bowel symptoms. The remainder of the inclusion and exclusion criteria were unchanged from the phase 2 trial. The primary endpoint was proptosis responder rate (percentage of patients with ≥2 mm reduction in the study eye without ≥2 mm increase in the fellow eye) at week 24 for teprotumumab *versus* placebo. Secondary outcomes included overall responder rate (the primary outcome of the phase 2 study) which was defined as the percentage of patients with both ≥2-point reduction in CAS AND ≥2 mm reduction in proptosis in the study eye in the absence of a corresponding worsening in the fellow eye, percentage of patients with a CAS 0 or 1, and diplopia improvement at week 24 and change in GO-QOL overall score through week 24. Unlike the phase 2 trial, this study included an extension. Specifically, those patients who did not achieve the primary

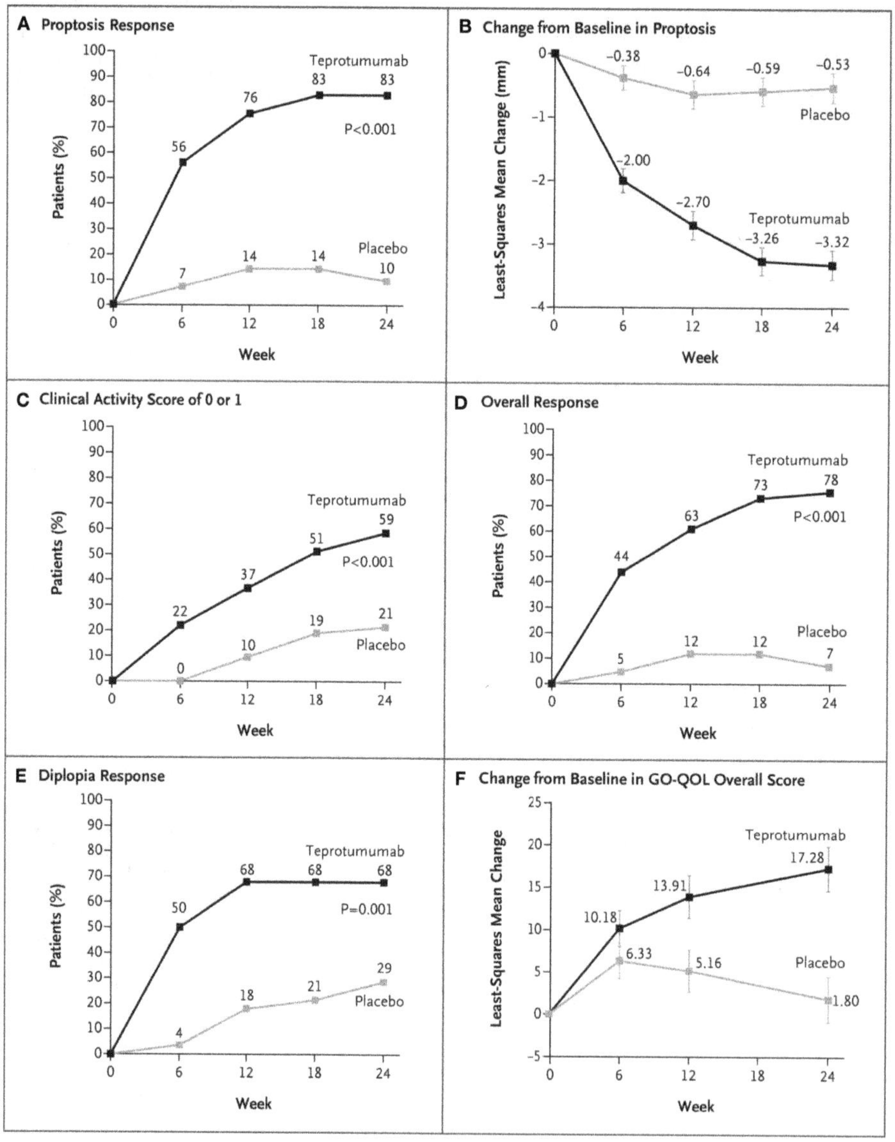

FIGURE 3 | **(A)** Proptosis responder analysis (percent of patients with ≥2 mm reduction in proptosis from baseline in the study eye). **(B)** Change from baseline in proptosis (least squares mean ± standard error). **(C)** Percent of patients with clinical activity score (CAS) of 0 or 1 in the study eye. **(D)** Overall responder rate (percent of patients with ≥2-point reduction in CAS and ≥2 mm reduction in proptosis from baseline in the study eye). **(E)** Diplopia response (percent of patients with improvement of at least one grade from baseline). **(F)** Change from baseline in transformed GO-QOL score (least squares mean ± standard error). From N. Engl. J. Med, Douglas R.S, Kahaly G.J., Patel A., Sile E.H.Z., Thompson R et al. Teprotumumab for the treatment of active thyroid eye disease. 382; 341-352.

outcome *i.e.* the proptosis non-responders, were eligible for participation in an open-label extension study (OPTIC-X (NCT03461211)]. This trial involved eight additional infusions of teprotumumab. Those patients not included in the extension were followed for 48 weeks. Those patients who responded during the initial treatment phase, regardless of treatment arm but then relapsed during follow-up could also enter the extension study.

Efficacy outcomes are shown in **Figure 2B**. The results from the trial revealed that 9.5% of patients receiving placebo achieved the primary response compared with 82.9% of those treated with teprotumumab at week 24 (delta 73.45%; 95% CI 58.89 to 88.01%; $p < 0.001$) (**Figure 3A**). A majority of patients responding did so at week 6. Mean proptosis response from baseline with teprotumumab at week 24 was −3.32 mm *versus* −0.53 in placebo or a mean difference from the placebo group of 2.79 mm (**Figure 3B**).

Secondary outcomes were achieved by significantly more patients receiving teprotumumab than those in the placebo cohort. CAS scores of 0 or 1 (**Figure 3C**) and over-all responders were also more numerous in the teprotumumab group at all study visits (**Figure 3D**). At baseline, both treatment groups included 28 patients with diplopia;

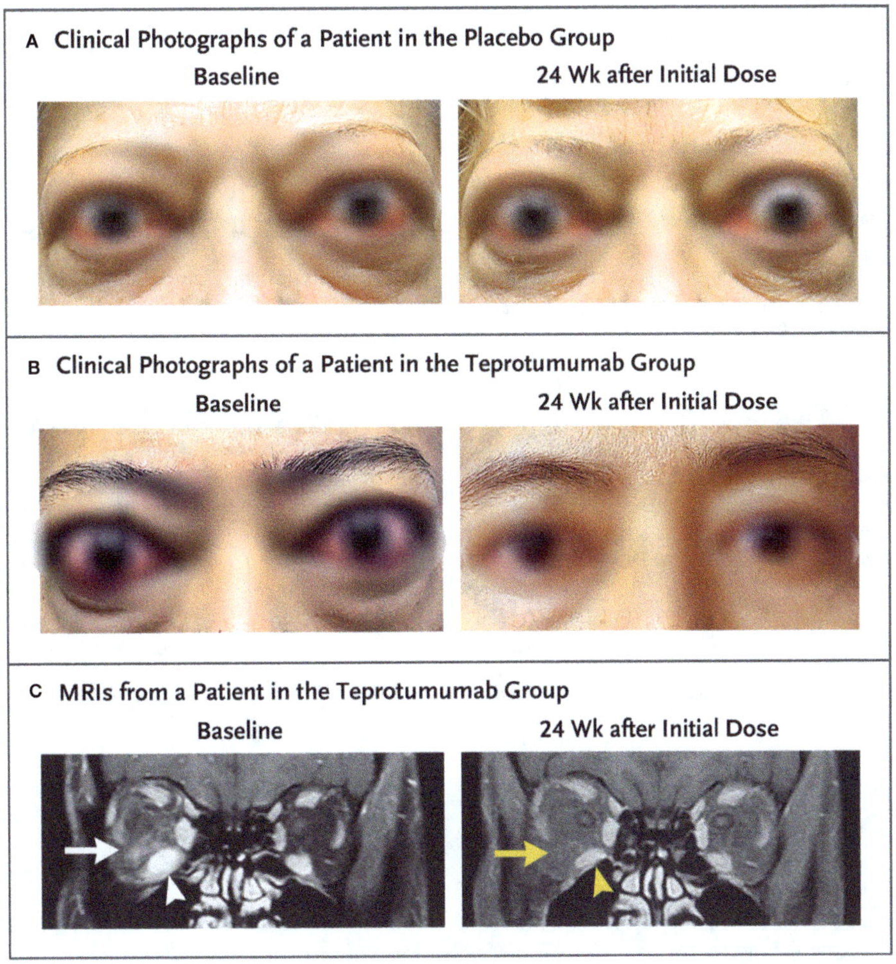

FIGURE 4 | Facial photographic images and MRIs at Baseline and 24 Weeks following treatment with either placebo or teprotumumab. **(A)** Clinical photographs of a patient receiving placebo. At baseline, the patient exhibits substantial proptosis (left eye, 29 mm and right eye, 27 mm) as well as multiple inflammatory signs (left eye Clinical Activity Score of 7 and right eye 5). At week 24, considerable proptosis and inflammatory signs remain. **(B)** Images of a teprotumumab-treated patient. Baseline proptosis (both eyes 24 mm), edema, upper and lower eyelid retraction, and multiple inflammatory signs (CAS 5 bilaterally). At week 24, considerable bilateral reductions in proptosis (−5 mm) and CAS (−4 points). **(C)** Coronal, contrast-enhanced, fat-saturated, T1-weighted MRIs in a single patient receiving teprotumumab at baseline and at week 24. Note marked enhancement of the inferior rectus muscle (white arrowhead) and orbital fat (white arrow) as well as inferior rectus muscle enlargement. At week 24, resolved inferior rectus muscle (yellow arrowhead) enhancement and orbital fat (yellow arrow). The muscle volume was reduced by 49% (yellow arrowhead). Proptosis reduction decreased from 23 mm at baseline to 18 mm at week 24. From N. Engl. J. Med, Douglas R.S, Kahaly G.J., Patel A., Sile E.H.Z., Thompson R. et al. Teprotumumab for the treatment of active thyroid eye disease. 382; 341–352.

improvement of ≥1 diplopia grade was experienced in 50.0% of patients receiving teprotumumab compared to 3.6% of those administered placebo at week 6. Diplopia improved with teprotumumab, regardless of disease severity at baseline when compared to placebo (**Figure 3E**) as did overall quality of life using the GO-QOL score (**Figure 3F**).

Additional assessments in the phase 3 trial were "before and after" facial photographs (**Figures 4A** and **4B**) and limited orbital imaging performed prior to and following treatment of six patients enrolled (off study protocol) at a single study site. Those imaging studies revealed decreased extraocular muscle volume with reduction of the inferior rectus muscle exhibiting the greatest change in 4/6 patients (**Figure 4C**). Orbital fat volume was reduced in two of these patients. Thus it would appear that teprotumumab affects both extraocular muscle and orbital fat compartments, in at least some patients with TAO.

CONCLUSIONS AND CONSIDERATION OF WHAT MIGHT LAY AHEAD FOR TEPROTUMUMAB IN TAO AND BEYOND

In aggregate, the two clinical trials demonstrate the substantial potential for IGF-IR inhibition in the treatment of active, moderate to severe TAO. Because both phase 2 and phase 3 trials excluded TAO of a duration longer than 9 months and did not allow enrollment of individuals with sight-threatening disease, neither study could inform the potential impact of teprotumumab in patients with either long-standing disease or compressive optic neuropathy. Thus, additional studies examining these patients will broaden our insights into the temporal dimensions of benefitand durability the drug can provide. Since its approval by the US FDA in January 2020 (9), case reports have revealed potential effectiveness in clinical stable TAO (74) and in worsening compressive optic neuropathy (75, 76). In addition, the impact of teprotumumab on thyroidfunctioninpatientsretaining intact thyroid glands should be assessed prospectively. Since other autoimmune diseases, including rheumatoid arthritis, are also associated with abnormalities in the IGF-I/IGF-IR pathway (61, 69), the potential therapeutic effects of IGF-IR inhibition may yield advances in treatments of those conditions as well.

AUTHOR CONTRIBUTIONS

The author confirms being the sole contributor of this work and has approved it for publication.

REFERENCES

1. Smith TJ, Hegedus L. Graves' Disease. *N Engl J Med* (2016) 375:1552–65. doi: 10.1056/NEJMra1510030
2. Smith TJ, Janssen J. Insulin-like Growth Factor-I Receptor and Thyroid-Associated Ophthalmopathy. *Endocr Rev* (2019) 40:236–67. doi: 10.1210/er.2018-00066
3. Pritchard J, Han R, Horst N, Cruikshank WW, Smith TJ. Immunoglobulin activation of T cell chemoattractant expression in fibroblasts from patients with Graves' disease is mediated through the insulin-like growth factor I receptor pathway. *J Immunol (Baltimore Md 1950)* (2003) 170:6348–54. doi: 10.4049/jimmunol.170.12.6348
4. Douglas RS, Gianoukakis AG, Kamat S, Smith TJ. Aberrant expression of the insulin-like growth factor-1 receptor by T cells from patients with Graves' disease may carry functional consequences for disease pathogenesis. *J Immunol (Baltimore Md: 1950)* (2007) 178:3281–7. doi: 10.4049/jimmunol.178.5.3281
5. Douglas RS, Naik V, Hwang CJ, Afifiyan NF, Gianoukakis AG, Sand D, et al. B cells from patients with Graves' disease aberrantly express the IGF-1 receptor: implications for disease pathogenesis. *J Immunol (Baltimore Md: 1950)* (2008) 181:5768–74. doi: 10.4049/jimmunol.181.8.5768
6. Pritchard J, Horst N, Cruikshank W, Smith TJ. Igs from patients with Graves' disease induce the expression of T cell chemoattractants in their fibroblasts. *J Immunol (Baltimore Md: 1950)* (2002) 168:942–50. doi: 10.4049/jimmunol.168.2.942
7. Tsui S, Naik V, Hoa N, Hwang CJ, Afifiyan NF, Sinha Hikim A, et al. Evidence for an association between thyroid-stimulating hormone and insulin-like growth factor 1 receptors: a tale of two antigens implicated in Graves' disease. *J Immunol (Baltimore Md: 1950)* (2008) 181:4397–405. doi: 10.4049/jimmunol.181.6.4397
8. Qu X, Wu Z, Dong W, Zhang T, Wang L, Pang Z, et al. Update of IGF-1 receptor inhibitor (ganitumab, dalotuzumab, cixutumumab, teprotumumab and figitumumab) effects on cancer therapy. *Oncotarget* (2017) 8:29501–18. doi: 10.18632/oncotarget.15704
9. Markham A. Teprotumumab: First Approval. *Drugs* (2020) 80:509–12. doi: 10.1007/s40265-020-01287-y
10. Bahn RS, Gorman CA, Woloschak GE, David CS, Johnson PM, Johnson CM. Human retroocular fibroblasts in vitro: a model for the study of Graves' ophthalmopathy. *J Clin Endocrinol Metab* (1987) 65:665–70. doi: 10.1210/jcem-65-4-665
11. Smith TJ, Bahn RS, Gorman CA. Hormonal regulation of hyaluronate synthesis in cultured human fibroblasts: evidence for differences between retroocular and dermal fibroblasts. *J Clin Endocrinol Metab* (1989) 69:1019–23. doi: 10.1210/jcem-69-5-1019
12. Smith TJ, Sempowski GD, Wang HS, Del Vecchio PJ, Lippe SD, Phipps RP. Evidence for cellular heterogeneity in primary cultures of human orbital fibroblasts. *J Clin Endocrinol Metab* (1995) 80:2620–5. doi: 10.1210/jcem.80.9.7673404
13. Smith TJ, Koumas L, Gagnon A, Bell A, Sempowski GD, Phipps RP, et al. Orbital fibroblast heterogeneity may determine the clinical presentation of thyroid-associated ophthalmopathy. *J Clin Endocrinol Metab* (2002) 87:385–92. doi: 10.1210/jcem.87.1.8164
14. Douglas RS, Afifiyan NF, Hwang CJ, Chong K, Haider U, Richards P, et al. Increased generation of fibrocytes in thyroid-associated ophthalmopathy. *J Clin Endocrinol Metab* (2010) 95:430–8. doi: 10.1210/jc.2009-1614
15. Young DA, Evans CH, Smith TJ. Leukoregulin induction of protein expression in human orbital fibroblasts: evidence for anatomical site-restricted cytokine-target cell interactions. *Proc Natl Acad Sci USA* (1998) 95:8904–9. doi: 10.1073/pnas.95.15.8904
16. Han R, Tsui S, Smith TJ. Up-regulation of prostaglandin E2 synthesis by interleukin-1beta in human orbital fibroblasts involves coordinate induction of prostaglandin-endoperoxide H synthase-2 and glutathione-dependent prostaglandin E2 synthase expression. *J Biol Chem* (2002) 277:16355–64. doi: 10.1074/jbc.M111246200

17. Han R, Chen B, Smith TJ. Jak2 dampens the induction by IL-1beta of prostaglandin endoperoxide H synthase 2 expression in human orbital fibroblasts: evidence for divergent influence on the prostaglandin E2 biosynthetic pathway. *J Immunol (Baltimore Md: 1950)* (2007) 179:7147–56. doi: 10.4049/jimmunol.179.10.7147
18. Hwang CJ, Afifiyan N, Sand D, Naik V, Said J, Pollock SJ, et al. Orbital fibroblasts from patients with thyroid-associated ophthalmopathy overexpress CD40: CD154 hyperinduces IL-6, IL-8, and MCP-1. *Invest Ophthalmol Vis Sci* (2009) 50:2262–8. doi: 10.1167/iovs.08-2328
19. Raychaudhuri N, Fernando R, Smith TJ. Thyrotropin regulates IL-6 expression in CD34+ fibrocytes: clear delineation of its cAMP-independent actions. *PLoS One* (2013) 8:e75100. doi: 10.1371/journal.pone.0075100
20. Wang HS, Cao HJ, Winn VD, Rezanka LJ, Frobert Y, Evans CH, et al. Leukoregulin induction of prostaglandin-endoperoxide H synthase-2 in human orbital fibroblasts. An in vitro model for connective tissue inflammation. *J Biol Chem* (1996) 271:22718–28. doi: 10.1074/jbc.271.37.22718
21. Cao HJ, Wang HS, Zhang Y, Lin HY, Phipps RP, Smith TJ. Activation of human orbital fibroblasts through CD40 engagement results in a dramatic induction of hyaluronan synthesis and prostaglandin endoperoxide H synthase-2 expression. Insights into potential pathogenic mechanisms of thyroid-associated ophthalmopathy. *J Biol Chem* (1998) 273:29615–25. doi: 10.1074/jbc.273.45.29615
22. Chen B, Tsui S, Boeglin WE, Douglas RS, Brash AR, Smith TJ. Interleukin-4 induces 15-lipoxygenase-1 expression in human orbital fibroblasts from patients with Graves disease. Evidence for anatomic site-selective actions of Th2 cytokines. *J Biol Chem* (2006) 281:18296–306. doi: 10.1074/jbc.M603484200
23. Pilling D, Fan T, Huang D, Kaul B, Gomer RH. Identification of markers that distinguish monocyte-derived fibrocytes from monocytes, macrophages, and fibroblasts. *PLoS One* (2009) 4:e7475. doi: 10.1371/journal.pone.0007475
24. Sorisky A, Pardasani D, Gagnon A, Smith TJ. Evidence of adipocyte differentiation in human orbital fibroblasts in primary culture. *J Clin Endocrinol Metab* (1996) 81:3428–31. doi: 10.1210/jcem.81.9.8784110
25. Koumas L, Smith TJ, Phipps RP. Fibroblast subsets in the human orbit: Thy-1+ and Thy-1- subpopulations exhibit distinct phenotypes. *Eur J Immunol* (2002) 32:477–85. doi: 10.1002/1521-4141(200202)32:2<477::AID-IMMU477>3.0.CO;2-U
26. Koumas L, Smith TJ, Feldon S, Blumberg N, Phipps RP. Thy-1 expression in human fibroblast subsets defines myofibroblastic or lipofibroblastic phenotypes. *Am J Pathol* (2003) 163:1291–300. doi: 10.1016/S0002-9440(10)63488-8
27. Fernando R, Lu Y, Atkins SJ, Mester T, Branham K, Smith TJ. Expression of thyrotropin receptor, thyroglobulin, sodium-iodide symporter, and thyroperoxidase by fibrocytes depends on AIRE. *J Clin Endocrinol Metab* (2014) 99:E1236–1244. doi: 10.1210/jc.2013-4271
28. Fernando R, Atkins S, Raychaudhuri N, Lu Y, Li B, Douglas RS, et al. Human fibrocytes coexpress thyroglobulin and thyrotropin receptor. *Proc Natl Acad Sci USA* (2012) 109:7427–32. doi: 10.1073/pnas.1202064109
29. Fernando R, Vonberg A, Atkins SJ, Pietropaolo S, Pietropaolo M, Smith TJ. Human fibrocytes express multiple antigens associated with autoimmune endocrine diseases. *J Clin Endocrinol Metab* (2014) 99:E796–803. doi: 10.1210/jc.2013-3072
30. Fang S, Huang Y, Liu X, Zhong S, Wang N, Zhao B, et al. Interaction Between CCR6+ Th17 Cells and CD34+ Fibrocytes Promotes Inflammation: Implications in Graves' Orbitopathy in Chinese Population. *Invest Ophthalmol Visual Sci* (2018) 59:2604–14. doi: 10.1167/iovs.18-24008
31. Fang S, Huang Y, Wang S, Zhang Y, Luo X, Liu L, et al. IL-17A Exacerbates Fibrosis by Promoting the Proinflammatory and Profibrotic Function of Orbital Fibroblasts in TAO. *J Clin Endocrinol Metab* (2016) 101:2955–65. doi: 10.1210/jc.2016-1882
32. Heufelder AE, Dutton CM, Sarkar G, Donovan KA, Bahn RS. Detection of TSH receptor RNA in cultured fibroblasts from patients with Graves' ophthalmopathy and pretibial dermopathy. *Thyroid* (1993) 3:297–300. doi: 10.1089/thy.1993.3.297
33. Li B, Smith TJ. PI3K/AKT pathway mediates induction of IL-1RA by TSH in fibrocytes: modulation by PTEN. *J Clin Endocrinol Metab* (2014) 99:3363–72. doi: 10.1210/jc.2014-1257
34. Lu Y, Atkins SJ, Fernando R, Trierweiler A, Mester T, Grisolia ABD, et al. CD34- Orbital Fibroblasts From Patients With Thyroid-Associated Ophthalmopathy Modulate TNF-alpha Expression in CD34+ Fibroblasts and Fibrocytes. *Invest Ophthalmol Vis Sci* (2018) 59:2615–22. doi: 10.1167/iovs.18-23951
35. Fernando R, Atkins SJ, Smith TJ. Slit2 May Underlie Divergent Induction by Thyrotropin of IL-23 and IL-12 in Human Fibrocytes. *J Immunol (Baltimore Md: 1950)* (2020) 204:1724–35. doi: 10.4049/jimmunol.1900434
36. Fernando R, Atkins SJ, Smith TJ. Intersection of Chemokine and TSH Receptor Pathways in Human Fibrocytes: Emergence of CXCL-12/CXCR4 Cross Talk Potentially Relevant to Thyroid-Associated Ophthalmopathy. *Endocrinology* (2016) 157:3779–87. doi: 10.1210/en.2016-1382
37. Smith TJ, Sempowski GD, Berenson CS, Cao HJ, Wang HS, Phipps RP. Human thyroid fibroblasts exhibit a distinctive phenotype in culture: characteristic ganglioside profile and functional CD40 expression. *Endocrinology* (1997) 138:5576–88. doi: 10.1210/endo.138.12.5563
38. Warner F. Ophthalmoplegia Externa complicating a case of Graves' Disease. *Med-Chirurgical Trans* (1883) 66:107–12. doi: 10.1177/095952878306600108
39. Zhou X, Zhou D, Wang J, Chen G. Treatment strategies for Graves' ophthalmopathy: a network meta-analysis. *Br J Ophthalmol* (2020) 104:551–6. doi: 10.1136/bjophthalmol-2018-313697
40. Wang Y, Smith TJ. Current concepts in the molecular pathogenesis of thyroid-associated ophthalmopathy. *Invest Ophthalmol Vis Sci* (2014) 55:1735–48. doi: 10.1167/iovs.14-14002
41. Oray M, Abu Samra K, Ebrahimiadib N, Meese H, Foster CS. Long-term side effects of glucocorticoids. *Expert Opin Drug Saf* (2016) 15:457–65. doi: 10.1517/14740338.2016.1140743
42. Smith TJ, Bartalena L. Will biological agents supplant systemic glucocorticoids as the first-line treatment for thyroid-associated ophthalmopathy? *Eur J Endocrinol* (2019) 181:D27–43. doi: 10.1530/EJE-19-0389
43. Bartalena L, Krassas GE, Wiersinga W, Marcocci C, Salvi M, Daumerie C, et al. Efficacy and safety of three different cumulative doses of intravenous methylprednisolone for moderate to severe and active Graves' orbitopathy. *J Clin Endocrinol Metab* (2012) 97:4454–63. doi: 10.1210/jc.2012-2389
44. Marcocci C, Bartalena L, Panicucci M, Marconcini C, Cartei F, Cavallacci G, et al. Orbital cobalt irradiation combined with retrobulbar or systemic corticosteroids for Graves' ophthalmopathy: a comparative study. *Clin Endocrinol* (1987) 27:33–42. doi: 10.1111/j.1365-2265.1987.tb00836.x
45. Pinchera A, Marcocci C, Bartalena L, Panicucci M, Marconcini C, Lepri A, et al. Orbital cobalt radiotherapy and systemic or retrobulbar corticosteroids for Graves' ophthalmopathy. *Horm Res* (1987) 26:177–83. doi: 10.1159/000180698
46. Nakahara H, Noguchi S, Murakami N, Morita M, Tamaru M, Ohnishi T, et al. Graves ophthalmopathy: MR evaluation of 10-Gy versus 24-Gy irradiation combined with systemic corticosteroids. *Radiology* (1995) 196:857–62. doi: 10.1148/radiology.196.3.7644656
47. Kim JW, Lee KH, Woo YJ, Kim J, Keum KC, Yoon JS. The Effect of Systemic Steroids and Orbital Radiation for Active Graves Orbitopathy on Postdecompression Extraocular Muscle Volume. *Am J Ophthalmol* (2016) 171:11–7. doi: 10.1016/j.ajo.2016.08.010
48. Bartalena L, Baldeschi L, Boboridis K, Eckstein A, Kahaly GJ, Marcocci C, et al. The 2016 European Thyroid Association/European Group on Graves' Orbitopathy Guidelines for the Management of Graves' Orbitopathy. *Eur Thyroid J* (2016) 5:9–26. doi: 10.1159/000443828
49. Tanda ML, Piantanida E, Masiello E, Cusini C, Bartalena L. Can combination of glucocorticoids with other immunosoppressive drugs reduce the cumulative dose of glucocorticoids for moderate-to-severe and active Graves' orbitopathy? *J Endocrinol Invest* (2019) 42:351–2. doi: 10.1007/s40618-019-01015-8
50. Salvi M, Covelli D. Combined immunosuppressants and less steroids in active graves' orbitopathy? *Clin Endocrinol* (2019) 90:525–7. doi: 10.1111/cen.13917
51. Marcocci C, Watt T, Altea MA, Rasmussen AK, Feldt-Rasmussen U, Orgiazzi J, et al. Fatal and non-fatal adverse events of glucocorticoid therapy for Graves' orbitopathy: a questionnaire survey among members of the European Thyroid Association. *Eur J Endocrinol* (2012) 166:247–53. doi: 10.1530/EJE-11-0779
52. Sisti E, Coco B, Menconi F, Leo M, Rocchi R, Latrofa F, et al. Intravenous glucocorticoid therapy for Graves' ophthalmopathy and acute liver damage: an epidemiological study. *Eur J Endocrinol* (2015) 172:269–76. doi: 10.1530/EJE-14-0712

53. Perez-Moreiras JV, Gomez-Reino JJ, Maneiro JR, Perez-Pampin E, Romo Lopez A, Rodríguez Alvarez FM, et al. Efficacy of Tocilizumab in Patients With Moderate-to-Severe Corticosteroid-Resistant Graves Orbitopathy: A Randomized Clinical Trial. *Am J Ophthalmol* (2018) 195:181–90. doi: 10.1016/j.ajo.2018.07.038
54. Salvi M, Covelli D. B cells in Graves' Orbitopathy: more than just a source of antibodies? *Eye (Lond)* (2019) 33:230–4. doi: 10.1038/s41433-018-0285-y
55. Pearce SHS, Dayan C, Wraith DC, Barrell K, Olive N, Jansson L, et al. Antigen-Specific Immunotherapy with Thyrotropin Receptor Peptides in Graves' Hyperthyroidism: A Phase I Study. *Thyroid* (2019) 29(7):1003–11. doi: 10.1089/thy.2019.0036
56. Oherle K, Acker E, Bonfield M, Wang T, Gray J, Lang I, et al. Insulin-like Growth Factor 1 Supports a Pulmonary Niche that Promotes Type 3 Innate Lymphoid Cell Development in Newborn Lungs. *Immunity* (2020) 52:275–94.e279. doi: 10.1016/j.immuni.2020.01.005
57. Sadagurski M, White MF. Integrating metabolism and longevity through insulin and IGF1 signaling. *Endocrinol Metab Clin North Am* (2013) 42:127–48. doi: 10.1016/j.ecl.2012.11.008
58. Jones JII, Clemmons DR. Insulin-like growth factors and their binding proteins: biological actions. *Endocr Rev* (1995) 16:3–34. doi: 10.1210/edrv-16-1-3
59. Hwa V, Oh Y, Rosenfeld RG. The insulin-like growth factor-binding protein (IGFBP) superfamily. *Endocr Rev* (1999) 20:761–87. doi: 10.1210/edrv.20.6.0382
60. De Meyts P, Whittaker J. Structural biology of insulin and IGF1 receptors: implications for drug design. *Nat Rev Drug Discov* (2002) 1:769–83. doi: 10.1038/nrd917
61. Smith TJ. Insulin-like growth factor-I regulation of immune function: a potential therapeutic target in autoimmune diseases? *Pharmacol Rev* (2010) 62:199–236. doi: 10.1124/pr.109.002469
62. Weightman DR, Perros P, Sherif IH, Kendall-Taylor P. Autoantibodies to IGF-1 binding sites in thyroid associated ophthalmopathy. *Autoimmunity* (1993) 16:251–7. doi: 10.3109/08916939309014643
63. Gianoukakis AG, Douglas RS, King CS, Cruikshank WW, Smith TJ. Immunoglobulin G from patients with Graves' disease induces interleukin-16 and RANTES expression in cultured human thyrocytes: a putative mechanism for T-cell infiltration of the thyroid in autoimmune disease. *Endocrinology* (2006) 147:1941–9. doi: 10.1210/en.2005-1375
64. Varewijck AJ, Boelen A, Lamberts SW, Fliers E, Hofland LJ, Wiersinga WM, et al. Circulating IgGs may modulate IGF-I receptor stimulating activity in a subset of patients with Graves' ophthalmopathy. *J Clin Endocrinol Metab* (2013) 98:769–76. doi: 10.1210/jc.2012-2270
65. Minich WB, Dehina N, Welsink T, Schwiebert C, Morgenthaler NG, Kohrle J, et al. Autoantibodies to the IGF1 receptor in Graves' orbitopathy. *J Clin Endocrinol Metab* (2013) 98:752–60. doi: 10.1210/jc.2012-1771
66. Krieger CC, Neumann S, Gershengorn MC. TSH/IGF1 receptor crosstalk: Mechanism and clinical implications. *Pharmacol Ther* (2020) 209:107502. doi: 10.1016/j.pharmthera.2020.107502
67. Smith TJ, Hoa N. Immunoglobulins from patients with Graves' disease induce hyaluronan synthesis in their orbital fibroblasts through the self-antigen, insulin-like growth factor-I receptor. *J Clin Endocrinol Metab* (2004) 89:5076–80. doi: 10.1210/jc.2004-0716
68. Atkins SJ, Lentz SII, Fernando R, Smith TJ. Disrupted TSH Receptor Expression in Female Mouse Lung Fibroblasts Alters Subcellular IGF-1 Receptor Distribution. *Endocrinology* (2015) 156:4731–40. doi: 10.1210/en.2015-1464
69. Pritchard J, Tsui S, Horst N, Cruikshank WW, Smith TJ. Synovial fibroblasts from patients with rheumatoid arthritis, like fibroblasts from Graves' disease, express high levels of IL-16 when treated with Igs against insulin-like growth factor-1 receptor. *J Immunol (Baltimore Md: 1950)* (2004) 173:3564–9. doi: 10.4049/jimmunol.173.5.3564
70. Pappo AS, Patel SR, Crowley J, Reinke DK, Kuenkele KP, Chawla SP, et al. R1507, a monoclonal antibody to the insulin-like growth factor 1 receptor, in patients with recurrent or refractory Ewing sarcoma family of tumors: results of a phase II Sarcoma Alliance for Research through Collaboration study. *J Clin Oncol* (2011) 29:4541–7. doi: 10.1200/jco.2010.28.15_suppl.10000
71. Ramalingam SS, Spigel DR, Chen D, Steins MB, Engelman JA, Schneider CP, et al. Randomized phase II study of erlotinib in combination with placebo or R1507, a monoclonal antibody to insulin-like growth factor-1 receptor, for advanced-stage non-small-cell lung cancer. *J Clin Oncol* (2011) 29:4574–80. doi: 10.1200/JCO.2011.36.6799
72. Smith TJ, Kahaly GJ, Ezra DG, Fleming JC, Dailey RA, Tang RA, et al. Teprotumumab for Thyroid-Associated Ophthalmopathy. *N Engl J Med* (2017) 376:1748–61. doi: 10.1056/NEJMoa1614949
73. Douglas RS, Kahaly GJ, Patel A, Sile S, Thompson EHZ, Perdok R, et al. Teprotumumab for the Treatment of Active Thyroid Eye Disease. *N Engl J Med* (2020) 382:341–52. doi: 10.1056/NEJMoa1910434
74. Ozzello DJ, Kikkawa DO, Korn BS. Early experience with teprotumumab for chronic thyroid eye disease. *Am J Ophthalmol Case Rep* (2020) 19:100744. doi: 10.1016/j.ajoc.2020.100744
75. Sears CM, Azad AD, Dosiou C, Kossler AL. Teprotumumab for Dysthyroid Optic Neuropathy: Early Response to Therapy. *Ophthalmic Plast Reconstr Surg* (2020). doi: 10.1097/IOP.0000000000001831
76. Slentz D, Smith TJ, Kim DS, Joseph SS. Teprotumumab For Optic Neuropathy in Thyroid Eye Disease. *Arch Ophthal (In Press)* (2020).

2

Microarray Data of Lacrimal Gland Implicates Dysregulated Protein Processing in Endoplasmic Reticulum in Graves' Ophthalmopathy

Wenling Tu[1,2†], *Jia Yao*[3†], *Zhanjun Mei*[1], *Xue Jiang*[1] *and Yuhong Shi*[1*]

[1] *Department of Nuclear Medicine, The Second Affiliated Hospital of Chengdu Medical College, China National Nuclear Corporation 416 Hospital, Chengdu, China,* [2] *School of Bioscience and Technology, Chengdu Medical College, Chengdu, China,* [3] *Research and Development Center, Chengdu SuAn Technology Co., Ltd, Chengdu, China*

***Correspondence:**
Yuhong Shi
shiyuhong89@hotmail.com

[†]*These authors share first authorship*

Graves' ophthalmopathy (GO) has become one of the most common orbital diseases. Although some evidences announced the potential mechanism of pathological changes in extraocular muscle and orbital adipose tissue, little is known about that in lacrimal enlargement of GO patients. Thus, gene expression profiles of lacrimal gland derived from GO patients and normal controls were investigated using the microarray datasets of GSE105149 and GSE58331. The raw data and annotation files of GSE105149 and GSE58331 were downloaded from Gene Expression Omnibus (GEO) database. Bioinformatics including differentially expressed genes (DEGs), Gene Ontology, Kyoto Encyclopedia of Gene and Genome (KEGG) pathway, protein-protein interaction (PPI) network construction, hub gene identification, and gene set variation analysis (GSVA) were successively performed. A total of 173 overlapping DEGs in GSE105149 and GSE58331 were screened out, including 20 up-regulated and 153 down-regulated genes. Gene Ontology, KEGG and GSVA analyses of these DEGs showed that the most significant mechanism was closely associated with endoplasmic reticulum (ER). Moreover, we identified 40 module genes and 13 hub genes which were also enriched in the ER-associated terms and pathways. Among the hub genes, five genes including *HSP90AA1*, *HSP90B1*, *DNAJC10*, *HSPA5*, and *CANX* may be involved in the dysfunction of protein processing in ER. Taken together, our observations revealed a dysregulated gene network which is essential for protein processing in ER in GO patients. These findings provided a potential mechanism in the progression of lacrimal enlargement in GO patients, as a new insight into GO pathogenesis.

Keywords: Graves' ophthalmopathy, lacrimal gland, protein processing in endoplasmic reticulum, hub gene, microarray data

INTRODUCTION

Graves' ophthalmopathy (GO), also known as thyroid eye disease (TED), is an orbital disease that is uniquely linked to Graves' disease (GD), generally present in 25%–50% of GD patients (1). The main clinical features of GO include proptosis, lacrimal gland enlargement, eyelid retraction, diplopia, and exposure keratopathy, even developing into irreversible vision loss in severe cases (2). It is generally agreed that GO is an autoimmune disease that results in orbital remodeling, enlargement and fibrosis (3). These pathological changes involves three distinct but related immune processes: inflammation, adipogenesis and glycosaminoglycan accumulation (4). Most investigators have hypothesized that orbital fibroblasts are the main targets of inflammatory cytokines released by infiltrated immune cells in the extraocular muscle and orbital adipose tissue (5). Moreover, activated orbital fibroblasts could secrete many cytokines, such as interleukins 1β, 6, 8, 16, TNF-α, RANTES and CD154 (6). These cytokines promote orbital trafficking of monocytes and macrophages, facilitate differentiation of orbital fibroblasts and stimulate accumulation of hyaluronic acid-rich stroma, leading to uncontrolled immune responses (4–6). Although several mechanisms have been proposed for the development of GO, the exact pathogenesis of GO has not yet been illustrated.

Recently, high-throughput technologies provided ample evidence on the potential biomarkers and molecular mechanisms of GO. For examples, microarray analysis revealed the potential role of CASQ2 to trigger autoimmunity events (7), and identified several adipogenesis-related genes and some genes involved in Wnt and IGF-1 signaling as being potentially implicated in pathogenesis (8–11). RNA-Seq also identified some meaningful genes (such as *PTX3*, *HOXB2*, *HOXB3*, *CCL2*, and *SERPINA1*) as potential biomarkers of GO (12–14). In addition, microRNA and protein sequencing found some blood circulating biomarkers that have the potential to diagnose GD, predict GO disease status and optimize patient management, such as hsa-miR-27a-3p, hsa-miR-22-3p, zonulin, haptoglobin, and lumican (15). All these accumulating findings improve our knowledge of the mechanisms underlying pathological changes in extraocular muscle and orbital adipose tissue of GO. Nevertheless, our understanding of the molecular mechanisms of lacrimal gland enlargement in GO is still limited.

In the present study, microarray analysis was performed to systematically investigate the key genes and pathways in lacrimal gland by mining the microarray datasets (GSE105149 and GSE58331) of GO and normal lacrimal samples. GSE105149 and GSE58331 were obtained from the public database GEO. These results would help to uncover a potential mechanism of lacrimal enlargement and offer new information for the pathogenesis of GO.

MATERIALS AND METHODS

Characteristics of the Microarray Data Sets

The Gene Expression Omnibus (GEO, http://www.ncbi.nlm.nih.gov/geo/) is a public functional genomics data repository. GEO has collected a large amount of omics data, such as high-throughput gene expression data, chips and microarrays. Microarray datasets of GSE105149 and GSE58331 were obtained by searching the keywords including Graves' ophthalmopathy, thyroid eye disease and thyroid-associated ophthalmopathy in GEO. The raw data and annotation files of GSE105149 and GSE58331 were downloaded from the GEO database. Rosenbaum JT et al. contributed to the generation of GSE105149 and GSE58331and provided many significant findings from different perspectives (16–21). GSE105149 was the microarray data of various lacrimal gland tissues, including sarcoidosis, granulomatosis with polyangiitis, thyroid eye disease, nonspecific orbital inflammation and healthy controls (16). Normal lacrimal samples from healthy individuals were obtained at the time of cosmetic surgery or blepharoplasty (16). GSE58331 was the microarray data of anterior orbit and lacrimal gland tissues, which were obtained from subjects with inflammatory diseases such as nonspecific orbital inflammation, sarcoidosis, granulomatosis with polyangiitis, IgG4-associated disease and thyroid eye disease as wells as from normal controls (17–21). Normal control tissues were obtained during surgeries such as blepharoplasty and enucleation on eyes with non-inflamed orbits (17–21). The diagnoses of all samples were based on the clinical and histopathological information submitted by orbital disease specialists and ocular pathologists (16–21). On account of GO or normal lacrimal gland as the inclusion criteria, the following samples were chosen in the present study: four TED lacrimal samples (GSM2823348, GSM2823349, GSM2823350, GSM2823351) and seven normal lacrimal samples (GSM2823306, GSM2823307, GSM2823308, GSM2823309, GSM2823310, GSM2823311, GSM2823312) were derived from GSE105149, and no sample was repeated; eight TED lacrimal samples (GSM1407195, GSM1407196, GSM1407199, GSM1407200, GSM1407202, GSM1407203, GSM1407204, GSM1407206) and seven normal lacrimal samples (GSM1407233, GSM1407235, GSM1407236, GSM1407237, GSM1407238, GSM1407240, GSM1407243) were obtained from GSE58331, in which eight TED samples were from four patients. Both microarrays have the same platform of GPL570 [HG-U133_Plus_2] Affymetrix Human Genome U133 Plus 2.0 Array.

Screening of the Differentially Expressed Genes

According to the raw data and annotation files, microarray probes were converted into corresponding gene symbols, and the expression value of one gene symbol corresponding to multiple probes was calculated by taking the average value. In addition, Z-score was chosen to normalize the converted data to extend the range of differential expression. The Limma R package (http://www.bioconductor.org/packages/release/bioc/html/limma.html) was used to detect differentially expressed genes (DEGs) between TED and normal lacrimal group. The cut-off criterion of DEGs was $P < 0.05$ and $|\log (\text{fold change})| \geq 1$. The false discovery rate (FDR) was not used to identify DEGs in the present study. Nonetheless, we calculated FDR and published it alongside the p-values to give a better idea of the robustness of DEGs.

Gene Ontology and Kyoto Encyclopedia of Genes and Genomes Pathway Analyses

Using the Database for Annotation, Visualization and Integrated Discovery (DAVID, https://david.ncifcrf.gov/), DEGs were mapped to Gene Ontology analysis to detect their possible functional processes from three terms of biological process (BP), molecular function (MF) and cellular component (CC). Moreover, Kyoto Encyclopedia of Genes and Genomes (KEGG) pathway analysis of DEGs was carried out to investigate their potential biological pathways by the KEGG Orthology-based Annotation System 2.0 (KOBAS 2.0, http://kobas.cbi.pku.edu.cn). $P < 0.05$ was considered as statistically significant difference.

Construction of Protein-Protein Interaction Network

DEGs were entered into the Search Tool for the Retrieval of Interacting Genes (STRING) database (https://string-db.org/) to construct a functional protein-protein interaction (PPI) network. An interaction with the composite score > 0.4 was considered statistically significant. Then, PPI network complex was visualized with Cytoscape software. The central node genes were screened out with the cut-off criteria of connectivity degree ≥10. Whereafter, the Molecular Complex Detection (MCODE) in Cytoscape software was utilized to identify densely connected regions from PPI network complex. The connected region with MCODE score >3 and node number >4 was considered to be the significant module.

Gene Set Variation Analysis

Gene set variation analysis (GSVA) is a nonparametric and unsupervised clustering approach to estimate the score of gene-set enriched pathways based on the expression profile of each sample (22). For GSVA analysis, we chose HALLMARK gene sets as the reference, t value > 2 and p value < 0.05 as the cut-off to identify significantly altered pathways. The GSVA R package (http://www.bioconductor.org/packages/release/bioc/html/GSVA.html) was used to calculate a pathway enrichment score between TED and normal lacrimal group. GSVA analysis for GSE105149, GSE58331, the combined data of GSE105149 and GSE58331 were performed, respectively.

RESULTS

Screening of the Common Molecular Origins Associated with GO Lacrimal Enlargement

Using P< 0.05 and |log (fold change) | ≥1 as the cut-off criterion, data from GSE105149 and GSE58331 were separately analyzed by the limma R package to identify DEGs. Representative heat maps showed different expression of all DEGs in the TED lacrimal samples relative to normal lacrimal samples (**Figure 1A**). 80 up-regulated and 440 down-regulated genes were present in the TED lacrimal samples of GSE105149, 868 up-regulated and 252 down-regulated genes were in the TED lacrimal samples of GSE58331. The overlap between the two microarray datasets contained 173 genes, including 20 up-regulated and 153 down-regulated genes in the TED lacrimal glands (**Figure 1B**, **Table S1**). Collectively, the common DEGs in two different gene expression profiles provided evidence on the common molecular origins of lacrimal gland enlargement in GO patients.

Investigation of the Potential Functions and Pathways in GO Lacrimal Enlargement

To investigate the mechanism, the overlapping DEGs were further measured through Gene Ontology and KEGG pathway analyses to explore the possible functions and pathways in the pathogenesis of GO lacrimal enlargement. Based on DAVID software, we observed a total of 81 Gene Ontology assignments, including 31 BPs, 9 MFs, and 41 CCs. The top five significant terms of Gene Ontology classification were illustrated in **Figures 2A–C**. In the BP category, most DEGs were involved in RNA splicing, protein folding in ER, cell-cell adhesion, mRNA processing and ER to Golgi vesicle-mediated transport. In the MF category, most DEGs may play roles in RNA binding, unfolded protein binding, peptidyl-prolyl cis-trans isomerase activity, cis-trans isomerase activity and nucleotide binding. In the CC category, a large percentage of the DEGs were associated with intracellular organelle lumen, nuclear lumen, cytosol, Golgi apparatus and ER. Furthermore, the KEGG analysis showed the dysfunction of protein processing in ER, phagosome and antigen processing and presentation pathways in GO lacrimal samples (**Figure 2D**). Taken together, these findings suggested that multiple functions and pathways were significantly associated with GO lacrimal enlargement.

Identification of the Most Significant Pathway and Hub Genes in GO Lacrimal Enlargement

To identify the most significant DEGs "hub genes" associated with GO lacrimal enlargement, we performed a PPI network construction of all the overlapping DEGs on the basis of the STRING database. Finally, 157 nodes and 282 edges were present in the PPI network complex (**Figure 3A**), in which 16 central node genes were selected with the cut-off criteria of connectivity degree ≥ 10 (**Figure 3B**). Subsequently, module analysis was performed by the plug-in MCODE in Cytoscape software in order to identify the significant modules from the PPI network complex. Then, 6 modules successfully emerged from the above PPI network complex, including 40 genes. According to the selection criteria of MCODE score > 3 and node number > 4, module a, module b, module c and module d were regarded as significant modules (**Figure 3C**). Among them, module A with the highest MCODE score and the maximum node number was considered as the most important module. Therefore, the common genes present in 16 central nodes and module A were

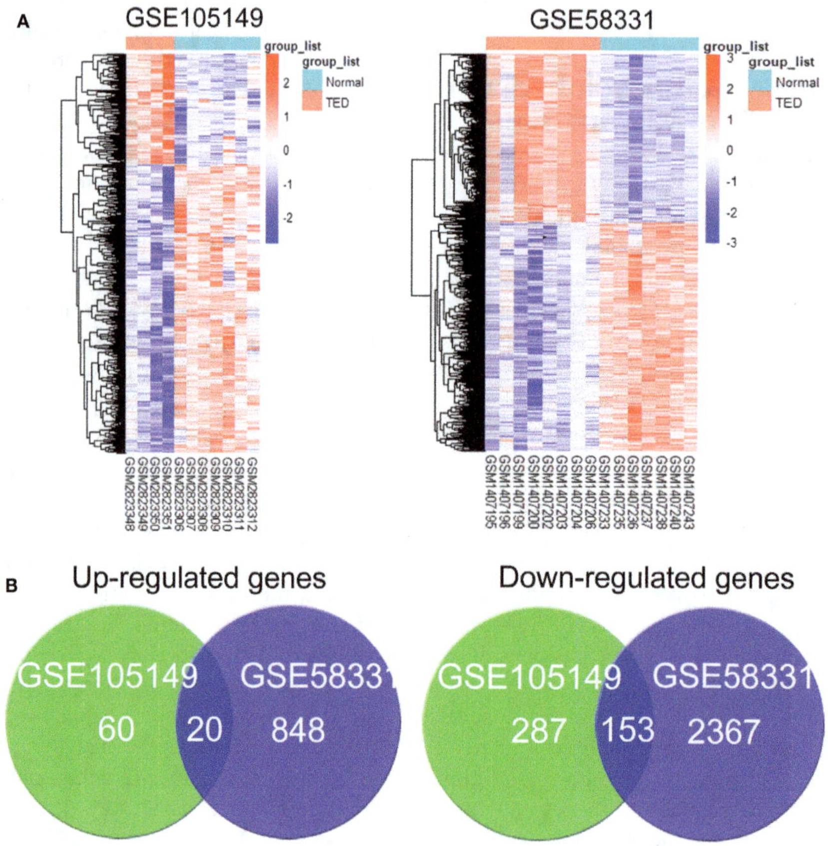

FIGURE 1 | Screening of the common differentially expressed genes associated with lacrimal enlargement in thyroid eye disease (TED). **(A)** hierarchical clustering heat maps showed different expression of all differentially expressed genes (DEGs) in the TED lacrimal samples relative to normal lacrimal samples. Red indicates that the expression of genes is relatively upregulated, and blue indicates that the expression of genes is relatively downregulated. **(B)** The DEGs were identified with the P-value <0.05 and |log (fold change)≥1 between thyroid eye disease (TED) and normal lacrimal samples from the mRNA expression profiling sets GSE105149 and GSE58331. Venn diagram showed the respective frequency of up-regulated and down-regulated genes in the TED lacrimal samples.

selected as hub genes, including *HSP90AA1*, *DNAJC10*, *HNRNPM*, *HNRNPD*, *HNRNPC*, *CANX*, *HSPA5*, *HSP90B1*, *SRSF11*, *DDX5*, *RBM25*, *HNRNPA2B1*, and *HSPA9* (**Figure 3C**, **Table 1**). Besides, function and pathway analyses of DEGs in the modules or hub genes were further carried out. The functional annotations of the genes involved in the modules were protein folding in ER, poly (A) RNA binding, focal adhesion (**Figures 4A–C**). Pathway analysis showed that the module genes mainly had a close relationship with protein processing in ER, spliceosome and pathogenic Escherichia coli infection (**Figure 4D**). Moreover, the 13 hub genes were significantly enriched in multiple functions such as protein folding in ER, poly (A) RNA binding and extracellular matrix (**Figures 5A–C**). And KEGG revealed that these hub genes were enriched in several pathways, especially protein processing in ER (**Figure 5D**).

According to Gene Ontology and KEGG pathway analyses for the entire DEGs set, 40 module genes and 13 hub genes, we observed that protein processing in ER was the most significant pathway, in which five hub genes including *HSP90AA1*, *HSP90B1*, *DNAJC10*, *HSPA5* and *CANX* were involved.

Differences in Pathway Activities between GO and Normal Lacrimal Gland

KEGG analysis requires relatively arbitrary selection of DEGs as input, only a small number of pathways were enriched in GO. In order to correct this selection to some extent, we applied GSVA analysis to investigate the critical pathways of GO. Since GSVA transforms data from a gene to a gene set based on the sample matrix in the coordinate frame, the enrichment pathway of each sample can be evaluated. As a result, GSVA analysis of TED versus normal lacrimal samples significantly revealed four up-regulated and five down-regulated signatures in the TED lacrimal samples of GSE105149 (**Figure 6A**), five up-regulated and 19 down-regulated signatures in the TED lacrimal samples of GSE58331 (**Figure 6B**). The common enriched signals in both GSE105149 and GSE58331 were KRAS_SIGNALING_DN, MYOGENESIS, MYC_TARGETS_V1, UNFOLDED_PROTEIN_RESPONSE, MTORC1_SIGNALING, PROTEIN_SECRETION and ANDROGEN_RESPONSE. In addition, the GSVA analysis of the combined data of GSE105149 and GSE58331 further supported the above results (**Figure 6C**). These results further supported the differences in pathway activities between GO and

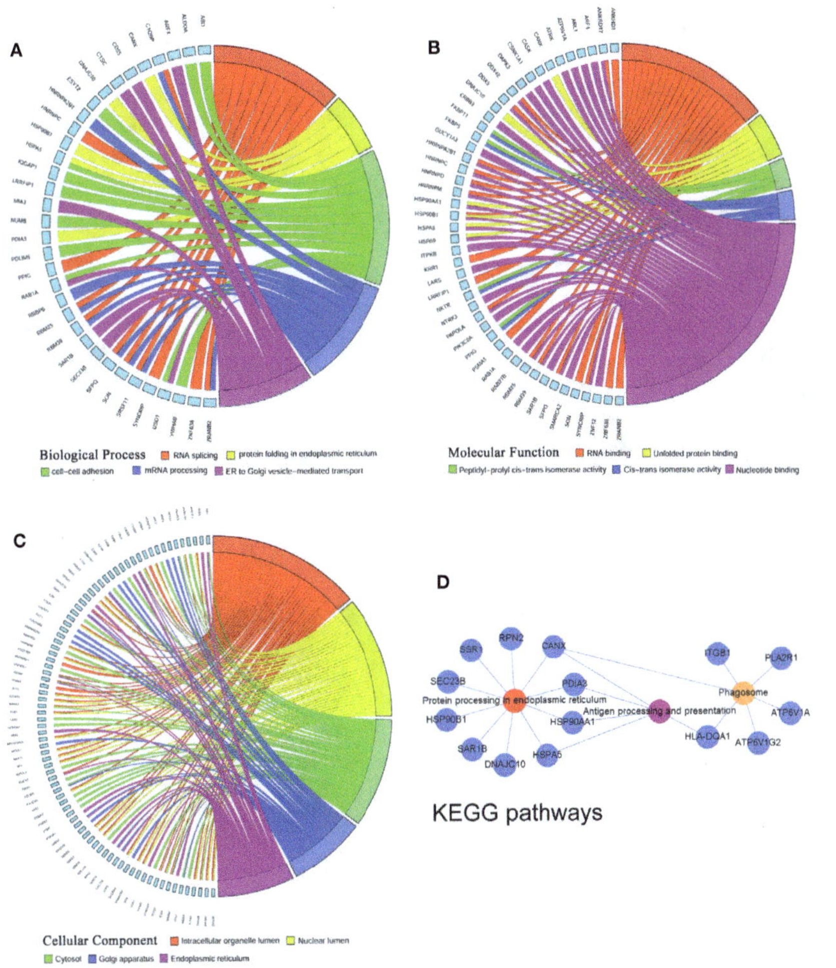

FIGURE 2 | Gene Ontology terms and Kyoto Encyclopedia of Genes and Genomes (KEGG) pathways of the common differentially expressed genes (DEGs) set. Circos plot represents the relationship between genes and the top 5 significant terms including biological process **(A)** cellular component **(B)** and molecular function **(C)**. Different colors from red, yellow, green, blue to purple indicate that the P values are sorted from minimum to maximum. **(D)** KEGG pathway analysis showed that DEGs were mainly enriched in pathways related to protein processing in endoplasmic reticulum, phagosome, and antigen processing and presentation. Different colors from red, yellow to purple indicate that the P values are sorted from minimum to maximum.

normal lacrimal gland, and provided novel or related pathways compared with KEGG pathway analysis.

DISCUSSION

Currently, our understanding of GO pathogenesis is mainly focused on the extraocular muscle and orbital adipose tissue. The molecular origins of lacrimal gland enlargement in GO has not yet been elucidated. In this work, two gene expression profiles from different cohort studies were analyzed to identify DEGs with common changes between lacrimal gland from patients with GO and that from normal groups. Further bioinformatics analysis was performed to investigate the significance of these DEGs, including Gene ontology analysis, KEGG pathway analysis, PPI network construction, hub gene identification and GSVA analysis.

We identified a total of 173 common DEGs which may be involved in the most significant function and pathway in ER, including BPs "Protein folding in ER" "ER to Golgi vesicle-mediated transport", MFs "Peptidyl-prolyl cis-trans isomerase activity" "Cis-trans isomerase activity" and CCs "Golgi apparatus" "ER" and pathways "Protein processing in ER" "Phagosome". As we known, ER is like a special factory for eukaryotic cells, in which at least one-third of molecules are synthesized, folded and transported (23). It maintains proper physiological proteostasis that the correctly folded molecules are modified and transported into the Golgi complexes, while the misfolded or unfolded molecules are trapped in the ER together with the molecular chaperone complex. When a large number of misfolded and unfolded molecules are accumulated, ER stress occurs and stimulates the unfolded protein response (UPR). Significantly, UPR intersects with different networks of inflammation, stress signals, and oxidative stress, in which NF-

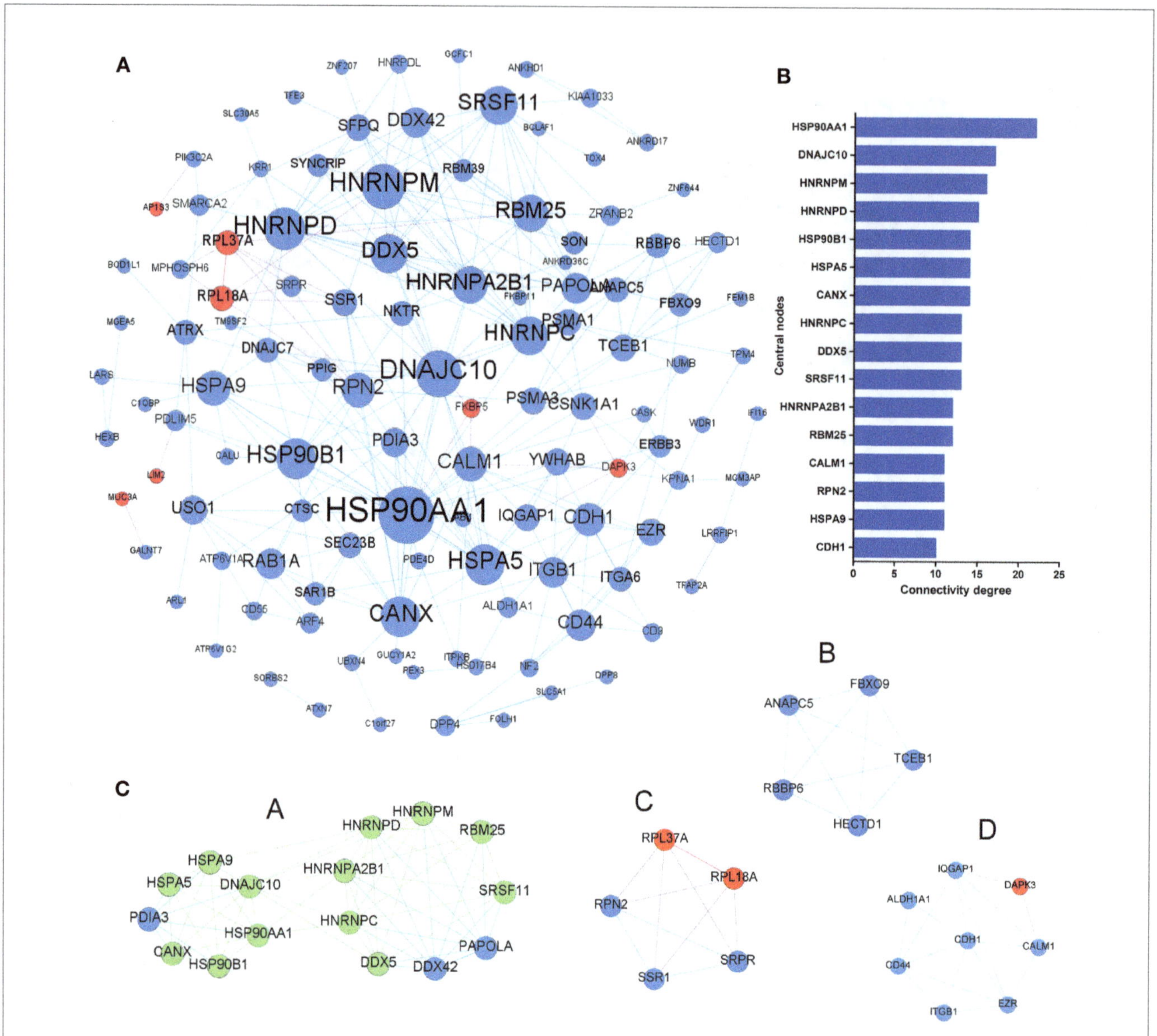

FIGURE 3 | Protein-protein interaction network of the common differentially expressed genes (DEGs) set. **(A)** The protein-protein interaction (PPI) network was visualized using Cytoscape software. The node size was proportional to the connectivity degree. The genes with no connectivity were not present in the network. **(B)** A total of 16 central node genes were screened out with the criteria of filtering degree ≥ 10 from the PPI network complex. **(C)** Module a, module b, module c, and module d were regarded as significant modules with the selection criteria of MCODE score > 3 and node number > 4. Red indicates that the expression of genes is relatively upregulated, and blue indicates that the expression of genes is relatively downregulated. In the module a, green indicates that the common genes present in 16 central nodes and module a were selected as hub genes.

kB and JNK-AP1 pathways are involved (24). Inflammation, as an important pathological change of GO, directly affects the severity and activity of GO. Clinically, glucocorticoids can effectively alleviate the condition of some active moderate to severe GO patients by controlling the inflammatory response (25). In addition, previous reports have confirmed the dysfunctions of NF-kB pathway and oxidative stress in the progression of GO (26–29). In this study, GSVA analysis also showed the dysregulation of protein secretion, oxidative phosphorylation, UPR and inflammatory response in lacrimal samples of GO. Therefore, these above evidences supported the ER and related signaling networks as potential mechanisms of GO lacrimal enlargement.

Protein processing in ER was identified as the most significant pathway associated with the pathogenesis of GO lacrimal enlargement, in which 5 hub genes including *HSP90AA1*, *HSP90B1*, *DNAJC10*, *HSPA5*, and *CANX* were involved. These proteins respectively encoding by *HSP90B1*, *DNAJC10*, *HSPA5*, and *CANX* are all located in the ER. Of them, HSP90AA1 has the highest connectivity in the PPI construction of DEGs, which

TABLE 1 | The hub genes associated with lacrimal gland enlargement in Graves' ophthalmopathy.

Gene symbol	GSE105149			GSE58331			Regulation
	False discoveryrate (FDR)	P value	Log (fold change)	False discoveryrate (FDR)	P value	Log (fold change)	
CANX	5.56E-02	2.59E-04	−1.02	3.25E-02	2.35E-03	−1.00	down
HSPA9	4.77E-02	1.22E-04	−1.07	3.24E-02	2.33E-03	−1.35	down
RBM25	1.11E-01	5.34E-03	−1.08	2.42E-02	8.83E-04	−1.58	down
HNRNPC	7.67E-02	1.53E-03	−1.11	3.46E-02	2.78E-03	−1.18	down
DNAJC10	5.80E-02	3.59E-04	−1.13	3.09E-02	2.03E-03	−1.57	down
DDX5	6.31E-02	5.59E-04	−1.14	4.36E-02	5.04E-03	−1.78	down
HNRNPM	3.95E-02	9.20E-06	−1.16	1.77E-02	1.57E-04	−1.45	down
HNRNPD	7.82E-02	1.65E-03	−1.26	3.61E-02	3.14E-03	−1.34	down
HSP90AA1	7.42E-02	1.11E-03	−1.27	2.51E-02	1.01E-03	−1.53	down
HSP90B1	5.43E-02	2.25E-04	−1.27	2.90E-02	1.68E-03	−1.16	down
HSPA5	7.43E-02	1.21E-03	−1.43	3.22E-02	2.30E-03	−1.34	down
HNRNPA2B1	5.01E-02	1.73E-04	−1.43	6.57E-02	1.17E-02	−1.29	down
SRSF11	6.10E-02	4.20E-04	−1.54	2.47E-02	9.66E-04	−1.42	down

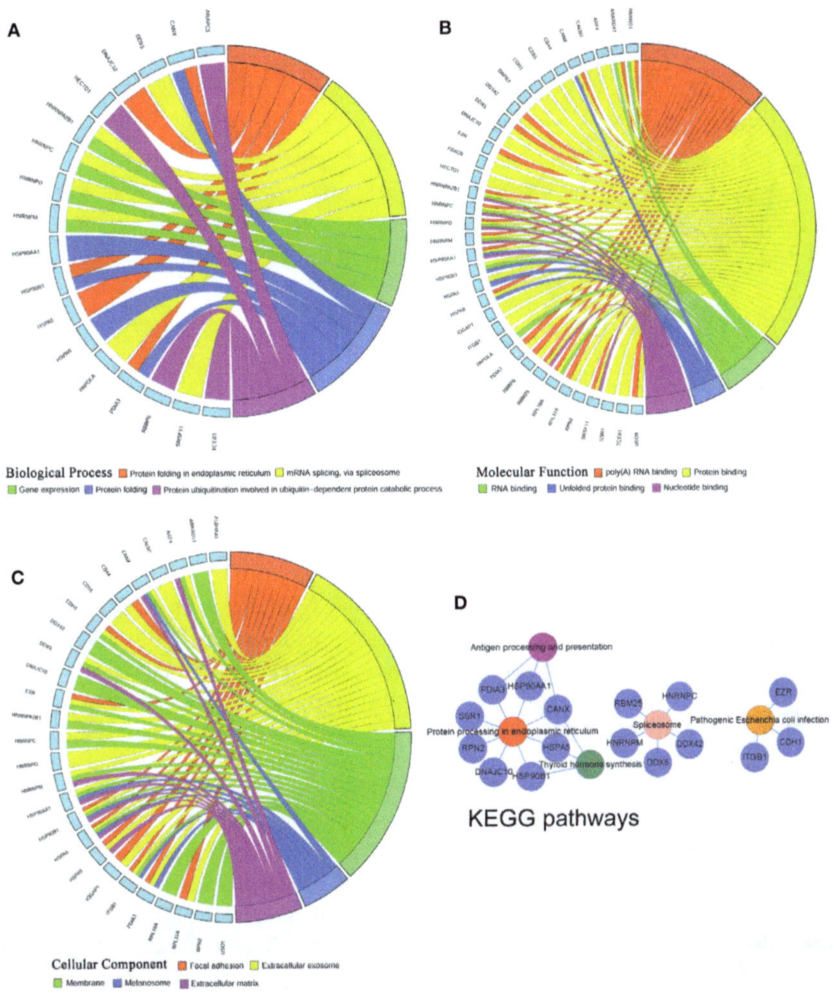

FIGURE 4 | Gene Ontology terms and Kyoto Encyclopedia of Genes and Genomes (KEGG) pathways of the module differentially expressed genes (DEGs) set. **(A)** Biological process, **(B)** Cellular component, **(C)** Molecular function, **(D)** KEGG pathways: Colors from red, pink, yellow, green to purple indicate that the P values are sorted from minimum to maximum.

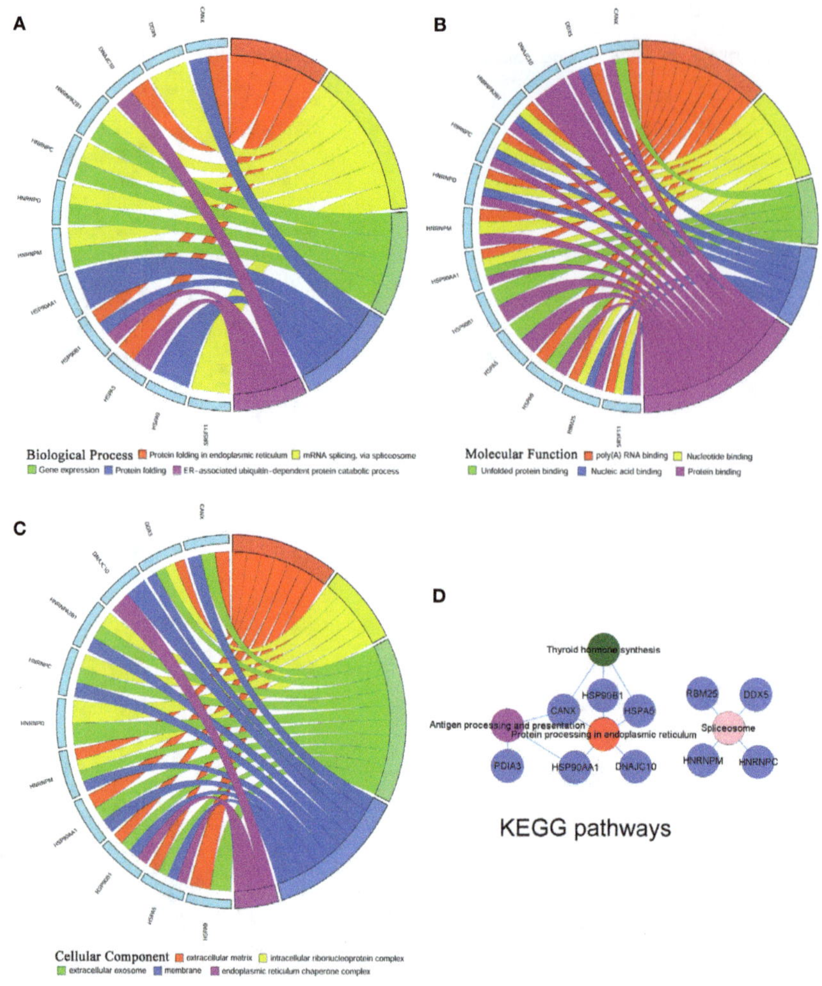

FIGURE 5 | Gene Ontology terms and Kyoto Encyclopedia of Genes and Genomes (KEGG) pathways of the hub differentially expressed genes (DEGs) set. **(A)** Biological process, **(B)** Cellular component, **(C)** Molecular function, **(D)** KEGG pathways: Colors from red, pink, green to purple indicate that the P values are sorted from minimum to maximum.

encodes the well-known cytoplasmic Hsp90α, a highly conserved molecular chaperone that facilitates folding, maturation, structural maintenance and appropriate modification of target molecules (known as clients) (30). These clients are enriched in vesicle-mediated transport, telomere maintenance, mitotic signal transduction, apoptosis, cell-cycle progression, innate immunity and targeted protein degradation (31). For example, the binding of Hsp90α to lipopolysaccharide (LPS) can mediate LPS-induced inflammation, including the secretion of TNF by monocytes (32). Interestingly, LPS-induced inflammation has been proved to affect the differentiation of orbital pre-adipocytes in GO (33). HSP90B1 encodes another Hsp90 isoform GRP94, an ER-resident molecular chaperone, which plays a vital role in the processing and transportation of secreting proteins (34). GRP94 shows many biochemical characteristics with other HSP90 family members, but also exhibits different activities, such as calcium binding, which is required for conditions in the ER (35). Studies have shown that GRP94 functions as a key molecular chaperone for various Toll-like receptors and integrins (36, 37), and also regulates innate and adaptive immunity (38). The absence of GRP94 in the hematopoietic system of mice leads to thrombocytopenia, prolonged bleeding, and massive platelets, which are clinically difficult to distinguish from human Bernard-soulier Syndrome (39). In addition, DNACJ10 and HSPA5 respectively encode the ER-resident proteins ERdj5 and BiP, which are crucial parts of ER-associated degradation (ERAD) complex involved in recognizing and degrading misfolded or unfolded molecules (40). ERAD is an essential quality-control system for ER molecules, in which the correctly folded molecules are transported to the secretion pathway and finally misfolded or unfolded molecules are translocated into the cytosol for proteasome degradation (41). Ushioda et al. confirmed that ERdj5 acts as a reductase that breaks the disulfide bonds of misfolded or unfolded molecules and facilitates ERAD by the

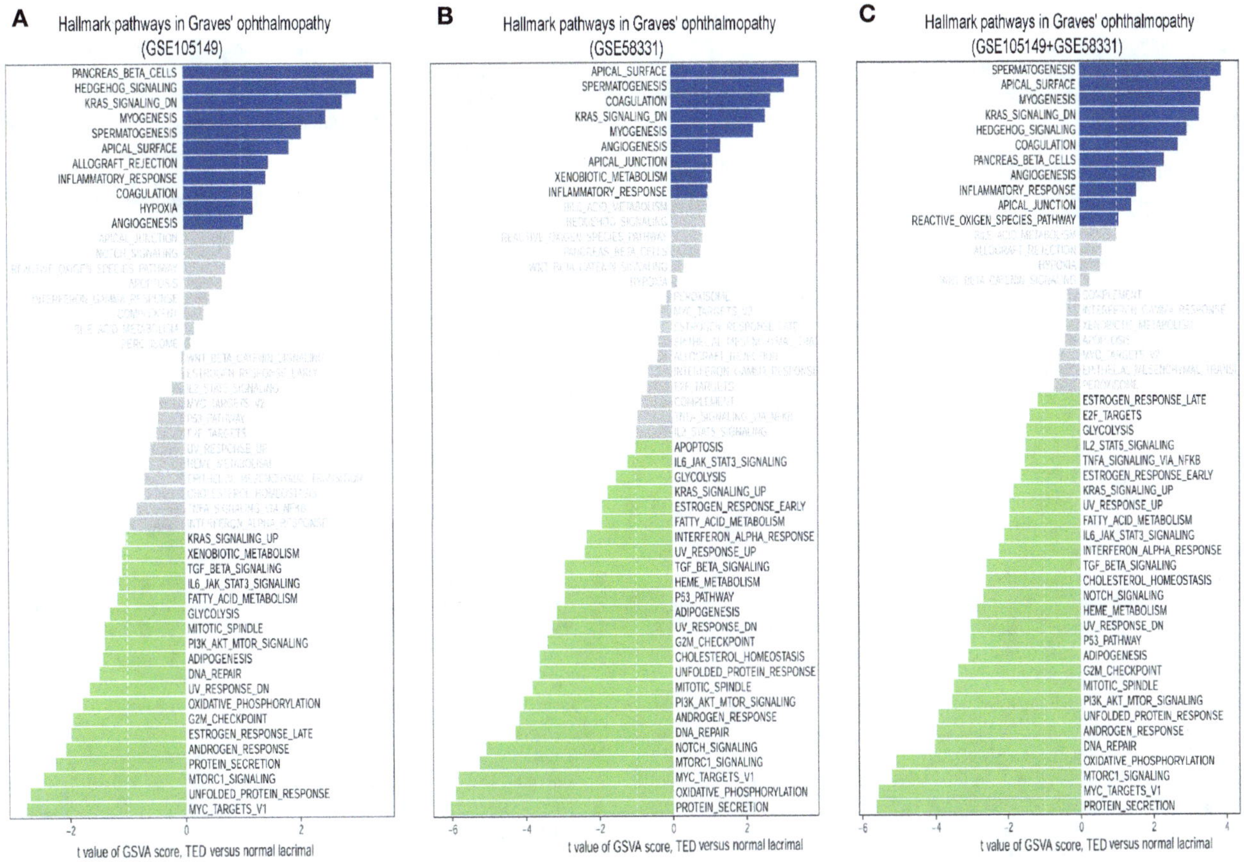

FIGURE 6 | Scores of gene set variation analysis (GSVA) for pathway activities between thyroid eye disease (TED) and normal lacrimal gland. **(A)** GSVA analysis of four TED versus seven normal lacrimal samples of GSE105149. **(B)** GSVA analysis of seven TED versus seven normal lacrimal samples of GSE58331. **(C)** The common GSVA analysis of 11 TED versus 14 normal lacrimal samples of GSE105149 and GSE58331. Shown are t values from a linear model, corrected for patient of origin. DN, down; v1, version.

physical and functional connections with BiP (42). Furthermore, studies suggested ERdj5 and BiP as the master regulator of calcium homeostasis and redox homeostasis in the ER (43). Similarly, Calnexin (CANX) is a key ER-resident chaperone to help folding and quality control, thus ensuring that only correctly folded and assembled molecules can further enter into the secretion pathway (44). All these findings further deepen our understanding of the important roles of *HSP90AA1*, *HSP90B1*, *DNAJC10*, *HSPA5* and *CANX* in protein processing in ER. Meanwhile, the observation that the down-regulated expression of these 5 hub genes in GO lacrimal samples, further indicated that ER dysfunction may contribute to the enlargement of GO lacrimal gland, and may extend to other pathological manifestations of GO.

In summary, our study presented a comprehensive bioinformatics analysis to identify potential key genes and pathways that may help to uncover the molecular mechanisms of the lacrimal gland enlargement in GO. Our findings firstly revealed that down-regulated expression of HSP90AA1, HSP90B1, DNAJC10, HSPA5, and CANX might generate the dysfunction of protein processing in ER, providing a novel explanation for the etiology and molecular events of the lacrimal enlargement in GO. When further molecular experiments confirmed the findings of the identified candidate genes and pathways in GO, the underlying molecular mechanisms of lacrimal gland enlargement in GO would be elucidated. All of these would contribute to a novel insight into GO pathogenesis.

AUTHOR CONTRIBUTIONS

WT and YS conceived the experiments. JY, ZM, and XJ analyzed the data. WT drafted the manuscript. All authors contributed to the article and approved the submitted version.

REFERENCES

1. Wang Y, Smith T. Current concepts in the molecular pathogenesis of thyroid-associated ophthalmopathy. *Invest Ophthalmol Vis Sci* (2014) 55(3):1735–48. doi: 10.1167/iovs.14-14002
2. Bartalena L, Baldeschi L, Boboridis K, Eckstein A, Kahaly GJ, Marcocci C, et al. The 2016 European Thyroid Association/European Group on Graves' Orbitopathy Guidelines for the Management of Graves' Orbitopathy. *Eur Thyroid J* (2016) 5(1):9–26. doi: 10.1159/000443828
3. Iyer S, Bahn R. Immunopathogenesis of Graves' ophthalmopathy: the role of the TSH receptor. *Best Pract Res Clin Endocrinol Metab* (2012) 26(3):281–9. doi: 10.1016/j.beem.2011.10.003
4. Bahn RS. Graves' ophthalmopathy. *N Engl J Med* (2010) 362(8):726–38. doi: 10.1056/NEJMra0905750
5. Bahn RS. Current Insights into the Pathogenesis of Graves' Ophthalmopathy. *Horm Metab Res* (2015) 47(10):773–8. doi: 10.1055/s-0035-1555762
6. Smith T J, Hegedus L. Graves' Disease. *N Engl J Med* (2016) 375(16):1552–65. doi: 10.1056/NEJMra1510030
7. Wescombe L, Lahooti H, Gopinath B, Wall JR. The cardiac calsequestrin gene (CASQ2) is up-regulated in the thyroid in patients with Graves' ophthalmopathy–support for a role of autoimmunity against calsequestrin as the triggering event. *Clin Endocrinol (Oxf)* (2010) 73(4):522–8. doi: 10.1111/j.1365-2265.2009.03753.x
8. Kumar S, Leontovich A, Coenen MJ, Bahn RS. Gene expression profiling of orbital adipose tissue from patients with Graves' ophthalmopathy: a potential role for secreted frizzled-related protein-1 in orbital adipogenesis. *J Clin Endocrinol Metab* (2005) 90(8):4730–5. doi: 10.1210/jc.2004-2239
9. Lantz M, Vondrichova T, Parikh H, Frenander C, Ridderstrale M, Asman P, et al. Overexpression of immediate early genes in active Graves' ophthalmopathy. *J Clin Endocrinol Metab* (2005) 90(8):4784–91. doi: 10.1210/jc.2004-2275
10. Ezra DG, Krell J, Rose GE, Bailly M, Stebbing J, Castellano L. Transcriptome-level microarray expression profiling implicates IGF-1 and Wnt signalling dysregulation in the pathogenesis of thyroid-associated orbitopathy. *J Clin Pathol* (2012) 65(7):608–13. doi: 10.1136/jclinpath-2012-200719
11. Khong JJ, Wang LY, Smyth GK, McNab AA, Hardy TG, Selva D, et al. Differential Gene Expression Profiling of Orbital Adipose Tissue in Thyroid Orbitopathy. *Invest Ophthalmol Vis Sci* (2015) 56(11):6438–47. doi: 10.1167/iovs.15-17185
12. Mou P, Chen Z, Jiang L, Cheng J, Wei R. PTX3: A Potential Biomarker in Thyroid Associated Ophthalmopathy. *BioMed Res Int* (2018) 2018):5961974. doi: 10.1155/2018/5961974
13. Tao W, Ayala-Haedo JA, Field MG, Pelaez D, Wester ST. RNA-Sequencing Gene Expression Profiling of Orbital Adipose-Derived Stem Cell Population Implicate HOX Genes and WNT Signaling Dysregulation in the Pathogenesis of Thyroid-Associated Orbitopathy. *Invest Ophthalmol Vis Sci* (2017) 58 (14):6146–58. doi: 10.1167/iovs.17-22237
14. Lee BW, Kumar VB, Biswas P, Ko AC, Alameddine RM, Granet DB, et al. Transcriptome Analysis of Orbital Adipose Tissue in Active Thyroid Eye Disease Using Next Generation RNA Sequencing Technology. *Open Ophthalmol J* (2018) 12:41–52. doi: 10.2174/1874364101812010041
15. Zhang L, Masetti G, Colucci G, Salvi M, Covelli D, Eckstein A, et al. Combining micro-RNA and protein sequencing to detect robust biomarkers for Graves' disease and orbitopathy. *Sci Rep* (2018) 8(1):8386. doi: 10.1038/s41598-018-26700-1
16. Rosenbaum JT, Choi D, Harrington CA, Wilson DJ, Grossniklaus HE, Sibley CH, et al. Gene Expression Profiling and Heterogeneity of Nonspecific Orbital Inflammation Affecting the Lacrimal Gland. *JAMA Ophthalmol* (2017) 135 (11):1156–62. doi: 10.1001/jamaophthalmol.2017.3458
17. Wong AJ, Planck SR, Choi D, Harrington CA, Troxell ML, Houghton DC, et al. IgG4 immunostaining and its implications in orbital inflammatory disease. *PloS One* (2014) 9(10):e109847. doi: 10.1371/journal.pone.0109847
18. Rosenbaum JT, Choi D, Wong A, Wilson DJ, Grossniklaus HE, Harrington CA, et al. The Role of the Immune Response in the Pathogenesis of Thyroid Eye Disease: A Reassessment. *PloS One* (2015) 10(9):e0137654. doi: 10.1371/journal.pone.0137654
19. Rosenbaum JT, Choi D, Wilson DJ, Grossniklaus HE, Sibley CH, Harrington CA, et al. Molecular diagnosis of orbital inflammatory disease. *Exp Mol Pathol* (2015) 98(2):225–9. doi: 10.1016/j.yexmp.2015.01.009
20. Rosenbaum JT, Choi D, Wilson DJ, Grossniklaus HE, Harrington CA, Sibley CH, et al. Parallel Gene Expression Changes in Sarcoidosis Involving the Lacrimal Gland, Orbital Tissue, or Blood. *JAMA Ophthalmol* (2015) 133 (7):770–7. doi: 10.1001/jamaophthalmol.2015.0726
21. Rosenbaum JT, Choi D, Wilson DJ, Grossniklaus HE, Harrington CA, Dailey RA, et al. Fibrosis, gene expression and orbital inflammatory disease. *Br J Ophthalmol* (2015) 99(10):1424–9. doi: 10.1136/bjophthalmol-2015-306614
22. Hanzelmann S, Castelo R, Guinney J. GSVA: gene set variation analysis for microarray and RNA-seq data. *BMC Bioinf* (2013) 14:7. doi: 10.1186/1471-2105-14-7
23. Wang M, Kaufman RJ. Protein misfolding in the endoplasmic reticulum as a conduit to human disease. *Nature* (2016) 529(7586):326–35. doi: 10.1038/nature17041
24. Hotamisligil GS. Endoplasmic reticulum stress and the inflammatory basis of metabolic disease. *Cell* (2010) 140(6):900–17. doi: 10.1016/j.cell.2010.02.034
25. Stan MN, Garrity JA, Bahn RS. The evaluation and treatment of graves ophthalmopathy. *Med Clin North Am* (2012) 96(2):311–28. doi: 10.1016/j.mcna.2012.01.014
26. Luo LH, Li DM, Wang YL, Wang K, Gao LX, Li S, et al. Tim3/galectin-9 alleviates the inflammation of TAO patients via suppressing Akt/NF-kB signaling pathway. *Biochem Biophys Res Commun* (2017) 491(4):966–72. doi: 10.1016/j.bbrc.2017.07.144
27. Li H, Yuan Y, Zhang Y, He Q, Xu R, Ge F, et al. Celastrol inhibits IL-1beta-induced inflammation in orbital fibroblasts through the suppression of NF-kappaB activity. *Mol Med Rep* (2016) 14(3):2799–806. doi: 10.3892/mmr.2016.5570
28. Choi W, Li Y, Ji YS, Yoon KC. Oxidative stress markers in tears of patients with Graves' orbitopathy and their correlation with clinical activity score. *BMC Ophthalmol* (2018) 18(1):303. doi: 10.1186/s12886-018-0969-x
29. Kau HC, Wu SB, Tsai CC, Liu CJ, Wei YH. Cigarette Smoke Extract-Induced Oxidative Stress and Fibrosis-Related Genes Expression in Orbital Fibroblasts from Patients with Graves' Ophthalmopathy. *Oxid Med Cell Longev* (2016) 2016:4676289. doi: 10.1155/2016/4676289
30. Taipale M, Jarosz DF, Lindquist S. HSP90 at the hub of protein homeostasis: emerging mechanistic insights. *Nat Rev Mol Cell Biol* (2010) 11(7):515–28. doi: 10.1038/nrm2918
31. Hartl FU, Bracher A, Hayer-Hartl M. Molecular chaperones in protein folding and proteostasis. *Nature* (2011) 475(7356):324–32. doi: 10.1038/nature10317
32. Triantafilou K, Triantafilou M, Dedrick RL. A CD14-independent LPS receptor cluster. *Nat Immunol* (2001) 2(4):338–45. doi: 10.1038/86342
33. Yi WS, Xu XL. Effects of LPS-induced inflammation on differentiation of orbital pre-adipocytes in thyroid-associated ophthalmopathy. *Zhonghua Yan Ke Za Zhi* (2011) 47(2):156–61.
34. Huck JD, Que NL, Hong F, Li Z, Gewirth DT. Structural and Functional Analysis of GRP94 in the Closed State Reveals an Essential Role for the Pre-N Domain and a Potential Client-Binding Site. *Cell Rep* (2017) 20(12):2800–9. doi: 10.1016/j.celrep.2017.08.079
35. Marzec M, Eletto D, Argon Y. GRP94: An HSP90-like protein specialized for protein folding and quality control in the endoplasmic reticulum. *Biochim Biophys Acta* (2012) 1823(3):774–87. doi: 10.1016/j.bbamcr.2011.10.013
36. Yang Y, Liu B, Dai J, Srivastava PK, Zammit DJ, Lefrancois L, et al. Heat shock protein gp96 is a master chaperone for toll-like receptors and is important in the innate function of macrophages. *Immunity* (2007) 26(2):215–26. doi: 10.1016/j.immuni.2006.12.005
37. Staron M, Yang Y, Liu B, Li J, Shen Y, Zuniga-Pflucker JC, et al. gp96, an endoplasmic reticulum master chaperone for integrins and Toll-like receptors, selectively regulates early T and B lymphopoiesis. *Blood* (2010) 115(12):2380–90. doi: 10.1182/blood-2009-07-233031
38. Randow F, Seed B. Endoplasmic reticulum chaperone gp96 is required for innate immunity but not cell viability. *Nat Cell Biol* (2001) 3(10):891–6. doi: 10.1038/ncb1001-891
39. Staron M, Wu S, Hong F, Stojanovic A, Du X, Bona R, et al. Heat-shock protein gp96/grp94 is an essential chaperone for the platelet glycoprotein Ib-IX-V complex. *Blood* (2011) 117(26):7136–44. doi: 10.1182/blood-2011-01-330464
40. Hagiwara M, Maegawa K, Suzuki M, Ushioda R, Araki K, Matsumoto Y, et al. Structural basis of an ERAD pathway mediated by the ER-resident protein disulfide reductase ERdj5. *Mol Cell* (2011) 41(4):432–44. doi: 10.1016/j.molcel.2011.01.021

41. Ellgaard L, Helenius A. Quality control in the endoplasmic reticulum. *Nat Rev Mol Cell Biol* (2003) 4(3):181–91. doi: 10.1038/nrm1052
42. Ushioda R, Hoseki J, Araki K, Jansen G, Thomas DY, Nagata K. ERdj5 is required as a disulfide reductase for degradation of misfolded proteins in the ER. *Science* (2008) 321(5888):569–72. doi: 10.1126/science.1159293
43. Ushioda R, Miyamoto A, Inoue M, Watanabe S, Okumura M, Maegawa KII, et al. Redox-assisted regulation of Ca2+ homeostasis in the endoplasmic reticulum by disulfide reductase ERdj5. *Proc Natl Acad Sci U.S.A.* (2016) 113 (41):E6055–63. doi: 10.1073/pnas.1605818113
44. Schrag JD, Bergeron JJ, Li Y, Borisova S, Hahn M, Thomas DY, et al. The Structure of calnexin, an ER chaperone involved in quality control of protein folding. *Mol Cell* (2001) 8(3):633–44. doi: 10.1016/s1097-2765(01) 00318-5

3

Mechanisms that Underly T Cell Immunity in Graves' Orbitopathy

Sijie Fang [1,2,3,4†], Yi Lu [1,2,3,4†], Yazhuo Huang [1,2,3,4†], Huifang Zhou [1,2] and Xianqun Fan [1,2*]*

[1] Department of Ophthalmology, Shanghai Ninth People's Hospital, Shanghai JiaoTong University School of Medicine, Shanghai, China, [2] Shanghai Key Laboratory of Orbital Diseases and Ocular Oncology, Shanghai Ninth People's Hospital, Shanghai JiaoTong University School of Medicine, Shanghai, China, [3] Shanghai Institute of Immunology, Shanghai JiaoTong University School of Medicine, Shanghai, China, [4] Department of Immunology and Microbiology, Shanghai JiaoTong University School of Medicine, Shanghai, China

***Correspondence:**
Xianqun Fan
fanxq@sjtu.edu.cn
Huifang Zhou
fangzzfang@163.com

[†] These authors have contributed equally to this work

Graves' orbitopathy (GO), also known as thyroid-associated ophthalmopathy, is the most common ocular abnormality of Graves' disease. It is a disfiguring, invalidating, and potentially blinding orbital disease mediated by an interlocking and complicated immune network. Self-reactive T cells directly against thyroid-stimulating hormone receptor-bearing orbital fibroblasts contribute to autoimmune inflammation and tissue remodeling in GO orbital connective tissues. To date, T helper (Th) 1 (cytotoxic leaning) and Th2 (antibody leaning) cell subsets and an emerging role of Th17 (fibrotic leaning) cells have been implicated in GO pathogenesis. The potential feedback loops between orbital native residential $CD34^-$ fibroblasts, $CD34^+$ infiltrating fibrocytes, and effector T cells may affect the T cell subset bias and the skewed pattern of cytokine production in the orbit, thereby determining the outcomes of GO autoimmune reactions. Characterization of the T cell subsets that drive GO and the cytokines they express may significantly advance our understanding of orbital autoimmunity and the development of promising therapeutic strategies against pathological T cells.

Keywords: Graves' orbitopathy, thyroid-associated ophthalmology, T cell immunity, effector T cell, orbital fibroblast, fibrocyte

INTRODUCTION

Graves' orbitopathy (GO), also known as thyroid-associated ophthalmopathy, is the ocular abnormality of Graves' disease (GD). The prevalence of GO in Europe is about 10/10,000 people, which is above the threshold for rarity in Europe (1). However, as the most common extrathyroidal complication, GO affects 25-30% of patients with Graves' hyperthyroidism and detailed orbital imaging has revealed orbital soft tissue changes in 70% of GD patients (2, 3). Patients with GO suffer from impaired visual function, facial disfigurement, and at worst, irreversible visual loss caused by corneal ulceration or dysthyroid optic neuropathy, which result in a poor quality of life and socio-economic status (4, 5). GO is a vexing autoimmune condition with both cellular and humoral immunities that form a sophisticated regulatory network, which leads to early orbital inflammation and late tissue remodeling (2, 4–6). Because of incomplete understanding of its precise pathogenesis, which partly results from the absence of suitable preclinical animal models, there is a lack of highly effective and well-tolerated therapies that target the most likely cause and glucocorticoids (GCs) are still the mainstay of treatment for active GO when inflammation is at peak (4, 5, 7, 8). Clinically, intravenous GC treatment has acceptable outcomes for most patients in the active phase. Nevertheless, a substantial number (20-30%) of active moderate-to-severe GO patients may not respond to GCs and adverse effects may occur after administration of high-dose or long-term GC use. Some patients may have disease progression despite GC treatment or relapse after steroid withdrawal (7, 8). Hence, a balance between benefits and risks of therapies for GO should be considered, which means developing more specific immunosuppressant strategies such as targeting T cells.

In the late 1980s, the role of T cell immunity was investigated in the orbital connective tissues of GO patients (9). Although thyroid-stimulating hormone receptor (TSHR) and its autoantibody play a major role in the pathological cascade of GO (2, 5), activation of humoral immunity, namely B cell immune responses, depends on defects in T cell immune modulation (10). The orbit is likely to have similar initial autoimmune reactions as those in the thyroid (5). It can be safely speculated that, among the various immune components that infiltrate the orbital connective tissues of GO patients, autoreactive T cells may act to establish and perpetuate the orbital inflammatory process. Recent studies have revealed that such disease-associated T cells include both T helper (Th) 1 (cytotoxic leaning) and Th2 (antibody leaning) subpopulations, and an emerging role of Th17 (fibrotic leaning) cells has also been implicated (6). The use of traditional non-specific immunosuppressants, such as cyclosporine that prevents interleukin (IL)-2 secretion by CD4$^+$ T cells and mycophenolate that inhibits T cell proliferation by depleting guanosine-tri-phosphate, appear to be effective as a step-down from GCs to achieve stable efficacy in the long term (11). In view of the above-mentioned facts, phenotypic and functional analyses of orbit-infiltrating T cells may provide better insights into the pathogenesis of GO.

In this review, we provide a detailed overview of the dysregulated T cell immunity in GO pathology. We include the early data as well as the latest research to reflect the developing course of understanding GO orbital autoimmunity. A selected listing of recommended studies on T cell pathogenesis in GO is summarized in **Table 1**. We highlight the integral role of pathological T cells that have deleterious effects on fibrocytes and orbital fibroblasts (OFs), and describe the development of targeted therapies for GO in an effective and safe manner.

CD4$^+$ AND CD8$^+$ T CELL IMMUNITIES IN GO

The first issue is whether cellular immunity is involved in GO inflammation. In an early study, Heufelder et al. reported the presence of CD3$^+$ cells that represent total T cells in orbital and pretibial connective tissues from two GD patients with both orbitopathy and dermopathy (12). The results provide evidence of T cells infiltrating the inflamed orbit. Phenotypic analysis of four peripheral blood mononuclear cell (PBMC) samples from four severe GO patients revealed the main subtype as CD4$^+$ T cells (CD4/CD8 ratios 1.9-2.5), which was similar to the phenotypes of four control PBMC samples, whereas their corresponding orbital connective tissue-derived T cell lines had equal amounts of CD4$^+$ and CD8$^+$ T cells (CD4/CD8 ratios 0.9-1.2) (38). The ratios of CD4/CD8 were unchanged in 153 GO T cell clones cultivated from the four orbital T cell lines and 166 and 236 T cell clones cultivated from the four PBMC samples of GO patients and control subjects, respectively (38). The relatively low ratios of CD4/CD8 in orbital connective tissue-derived T cell lines and clones indicate that there is a disorder of cellular immune function in GO orbits. Grubeck-Loebenstein et al. established and characterized six T cell lines from orbital connective tissues of two severe GO patients and found they were predominantly CD8$^+$CD45RO$^+$ T cells (77%-96%) (39). The above two studies imply that a cytolytic T cell immunity triggered by CD8$^+$ T cells may contribute to orbital inflammation in GO in a major histocompatibility complex (MHC) class I dependent manner. But the results cannot tell whether there exists a more efficient and unique antigen-presenting process to activate orbit-specific T cells. Stover et al. screened 64 orbital connective tissue-derived T cell clones expanded from two GO patients and reported an obvious predominance of the CD4$^+$ T cell population (CD4/CD8 ratio 8.2) that contrasted with six PBMC samples (CD4/CD8 ratio 2.1) (39). In another study, the same research group analyzed 10 of 17 T cell lines derived from orbital connective tissues of six severe GO patients and found mainly CD4$^+$ T cells (six of 10 strains) with a similar CD4$^+$/CD8$^+$ T cell distribution (40). The studies supporting the role of CD4$^+$ T cells suggest an MHC class II pathway primed by a specialized antigenic determinant within the thyroid and at the involved orbital connective tissues. Pappa et al. investigated the extraocular muscles (EOMs) of 10 GO patients who underwent corrective strabismus surgery and examined six EOM-derived T cell lines from four patients. Five were CD4$^+$CD45RO$^+$ T cells (85%-97%) and CD8$^+$ T cells (68%) were dominant in only one strain. The same status was found in the four corresponding PBMC samples (three were mostly CD4$^+$ cells (89%-98%)) of each patient. They further reported detectable T cell receptor (TCR) gene expression in 10 out of 12 EOMs collected from the other five patients and in all five EOMs collected from three control subjects (41). The discrepancy of CD4$^+$ and CD8$^+$ T cell subsets in the above findings may lie in the small number of patients, the heterogeneity of patients involved in the different studies, and the different research methods. Notably, the T cell lines or clones in the above studies were cultured tissue- or peripheral blood-derived T cells expanded for several days to weeks, which may affect the initial status of these T cells to a certain extend. For example, CD8$^+$ T cells may have more rapid expansion and CD4$^+$ T cells gradually die during culture. Förster et al. established 18 T cell lines from orbital connective tissues of six severe GO patients and reported that 10 were predominantly the CD4$^+$ phenotype, whereas three were mostly CD8$^+$ cells (42). Intriguingly, in their study, even two independent T cell lines derived from the same patient had distinct T cell phenotypes (CD4 or CD8). This indicates that both CD4$^+$ and CD8$^+$ T cells

TABLE 1 | Recommended Studies on T cell Pathogenesis in GO.

Reference	Study subjects	Main findings
T cell immunity and TCR repertoires		
Heufelder et al. (12)	Biopsies of thyroid glands, orbital connective tissues, pretibial skins, and PBMCs from two GD patients with both orbitopathy and dermopathy and two non-GO controls	Both orbital connective tissues and pretibial connective tissues were infiltrated by $CD3^+$ T cells; Marked similarities of intrathyroidal, orbital, and pretibial TCR gene repertoires were found, which indicate apparent TCR restriction and T cell oligoclonality.
Pappa et al. (13)	Biopsies of EOMs from five early active GO patients, nine late stable GO patients, and 14 non-GO patients	$CD4^+$ and $CD8^+$ T cells and macrophages were significantly present in EOMs of active GO compared with both stable GO and controls; Increased HLA-DR expression on OFs, but not EOM fibres, was observed in both active and stable GO.
Rotondo Dottore et al. (14)	Biopsies of orbital connective tissues from 20 consecutive GO patients	A positive correlation was found between $CD3^+$ T and $CD20^+$ B cells infiltrating orbital connective tissues with GO clinical activity.
Wang et al. (15)	Biopsies of thyroid glands and PBMCs from six GD patients; PBMCs from 43 GO patients and 57 stable GD patients	A model for prediction of GO progression in GD cohort with high sensitivity and specificity.
Aniszewski et al. (16)	117 $CD4^+$ T cell clones expanded from orbital connective tissues of 6 GO patients	Th1 immune response predominated in early active GO and Th2 immune response predominated in late stable GO.
Effector T cell, OF, and fibrocyte interaction		
Feldon et al. (17)	GO and control OFs; autologous T cells from PBMCs	Autologous T cells promoted the proliferation of GO OFs dependent on MHC class II and CD40-CD40L pathways.
Hwang et al. (18)	GO and control OFs	GO OFs expressed elevated levels of CD40 that could be further up-regulated by IFN-γ; CD40-CD40L combination led to IL-6, IL-8, and MCP-1 production in GO OFs; $CD90^+$ GO OFs expressed more CD40 than $CD90^-$ GO OFs.
van Steensel et al. (19)	Biopsies of orbital connective tissues from GO patients and controls; GO OFs	Mast cells, monocytes, and macrophages expressed increased levels of PDGF-A and PDGF-B in GO orbital connective tissues; PDGF-AB and PDGF-BB promoted proliferation and hyaluronan and IL-6 production by GO OFs.
Tsui et al. (20)	Biopsies of thyroid glands and orbital connective tissues; GO and control OFs; thyrocytes	TSHR levels were higher on thyrocytes than GO and control OFs; Differentiation of GO OFs, but not control OFs, into adipocytes led to increased TSHR expression; IGF-1R levels were higher on GO OFs than control OFs; TSHR and IGF-1R colocalized to the perinuclear and cytoplasmic areas of both GO OFs and thyrocytes.
Cao et al. (21)	GO and control OFs	CD40-CD40L combination led to the synthesis of hyaluronan and PGE_2 in GO OFs; PGE_2 production in GO OFs was caused by increased expression of PGSH-2 at both transcriptional and translational levels regulated by IL-1α expression
Koumas et al. (22)	GO OFs; myometrial fibroblasts	$CD90^+$ myometrial fibroblasts and GO OFs were capable of myofibroblast differentiation by TGF-β or platelet concentrate supernatant treatment; $CD90^-$ myometrial fibroblasts and GO OFs were capable of lipofibroblast differentiation by 15-deoxy-$\Delta^{12,14}$-PGJ_2 or ciglitazone treatment.
Antonelli et al. (23)	Sera from consecutive subjects including 60 GD patients, 60 GO patients, and 60 controls; GO thyrocytes, OFs, and induced preadipocytes; Control fibroblasts and induced preadipocytes from dermal tissues of the same patients	CXCL10 was higher in GD and GO patients than controls; CXCL10 was significantly higher in active GO patients than inactive GO patients; IFN-γ and TNF-α synergistically induced CXCL10 production in GO thyrocytes, OFs, and preadipocytes, which was suppressed by PPAR-γ agonist.
Antonelli et al. (24)	GO thyrocytes, OFs, and induced preadipocytes; Control fibroblasts and induced preadipocytes from dermal tissues of the same patients	IFN-γ and TNF-α synergistically induced CXCL9 and CXCL11 production in GO thyrocytes, OFs, and preadipocytes, which was suppressed by PPAR-γ agonist.
Han et al. (25)	GO and control OFs	IFN-γ and IL-4 attenuated IL-1β-provoked PGE_2 production by suppressing PGHS-2 gene promoter activity but enhanced IL-1β-initiated hyaluronan production by up-regulating hyaluronan synthase-2 gene expression in GO OFs.
Han et al. (26)	GO and control OFs	IFN-γ and IL-4 attenuated IL-1β-induced TIMP-1 production by suppressing TIMP-1 gene promoter activity in GO OFs.
Huber et al. (27)	Whole blood from 216 GD patients and 368 healthy controls	rs2201841 was strongly associated with GO development, especially AA and CC genotypes of *Il23r*.
Douglas et al. (28)	Biopsies of orbital connective tissues; PBMCs from 70 GD patients (including 51 GO patients) and 25 healthy controls; GO and control OFs; thyrocytes; fibrocytes	$CD34^+CXCR4^+$Collagen I^+TSHR^+ fibrocytes were increased in PBMCs of GD patients; TSH induced fibrocytes to produce IL-6 and TNF-α; Increased fibrocytes were found in orbital connective tissues of GO patients.
Gillespie et al. (29)	PBMCs from 31 GO patients and 19 healthy controls; GO OFs; GO and control fibrocytes	Fibrocytes expressed higher levels of TSHR than GO OFs; GO fibrocytes expressed higher levels of TSHR than control fibrocytes; TSH or M22 greatly stimulated the production of various cytokines and chemokines such as IL-8, RANTES, and MCP-1 in both GO and control fibrocytes.
Fang et al. (30)	Biopsies of orbital connective tissues; PBMCs from 34 GO patients and 36 healthy controls; GO and control OFs; *in vitro*-differentiated Th17 cells	GO peripheral Th17 cells produced IFN-γ and IL-22 and were related to clinical activity score; IL-17A enhanced TGF-β–induced fibrosis in $CD90^+$ OFs but inhibited 15-deoxy-$\Delta^{12,14}$-PGJ_2–induced adipogenesis in $CD90^-$ OFs; Th17 cells stimulated proinflammatory cytokine expression of GO OFs and GO OFs promoted Th17 cell differentiation by PGE_2 production.

(Continued)

TABLE 1 | Continued

Reference	Study subjects	Main findings
Fang et al. (31)	21 GO orbital connective tissues and 38 control orbital connective tissues; CD34$^+$ GO OFs; *in vitro*-differentiated Th17 cells	GO orbital microenvironment was composed of T cells, B cells, natural killer cells, dendritic cells, macrophages, plasma cells, and CD34$^+$ OFs; Orbit-infiltrating Th17 cells displayed a Th1-like phenotype and expressed high levels of IL-1R and IL-23R; CD34$^+$ OFs enhanced IL-1R and IL-23R expression on Th17 cells by PGE$_2$-EP2/EP4-cAMP signaling.
Fang et al. (32)	PBMCs from 16 active and 14 stable GO patients and 20 healthy controls; GO and control fibrocytes; *in vitro*-differentiated Th17 cells	IL-17A stimulated cytokine production in both GO and control fibrocytes; Autologous Th17 cells promoted inflammatory and antigen-presenting functions of GO fibrocytes; GO fibrocytes enhanced Th17 cell phenotype and recruited Th17 cells by MIP-3 and CCR6 combination.
Fang et al. (33)	Biopsies of orbital connective tissues; Sera and PBMCs from consecutive subjects including 37 GO patients, 38 GD patients, and 32 healthy controls	Increased CXCR3$^+$ IFN-γ-producing Th17.1 cells were positively correlated with GO activity and associated with the development of very severe GO; In GC-resistant, very severe GO patients, CXCR3$^+$ IFN-γ-producing Th17.1 cells remained at high levels in blood and orbital connective tissues, which were positively correlated with elevated triglycerides.
Fernando et al. (34)	GO OFs; GO and control fibrocytes	TSH and M22 induced IL-23, but not IL-12, expression in fibrocytes, while they induced IL-12 production in GO OFs; The shift from IL-23 expression in fibrocytes to that of IL-12 in CD34$^+$ GO OFs was regulated by Slit2.
GO animal model		
Moshkelgosha et al. (35)	hTSHR-A subunit plasmid-immunized BALB/c mice	TSHR was the pathogenic antigen in GO; Interstitial inflammation of extraocular muscles with CD3$^+$ T cells, F4/80$^+$ macrophages, and mast cells, accompanied by glycosaminoglycan deposition was observed in murine orbits.
Zhang et al. (36)	hTSHR-A subunit-expressing adenovirus-immunized BALB/c mice	Fibrosis and adipogenesis accompanied by CD4$^+$ T cell infiltration were seen in murine periorbital fat tissues; Increased frequencies of Th1 cells and decreased frequencies of Th2 cells and regulatory T cells were shown in the splenocytes of GO mice.
Masetti et al. (37)	hTSHR-A subunit plasmid-immunized BALB/c mice	*Bacteroides* and *Bifidobacterium* counts were more abundant in mice in Center 1, while *Lactobacillus* counts were more abundant in mice in Center 2; Significantly higher yeast counts were found in Center 1 TSHR-immunized mice; A significant positive correlation was found between the presence of *Firmicutes* and orbital adipogenesis in Center 2 TSHR-immunized mice.

are involved in GO pathogenesis. However, the phenotypic analysis was also based on T cell lines cultured *in vitro*. Therefore, direct *in vivo* T cell examination is needed to avoid biases and better reflect the real orbital immunity in GO inflammation.

Subsequently, an *in situ* study by immunohistochemistry demonstrated that both CD4$^+$ and CD8$^+$ T cells had infiltrated the EOMs in early active GO, which were much less evident in late inactive GO and control subjects (13). A recent study examined 26 GO patients and seven control subjects by immunohistochemistry, which showed that TCR expression was strong and diffuse in severe patients, although the orbital TCR detectable rate was similar in both active severe and inactive mild GO. Active severe GO patients had a higher CD3 detectable rate compared with inactive mild GO patients. Additionally, no expression of TCR or CD3 was found in control orbits (43). These data support the idea that GO orbital connective tissues are variably infiltrated by lymphocytes during active disease when medications are more effective than in the inactive disease.

We used flow cytometric analysis and found no differences in the frequency of circulating CD4$^+$ and CD8$^+$ T cells or the ratios of CD4/CD8 between GO patients and control subjects (44). In agreement with the above immunohistochemistry studies, infiltrated CD4$^+$ and CD8$^+$ T cells extended throughout the orbital connective tissues of GO patients, especially in the active phase, compared with control subjects (44, 45). Rotondo Dottore et al. confirmed that the total number of orbit-infiltrating T cells was correlated positively with the GO clinical activity score in simple and multiple linear regression models (14). Studies in GO murine models also supported T cell-mediated inflammation in the orbit *in vivo*. CD3$^+$ total T cells were found to infiltrate into the orbital muscles and periorbital tissues of human (h) TSHR-A subunit plasmid-immunized BALB/c mice (35, 46). The same phenomenon was found in mouse TSHR-A subunit plasmid-immunized BALB/c mice (47). Intriguingly, increased CD4$^+$ T cell subsets were reported in periorbital fat of SKG mice after intraperitoneal administration of zymosan A compared with wild type mice (48). A recent study used an adenovirus that expressed the hTSHR-A subunit to induce GO in BALB/c mice and also observed CD4$^+$ T cell infiltration in periorbital fat tissues (36). Collectively, these data shed light on the presence and type of T cells in GO, which suggest a complex inflammatory microenvironment in the orbit.

SELF-REACTIVE T CELLS DIRECTED AGAINST OFS

The second issue is whether T cells in GO recognize autoantigens, i.e., a primary GO immune response leads to the development of antigen-specific T cell responsiveness and clonal proliferation in the orbit. This will determine whether T cell immunity is specifically directed against orbital antigens. Heufelder et al. reported that in the two GD patients with both orbitopathy and dermopathy the vast majority of TCRs in the orbital and pretibial connective tissues were αβ chains and not γδ chians (12). Although expression of a broad spectrum of both TCR Vα and Vβ genes was observed in the PBMCs of patients, marked restriction of TCR Vα and Vβ gene expression was found in thyroid glands and orbital and pretibial connective tissues compared with PBMCs. Furthermore, thyroid, orbital, and pretibial tissues from two control subjects did not express restricted TCR transcripts (12). These data imply the potential GO-specific oligoclonal expression of the TCR gene repertoire. To further characterize the limited variability of antigen receptors on extrathyroidal T cells in GO, Heufelder et al. examined the TCR V gene repertoire *in situ* in orbital connective tissues and EOMs from eight early severe GO patients and observed apparent TCR Vα and Vβ gene restriction compared with matched PBMCs. Loss of TCR gene restriction was observed in four late GO patients and no TCR gene restriction was found in samples from three non-GO control subjects (49, 50). These findings suggest that oligoclonality of T cell immunity may be lost during GO, which indicates that antigen specificity of orbit-infiltrating T cells occurs in the early active phase of GO. This is important because an early adaptive immune response implies organ-specific autoimmunity in orbital connective tissues independent of the thyroid. Development of diversity or polyclonality of the TCR gene repertoire indicates that orbital inflammation is at the burnout stage. Heufelder summarized data from three severe active GO patients with GD and dermopathy and reported not only marked TCR restriction, but also several conserved junctional motifs shared by T cells in the orbit, thyroid, and pretibial tissue despite obvious heterogeneity of the TCR genes in each patient (12, 51). This highlights the presence of certain oligoclonal T cell populations stimulated by the analogous antigenic determinants shared by the thyroid and the involved extrathyroidal compartments. A recent interesting study proposed a novel TCR clonal expansion and chaos score to predict GO development in GD by characterizing complementarity determining region 3 of the TCR Vβ gene repertoire in PBMCs, which indicates specific GO TCR signatures distinctive from GD (15). These selected TCR-bearing T cells are self-reactive and recruited to the orbit at GO attack, which lead to orbital inflammation.

The next issue is unraveling the specific cell type or protein that triggers GO self-reactive T cell expansion. Genetic immunization with mouse TSHR-A subunit breaks self-tolerance and induces GO-like pathology in BALB/c mice (47). Splenic T cells from BALB/c mice that have received hTSHR-A subunit prepared as a maltose-binding protein fusion induce orbital pathology in naïve recipient BALB/c mice marked by the presence of $CD3^+$ total T cells (52). Furthermore, splenic T cells from hTSHR-A subunit plasmid-primed GO BALB/c mice show proliferative responses to purified TSHR antigen (53). These data from animal models provide a clue to potential TSHR-specific T cell responses that may also occur in the GO patient orbit. Arnold et al. reported occasional proliferation responses to EOM antigens in 10 circulating T cell lines from 10 severe GO patients. Additionally, these T cells hardly produced interferon (IFN)-γ under EOM antigen stimulation (54). Similarly, in the *in vitro* model presented by Grubeck-Loebenstein et al., six T cell lines from orbital connective tissues did not proliferate in response to EOM antigen stimulation, but all had apparent proliferation after autologous OF treatment (39). In the *in vitro* model of Otto et al., the established 17 orbital T cell lines responded significantly to autologous orbital connective tissue proteins (6-10 and 19-26 kDa). A similar phenomenon was seen in most GO PBMCs that were more sensitive to autologous proteins from OFs than myoblasts. Moreover, orbital T cell lines hardly responded to allogeneic orbital proteins (40). Conversely, the authors demonstrated that 18 established T cell lines were barely able to respond to TSHR (2/18), thyroidal peroxidase (2/18) or thyroglobulin (none) (42). The results suggest the primary antigen role of TSHR and antigen-specific T cell clones in GO patients. However, the relatively low proliferation rate is confusing. It is important to note that although irradiated autologous PBMCs were added as feeders to help T cell to clone in these two studies, the antigen-induced T cell-specific proliferative response is acted in an antigen-presenting cell (APC)-dependent manner. The same research group used PBMCs from 16 GO patients and 12 controls and confirmed that incubation of GO PBMCs with OFs from the same patients led to marked T cell proliferation compared with control OFs. Similarly, compared with control OFs, GO OFs also had increased proliferation responses to stimulation by autologous PBMCs (55). This implies that OFs express GO autoantigens, and we hypothesize that GO OFs may function as facultative APCs to stimulate the proliferation of antigen-specific T cells, which has been confirmed by the fact that autologous T cells also stimulate the proliferation of GO OFs, but not eyelid-derived fibroblasts, *via* MHC class II and CD40-CD40 ligand (CD40L) signaling (17). We and other groups have shown that GO orbital connective tissues express higher gene and protein levels of MHC II and CD40 than control subjects (18, 30, 43, 56). Moreover, MHC II^+ cells and $CD40^+$ cells are local fibroblast-shaped cells and invading mononuclear cells such as macrophages in orbital connective tissues (18, 56). Even in stable GO, orbital connective tissues are activated to persistently express MHC II (56). Similarly, murine OFs derived from hTSHR-A subunit plasmid-primed BALB/c mice showed strong expression of CD40, TSHR, and insulin-like grow factor 1 receptor (IGF-1R) (57). Taken together, these findings have revealed sensitized and orbital connective tissue-specific T cells in circulation and the orbit of GO patients and provided evidence for self-reactive T cell populations directed against OFs.

PRIMARY IMMUNE REACTION IN THE ORBIT

The third issue is how T cells and OFs communicate with each other, which causes a series of pathophysiological changes in the GO process. Evidence for both T and B cells infiltrating GO orbital connective tissues was shown as early as 2012 (58). Many other *in situ* immunohistochemistry studies have demonstrated the presence of $CD4^+$ T cells (44, 45, 56, 59), $CD20^+$ B cells

(14, 60, 61), CD14$^+$ monocytes (19, 56), CD68$^+$ macrophages (19, 59, 62), and CD117$^+$ mast cells (19, 63) as the main invading immune components in the GO orbit. Using single cell sequencing analysis, we showed that various genes are expressed in GO orbital connective tissues, which can be classified into six independent cell types: APCs, lymphocytes including T and B cells, OFs, adipocytes, endothelial cells, and myocytes (31). This indicates an extremely complicated local orbital microenvironment, in which infiltrating immune cells and non-immune stromal cells interact with each other. The presence of APCs in the orbit further supports the idea that a primary GO autoimmune reaction occurs within the extrathyroidal compartment, although it resembles the process in the thyroid. OFs that express TSHR and IGF-1R (20, 31) detect danger signals to guide the property and intensity of the GO-adaptive immune response (64, 65). TSHR has been recognized as an autoantigen, but might not be the only one that activates GO self-reactive T cells. More work is needed to explain why GO occurs in patients with Hashimoto's thyroiditis with no evident TSHR autoimmune reactivity (2, 8). Although IGF-1R might be another autoantigen, GO pathology does not involve directly stimulating IGF-1R antibodies (5, 8). Serum antibodies against the IGF-1R are greater in GD patients, regardless of the presence of GO, suggesting a less pathogenic role of IGF-1R antibodies in GO (66, 67). In fact, a functional and physical crosstalk between TSHR and IGF-1R seems to be more important (5, 8). Defects in immune modulation lead to the breakdown of self-tolerance to thyroid or orbital connective tissues. Then, antigen-presenting cells (OFs themselves, fibrocytes, B cells, macrophages, or dendritic cells in the vicinity) recognize the exposed TSHR epitopes on the OF surface and then process and present the TSHR peptides to T cells, which leads to T cell clonal expansion and migration into orbital connective tissues (5, 6, 64). It should be noted that self-reactive B cells are likely to participate in GO antigen-presenting process. In recent onset GD patients, autoreactive B cells in PBMCs expressed CD86 and no longer appeared anergic, which indicates the activation and differentiation of B cells into plasma cells, leading to autoantibody production (68). Hence, it is reasonable to postulate that the same immune response occurs in orbital connective tissues in GO, where high levels of TSHR autoantibodies are detected in the sera of patients and may precede the onset of eye disease. A vital role of rituximab in the treatment of GO may lie in the blockade of antigen-presenting function of these activated self-reactive B cells (69). In addition, the over-reactive immune process has many other complicated mechanisms including thymic and peripheral T cell deletions and T cell anergy (5, 6, 70). Activated T cells provide the second signal for self-reactive B cell activation *via* the interaction of CD40L on the T cell surface with CD40 on the B cell surface. Moreover, the combination of B7 on the B cell surface and CD28 on the T cell surface provides the second signal for further activation of self-reactive T cells (5, 64, 71). Autoantibodies against TSHR are produced by plasma cells differentiated from activated B cells and autoantibody class switching (IgM to IgG and IgE) is aided by IL-4 secreted by activated T cells (mainly Th2 cells) (5, 64, 71). Autoantibodies, including stimulating, neutralizing, and blocking IgG (72), target the TSHR on OFs, which may promote cytokine and chemoattractant production, deposition of extracellular matrix (ECM) such as hyaluronan, and pathological OF differentiation into adipocytes and myofibroblasts (73). Potential cross-talk of TSHR with IGF-1R on OFs helps to augment the expression of inflammatory molecules and hyaluronan synthesis (74, 75). The above pathological processes are largely due to the cell contact between OFs and T cells and cytokines produced by various T cell types (**Figure 1**).

An important intercellular communication in GO is CD40-CD40L signaling (**Figure 2**). CD40 is a mitogenic receptor that belongs to the tumor necrosis factor (TNF)-α receptor superfamily (76). CD40 is constitutively expressed by human fibroblasts derived from different tissue sources including OFs (18, 76), which facilitates fibroblast proliferation (76). GO OFs express elevated CD40 at gene and protein levels compared with control OFs (18, 77). When delineated by the cell surface marker CD90, CD90$^+$ GO OFs had considerably greater CD40 expression than that on CD90$^-$ subsets as well as both control OF subsets (18). The combination of CD40 on OFs with CD40L on T cells leads to the three following pathological effects: (1) The release of inflammatory cytokines that induce acute and chronic orbital inflammation. Activation of GO OFs by CD40 engagement elevates IL-6 and IL-8 protein levels comparable with those produced by CD40-activated control OFs (77). Additionally, GO OFs primed with IFN-γ appear to be more responsive to CD40 activation than control OFs with regard to macrophage chemoattractant protein-1 (MCP-1) expression (18). Intriguingly, overproduction of IL-6 and IL-8 has been observed in CD90$^+$ GO OFs compared with CD90$^-$ GO OFs after priming with IFN-γ (18). Conversely, CD40-CD40L signaling stimulates relatively low IL-6 and IL-8 production in both control OF subsets even when pre-incubated with IFN-γ (18). Hence, the higher expression of CD40 on CD90$^+$ GO OFs may be critical to generate IL-6 and IL-8 in response to CD40L. Moreover, time-dependent secretion of prostaglandin (PG) E_2 from GO OFs induced by CD40 engagement has been attributed to the up-regulation of IL-1α production, which enhances the expression of prostaglandin endoperoxide H synthase-2 (PGSH-2 or COX-2) at both transcriptional and translational levels (21). (2) Up-regulation of adhesion molecules promotes immune cell recruitment to orbital connective tissues. GO orbital connective tissues expressed higher levels of intercellular adhesion molecule-1 (ICAM-1) and vascular cell adhesion molecule-1 (VCAM-1) compared with control subjects (30). The gene and protein expressions of ICAM-1 (78), VCAM-1, and E-selectin (79) were increased by CD40 activation in both GO and control OFs in dose- and time-dependent manners, with a more obvious effect on the former. Moreover, sphingolipids were induced in GO OFs, but not control OFs, which attracted T cells to migrate (80). (3) Synthesis of hyaluronan leads to the edema of orbital connective tissues and late-stage tissue remodeling. These phenomena are independent of PGE_2 synthesis in GO OFs (21). Signal transductions for the pathways involved in the

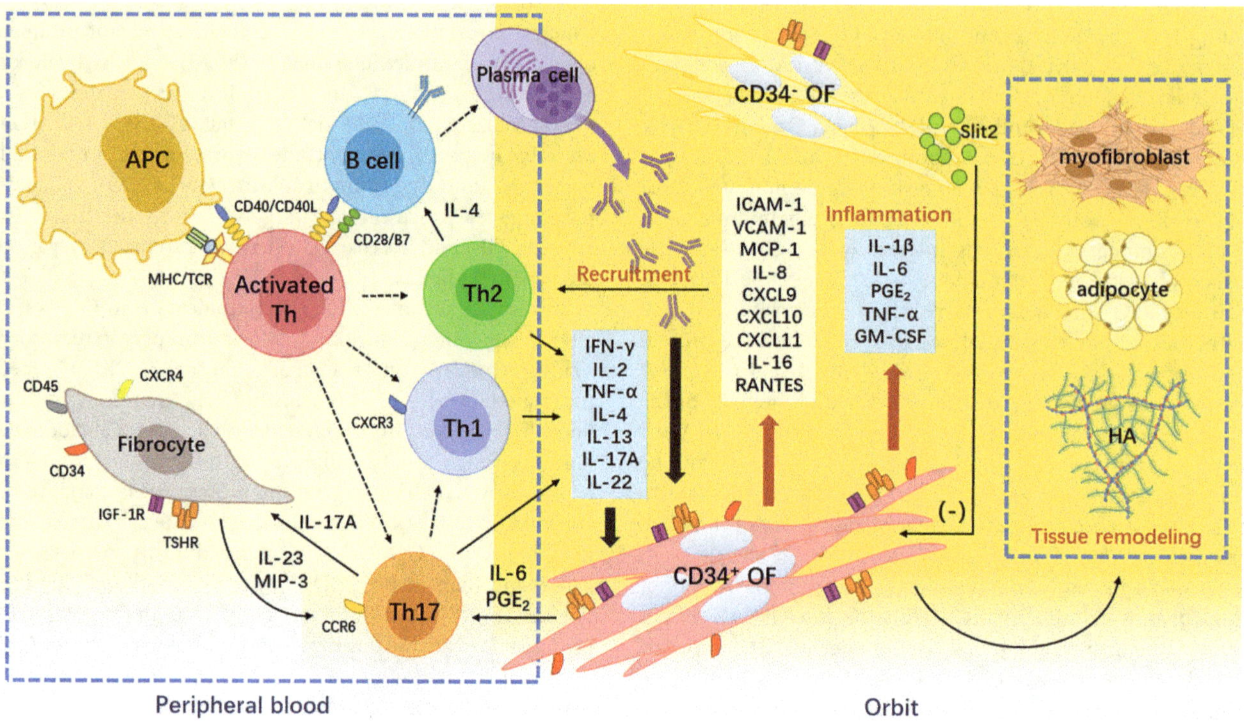

FIGURE 1 | Pathogenesis of Graves' orbitopathy. Breakdown of self-tolerance to thyroid-stimulating hormone receptor (TSHR) leads to the recognition of TSHR epitopes by antigen-presenting cells and B cells. They process the TSHR peptides to activate naïve T helper (Th) cells. Activated and expanded naïve Th cells differentiate into different subsets including interferon (IFN)-γ-producing Th1 cell, interleukin (IL)-4-producing Th2 cells, and IL-17A-producing Th17 cells. These cytokines together with autoantibodies produced by plasms cells derived from self-reactive B cells stimulate orbital fibroblasts (OFs), thereby initiating inflammatory responses in the orbit. IFN-γ is cytotoxic, IL-4 helps B cell expansion and autoantibody class switching, and IL-17A is proinflammatory and profibrotic. Meanwhile, peripheral $CD34^+$ fibrocytes infiltrate orbital connective tissues and transition into $CD34^+$ OFs. Upon IFN-γ and IL-17A stimulation, these $CD34^+$ cells not only robustly produce chemokines such as C-X-C motif ligand 9/10/11 attracting C-X-C chemokine receptor 3^+ Th1 cell and macrophage inflammatory protein-3 attracting C-C chemokine receptor 6^+ Th17 cells but also secrete a large amount of cytokines such as IL-1β and prostaglandin E_2 that exacerbate orbital inflammation. $CD34^+$ OFs ultimately synthesize hyaluronic acid and differentiate into adipocytes or myofibroblasts that cause orbital tissue remodeling. The orbital native residential $CD34^-$ OFs express immunomodulatory molecules such as Slit2 to restrain the activities of the infiltrating $CD34^+$ OFs.

CD40-CD40L combination mentioned above mainly include nuclear translocation of nuclear factor-κB, mitogen-activated protein kinases, and phosphatidylinositol-3-kinase. Further studies are needed to examine in more depth the cognate interactions between GO OFs and infiltrating T cells *via* CD40-CD40L communication.

Furthermore, T cell-OF interaction triggers the differentiation of OFs into adipocytes (8). Feldon et al. reported that GO orbital connective tissues and GO OFs highly expressed peroxisome proliferator-activated receptor (PPAR)-γ mRNA and proteins (81). In an autologous periphery T cell-OF coculture system, activated T cells drove the differentiation of GO OFs into orbital adipocytes. These activated T cells not only expressed up-regulated levels of PGSH-2 but also synthesized PGD_2 and related PGJ_2 that are PPAR-γ ligands (81). This PPAR-γ-dependent adipogenic process of GO OFs provides evidence for how inflammation-provoking T cells regulate adipogenesis of orbital connective tissues and an interesting clue to the many faces of T cell immunity in GO.

PARADIGM OF TH1/TH2 IMMUNE RESPONSES

Previous studies have shown that both Th1 and Th2 cell subsets are involved in GO autoimmunity. In a study by De carli et al., 153 orbital T cell clones expanded from four severe GO patients exhibited remarkably high proportions of both $CD4^+$ and $CD8^+$ T cell phenotypes with a Th1-like cytokine profile including IFN-γ (82% in CD4; 88% in CD8), IL-2 (79% in CD4; 81% in CD8), and TNF-α (90% in CD4; 88% in CD8), but not IL-4 (4% in CD4; 0% in CD8) or IL-5 (1% in CD4; 0% in CD8), compared with T cell clones expanded from PBMCs of both GO patients and control subjects (38). Förster et al. examined cytokine gene expression in 18 orbital T cell lines from six severe GO patients and detected expression of Th1 cytokine genes *Ifng* (10/18), *Tnfa* (12/18), and *Il2* (17/18) as well as Th2 cytokine genes *Il4* (12/18) and *Il5* (17/18). Other expressed cytokine genes were *Il6* (13/18), *Il10* (4/18), and *Tnfb* (15/18) (42). Using orbital T cell clones expanded from three severe GO patients, Yang et al. observed expression of *Ifng*

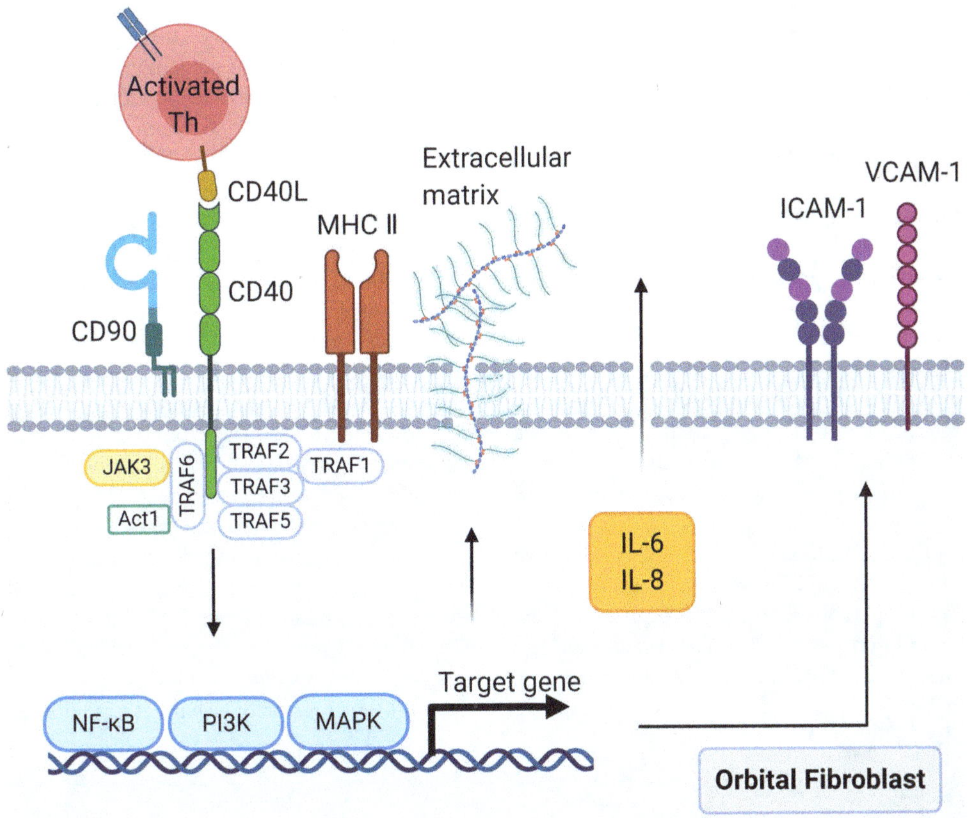

FIGURE 2 | The CD40-CD40 ligand signaling in orbital fibroblasts. When CD40 ligand on self-reactive T cells combines with CD40 on orbital fibroblasts, the nuclear translocation of nuclear factor-κB, mitogen activated protein kinases, and phosphatidylinositol-3-kinase signaling pathways will be activated, leading to the synthesis of cytokines interleukin-6 and interleukin-8, costimulatory molecules intercellular adhesion molecule-1 and vascular cell adhesion molecule-1, and extracellular matrix.

and *Il2* in eight out of 14 $CD4^+$ T cell clones and four out of six $CD8^+$ T cell clones. The authors also assessed cytokine secretion in 38 $CD4^+$ and 10 $CD8^+$ strains, including the T cell clones for gene expression examination, and reported detectable levels of IFN-γ in most T cell clones (36/38 in CD4; 9/10 in CD8), of which some secreted IL-2 (8/36 in CD4; 5/10 in CD8). No Th2 cytokine gene profile and only three IL-4-secreting and five IL-10-secreting T cell clones were found (82). These results indicate that the great majority of orbit-infiltrating T cells express a Th1-like cytokine profile at both transcriptional and translational levels. In a study by Pappa et al., nine EOM-derived T cell lines from four GO patients were all positive for Th1 cytokine IFN-γ and IL-2. Other tested cytokines included TNF-β (5/9) and transforming growth factor (TGF)-β (9/9). They also found that Th2 cytokine IL-4 was positive in three out of five examined T cell lines (among the nine T cell lines) and IL-10 was positive in four out of five. However, the detectable rates of cytokines genes *Il1a*, *Il2*, *Il4*, *Il6*, *Il8*, *Il10*, *Il5*, and *Tnfa* varied among another 12 different EOMs of a further five patients. Expression of *Ifng*, *Il13*, *Il1b*, and *Il12p40* was not detected in these EOMs. *Il6* and *Il8* were the only cytokine genes expressed in two out of five EOMs from three control subjects (41). It should be considered that gene and protein expressions are not complete coincident. Furthermore, apart from the technical problems related to the lymphocyte number and sample size, the various pre-surgery treatments that each patient had received and whether T cell clones were consecutively included or selected from independent patient cohorts will introduce biases and affect the results.

An important study by Aniszewski et al. examined cytokine production of 57 $CD4^+$ T cell clones expanded from six GO patients and explicitly showed that T cell clones from recent onset GO (less than 2 years) mainly produced IFN-γ (47%) compared with IL-4 (23%), whereas those from remote onset GO (more than 2 years) dominantly produced IL-4 (75%) compared with IFN-γ (0%) (16). These findings suggest that the Th1 immune response may predominate in early active GO and the Th2 immune response is likely to play a role in late inactive GO. Unfortunately, all T cell strains examined were cultured and expanded *in vitro* for many days and only four T cell clones were matched for late GO, which drew criticism of the study design in which conclusions were made on the basis of data that may result in inaccurate estimates of T cell populations that invaded *in situ* within the orbit. Additionally, short duration GO is not exactly the same as active GO and longer duration GO does not mean that orbital inflammation is apparently absorbed.

By directly investigating the cytokine gene expression of EOMs *in vivo* from 14 GO patients and orbital connective tissues from 29 GO patients, expression of *Ifng* (13/14), *Tnfα* (5/14), *Il1b* (8/14), and *Il6* (9/14) was mainly detected in EOMs, while they were less often expressed in orbital connective tissues in which *Il4* (7/29) and *Il0* (11/29) were more frequently expressed (83). Notably, the mean GO duration of the patients involved in the study was 2 years, which may account for the lower expression of *Ifng* and relatively higher expression of *Il4* in orbital connective tissues. Additionally, we cannot neglect the fact that all patients had undergone orbital irradiation before tissues were obtained and half had received high-dose GCs. Wakelkamp et al. investigated cytokine gene expression in orbital connective tissues from 17 GO patients, of whom six had untreated active disease and underwent emergency decompression surgeries. The other 11 patients were in the inactive phase and underwent rehabilitative surgeries. Compared with inactive GO patients, active GO patients had increased expression levels of *Il1b*, *Il6*, *Il8*, and *Il10*. Expression of Th1 cytokine genes *Ifng*, *Il2*, and *Il12p40* was also higher in active orbital connective tissues. However, expression of Th2 cytokine genes *Il5* and *Il13* was comparable in both patient groups and *Il4* expression was not found in the study (84). These data imply the importance of the Th1, but not Th2, immune response and many other proinflammatory cytokines in the autoimmune environment in the active GO orbit, although the gene expression results need to be supported at the protein level. Furthermore, the source of the examined cytokines cannot be identified in the bulk sequencing data.

Many recent studies have confirmed that orbital connective tissues from GO exhibit strong immunostaining for IFN-γ in the infiltrating cells, especially in the active phase (33, 45, 61). Using *in vivo* flow cytometric analysis, we demonstrated an increased frequency of $CD3^{+}CD8^{-}$ IFN-γ-producing T cells in both GO peripheral blood and orbital connective tissues compared with control subjects (31, 45). In hTSHR-A subunit plasmid-primed GO BALB/c mice, splenic T cells secreted IFN-γ (53). An increased frequency of $CD4^{+}$ IFN-γ-producing T cells derived from splenocytes has also been observed in hTSHR-A subunit-expressing adenovirus-immunized GO BALB/c mice (36). In an SKG murine model of GO, expression of *Ifng*, *Tnfa*, and *Il2* was augmented in periorbital tissues and their protein levels were elevated in sera compared with wild type mice (48).

However, the pathological effects of IFN-γ on OFs are not fully understood (**Figure 3**). An essential function of IFN-γ in GO is acting as the "sinister partner" of CD40-CD40L signaling to exacerbate orbital inflammation. IFN-γ not only up-regulates CD40 on human fibroblasts derived from lung, skin, and gingiva, but also shifts fibroblasts to the G0/G1 phase of the cell cycle (76). Expression of CD40 was further augmented by IFN-γ in

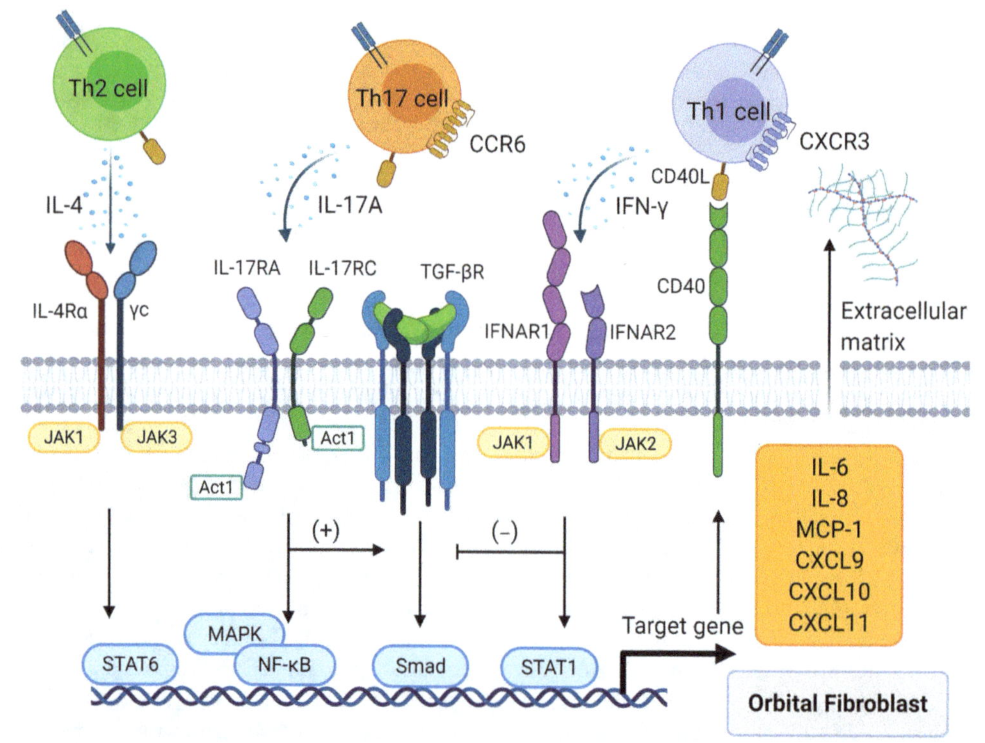

FIGURE 3 | The effects of T cell cytokines on orbital fibroblasts (OFs). T helper (Th) 1 cytokine interferon-γ, Th2 cytokine interleukin (IL)-4, and Th17 cytokine IL-17A result in the production of IL-6, IL-8, macrophage chemoattractant protein-1, C-X-C motif ligand 9/10/11, and extracellular matrix in OFs. Interferon–γ interferes with transforming growth factor-β induced fibrosis in OFs while IL-17A strengthens this process.

both GO and control OFs regardless of CD90 expression (18, 77, 85). Additionally, MHC II expression was increased in both GO and control OFs after IFN-γ stimulation (17, 77, 85) with a more potent effect on $CD90^-$ GO OFs (85). High-dose IFN-γ (1000 U/ml) alone was a potent stimulant of MCP-1 in GO and non-GO OFs as well as GO OF-differentiated adipocytes (86, 87) and induced IL-8 secretion with long term incubation (24 hours) (86). However, low- and medium-dose IFN-γ (100-500 U/ml) alone did not up-regulate IL-6 or IL-8 expression in GO and control OFs as well as their corresponding subsets (77, 85, 88), but greatly promoted IL-6 and IL-8 production provoked by CD40-CD40L signaling in mixed GO and control OF populations (77) as well as pure $CD90^+$ and $CD90^-$ GO OF subsets (18, 85).

Another major pathological role of IFN-γ is establishment of a positive inflammatory feedback loop that maintains Th1 immune response in GO. The serum levels of chemokine C-X-C motif ligand (CXCL) 10 were higher in GO patients than control subjects, especially in active disease (23). Dose-dependent secretion of CXCL9, CXCL10, and CXCL11 after IFN-γ treatment has been observed in GO OFs as well as GO OF-differentiated adipocytes (23, 24). Although TNF-α alone did not induce secretion of the chemokines in GO OFs and adipocytes, IFN-γ further promoted MCP-1, CXCL9, CXCL10, and CXCL11 release stimulated by TNF-α in these cells (23, 24, 87). The proinflammatory effect that IFN-γ with TNF-α synergistically exerts on GO OFs and adipocytes is suppressed in a dose-dependent manner by PPAR-α agonists fenofibrate, gemfibrozil, or ciprofibrate, and PPAR-γ agonists rosiglitazone or pioglitazone (23, 24, 87, 89). A study regarding the role of circulating CXCL9 and CXCL10 as potential markers for GO activity revealed that GC treatment and teleradiotherapy significantly decreased CXCL9 and CXCL10 serum concentrations compared with basal values in GO patients. A positive correlation between CXCL9 and CXCL10 was also found in this study (90). Because C-X-C chemokine receptor (CXCR) 3 is particularly expressed on Th1 cells, which binds CXCL9, CXCL10, and CXCL11 (91), the above studies reflect an accurately self-modulated Th1 immunity-mediated inflammatory network in GO.

Furthermore, IFN-γ results in the accumulation of ECM in GO. IFN-γ enhances hyaluronan synthesis activated by CD40-CD40L signaling in GO OFs and strengthens IL-1β-induced hyaluronan synthesis in GO OFs by promoting expression of the hyaluronan synthase-2 gene (21, 25). It does not directly induce PGE_2 secretion in GO OFs or contribute to PGE_2 levels initiated by CD40-CD40L signaling (21). However, IFN-γ acts synergistically with CD40-CD40L signaling to elicit a dramatic increase in PGE_2 production in $CD90^+$ GO OFs and $CD90^-$ GO OFs *via* up-regulation of PGSH-2 proteins (85). Conversely, IFN-γ attenuates IL-1β-provoked PGE_2 production in GO OFs *via* down-regulation of PGHS-2 mediated by decreased *Pghs-2* promoter activity and weakened PGHS-2 mRNA stability. This process is regulated by Janus kinase 2 signaling (25). The different modulation of PGE_2 production by IFN-γ in combination with other molecular signals indicates a potential role of Th1 cell immunity and its related cytokines in regulating tissue reactivity and remodeling in the orbit. It is recognized that $CD90^+$ OFs tend to differentiate into myofibroblasts, a hallmark of late GO fibrosis, whereas $CD90^-$ OFs tend to differentiate into adipocytes (2, 6, 22). IFN-γ blocks TGF-β-induced α-smooth muscle actin (SMA) expression in $CD90^+$ GO OFs, which inhibits myofibroblast differentiation (22). Similarly, high levels of tissue inhibitor of metalloproteinase (TIMP)-1 gene and protein expression associated with fibrosis have been observed in IL-1β-treated GO OFs in a dose- and time-dependent manner, which was attenuated by IFN-γ *via* down-regulation of *Timp1* promoter activity (26). This suggests that IFN-γ is more of a kind of proinflammatory factor that causes tissue damage and degeneration, and proves that the Th1 immune reaction is predominantly involved in early active GO.

The pathological effects of Th2 cytokines on OFs have yet to be examined carefully (**Figure 3**). Studies in GO murine models have not been able to duplicate Th2-dominated immune responses. A decreased frequency of $CD4^+$ IL-4-producing splenic T cells has been observed in hTSHR-A subunit-expressing adenovirus-immunized GO BALB/c mice (36). However, compared with wild type mice, expression of *Il4*, *Il5*, and *Il13* was increased in periorbital tissues of GO SKG mice (48). In another study, serum IL-4 remained at a higher level in hTSHR-A subunit plasmid-immunized GO BALB/c mice than in normal mice with extension of the immune time when IL-6, TNF-α, and granulocyte-macrophage colony stimulating factor were gradually declining (92). These results imply a possible role of Th2 cell-triggered immune responses in orbital connective tissues of stable GO. We used flow cytometry to confirm that the frequencies of $CD3^+CD8^-$ IL-13-producing T cells and $CD3^+CD8^-GATA3^+$ T cells were augmented in orbital connective tissues from GO patients. Both IL-13 and GATA3 were significantly related to GO development in a multivariate logistic regression model (31). These results suggest an indispensable and major role of Th2 immunity in GO inflammation. Although IL-4 cannot up-regulate CD40 expression in fibroblasts (76), it has many similar effects in regulating the biological behaviors of GO OFs. IL-4 suppresses *Timp1* promoter activation by IL-1β, which reduces the levels of TIMP-1 gene and protein expression in GO OFs (26). IL-4 also suppresses *Pghs-2* promoter activation by IL-1β, thereby inhibiting secretion of PGE_2 from GO OFs (25). However, IL-4 promotes IL-1β-initiated hyaluronan synthesis in GO OFs by up-regulating hyaluronan synthase-2 gene expression (25). The identical functions of IFN-γ and IL-4 suggest transition from Th1 to Th2 cells to maintain the delicate balance between ECM production and degradation in orbital connective tissues as GO progresses from the early to late stage. In view of the major involvement of Th2 cell immunity in tissue fibrosis (93), more research on the relationship between Th2 cytokines IL-4, IL-5, and IL-13 and GO tissue remodeling is needed.

EMERGING ROLE OF THE TH17 IMMUNE RESPONSE

The first evidence regarding the possible role of Th17 cells in GO pathogenesis was published in 2008. A total of 216 GD patients and 368 control subjects were genotyped for single nucleotide polymorphisms of *Il23r*. rs2201841 was strongly associated with GO, especially AA ($P=1.0\times10^{-4}$; OR=2.4) and CC ($P=1.4\times10^{-4}$; OR=2.36) genotypes (27). This indicates that *Il23r* variants may increase susceptibility to GO by regulating the expression or function of IL-23R on Th17 cells. Soon after, Kim et al. reported significantly higher detectable rates and serum levels of IL-17A in GO patients than those in control subjects, especially in the active phase (94). This was confirmed by another study in which serum IL-17A was higher in both active and inactive GO patients than in control subjects, despite its relative reduction compared with GD patients without eye disease (95). Additionally, Wei et al. observed the highest levels of serum IL-17A in active GO patients compared with those in both inactive GO and GD patients (96). Other studies that focused on lacrimal glands and the ocular surface have revealed elevated IL-17A levels in the tears of active and inactive GO patients (97–99). An orbital magnetic resonance scan showed that the axial lacrimal gland area was positively correlated with IL-17A concentrations in GO patient tears (99). Both serum and tear IL-17A levels have been positively correlated with the GO clinical activity score (94, 96, 99). We also observed up-regulated serum levels of IL-17A, but not IL-17F, in GO patients (44). More importantly, IL-23 (44, 94), IL-6 (44, 95, 97–99), and IL-1β (44, 97–99) concentrations were elevated in both sera and tears from active and inactive GO patients and more enriched in active phase, which are crucial factors for the differentiation of Th17 cells (100, 101). Analogously, the expression of IL-17A, IL-23, IL-6, and IL-1β increases diffusely around small vessels or fibroblasts and adipocytes within GO orbital connective tissues (44). These cytokines may construct a suitable microenvironment for the survival and activation of Th17 cells both systemically and locally in GO. We found that $CD3^+$ IL-17A-producing T cells were increased among GO PBMCs compared with controls. Furthermore, both $CD3^+CD8^-$ (Th17) and $CD3^+CD8^+$ (Tc17) IL-17A-producing subsets are augmented in GO peripheral blood (44, 45). The $CD3^+CD8^-$ T cells in GO also express a higher proportion of retinoic acid receptor related orphan receptor (ROR)-γt, the key transcription factor for Th17 cells (44). Intriguingly, most Th17 and Tc17 cells are $CD45RO^+$ memory T cells (30, 44, 45), which indicates that these IL-17A-producing T cells might have been exposed to autoantigens such as TSHR and activated in the very early phase of GO or even in the GD stage. This is supported by the fact that the frequency of peripheral Th17 cells is higher in new-onset and intractable GD patients (102–104). More importantly, IL-17A-producing and RORγt-bearing Th17 cells were recruited at a higher fraction in GO orbital connective tissues, which were significantly associated with GO occurrence in a multivariate logistic regression model (31).

Th17 cells facilitate the inflammatory state of OFs in GO autoimmunity (**Figure 3**). In our *in vitro* model, IL-17A promoted transcriptional and translational expression of IL-6, IL-8, and MCP-1 in GO OFs in a dose- and time-dependent manner compared with fibroblasts derived from eyelid tissues. However, IL-17A did not affect the production of IL-23, IL-1β, or TGF-β in GO OFs (44). IL-17A alone did not stimulate RANTES (regulated upon activation, normal T-cell expressed and secreted) production, but strongly induced its mRNA and protein expression in the presence of CD40-CD40L signaling in both GO and control OFs in a dose- and time-dependent manner (45). In a Th17 cell-OF coculture system, Th17 cells promoted the secretion of IL-6, IL-8, MCP-1, macrophage inflammatory protein (MIP)-3, TNF-α, and granulocyte-macrophage colony stimulating factor from both $CD90^+$ and $CD90^-$ OFs (30). In recent years, circulating fibrocytes have been recognized to participate in GO inflammation and tissue remodeling (105, 106). These cells express CD45, CD34, CXCR4, collagen I, thyroglobulin, TSHR, and IGF-1R, and were far more frequent in the circulation of GD and GO patients than in control subjects and were highly detected in GO orbital connective tissues, but were absent in control orbits (28, 29, 107). Both GO and control fibrocytes secreted TNF-α, IL-6, IL-8, IL-12, MCP-1, RANTES, MIP-1a, MIP-1b, CXCL10, and granulocyte colony-stimulating factor when stimulated by TSH or M22, a monoclonal TSHR-activating antibody (28, 29, 108). We found that GO and control fibrocytes synthesized IL-6, IL-8, and MCP-1 robustly in response to IL-17A, while GO fibrocytes had higher levels of basal and induced secretion of these cytokines than control fibrocytes (32). In a Th17 cell-fibrocyte coculture system, we found that expression of *Il6*, *Il8*, *Mcp1*, *Mip3a*, *Tnfa*, *Cxcl9*, and *Cxcl10* was augmented in GO fibrocytes and their proteins had accumulated in the culture supernatants (32). Both fibrocytes and OFs as well as OF subsets delineated by CD90 express IL-17RA (30, 32, 44), which suggests consecutive stimulation by Th17 cells from peripheral circulation to local orbital connective tissues in GO.

Th17 cells also modulate the fibrosis and adipogenesis balance in GO OFs. IL-17A directly leads to various ECM depositions in orbital connective tissues. Compared with control OFs, the gene and protein synthesis of fibronectin, collagen I, collagen III, TIMP-1, TIMP-2, matrix metalloproteinase (MMP)-1, and MMP-2 was greatly induced by IL-17A treatment of GO OFs in a dose- and time-dependent manner (44). Up-regulation of α-SMA gene and protein expression has been observed in IL-17A-treated GO OFs, which demonstrates differentiation of OFs into myofibroblasts (44). Unexpectedly, when we used pure $CD90^+$ and $CD90^-$ GO OF subsets, IL-17A exerted distinct effects on the two cell types. Low-dose IL-17A (10 ng/ml) was sufficient to enhance the fibrotic process marked by increased protein levels of α-SMA, fibronectin, collagen I, TIMP-1, and MMP-2 in GO OFs provoked by TGF-β. However, both low- and high (100 ng/ml)-dose IL-17A interfered with adipogenic differentiation of $CD90^-$ OFs induced by 15-deoxy-$\Delta^{12,14}$-PGJ_2. The protein levels of perilipin A, adipocyte differentiation-related protein, adiponectin, and PPAR-γ were down-regulated in $CD90^-$ OFs in the presence of IL-17A (30). IL-17A promoted phosphorylation of JNK/c-Jun in $CD90^+$ OFs, but impeded phosphorylation of CEBP/α in $CD90^-$ OFs. Additionally, in $CD90^+$ OFs, proteomics analysis has revealed that IL-17A enhances the production of ECM and proteins that are positive regulators for TGF-β and JNK cascade, but prevents adipocyte differentiation of $CD90^-$ OFs by up-regulating proteins involved in fatty acid oxidation, degradation, and efflux processes (30). Owing to the considerably high proportion of the $CD90^+$

phenotype among GO OFs (30, 109), these findings suggest that GO OFs have a repertoire of differentiation that is more skewed towards myofibroblasts under IL-17A stimulation.

However, GO OFs regulate the phenotype and function of Th17 cells. In a Th17 cell-OF coculture system, both CD90$^+$ and CD90$^-$ GO OFs enhanced the secretion of IL-17A from Th17 cells. Other supernatant-enriched cytokines included IL-22 and IL-21. An increased frequency of IL-17A$^+$RORγt$^+$ Th17 cells was shown by flow cytometry in the coculture system, which was repressed by down-regulating PGE_2 released from CD90$^+$ and CD90$^-$ GO OFs (30). The molecular mechanisms were possibly mediated by up-regulating IL-23R and IL-1R expression on Th17 cells, which was caused by PGE_2-EP2/EP4 signaling that led to intracellular cAMP formation and subsequent phosphorylation of cAMP-responsive element-binding protein (31). These *in vitro* findings are consistent with the observation that GO orbital connective tissues contain a level of PGE_2 and orbit-infiltrating Th17 cells express more IL-23R and IL-1R (31). Moreover, the Th17 cell-OF interaction results in a dramatic elevation of the expression of CD40, MHC II, ICAM-1, and VCAM-1 on CD90$^+$ and CD90$^-$ GO OFs, particularly on those that are also CD34$^+$ (30). Such CD34$^+$ OFs may originate putatively from CD34$^+$ fibrocyte progenitors (106). Flow cytometric analysis has shown that CD34$^+$ GO OFs have higher levels of IL-17RA than native residential CD34$^-$ subsets, which might account for the overexpressed CD40 and MHC II on CD34$^+$ cells (31). Moreover, Th17 cell-fibrocyte interplay not only enhances IL-17A production in Th17 cells, but also significantly promotes CD40 and MHC II expression on GO fibrocytes (32).

How are Th17 cells recruited into orbital connective tissues in GO? Both peripheral and orbit-infiltrating Th17 cells express C-C chemokine receptor (CCR) 6, a MIP-3 receptor (30–32). Therefore, the MIP-3 released by GO fibrocytes might be a strong attractant that directs Th17 cells to sites of inflamed orbital connective tissues. Guo et al. demonstrated that orbit-infiltrating T cells in GO express CD44 (110), a specific cell surface receptor for hyaluronan (111). CD44 is highly elevated on activated T cells (112, 113) and particularly on CCR6$^+$ IL-17A-producing Th17 cells in our study (30). However, T cell subsets with low expression of CD44 hardly secrete IL-17A in GO patients (30). Thus, with increased pericellular hyaluronan deposition, CD44 may facilitate Th17 cell attachment to GO OFs.

In recent years, the concept of Th17 cell plasticity has become prominent. Th17 cells acquire much more complex functional phenotypes than previously thought. Although they can shift phenotype within their lineage, Th17 cells have a dynamic ability to trans-differentiate into other CD4$^+$ T cell subsets such as Th1 and Th2 cells (100, 114, 115). IFN-γ- and IL-22-producing Th17 cells are detected at significantly higher levels among GO PBMCs, especially in active patients (30, 45). These so called pathogenic Th17 cells express both RORγt and Tbet. They infiltrate into GO orbital connective tissues and more likely produce IFN-γ instead of IL-17A (31). TSH and M22 robustly induced gene and protein expression of IL-23 in GO fibrocytes, but not IL-12, which was significantly produced by GO OFs under the same conditions (34). However, pure CD34$^+$ OFs preferentially expressed *Il23p19*, while their homologous CD34$^-$ OFs greatly expressed *Il12p35* (34). The distinct roles of CD34$^+$ and CD34$^-$ OFs reflect the potential shift from a non-pathogenic to pathogenic state of circulating Th17 cells into orbit-infiltrating Th17 cells, which is consistent with the TSHR signaling that drives the specific cytokine milieu by CD34$^+$ fibrocytes that masquerade as CD34$^+$ OFs within orbital connective tissues. The expression of IL-23 by CD34$^+$ fibrocyte/OF lineages might play a prominent part in reinforcing the highly IL-23R-bearing Th17 phenotype in GO orbits (31) by endowing Th17 cells with "pathogenic" effector functions. We recently reported an increase in peripheral classic CD3$^+$CD8$^-$CXCR3$^+$CCR6$^-$ Th1 cells in active moderate-to-severe GO patients and GD patients, which were decreased in active very severe GO patients. Conversely, we found that classic CD3$^+$CD8$^-$CXCR3$^-$CCR6$^+$ Th17 and non-classic CD3$^+$CD8$^-$CXCR3$^+$CCR6$^+$ Th17.1 cells were elevated among PBMCs from active very severe GO patients compared with both active moderate-to-severe GO and GD patients. Intriguingly, the non-classic Th17.1 cells favored IFN-γ production in active very severe GO patients, but preferentially secreted IL-17A in active moderate-to-severe GO patients. Moreover, the peripheral Th17.1 cells expressed higher levels of RORγt in active moderate-to-severe GO patients, whereas they had augmented levels of Tbet in active very severe GO patients, which was in concert with the different cytokine production phenotypes of these two patient cohorts. Very severe GO patients who did not respond to intravenous GC treatment had a sustained higher frequency of circulating and orbit-infiltrating Th17.1 cells (33). Therefore, we speculate an immunological transition process from Th1 cell immunity to Th17 cell immunity may indicate the development of very severe eye disease in GD. The overactivity of Th17.1 cells may serve as a hallmark for the not yet subsided inflammatory storm in orbital connective tissues. Evidence from animal models is indicating that IL-17A and IFN-γ double-producing Th17 cells are pathogenic drivers of various human autoimmune diseases such as multiple sclerosis, diabetes type 1, uveitis, dry eye, rheumatoid arthritis, and inflammatory bowel disease (100, 114). Unfortunately, no convincing evidence of detectable Th17 cells has been observed in current GO murine models (36, 53), which makes it difficult to prove our hypothesis. The distinctive genetic backgrounds of BALB/c and C57BL/6J mice may partially be responsible for their susceptibility to GD and GO as well as the different T cell responses under autoimmune disease conditions (116). In this regard, a role of the gut microbiota that influence the immunological responses of induced GO murine models cannot be neglected (37, 117). For example, the YCH46 strain of *Bacteroides fragilis* reduces Th17 cell numbers by releasing propionic acid in GD patients (118). An interesting study reported correlations between murine GO manifestation and gut microbial taxonomies. Significant differences in the diversity and spatial organization of the gut microbiota of hTSHR-A subunit plasmid-immunized BALB/c mice were shown in two centers from different countries (37). Thus, the impact of different regions is also a source of potentially conflicting results, since the microbiome changes across different countries. Disease-associated gut microbiota may contribute to the induced immune responses in GO murine models. Despite the confounding deviation from real human GO, future animal models will certainly be developed from existing experience and provide researchers with novel points of study to investigate the immunopathogenesis of GO.

FUTURE PERSPECTIVES

To date, immunomodulation therapy has been widely used for treatment of GO. Traditional non-specific immunosuppressants are effective in combination with GC treatment as alternative options for active moderate-to-severe GO (8, 11). Azathioprine and methotrexate interfere with purine synthesis that is necessary for lymphocyte proliferation. Mycophenolate, which inhibits inosine monophosphate dehydrogenase, and cyclosporine, which prevents IL-2 secretion, also exert anti-proliferative effect on lymphocytes (8, 11). However, none of these therapeutic approaches appear to alter the natural course of GO, which makes development of more specific drugs critical to address an important unmet medical need. Considering the complexity of GO pathogenesis, there remain many ambiguous aspects of the pathological T cell activities within orbital connective tissues. For example, T cell migration and activation induced by autoantigens, autoantibodies, and immunomodulatory proteins. Activating TSHR on thymocytes enhances thymic output and therefore the functional T cell repertoire in the periphery (119). A larger proportion of peripheral $CD3^+CD45RO^+IGF\text{-}1R^+$ T cells is seen in GO patients compared with control subjects. IGF-1R, which increases upon TCR stimulation, not only inhibits Fas-mediated apoptosis, but also supports the expansion of memory T cells in GO (120). Furthermore, the proportion of peripheral $IGF\text{-}1R^+$ T cells declines with clinical improvement in GO patients after rituximab treatment (121). Autoantibodies from GO patients up-regulate T cell chemoattractant IL-16 and RANTES from GO OFs (122). Moreover, T cell immunoglobulin domain and mucin domain 3, which restrains cytokine production in effector T cells except Th2 cells, is down-regulated in peripheral Th1 and Th17 cells in GO patients (123, 124). Slit2 from residential $CD34^-$ OFs might inhibit production of IL-6 from GO $CD34^+$ OFs, thereby ameliorating orbital inflammation and repressing Th17 cell differentiation (125). These findings offer new insights to explore novel approaches for therapy of GO. Existing evidence for the efficacy and relative safety of rituximab against $CD20^+$ B cells, tocilizumab against IL-6, etanercept, infliximab, and adalimumab against TNF-α is encouraging (7, 71, 126). The impressive results of teprotumumab have provided the unprecedented possibility for monoclonal antibodies in combination with GCs for GO therapy, although more evidence must be provided. Trials of utilizing belimumab against BAFF (EUDRACT 2015–002127–26), K1-70 against TSHR (NCT02904330), and iscalimab against CD40 (NCT02713256) are currently underway. Blocking the IL-23/IL-17A axis as a therapeutic strategy for GO is also promising considering its effectiveness in other autoimmune diseases such as psoriasis and mandatory spondylitis (71). Notably, a recent interesting study had the first attempt of antigen-specific immunotherapy with ATX-GD-59 that contains two TSHR peptides 9B-N and 5D-K1 in GD, which suggests that ATX-GD-59 is a safe and well-tolerated treatment (127). This antigen-specific method blocks the activation of APCs by binding with HLA-DR molecules, thereby inhibiting the subsequent cascade reactions of self-reactive T and B cells, which truly represents the needed breakthrough for targeted and effective therapy with less prone to general side effects. Novel biological agent identification on the basis of advances in GO pathogenesis is time-consuming but rewarding, which ultimately benefits patients with this debilitating disease.

AUTHOR CONTRIBUTIONS

SF and YH wrote the paper. YL constructed all the figures. HZ revised the paper. XF was responsible for the writing idea and framework of the paper. All authors contributed to the article and approved the submitted version.

FUNDING

This work was supported by the National Natural Science Foundation of China (81930024, 81761168037, 81770974, 81800695, 82071003, 82000879, 81570883, 81600766, 31701046, 31600971, and 31500714), the National Key R&D Program of China (2018YFC1106100, 2018YFC1106101), the Shanghai Sailing Program (18YF1412300), the Research Grant of the Shanghai Science and Technology Committee (20DZ2270800, 17DZ2260100, 19410761100, and 19DZ2331400), the Clinical Research Plan of SHDC (SHDC2020CR3051B), the Project of Medical Robots (IMR-NPH202002) From the Clinical Joint Research Center of the Institute of Medical Robots, Shanghai JiaoTong University-Shanghai Ninth People's Hospital, the Collaborative Research Project of Translational Medicine Collaborative Innovation Center, Shanghai JiaoTong University School of Medicine (TM201718), the Shanghai Municipal Education Commission—Gaofeng Clinical Medicine Grant Support (20152228), the Shanghai JiaoTong University Translational Medicine Crossed Research Grant (ZH2018ZDA12, ZH2018QNA07), the Sample Database Project of Shanghai Ninth People's Hospital (YBKB201901), and the Joint Innovation Team for Young Physicians of Shanghai Ninth People's Hospital (QC202002).

ACKNOWLEDGMENTS

We thank Mitchell Arico from Liwen Bianji, Edanz Group China (www.liwenbianji.cn/ac), for editing the English text of a draft of this manuscript.

REFERENCES

1. Perros P, Hegedüs L, Bartalena L, Marcocci C, Kahaly GJ, Baldeschi L, et al. Graves' orbitopathy as a rare disease in Europe: a European Group on Graves' Orbitopathy (EUGOGO) position statement. *Orphanet J Rare Dis* (2017) 12(1):72. doi: 10.1186/s13023-017-0625-1
2. Smith TJ, Hegedüs L. Graves' Disease. *N Engl J Med* (2016) 375(16):1552–65. doi: 10.1056/NEJMra1510030
3. Lanzolla G, Marcocci C, Marinò M. Oxidative Stress in Graves Disease and Graves Orbitopathy. *Eur Thyroid J* (2020) 9(suppl 1):40–50. doi: 10.1159/000509615
4. Wiersinga WM. Advances in treatment of active, moderate-to-severe Graves' ophthalmopathy. *Lancet Diabetes Endocrinol* (2017) 5(2):134–42. doi: 10.1016/S2213-8587(16)30046-8
5. Davies TF, Andersen S, Latif R, Nagayama Y, Barbesino G, Brito M, et al. Graves' disease. *Nat Rev Dis Primers* (2020) 6(1):52. doi: 10.1038/s41572-020-0184-y
6. Huang Y, Fang S, Li D, Zhou H, Li B, Fan X. The involvement of T cell pathogenesis in thyroid-associated ophthalmopathy. *Eye (Lond)* (2019) 33 (2):176–82. doi: 10.1038/s41433-018-0279-9
7. Genere N, Stan MN. Current and Emerging Treatment Strategies for Graves' Orbitopathy. *Drugs* (2019) 79(2):109–24. doi: 10.1007/s40265-018-1045-9
8. Taylor PN, Zhang L, Lee RWJ, Muller I, Ezra DG, Dayan CM, et al. New insights into the pathogenesis and nonsurgical management of Graves orbitopathy. *Nat Rev Endocrinol* (2020) 16(2):104–16. doi: 10.1038/s41574-019-0305-4
9. Weetman AP, Cohen S, Gatter KC, Fells P, Shine B. Immunohistochemical analysis of the retrobulbar tissues in Graves' ophthalmopathy. *Clin Exp Immunol* (1989) 75(2):222–7.
10. Crotty S. A brief history of T cell help to B cells. *Nat Rev Immunol* (2015) 15 (3):185–9. doi: 10.1038/nri3803
11. Strianese D, Rossi F. Interruption of autoimmunity for thyroid eye disease: B-cell and T-cell strategy. *Eye (Lond)* (2019) 33(2):191–9. doi: 10.1038/s41433-018-0315-9
12. Heufelder AE, Wenzel BE, Scriba PC. Antigen receptor variable region repertoires expressed by T cells infiltrating thyroid, retroorbital, and pretibial tissue in Graves' disease. *J Clin Endocrinol Metab* (1996) 81(10):3733–9. doi: 10.1210/jcem.81.10.8855831
13. Pappa A, Lawson JM, Calder V, Fells P, Lightman S. T cells and fibroblasts in affected extraocular muscles in early and late thyroid associated ophthalmopathy. *Br J Ophthalmol* (2000) 84(5):517–22. doi: 10.1136/bjo.84.5.517
14. Rotondo Dottore G, Torregrossa L, Caturegli P, Ionni I, Sframeli A, Sabini E, et al. Association of T and B Cells Infiltrating Orbital Tissues With Clinical Features of Graves Orbitopathy. *JAMA Ophthalmol* (2018) 136(6):613–9. doi: 10.1001/jamaophthalmol.2018.0806
15. Wang Y, Liu Y, Yang X, Guo H, Lin J, Yang J, et al. Predicting the early risk of ophthalmopathy in Graves' disease patients using TCR repertoire. *Clin Transl Med* (2020) 10(7):e218. doi: 10.1002/ctm2.218
16. Aniszewski JP, Valyasevi RW, Bahn RS. Relationship between disease duration and predominant orbital T cell subset in Graves' ophthalmopathy. *J Clin Endocrinol Metab* (2000) 85(2):776–80. doi: 10.1210/jcem.85.2.6333
17. Feldon SE, Park DJ, O'Loughlin CW, Nguyen VT, Landskroner-Eiger S, Chang D, et al. Autologous T-lymphocytes stimulate proliferation of orbital fibroblasts derived from patients with Graves' ophthalmopathy. *Invest Ophthalmol Vis Sci* (2005) 46(11):3913–21. doi: 10.1167/iovs.05-0605
18. Hwang CJ, Afifiyan N, Sand D, Naik V, Said J, Pollock SJ, et al. Orbital fibroblasts from patients with thyroid-associated ophthalmopathy overexpress CD40: CD154 hyperinduces IL-6, IL-8, and MCP-1. *Invest Ophthalmol Vis Sci* (2009) 50(5):2262–8. doi: 10.1167/iovs.08-2328
19. van Steensel L, Paridaens D, van Meurs M, van Hagen PM, van den Bosch WA, Kuijpers RW, et al. Orbit-infiltrating mast cells, monocytes, and macrophages produce PDGF isoforms that orchestrate orbital fibroblast activation in Graves' ophthalmopathy. *J Clin Endocrinol Metab* (2012) 97(3): E400–8. doi: 10.1210/jc.2011-2697
20. Tsui S, Naik V, Hoa N, Hwang CJ, Afifiyan NF, Sinha Hikim A, et al. Evidence for an association between thyroid-stimulating hormone and insulin-like growth factor 1 receptors: a tale of two antigens implicated in Graves' disease. *J Immunol* (2008) 181(6):4397–405. doi: 10.4049/jimmunol.181.6.4397
21. Cao HJ, Wang HS, Zhang Y, Lin HY, Phipps RP, Smith TJ. Activation of human orbital fibroblasts through CD40 engagement results in a dramatic induction of hyaluronan synthesis and prostaglandin endoperoxide H synthase-2 expression. Insights into potential pathogenic mechanisms of thyroid-associated ophthalmopathy. *J Biol Chem* (1998) 273(45):29615–25. doi: 10.1074/jbc.273.45.29615
22. Koumas L, Smith TJ, Feldon S, Blumberg N, Phipps RP. Thy-1 expression in human fibroblast subsets defines myofibroblastic or lipofibroblastic phenotypes. *Am J Pathol* (2003) 163(4):1291–300. doi: 10.1016/S0002-9440(10)63488-8
23. Antonelli A, Rotondi M, Ferrari SM, Fallahi P, Romagnani P, Franceschini SS, et al. Interferon-gamma-inducible alpha-chemokine CXCL10 involvement in Graves' ophthalmopathy: modulation by peroxisome proliferator-activated receptor-gamma agonists. *J Clin Endocrinol Metab* (2006) 91(2):614–20. doi: 10.1210/jc.2005-1689
24. Antonelli A, Ferrari SM, Fallahi P, Frascerra S, Santini E, Franceschini SS, et al. Monokine induced by interferon gamma (IFNgamma) (CXCL9) and IFNgamma inducible T-cell alpha-chemoattractant (CXCL11) involvement in Graves' disease and ophthalmopathy: modulation by peroxisome proliferator-activated receptor-gamma agonists. *J Clin Endocrinol Metab* (2009) 94(5):1803–9. doi: 10.1210/jc.2008-2450
25. Han R, Smith TJ. T helper type 1 and type 2 cytokines exert divergent influence on the induction of prostaglandin E2 and hyaluronan synthesis by interleukin-1beta in orbital fibroblasts: implications for the pathogenesis of thyroid-associated ophthalmopathy. *Endocrinology* (2006) 147(1):13–9. doi: 10.1210/en.2005-1018
26. Han R, Smith TJ. Induction by IL-1 beta of tissue inhibitor of metalloproteinase-1 in human orbital fibroblasts: modulation of gene promoter activity by IL-4 and IFN-gamma. *J Immunol* (2005) 174 (5):3072–9. doi: 10.4049/jimmunol.174.5.3072
27. Huber AK, Jacobson EM, Jazdzewski K, Concepcion ES, Tomer Y. Interleukin (IL)-23 receptor is a major susceptibility gene for Graves' ophthalmopathy: the IL-23/T-helper 17 axis extends to thyroid autoimmunity. *J Clin Endocrinol Metab* (2008) 93(3):1077–81. doi: 10.1210/jc.2007-2190
28. Douglas RS, Afifiyan NF, Hwang CJ, Chong K, Haider U, Richards P, et al. Increased generation of fibrocytes in thyroid-associated ophthalmopathy. *J Clin Endocrinol Metab* (2010) 95(1):430–8. doi: 10.1210/jc.2009-1614
29. Gillespie EF, Papageorgiou KI, Fernando R, Raychaudhuri N, Cockerham KP, Charara LK, et al. Increased expression of TSH receptor by fibrocytes in thyroid-associated ophthalmopathy leads to chemokine production. *J Clin Endocrinol Metab* (2012) 97(5):E740–6. doi: 10.1210/jc.2011-2514
30. Fang S, Huang Y, Zhong S, Li Y, Zhang Y, Li Y, et al. Regulation of Orbital Fibrosis and Adipogenesis by Pathogenic Th17 Cells in Graves Orbitopathy. *J Clin Endocrinol Metab* (2017) 102(11):4273–83. doi: 10.1210/jc.2017-01349
31. Fang S, Huang Y, Wang N, Zhang S, Zhong S, Li Y, et al. Insights Into Local Orbital Immunity: Evidence for the Involvement of the Th17 Cell Pathway in Thyroid-Associated Ophthalmopathy. *J Clin Endocrinol Metab* (2019) 104(5):1697–711. doi: 10.1210/jc.2018-01626
32. Fang S, Huang Y, Liu X, Zhong S, Wang N, Zhao B, et al. Interaction Between CCR6+ Th17 Cells and CD34+ Fibrocytes Promotes Inflammation: Implications in Graves' Orbitopathy in Chinese Population. *Invest Ophthalmol Vis Sci* (2018) 59(6):2604–14. doi: 10.1167/iovs.18-24008
33. Fang S, Zhang S, Huang Y, Wu Y, Lu Y, Zhong S, et al. Evidence for Associations Between Th1/Th17 "Hybrid" Phenotype and Altered Lipometabolism in Very Severe Graves Orbitopathy. *J Clin Endocrinol Metab* (2020) 105(6):dgaa124. doi: 10.1210/clinem/dgaa124
34. Fernando R, Atkins SJ, Smith TJ. Slit2 May Underlie Divergent Induction by Thyrotropin of IL-23 and IL-12 in Human Fibrocytes. *J Immunol* (2020) 204 (7):1724–35. doi: 10.4049/jimmunol.1900434
35. Moshkelgosha S, So PW, Deasy N, Diaz-Cano S, Banga JP. Cutting edge: retrobulbar inflammation, adipogenesis, and acute orbital congestion in a preclinical female mouse model of Graves' orbitopathy induced by thyrotropin receptor plasmid-in vivo electroporation. *Endocrinology* (2013) 154(9):3008–15. doi: 10.1210/en.2013-1576

36. Zhang M, Ding X, Wu LP, He M, Chen Z, Shi B, et al. A Promising Mouse Model of Graves' Orbitopathy Induced by Adenovirus Expressing Thyrotropin Receptor A Subunit. *Thyroid* (2020). doi: 10.1089/thy.2020.0088
37. Masetti G, Moshkelgosha S, Köhling HL, Covelli D, Banga JP, Berchner-Pfannschmidt U, et al. INDIGO consortium. Gut microbiota in experimental murine model of Graves' orbitopathy established in different environments may modulate clinical presentation of disease. *Microbiome* (2018) 6(1):97. doi: 10.1186/s40168-018-0478-4
38. de Carli M, D'Elios MM, Mariotti S, Marcocci C, Pinchera A, Ricci M, et al. Cytolytic T cells with Th1-like cytokine profile predominate in retroorbital lymphocytic infiltrates of Graves' ophthalmopathy. *J Clin Endocrinol Metab* (1993) 77(5):1120–4. doi: 10.1210/jcem.77.5.8077301
39. Grubeck-Loebenstein B, Trieb K, Sztankay A, Holter W, Anderl H, Wick G. Retrobulbar T cells from patients with Graves' ophthalmopathy are CD8+ and specifically recognize autologous fibroblasts. *J Clin Invest* (1994) 93 (6):2738–43. doi: 10.1172/JCI117289
40. Otto EA, Ochs K, Hansen C, Wall JR, Kahaly GJ. Orbital tissue-derived T lymphocytes from patients with Graves' ophthalmopathy recognize autologous orbital antigens. *J Clin Endocrinol Metab* (1996) 81(8):3045–50. doi: 10.1210/jcem.81.8.8768872
41. Pappa A, Calder V, Ajjan R, Fells P, Ludgate M, Weetman AP, et al. Analysis of extraocular muscle-infiltrating T cells in thyroid-associated ophthalmopathy (TAO). *Clin Exp Immunol* (1997) 109(2):362–9. doi: 10.1046/j.1365-2249.1997.4491347.x
42. Förster G, Otto E, Hansen C, Ochs K, Kahaly G. Analysis of orbital T cells in thyroid-associated ophthalmopathy. *Clin Exp Immunol* (1998) 112(3):427–34. doi: 10.1046/j.1365-2249.1998.00613.x
43. Pawlowski P, Wawrusiewicz-Kurylonek N, Eckstein A, Reszec J, Luczynski W, Johnson K, et al. Disturbances of modulating molecules (FOXP3, CTLA-4/CD28/B7, and CD40/CD40L) mRNA expressions in the orbital tissue from patients with severe graves' ophthalmopathy. *Mediators Inflamm* (2015) 2015:340934. doi: 10.1155/2015/340934
44. Fang S, Huang Y, Wang S, Zhang Y, Luo X, Liu L, et al. IL-17A Exacerbates Fibrosis by Promoting the Proinflammatory and Profibrotic Function of Orbital Fibroblasts in TAO. *J Clin Endocrinol Metab* (2016) Aug101 (8):2955–65. doi: 10.1210/jc.2016-1882
45. Fang S, Huang Y, Zhong S, Zhang Y, Liu X, Wang Y, et al. IL-17A Promotes RANTES Expression, But Not IL-16, in Orbital Fibroblasts Via CD40-CD40L Combination in Thyroid-Associated Ophthalmopathy. *Invest Ophthalmol Vis Sci* (2016) 57(14):6123–33. doi: 10.1167/iovs.16-20199
46. Plöhn S, Hose M, Schlüter A, Michel L, Diaz-Cano S, Hendgen-Cotta UB, et al. Fingolimod Improves the Outcome of Experimental Graves' Disease and Associated Orbitopathy by Modulating the Autoimmune Response to the Thyroid-Stimulating Hormone Receptor. *Thyroid* (2019) 29(9):1286–301. doi: 10.1089/thy.2018.0754
47. Schlüter A, Horstmann M, Diaz-Cano S, Plöhn S, Stähr K, Mattheis S, et al. Genetic immunization with mouse thyrotrophin hormone receptor plasmid breaks self-tolerance for a murine model of autoimmune thyroid disease and Graves' orbitopathy. *Clin Exp Immunol* (2018) 191(3):255–67. doi: 10.1111/cei.13075
48. Park S, Park DY, Kim J, Woo KI, Kim YD, Han J, et al. Enhanced orbital adipogenesis in a mouse model of T-cell-mediated autoimmunity, zymosan A-treated SKG mice: Implications for Graves' ophthalmopathy. *Sci Rep* (2020) 10(1):7329. doi: 10.1038/s41598-020-64402-9
49. Heufelder AE, Herterich S, Ernst G, Bahn RS, Scriba PC. Analysis of retroorbital T cell antigen receptor variable region gene usage in patients with Graves' ophthalmopathy. *Eur J Endocrinol* (1995) 132(3):266–77. doi: 10.1530/eje.0.1320266
50. Heufelder AE, Schworm HD, Wenzel BE, Garrity JA, Bahn RS. Molecular analysis of antigen receptor variable region repertoires in T lymphocytes infiltrating the intrathyroidal and extrathyroidal manifestations in patients with Graves' disease. *Exp Clin Endocrinol Diabetes* (1996) 104 Suppl 4:84–7. doi: 10.1055/s-0029-1211709
51. Heufelder AE. T-cell restriction in thyroid eye disease. *Thyroid* (1998) 8 (5):419–22. doi: 10.1089/thy.1998.8.419
52. Many MC, Costagliola S, Detrait M, Denef F, Vassart G, Ludgate MC. Development of an animal model of autoimmune thyroid eye disease. *J Immunol* (1999) 162(8):4966–74.
53. Berchner-Pfannschmidt U, Moshkelgosha S, Diaz-Cano S, Edelmann B, Görtz GE, Horstmann M, et al. Comparative Assessment of Female Mouse Model of Graves' Orbitopathy Under Different Environments, Accompanied by Proinflammatory Cytokine and T-Cell Responses to Thyrotropin Hormone Receptor Antigen. *Endocrinology* (2016) 157(4):1673–82. doi: 10.1210/en.2015-1829
54. Arnold K, Tandon N, McIntosh RS, Elisei R, Ludgate M, Weetman AP. T cell responses to orbital antigens in thyroid-associated ophthalmopathy. *Clin Exp Immunol* (1994) 96(2):329–34. doi: 10.1111/j.1365-2249.1994.tb06562.x
55. Stover C, Otto E, Beyer J, Kahaly G. Cellular immunity and retrobulbar fibroblasts in Graves' ophthalmopathy. *Thyroid* (1994) Summer4(2):161–5. doi: 10.1089/thy.1994.4.161
56. Eckstein AK, Quadbeck B, Tews S, Mann K, Krüger C, Mohr CH, et al. Thyroid associated ophthalmopathy: evidence for CD4(+) gammadelta T cells; de novo differentiation of RFD7(+) macrophages, but not of RFD1(+) dendritic cells; and loss of gammadelta and alphabeta T cell receptor expression. *Br J Ophthalmol* (2004) 88(6):803–8. doi: 10.1136/bjo.2003.035915
57. Görtz GE, Moshkelgosha S, Jesenek C, Edelmann B, Horstmann M, Banga JP, et al. Pathogenic Phenotype of Adipogenesis and Hyaluronan in Orbital Fibroblasts From Female Graves' Orbitopathy Mouse Model. *Endocrinology* (2016) 157(10):3771–8. doi: 10.1210/en.2016-1304
58. Salvi M, Vannucchi G, Currò N, Introna M, Rossi S, Bonara P, et al. Small dose of rituximab for graves orbitopathy: new insights into the mechanism of action. *Arch Ophthalmol* (2012) 130(1):122–4. doi: 10.1001/archopthalmol.2011.1215
59. Pawlowski P, Poplawska I, Mysliwiec J, Dik WA, Eckstein A, Berchner-Pfannschmidt U, et al. Search of reference biomarkers reflecting orbital tissue remodeling in the course of Graves' orbitopathy. *Folia Histochem Cytobiol* (2020) 58(1):37–45. doi: 10.5603/FHC.a2020.0003
60. Khanna D, Chong KK, Afifiyan NF, Hwang CJ, Lee DK, Garneau HC, et al. Rituximab treatment of patients with severe, corticosteroid-resistant thyroid-associated ophthalmopathy. *Ophthalmology* (2010) 117(1):133–139.e2. doi: 10.1016/j.ophtha.2009.05.029
61. Tang F, Chen X, Mao Y, Wan S, Ai S, Yang H, et al. Orbital fibroblasts of Graves' orbitopathy stimulated with proinflammatory cytokines promote B cell survival by secreting BAFF. *Mol Cell Endocrinol* (2017) 446:1–11. doi: 10.1016/j.mce.2017.01.014
62. Chen MH, Chen MH, Liao SL, Chang TC, Chuang LM. Role of macrophage infiltration in the orbital fat of patients with Graves' ophthalmopathy. *Clin Endocrinol (Oxf)* (2008) 69(2):332–7. doi: 10.1111/j.1365-2265.2008.03219.x
63. Virakul S, Phetsuksiri T, van Holten-Neelen C, Schrijver B, van Steensel L, Dalm VASH, et al. Histamine induces NF-κB controlled cytokine secretion by orbital fibroblasts via histamine receptor type-1. *Exp Eye Res* (2016) 147:85–93. doi: 10.1016/j.exer.2016.05.005
64. Lehmann GM, Feldon SE, Smith TJ, Phipps RP. Immune mechanisms in thyroid eye disease. *Thyroid* (2008) 18(9):959–65. doi: 10.1089/thy.2007.0407
65. Ichim TE, O'Heeron P, Kesari S. Fibroblasts as a practical alternative to mesenchymal stem cells. *J Transl Med* (2018) 16(1):212. doi: 10.1186/s12967-018-1536-1
66. Lanzolla G, Ricci D, Nicolì F, Sabini E, Sframeli A, Brancatella A, et al. Putative protective role of autoantibodies against the insulin-like growth factor-1 receptor in Graves' Disease: results of a pilot study. *J Endocrinol Invest* (2020) 43(12):1759–68. doi: 10.1007/s40618-020-01341-2
67. Marinò M, Rotondo Dottore G, Ionni I, Lanzolla G, Sabini E, Ricci D, et al. Serum antibodies against the insulin-like growth factor-1 receptor (IGF-1R) in Graves' disease and Graves' orbitopathy. *J Endocrinol Invest* (2019) 42 (4):471–80. doi: 10.1007/s40618-018-0943-8
68. Smith MJ, Rihanek M, Coleman BM, Gottlieb PA, Sarapura VD, Cambier JC. Activation of thyroid antigen-reactive B cells in recent onset autoimmune thyroid disease patients. *J Autoimmun* (2018) 89:82–9. doi: 10.1016/j.jaut.2017.12.001
69. Salvi M, Covelli D. B cells in Graves' Orbitopathy: more than just a source of antibodies? *Eye (Lond)* (2019) 33(2):230–4. doi: 10.1038/s41433-018-0285-y
70. Weyand CM, Goronzy JJ. The immunology of rheumatoid arthritis. *Nat Immunol* (2020) 22(1):10–8. doi: 10.1038/s41590-020-00816-x

71. Huang Y, Fang S, Zhang S, Zhou H. Progress in the pathogenesis of thyroid-associated ophthalmopathy and new drug development. *Taiwan J Ophthalmol* (2020) 10(3):174–80. doi: 10.4103/tjo.tjo_18_20
72. Kahaly GJ, Diana T. TSH Receptor Antibody Functionality and Nomenclature. *Front Endocrinol (Lausanne)* (2017) 8:28. doi: 10.3389/fendo.2017.00028
73. Dik WA, Virakul S, van Steensel L. Current perspectives on the role of orbital fibroblasts in the pathogenesis of Graves' ophthalmopathy. *Exp Eye Res* (2016) 142:83–91. doi: 10.1016/j.exer.2015.02.007
74. Smith TJ, Janssen JA. Building the Case for Insulin-Like Growth Factor Receptor-I Involvement in Thyroid-Associated Ophthalmopathy. *Front Endocrinol (Lausanne)* (2017) 7:167. doi: 10.3389/fendo.2016.00167
75. Krieger CC, Neumann S, Gershengorn MC. TSH/IGF1 receptor crosstalk: Mechanism and clinical implications. *Pharmacol Ther* (2020) 209:107502. doi: 10.1016/j.pharmthera.2020.107502
76. Fries KM, Sempowski GD, Gaspari AA, Blieden T, Looney RJ, Phipps RP. CD40 expression by human fibroblasts. *Clin Immunol Immunopathol* (1995) 77(1):42–51. doi: 10.1016/0090-1229(95)90135-3
77. Sempowski GD, Rozenblit J, Smith TJ, Phipps RP. Human orbital fibroblasts are activated through CD40 to induce proinflammatory cytokine production. *Am J Physiol* (1998) 274(3):C707–14. doi: 10.1152/ajpcell.1998.274.3.C707
78. Zhao LQ, Wei RL, Cheng JW, Cai JP, Li Y. The expression of intercellular adhesion molecule-1 induced by CD40-CD40L ligand signaling in orbital fibroblasts in patients with Graves' ophthalmopathy. *Invest Ophthalmol Vis Sci* (2010) 51(9):4652–60. doi: 10.1167/iovs.09-3789
79. Wang H, Zhu LS, Cheng JW, Cai JP, Li Y, Ma XY, et al. CD40 ligand induces expression of vascular cell adhesion molecule 1 and E-selectin in orbital fibroblasts from patients with Graves' orbitopathy. *Graefes Arch Clin Exp Ophthalmol* (2015) 253(4):573–82. doi: 10.1007/s00417-014-2902-1
80. Plöhn S, Edelmann B, Japtok L, He X, Hose M, Hansen W, et al. CD40 Enhances Sphingolipids in Orbital Fibroblasts: Potential Role of Sphingosine-1-Phosphate in Inflammatory T-Cell Migration in Graves' Orbitopathy. *Invest Ophthalmol Vis Sci* (2018) 59(13):5391–7. doi: 10.1167/iovs.18-25466
81. Feldon SE, O'loughlin CW, Ray DM, Landskroner-Eiger S, Seweryniak KE, Phipps RP. Activated human T lymphocytes express cyclooxygenase-2 and produce proadipogenic prostaglandins that drive human orbital fibroblast differentiation to adipocytes. *Am J Pathol* (2006) 169(4):1183–93. doi: 10.2353/ajpath.2006.060434
82. Yang D, Hiromatsu Y, Hoshino T, Inoue Y, Itoh K, Nonaka K. Dominant infiltration of T(H)1-type CD4+ T cells at the retrobulbar space of patients with thyroid-associated ophthalmopathy. *Thyroid* (1999) 9(3):305–10. doi: 10.1089/thy.1999.9.305
83. Hiromatsu Y, Yang D, Bednarczuk T, Miyake I, Nonaka K, Inoue Y. Cytokine profiles in eye muscle tissue and orbital fat tissue from patients with thyroid-associated ophthalmopathy. *J Clin Endocrinol Metab* (2000) 85 (3):1194–9. doi: 10.1210/jcem.85.3.6433
84. Wakelkamp IM, Bakker O, Baldeschi L, Wiersinga WM, Prummel MF. TSH-R expression and cytokine profile in orbital tissue of active vs. inactive Graves' ophthalmopathy patients. *Clin Endocrinol (Oxf)* (2003) 58(3):280–7. doi: 10.1046/j.1365-2265.2003.01708.x
85. Koumas L, Smith TJ, Phipps RP. Fibroblast subsets in the human orbit: Thy-1+ and Thy-1- subpopulations exhibit distinct phenotypes. *Eur J Immunol* (2002) 32(2):477–85. doi: 10.1002/1521-4141(200202)32:2<477::AID-IMMU477>3.0.CO;2-U
86. Elner VM, Burnstine MA, Kunkel SL, Strieter RM, Elner SG. Interleukin-8 and monocyte chemotactic protein-1 gene expression and protein production by human orbital fibroblasts. *Ophthalmic Plast Reconstr Surg* (1998) 14(2):119–25. doi: 10.1097/00002341-199803000-00008
87. Antonelli A, Ferrari SM, Frascerra S, Ruffilli I, Pupilli C, Bernini G, et al. β (CCL2) and α (CXCL10) chemokine modulations by cytokines and peroxisome proliferator-activated receptor-α agonists in Graves' ophthalmopathy. *J Endocrinol* (2012) 213(2):183–91. doi: 10.1530/JOE-11-0488
88. Chen B, Tsui S, Smith TJ. IL-1 beta induces IL-6 expression in human orbital fibroblasts: identification of an anatomic-site specific phenotypic attribute relevant to thyroid-associated ophthalmopathy. *J Immunol* (2005) 175 (2):1310–9. doi: 10.4049/jimmunol.175.2.1310
89. Antonelli A, Ferrari SM, Frascerra S, Ruffilli I, Gelmini S, Minuto M, et al. Peroxisome proliferator-activated receptor-α agonists modulate CXCL9 and CXCL11 chemokines in Graves' ophthalmopathy fibroblasts and preadipocytes. *Mol Cell Endocrinol* (2012) 349(2):255–61. doi: 10.1016/j.mce.2011.11.001
90. Mysliwiec J, Palyga I, Kosciuszko M, Kowalska A, Gorska M. Circulating CXCL9 and CXCL10 as markers of activity of Graves' orbitopathy during treatment with corticosteroids and teleradiotherapy. *Horm Metab Res* (2012) 44(13):957–61. doi: 10.1055/s-0032-1316352
91. Fallahi P, Ferrari SM, Ragusa F, Ruffilli I, Elia G, Paparo SR, et al. Th1 Chemokines in Autoimmune Endocrine Disorders. *J Clin Endocrinol Metab* (2020) 105(4):dgz289. doi: 10.1210/clinem/dgz289
92. Park M, Banga JP, Kim GJ, Kim M, Lew H. Human placenta-derived mesenchymal stem cells ameliorate orbital adipogenesis in female mice models of Graves' ophthalmopathy. *Stem Cell Res Ther* (2019) 10(1):246. doi: 10.1186/s13287-019-1348-0
93. Gieseck RL3, Wilson MS, Wynn TA. Type 2 immunity in tissue repair and fibrosis. *Nat Rev Immunol* (2018) 18(1):62–76. doi: 10.1038/nri.2017.90
94. Kim SE, Yoon JS, Kim KH, Lee SY. Increased serum interleukin-17 in Graves' ophthalmopathy. *Graefes Arch Clin Exp Ophthalmol* (2012) 250 (10):1521–6. doi: 10.1007/s00417-012-2092-7
95. Shen J, Li Z, Li W, Ge Y, Xie M, Lv M, et al. Th1, Th2, and Th17 Cytokine Involvement in Thyroid Associated Ophthalmopathy. *Dis Markers* (2015) 2015:609593. doi: 10.1155/2015/609593
96. Wei H, Guan M, Qin Y, Xie C, Fu X, Gao F, et al. Circulating levels of miR-146a and IL-17 are significantly correlated with the clinical activity of Graves' ophthalmopathy. *Endocr J* (2014) 61(11):1087–92. doi: 10.1507/endocrj.ej14-0246
97. Huang D, Xu N, Song Y, Wang P, Yang H. Inflammatory cytokine profiles in the tears of thyroid-associated ophthalmopathy. *Graefes Arch Clin Exp Ophthalmol* (2012) 250(4):619–25. doi: 10.1007/s00417-011-1863-x
98. Ujhelyi B, Gogolak P, Erdei A, Nagy V, Balazs E, Rajnavolgyi E, et al. Graves' orbitopathy results in profound changes in tear composition: a study of plasminogen activator inhibitor-1 and seven cytokines. *Thyroid* (2012) 22 (4):407–14. doi: 10.1089/thy.2011.0248
99. Huang D, Luo Q, Yang H, Mao Y. Changes of lacrimal gland and tear inflammatory cytokines in thyroid-associated ophthalmopathy. *Invest Ophthalmol Vis Sci* (2014) 55(8):4935–43. doi: 10.1167/iovs.13-13704
100. Stadhouders R, Lubberts E, Hendriks RW. A cellular and molecular view of T helper 17 cell plasticity in autoimmunity. *J Autoimmun* (2018) 87:1–15. doi: 10.1016/j.jaut.2017.12.007
101. Stockinger B, Omenetti S. The dichotomous nature of T helper 17 cells. *Nat Rev Immunol* (2017) 17(9):535–44. doi: 10.1038/nri.2017.50
102. Nanba T, Watanabe M, Inoue N, Iwatani Y. Increases of the Th1/Th2 cell ratio in severe Hashimoto's disease and in the proportion of Th17 cells in intractable Graves' disease. *Thyroid* (2009) 19(5):495–501. doi: 10.1089/thy.2008.0423
103. Qin J, Zhou J, Fan C, Zhao N, Liu Y, Wang S, et al. Increased Circulating Th17 but Decreased CD4+Foxp3+ Treg and CD19+CD1dhiCD5+ Breg Subsets in New-Onset Graves' Disease. *BioMed Res Int* (2017) 2017:8431838. doi: 10.1155/2017/8431838
104. Vitales-Noyola M, Ramos-Levi AM, Martínez-Hernández R, Serrano-Somavilla A, Sampedro-Nuñez M, González-Amaro R, et al. Pathogenic Th17 and Th22 cells are increased in patients with autoimmune thyroid disorders. *Endocrine* (2017) 57(3):409–17. doi: 10.1007/s12020-017-1361-y
105. Smith TJ. TSH-receptor-expressing fibrocytes and thyroid-associated ophthalmopathy. *Nat Rev Endocrinol* (2015) 11(3):171–81. doi: 10.1038/nrendo.2014.226
106. Smith TJ. Potential Roles of CD34+ Fibrocytes Masquerading as Orbital Fibroblasts in Thyroid-Associated Ophthalmopathy. *J Clin Endocrinol Metab* (2019) 104(2):581–94. doi: 10.1210/jc.2018-01493
107. Fernando R, Atkins S, Raychaudhuri N, Lu Y, Li B, Douglas RS, et al. Human fibrocytes coexpress thyroglobulin and thyrotropin receptor. *Proc Natl Acad Sci U S A* (2012) 109(19):7427–32. doi: 10.1073/pnas.1202064109
108. Fernando R, Atkins SJ, Smith TJ. Intersection of Chemokine and TSH Receptor Pathways in Human Fibrocytes: Emergence of CXCL-12/CXCR4

Cross Talk Potentially Relevant to Thyroid-Associated Ophthalmopathy. *Endocrinology* (2016) 157(10):3779–87. doi: 10.1210/en.2016-1382

109. Smith TJ, Padovani-Claudio DA, Lu Y, Raychaudhuri N, Fernando R, Atkins S, et al. Fibroblasts expressing the thyrotropin receptor overarch thyroid and orbit in Graves' disease. *J Clin Endocrinol Metab* (2011) 96(12):3827–37. doi: 10.1210/jc.2011-1249
110. Guo N, Woeller CF, Feldon SE, Phipps RP. Peroxisome proliferator-activated receptor gamma ligands inhibit transforming growth factor-beta-induced, hyaluronan-dependent, T cell adhesion to orbital fibroblasts. *J Biol Chem* (2011) 286(21):18856–67. doi: 10.1074/jbc.M110.179317
111. Toole BP. Hyaluronan: from extracellular glue to pericellular cue. *Nat Rev Cancer* (2004) 4(7):528–39. doi: 10.1038/nrc1391
112. Katoh S, Matsumoto N, Kawakita K, Tominaga A, Kincade PW, Matsukura S. A role for CD44 in an antigen-induced murine model of pulmonary eosinophilia. *J Clin Invest* (2003) 111(10):1563–70. doi: 10.1172/JCI16583
113. Schumann J, Stanko K, Schliesser U, Appelt C, Sawitzki B. Differences in CD44 Surface Expression Levels and Function Discriminates IL-17 and IFN-γ Producing Helper T Cells. *PloS One* (2015) 10(7):e0132479. doi: 10.1371/journal.pone.0132479
114. Sungnak W, Wang C, Kuchroo VK. Multilayer regulation of CD4 T cell subset differentiation in the era of single cell genomics. *Adv Immunol* (2019) 141:1–31. doi: 10.1016/bs.ai.2018.12.001
115. Agalioti T, Villablanca EJ, Huber S, Gagliani N. TH17 cell plasticity: The role of dendritic cells and molecular mechanisms. *J Autoimmun* (2018) 87:50–60. doi: 10.1016/j.jaut.2017.12.003
116. Horie I, Abiru N, Saitoh O, Ichikawa T, Iwakura Y, Eguchi K, et al. Distinct role of T helper Type 17 immune response for Graves' hyperthyroidism in mice with different genetic backgrounds. *Autoimmunity* (2011) 44(2):159–65. doi: 10.3109/08916931003777247
117. Moshkelgosha S, Masetti G, Berchner-Pfannschmidt U, Verhasselt HL, Horstmann M, Diaz-Cano S, et al. Gut Microbiome in BALB/c and C57BL/6J Mice Undergoing Experimental Thyroid Autoimmunity Associate with Differences in Immunological Responses and Thyroid Function. *Horm Metab Res* (2018) 50(12):932–41. doi: 10.1055/a-0653-3766
118. Su X, Yin X, Liu Y, Yan X, Zhang S, Wang X, et al. Gut Dysbiosis Contributes to the Imbalance of Treg and Th17 Cells in Graves' Disease Patients by Propionic Acid. *J Clin Endocrinol Metab* (2020) 105(11):dgaa511. doi: 10.1210/clinem/dgaa511
119. van der Weerd K, van Hagen PM, Schrijver B, Heuvelmans SJ, Hofland LJ, Swagemakers SM, et al. Thyrotropin acts as a T-cell developmental factor in mice and humans. *Thyroid* (2014) 24(6):1051–61. doi: 10.1089/thy.2013.0396
120. Douglas RS, Gianoukakis AG, Kamat S, Smith TJ. Aberrant expression of the insulin-like growth factor-1 receptor by T cells from patients with Graves' disease may carry functional consequences for disease pathogenesis. *J Immunol* (2007) 178(5):3281–7. doi: 10.4049/jimmunol.178.5.3281
121. McCoy AN, Kim DS, Gillespie EF, Atkins SJ, Smith TJ, Douglas RS. Rituximab (Rituxan) therapy for severe thyroid-associated ophthalmopathy diminishes IGF-1R(+) T cells. *J Clin Endocrinol Metab* (2014) 99(7):E1294–9. doi: 10.1210/jc.2013-3207
122. Pritchard J, Horst N, Cruikshank W, Smith TJ. Igs from patients with Graves' disease induce the expression of T cell chemoattractants in their fibroblasts. *J Immunol* (2002) 168(2):942–50. doi: 10.4049/jimmunol.168.2.942
123. Luo LH, Li DM, Wang YL, Wang K, Gao LX, Li S, et al. Tim3/galectin-9 alleviates the inflammation of TAO patients via suppressing Akt/NF-kB signaling pathway. *Biochem Biophys Res Commun* (2017) 491(4):966–72. doi: 10.1016/j.bbrc.2017.07.144
124. Zhao J, Lin B, Deng H, Zhi X, Li Y, Liu Y, et al. Decreased Expression of TIM-3 on Th17 Cells Associated with Ophthalmopathy in Patients with Graves' Disease. *Curr Mol Med* (2018) 18(2):83–90. doi: 10.2174/1566524018666180705105753
125. Fernando R, Grisolia ABD, Lu Y, Atkins S, Smith TJ. Slit2 Modulates the Inflammatory Phenotype of Orbit-Infiltrating Fibrocytes in Graves' Disease. *J Immunol* (2018) 200(12):3942–9. doi: 10.4049/jimmunol.1800259
126. Strianese D. Update on Graves disease: advances in treatment of mild, moderate and severe thyroid eye disease. *Curr Opin Ophthalmol* (2017) 28 (5):505–13. doi: 10.1097/ICU.0000000000000402
127. Pearce SHS, Dayan C, Wraith DC, Barrell K, Olive N, Jansson L, et al. Antigen-Specific Immunotherapy with Thyrotropin Receptor Peptides in Graves' Hyperthyroidism: A Phase I Study. *Thyroid* (2019) 29(7):1003–11. doi: 10.1089/thy.2019.0036

4

Therapy with Different Dose Regimens of Rituximab in Patients with Active Moderate-to-Severe Graves' Orbitopathy

Irene Campi[1], Guia Vannucchi[1], Ilaria Muller[2,3,4], Elisa Lazzaroni[2], Nicola Currò[5], Martina Dainese[2], Benedetta Montacchini[2], Danila Covelli[2], Claudio Guastella[6], Lorenzo Pignataro[6], Laura Fugazzola[1,7], Maura Arosio[2,3] and Mario Salvi[2]*

[1] Department of Endocrine and Metabolic Diseases, Istituto Auxologico Italiano IRCCS, Milan, Italy, [2] Graves' Orbitopathy Center, Endocrinology, Fondazione IRCCS Cà Granda, Ospedale Maggiore Policlinico Milan, Milan, Italy, [3] Department of Clinical Sciences and Community Health, University of Milan, Milan, Italy, [4] Division of Infection and Immunity, School of Medicine, Cardiff University, Cardiff, United Kingdom, [5] Ophthalmology, Fondazione IRCCS Cà Granda, Ospedale Maggiore Policlinico Milan, Milan, Italy, [6] Otolaryngology, University of Milan and Fondazione IRCCS Cà Granda, Milan, Italy, [7] Department of Pathophysiology and Transplantation, University of Milan, Milan, Italy

***Correspondence:**
Mario Salvi
mario@mariosalvinet.it

Background: Immunosuppressive therapy of Graves' orbitopathy (GO) is indicated during the active phase of disease. Intravenous steroids (IVGC) are effective in about 70% of patients, although unresponsiveness or relapse are observed. In previous studies, rituximab (RTX) has been shown to be effective in inactivating moderate-to-severe GO when used early in the disease, but its optimal dosage has never been studied in randomized clinical trials. Aim of this study was to compare the efficacy and safety of different doses of RTX, based on a *post-hoc* analysis of two open label studies and one prospective trial randomized to IVGC.

Methods: of 40 patients (35 women, 5 men), with active moderate-to-severe GO treated with RTX, 14 received a single dose of 100 mg (Group 1), 15 a single dose of 500 mg (Group 2) and 11 two 1000 mg doses, administered one week apart (Group 3). Thyroid function, TSH-receptor antibodies (TRAb) and peripheral CD19+ cells were measured. Primary endpoint was disease inactivation, measured as a decrease of the Clinical Activity Score (CAS) of at least two points. Secondary endpoints were improvement of proptosis, diplopia, quality of life and safety.

Results: Baseline CAS decreased significantly in all groups ($P<0.0001$), independently of GO duration or whether patients had newly occurring or relapsing GO after IVGC. Proptosis did not significantly change. There was an inverse correlation between the Gorman score for diplopia and RTX dose ($P<0.01$). The appearance score of the GO-QoL improved in Group 1 ($P=0.015$), and the visual function score, in Group 2 ($P=0.04$). A reduction of serum TRAb was observed in Group 1 ($P=0.002$) and Group 2 ($P<0.0002$), but not in Group 3. CD19+ cell decreased in all groups ($P<0.01$), independently of the dose.

Conclusions: We studied the optimal dosage of RTX in the treatment of active moderate-to-severe GO. In this analysis, we considered the efficacy of RTX in inactivating GO, in changing its natural course, its effect on disease severity and on the patients' quality of life. Based on our clinical findings, and balancing the cost of therapy, a single 500 mg dose regimen is suggested in the majority of patients.

Keywords: Graves' disease, Graves' orbitopathy, Rituximab, B lymphocytes, TSH-receptor antibodies

INTRODUCTION

Graves' disease (GD) is a thyroid autoimmune disorder in which anti-thyrotropin (TSH) receptor autoantibodies (TRAb) with stimulating activity induce hyperthyroidism. Graves' orbitopathy (GO), characterized by inflammation and remodelling of orbital tissues, is the main extra-thyroidal manifestation of GD. Moderate-to-severe GO determines major facial disfigurement, psychosocial impact and, rarely progression to sight loss (1, 2). Typically, GO has a diphasic course (3) with an inflammatory and progressive phase, followed by stabilization and subsequent scarring due to tissue fibrosis. Medical treatment, based on immunosuppression, is indicated during the active phase of GO. Intravenous steroids have been shown to be effective in about 70% of patients, although unresponsiveness and disease relapse are observed in a good proportion of patients (20-30%) (4).

Rituximab (RTX) is a human/mouse chimeric monoclonal antibody that binds the CD20 antigen on the surface of B cells and induces rapid depletion of B cells in both periphery and lymphoid organs. Clinically approved indications for the use of RTX in autoimmune disease are currently rheumatoid arthritis and ANCA-related vasculitis (5). In previous studies (6), RTX has been shown to be effective in inactivating moderate-to-severe GO when used early in the disease, but may have little effect in longer duration disease (7). The clinical effect of RTX in GO is quite rapid, since disease generally inactivates within 4 - 6 weeks after the first infusion (8). RTX induces B-cell lysis and may activate anaphylatoxins and other inflammatory cytokines with subsequent recruitment of phagocytes within the orbital tissue and depletion of inflammatory cells yielding tissue fibrosis (9, 10). This may explain why, after B cells repopulation, reactivation of GO was only observed rarely.

RTX therapy is not devoid of side effects: infections may arise due to hypogammaglobulinemia, although they are also commonly associated to therapy with steroids or other immunosuppressive drugs (11). Acute infusion reactions related to the release of cytokines produced by macrophages, monocytes, lymphocytes and NK cells, can be observed in 10-30% of patients at the first infusion (12). These effects may be associated to larger doses of RTX and significant lymphocytic infiltrates in target organs (13).

The optimal dosage of RTX in GO has never been studied in randomized, dose finding clinical trials. Standard dosing in rheumatoid arthritis and other autoimmune diseases consists of two i.v. administrations of 1000 mg with a 2-week interval. This dose was also initially used in most open studies (8) and in individual case reports (10) in patients with GO. Rapid and complete B lymphocyte depletion was shown to occur already after very low dosages (25-100 mg) of i.v. RTX (9). In a prospective randomized clinical study it was shown that the efficacy of a single 500 mg RTX dose was comparable to two 1000 mg doses (7) in inactivating GO and more effective than i.v. methylprednisolone (6). Later observation that in GO total peripheral (and orbital) B cell depletion was occurring even after low doses of RTX (100 mg) (9), has allowed us to reduce the therapeutic dose to a single infusion of 100 mg RTX (14).

Aim of the present study was to compare the efficacy and safety of different doses of RTX, employed prospectively in two open label studies (14, 15) and in one trial in which RTX was randomized to i.v. steroid therapy (6), in active GO.

PATIENTS AND METHODS

Patients

Forty patients, 35 women and 5 men, 32-81 years of age (mean ± SE 58.7 ± 2.7 yr), with active moderate to severe GO were grouped based on the RTX dose that they received (**Table 1**). Of these patients, 14 were treated with a single dose of 100 mg (Group 1), 15 with a single dose of 500 mg (Group 2) and 11 with two 1000 mg doses of RTX, administered one week apart (Group 3). Of the 40 patients included in the study, 34 had GD, 11 in group 1, 12 in group 2 and 11 in group 3, five had Hashimoto's thyroiditis, of whom three in Group 1 and two in Group 2, and one had euthyroid GO (Group 2). Thirty of 34 GD patients were euthyroid or subclinical hypothyroid because slightly overtreated with methimazole and four slightly hyperthyroid at the time of treatment. Nineteen patients were smokers, not significantly distributed in the three groups (**Table 1**). All patients had mean GO duration of 11 ± 3 months. Nineteen patients were previously treated with corticosteroid therapy, nine in Group 1, six in Group 2 and four in Group 3. Glucocorticoids were discontinued at least three months before RTX administration. Patients were followed-up to 76-weeks follow-up to assess the need of rehabilitative surgery.

RTX Administration Schedule

RTX dosing and treatment schedule were adapted based on the experience achieved with this drug throughout the years. The dose of RTX initially employed in the treatment of active moderate-to-severe GO was based on previous work in autoimmunity (6, 16, 17) and consisted of a single dose of 100 mg and 500 mg (Group 1 and Group 2, respectively) or 1000 mg twice at two weeks interval (Group 3).

All patients, one hour prior to RTX infusion, received oral paracetamol (1 gr), chlorphenamine (10 mg) and i.v. hydrocortisone (100 mg) to prevent possible infusion reactions.

TABLE 1 | Baseline clinical characteristics of patients with moderate-to-severe GO treated with different doses of RTX.

Group (dose of RTX)	GROUP 1 (100 mg)	GROUP 2 (500 mg)	GROUP 3 (1000 mg x2)	P
Number of patients	14	15	11	
Age * (years)	55.6 ± 3.3	56.9 ± 3.1	63.5 ± 1.6	0.09
Gender (F/M)	12/2	14/1	9/2	0.67
Smoker (Yes/No)	5/9	8/7	6/5	0.55
FT4 (pmol/L) *	11.9 ± 1.0	11.7 ± 1.0	9.8 ± 1.4	0.15
TRAb (mU/mL) *	27.6 ± 13.8	12.7 ± 3.0	11.6 ± 4.1	0.93
GO duration (months) *	4.9 ± 1.6	6.3 ± 1.5	10.7 ± 3.0	0.14
New onset/relapse (%)	4/10 (30)	9/6 (60)	7/4 (64)	0.14
CAS *	4.6 ± 0.3	4.3 ± 0.2	4.4 ± 0.3	0.73
Proptosis right eye (mm) *	23.8 ± 0.7	23.0 ± 0.6	21.4 ± 0.9	0.13
Proptosis left eye (mm) *	23.6 ± 1.0	22.6 ± 0.7	21.3 ± 0.9	0.21
Gorman score N (0/1/2/3)	4/4/2/4	3/4/7/1	4/2/4/1	0.45
$CD19^+$ cells * (cells/mm^3)	293.5 ± 24.7	236.5 ± 31.2	269.7 ± 50.4	0.21
GO-QoL Appearance * (%)	56.6 ± 6.3	61.0 ± 6.7	69.0 ± 13.0	0.69
GO-QoL Function *(%)	56.4 ± 9.7	42.3 ± 7.3	77.0 ± 14.6	0.18
Thyroid status (0 = Euthyroid, 1 = Hyperthyroid, 2 = Hypothyroid)	11/1/2	12/2/1	5/1/5	0.15
Thyroid diagnosis N (GD/HT/EGO)	11/3/0	12/2/1	11/0/0	0.66**
Thyroid disease duration	33.9 ± 9.3	44.1 ± 14.9	50.8 ± 35.6	0.68
N of GD patients treated with RAI/TX before RTX (on L-T4)	4 (3)	2 (2)	2 (1)	0.58

*All values are expressed as mean ± SE.
**in the Chi-Square analysis HT and EGO were added together.
CAS, clinical activity score; EGO, euthyroid Graves' orbitopathy; GD, Graves' disease; GO, Graves' orbitopathy; HT, Hashimoto' thyroiditis; L-T4, levothyroxine; QOL, quality of life; RAI, radioiodine treatment; RTX, rituximab; TX, total thyroidectomy.
Patients were defined as euthyroid (0) hyperthyroid (1) or hypothyroid (2) in case of normal, elevated or low FT3 and/or FT4, independently on TSH serum levels.

Patients with severe chronic diseases, ongoing infections or neoplastic diseases were excluded from treatment. RTX was also not administered in patents with known significant coronary artery disease, cardiac arrhythmias, congestive heart failure, active infection, primary or secondary immunodeficiency, history of hypersensitivity, known anaphylaxis to mouse-derived proteins, positive Purified Protein Derivative (PPD) test without documentation of treatment for tuberculosis (TB) infection and denied consent to HIV testing. During treatment and follow-up, complete blood count, serum glucose, aminotransferases and gamma glutamyltransferase were closely monitored. Side effects were classified as major (diabetes mellitus, depressive syndrome, increase of aminotransferases levels 5 times or above the upper normal limit) and minor (dyspepsia, laryngeal itching, rhinorrhea, insomnia).

Biochemical Analysis

Serum free-thyroxine (FT4), free-triiodothyronine (FT3) and TSH concentrations were measured using an electro-chemiluminescent immunoassay (ECLIA, Roche Diagnostics) and normal ranges were 8-17 pg/ml, 2-5 pg/ml and 0.26-5.2 mU/L, respectively. Serum TRAb were measured as TSH binding inhibitory immunoglobulins (TBII), using a 2nd generation TRAK human lumitest (Thermofisher, AG, Henningsdorf/Berlin, Germany; n.v.<1.5 U/L). Lymphocyte subpopulations were measured at baseline and at each follow-up examination.

Cytofluorimetric Analysis

The pattern of peripheral blood lymphocytes was studied before RTX and subsequently during the study period and the follow-up. We tested the standard immunophenotypic panel (CD3+, CD3+4+, CD3+8+, CD3+DR+, CD20+, CD19+5+, CD56+16+3) on aliquots of around 10^5 lymphocytes, submitted to triple staining procedures for immunogating with CD45, and the pairs of monoclonal antibodies to subpopulations of T, B and NK cells, subsequently processed in the flow cytometer (BD Facsan, Cell-quest software).

Study Endpoints and Clinical Assessment

Primary endpoint of the study was GO inactivation, defined as a reduction of 2 points of CAS, or a CAS of 3/10 or less, at 12 and 24 weeks after treatment with any RTX dose, when compared to baseline. The analysis of efficacy was also carried out after stratifying patients for disease duration of more or less of six months at the time of intervention.

Secondary endpoints at 24 weeks were: 1) changes of the severity of GO: significant improvement was considered a 2 mm reduction of proptosis, and of at least one class of the Gorman's score for diplopia (18); 2) improvement of the quality of life (QoL), assessed with a specific and validated questionnaire for GO (GO-QoL) (19): an increase of at least 6 points of the score of the questionnaire at 24 weeks was considered significant; 3) decrease of serum levels of TRAb; 4) decrease of peripheral B-cell lymphocytes; 5) occurrence of any major adverse events.

Statistical Analysis

This was a *post-hoc* analysis of three prospective trials, one randomized to intravenous steroids and two open label. All values are expressed as mean ± standard error (SE) or ± standard deviation (SD), as specified. Analysis by Fischer exact test, Wilcoxon and Mann-Whitney test were applied, as appropriate, and performed using SPSS 8.0 for Windows.

Statistical significance was defined as $P < 0.05$. An ANOVA or Friedman model was used to study the changes of the CAS values during treatment and follow-up. A *per protocol* analysis of the data was carried out and patients undergoing surgical orbital decompression during the observation period up to 24 weeks, were not included in the analysis of the disease outcomes.

RESULTS

Disease Inactivation and Relapse

There were no significant differences in baseline clinical and immunological features in the patients of the three groups of the study (**Table 1**).

In Group 1, baseline CAS value was 4.6 ± 0.3 and decreased to 2.1 ± 0.4 at 12 weeks (P<0.05) and to 1.1 ± 0.2 at 24 weeks (P<0.0001). In Group 2, baseline CAS was 4.3 ± 0.2 and decreased to 1.4 ± 0.4 (P<0.001) and to 0.5 ± 0.3 (P<0.0001) at 12 and 24 weeks, respectively. In Group 3, baseline CAS was 4.4 ± 0.3, 1.8 ± 0.4 (P<0.05) and 0.7 ± 0.2 (P<0.0001) at 12 and 24 weeks, respectively (**Table 2**).

There was no difference in the CAS reduction at 12 weeks in the three Groups of patients (2.6 ± 0.4 in Group 1, 2.9 ± 0.4 in Group 2, 2.6 ± 0.4 points in Group 3; P=N.S). No difference was also observed at 24 weeks (3.6 ± 0.3 in Group 1, 3.8 ± 0.3 in Group 2 and 3.6 ± 0.4 in Group 3; P=N.S; **Figure 1**). GO inactivation was not significantly associated to disease duration (more or less than 6 months) independently of the dose employed (not shown, P=N.S). Response to RTX therapy was not different whether patients had newly occurring GO or relapse after previous steroid therapy (not shown, P=N.S.).

No patient showed disease reactivation at 24 weeks and during follow-up to 76 weeks. Two patients treated with 100 mg RTX, despite an initial response to treatment, eventually developed dysthyroid optic neuropathy (DON) and required prompt surgical orbital decompression.

Disease Severity and Quality of Life

Mean proptosis values did not significantly change at 24 weeks in any of the 3 groups after RTX (**Table 3**).

Patients receiving 500 mg of RTX tended to have more improved or stable diplopia (Chi-square P<0.06; **Figure 2**), and this finding was confirmed by the observation of a significant inverse correlation of the Gorman score with the dose of RTX (r -0.43, P< 0.01).

In Group 1 the appearance score of the GO-QoL questionnaire improved in 6/14 patients and the visual function score in 4/14 (**Table 3**), with significant increase of the overall appearance score (P=0.015, **Figure 3A**), but not of the function score (**Figure 3B**). In Group 2 improvement of the appearance score was observed in 7/15 patients and in one of the visual function score, although improvement was significant only for the overall visual function score (P=0.04, **Figure 3B**), and not of the appearance score (**Figure 3A**). In Group 3 analysis of the overall score was not performed due to the low number of patients who completed the questionnaire.

Thyroid Function and Serum TRAb

All but one patients at 24 weeks were euthyroid (P=0.04, not shown). Detailed data on baseline treatments for the thyroid diseases are reported in **Table 1**. A significant reduction of serum TRAb levels at 24 weeks was observed after RTX in Group 1 (P=0.002) and Group 2 (P<0.0002), but not in Group 3 patients (P=NS; **Figure 4**).

Lymphocytes Depletion

Peripheral lymphocyte subpopulations were studied at 24 weeks in order to assess how different RTX doses affect CD19+ cell depletion. A significant reduction in CD19 cell numbers was observed in all three groups (P< 0.01), independently of the RTX dose employed (**Figure 5**). At 24 weeks, the number of CD 19+ cells in patients of Group 1 were 75.1 ± 15.3, significantly higher than in patients of Group 2 (27.1 ± 7.1; P=0.05) Group 3 (7.5 ± 4.3; P=0.0001), while the difference is not statistically significant between patients of Group 2 and Group 3 (**Table 3**).

Overall, rehabilitative surgery (evaluated at 76 weeks post-treatment with RTX) was performed in 20 patients. Ten patients underwent orbital decompressions, of whom eight elective and two emergency (DON), six patients strabismus surgery and four eyelid surgery. The distribution of surgical procedures among patients was not related to the RTX dose employed.

We did not observe any significant changes in the CD4+ or CD8+ T lymphocytes levels following RTX infusion, in any Groups (**Supplementary Figure 1**). Interestingly, we observed a slightly increase in the number of natural killer cells (NK) in Group 1 and 2 after RTX. This difference reached the statistical significance only at 8 weeks in Group 1 and at 32 and 40 weeks in Group 2 compared to baseline values. On the contrary, the number of NK cells remained stable in Group 3 (**Supplementary Figure 1**).

TABLE 2 | Clinical activity score (CAS) at baseline and 12 and 24 weeks after treatment with different doses of RTX.

	Baseline	12 weeks	P*	24 weeks	P*0 vs 24 weeks	P *12 vs 24 weeks
GROUP 1 100 mg	4.6 ± 0.3	2.1 ± 0.4	*<0.05*	1.1 ± 0.2	*<0.0001*	*NS*
GROUP 2 500 mg	4.3 ± 0.2	1.4 ± 0.4	*<0.001*	0.5 ± 0.3	*<0.0001*	*NS*
GROUP 3 1000 mg X2	4.4 ± 0.3	1.8 ± 0.4	*<0.05*	0.7 ± 0.2	*<0.0001*	*NS*

**Friedman TEST.*
All values are expressed as mean ± SE. NS, not significant.

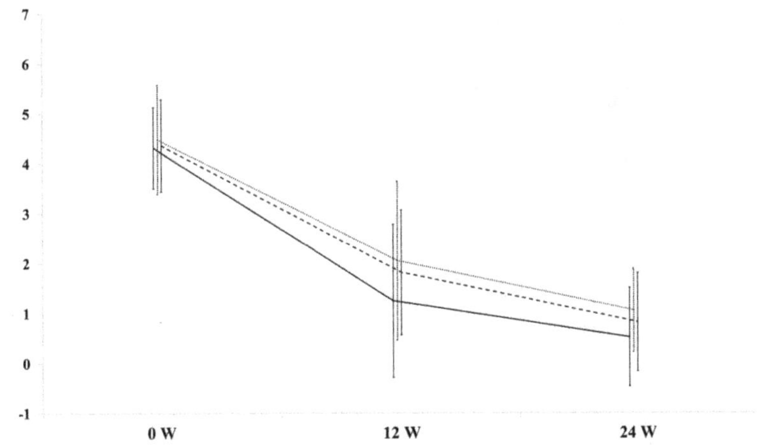

FIGURE 1 | Decrease of the Clinical Activity Score (CAS) at 12 and 24 weeks after rituximab (RTX) in patients with Graves' orbitopathy (GO). Dotted line= Group 1 (RTX 100 mg); solid line=Group 2 (RTX 500 mg); long dash line=Group 3 (RTX 1000 mg x 2).

Adverse Events

Minor adverse reactions such as itching of the throats and stuffiness of nose with rhinorrhea, were experienced by many patients. In these cases, resolution of the symptoms occurred after slowing down the rate of RTX infusion. In two patients of Group 1 a major adverse event known as the syndrome of release of cytokines occurred early during RTX infusion. This was characterized by orbital edema and progressive decline of vision rapidly occurring 30 minutes after the beginning of the infusion. This reaction was controlled by the administration of 100 mg of i.v. hydrocortisone with complete recovery of vision after 3 hours (9). Two patients treated with 100 mg RTX developed DON, possibly present at a subclinical stage at the time of treatment. This event is to be considered treatment failure, rather than an adverse event.

Cost of Treatment

The cost of RTX therapy depends the dose employed. The actual cost of one single 100 mg dose is of € 338, that of one 500 mg dose is € 1,698 and that of a two-dose cycle of 1000 mg is € 2.154, as released by the manufacturer in Europe (Roche Ltd.)

DISCUSSION

The first and most important finding of this study is that doses of RTX ranging from 100 to 2000 mg invariably induce inactivation of moderate-to-severe GO with only some differences in the clinical response, especially on diplopia, quality of life assessment and CD 19+ cells repopulation. This study is based on a *post-hoc* analysis of data collected from one prospective RCT and two open label studies that have employed different protocols and dosing of RTX administration.

Our findings show that any of the three RTX dosages used (100 mg, 500 mg and 1000 mg x 2) is equally effective in inactivating the disease in >95% of patients at 12 and 24 weeks after infusion. Efficacy of RTX has been known to be associated to the duration of B cell depletion in the circulation (14). In this

TABLE 3 | Clinical outcome of patients with moderate severe GO assessed 24 weeks after therapy with different doses of RTX.

	GROUP 1 (100 mg)	GROUP 2 (500 mg)	GROUP 3 (1000 mg x2)	P*
Number of patient	14	15	11	
TRAb (mU/L)	14.9 ± 7.5	5.98 ± 1.98	10.5 ± 4.0	*0.48*
CAS	1.07 ± 0.2	0.5 ± 0.3	0.7 ± 0.2	*0.14*
Proptosis right eye (mm)	22.6 ± 0.8	22.97 ± 0.7	22.05 ± 1.4	*0.73*
Proptosis left eye (mm)	23.0 ± 0.9	22.7 ± 0.6	21.5 ± 1.1	*0.58*
Δ Proptosis right eye (mm)**	-1.2 ± 0.4	-0.08 ± 0.3	0.64 ± 1.1	*0.08*
Δ Proptosis left eye (mm)**	-0.6 ± 0.6	0.10 ± 0.2	0.2 ± 0.5	*0.50*
GO-QoL Appearance (%)	71.6 ± 4.6	59.8 ± 6.4	83.2 ± 5.97	*0.18*
GO-QoL Functions (%)	52.0 ± 9.8	58.9 ± 9.2	72.3 ± 16.8	*0.66*
$CD19^+$ cells (cells/mm^3)	75.1 ± 15.3	27.1 ± 7.1	7.5 ± 4.3	*G1 vs G2 P<0.05; G1 vs G3 P<0.0001; G2 vs G3 P = NS*

All values are expressed as mean ± SE
**Mann-Whitney test*
***Difference in between proptosis at 0 and 24 weeks.*
GO, Graves' orbitopathy; CAS, clinical activity score; GO-QoL, quality of life questionnaire; NS, not significant.

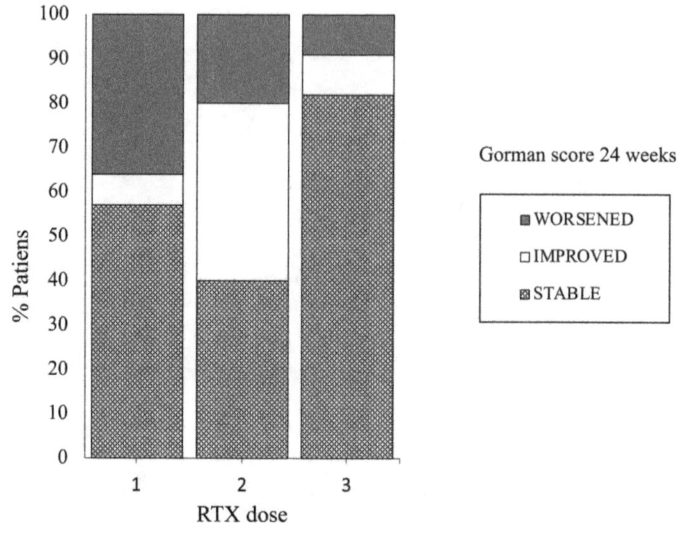

FIGURE 2 | Proportions of patients with GO with modifications of the Gorman score for diplopia after treatment with three different doses of RTX: 1= Group 1 (RTX 100 mg); 2= Group 2 (RTX 500 mg); 3 Group 3 (RTX 1000 mg x 2). Chi Square test.

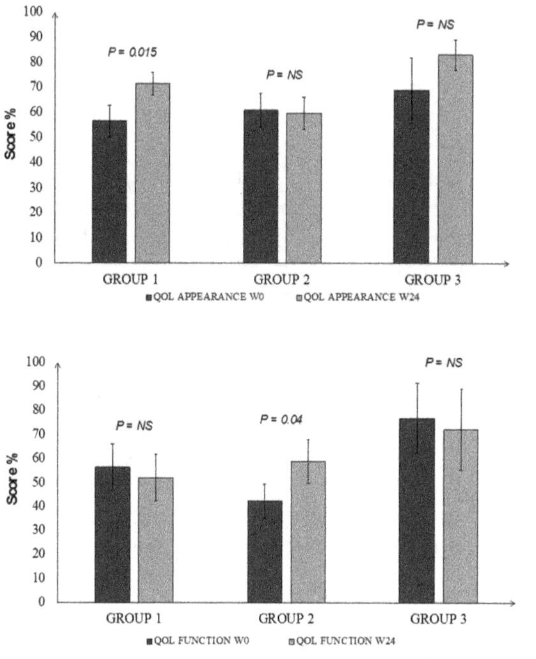

FIGURE 3 | Changes in the baseline score of the Quality of Life assessment of patients with GO at 24 weeks after treatment with different doses of RTX. Panel **(A)** (upper): appearance score, Panel **(B)** (lower): function score. Group 1 = 100 mg; Group 2 = 500 mg; group 3 = 1000 mg x 2; baseline values are in dark grey and values at 24 weeks in light grey. Wilcoxon matched pair test.

study we show that peripheral CD19+ cells begin repopulating only slightly earlier than 24 weeks in patients treated with the very low dose (100 mg), but later in those administered either 500 or 2000 mg. B cell return in the circulation, though, does not modify the disease outcome or favor disease relapse during follow-up (up to 12 months) (6, 14, 20). Based on these observations, we believe that in moderate-severe GO lower doses of RTX, which are generally burdened by a lower risk of adverse events such as reactivation of infections (12) or the induction of other autoimmune processes after depletion of B cells (21), should be preferred.

We studied whether RTX induced inactivation may depend on GO duration of less or more than 6 months, as previous studies have suggested that in GO of longer duration RTX might be less effective (7, 17). We did not find differences in the therapeutic response based on the duration of disease with any of the doses employed. We suggest that efficacy of RTX treatment is likely more related to the early inflammatory phase of GO, than to disease duration. We observed no difference in the response of patients with newly diagnosed GO or of those with relapsing disease after a complete cycle of intravenous steroids, who invariably had longer disease duration (up to 66 months). This findings, besides confirming that disease activity rather than duration is important for the effect of RTX in GO, also suggest that this modality of therapy can be proposed as second line treatment when steroids fail (1, 2).

The therapeutic outcome on parameters of disease severity, especially those related to muscle involvement, appear to be of importance, as the presence of diplopia in inactive GO has an impact on the quality of life of patients. While there were no significant changes in the degree of proptosis with any of the three dosages used, we did observe a significant improvement of the Gorman score for diplopia when higher RTX doses (Group 2 and Group 3) were employed. A possible explanation for this is that higher doses might be more effective than lower doses in preventing the orbital tissue fibrosis that follows the active disease phase.

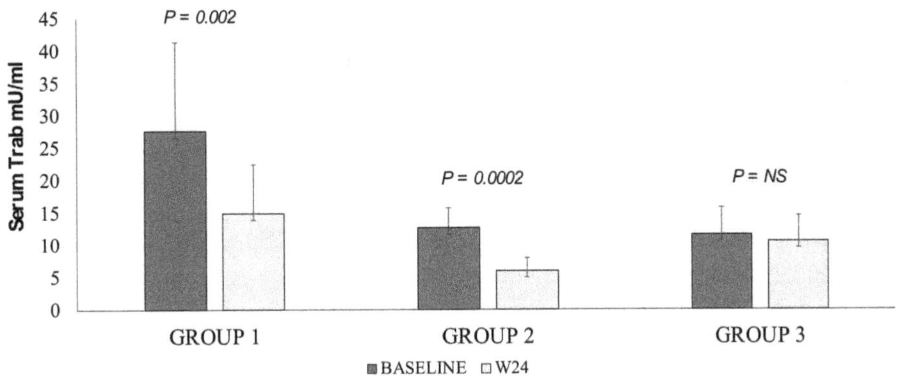

FIGURE 4 | Changes of serum TRH receptor antibody levels at 24 weeks in patients with GO treated with different doses of RTX. Group 1 = 100 mg; Group 2 = 500 mg; group 3 = 1000 mg x 2. Baseline values are in dark grey and values at 24 weeks in light grey. Paired T test.

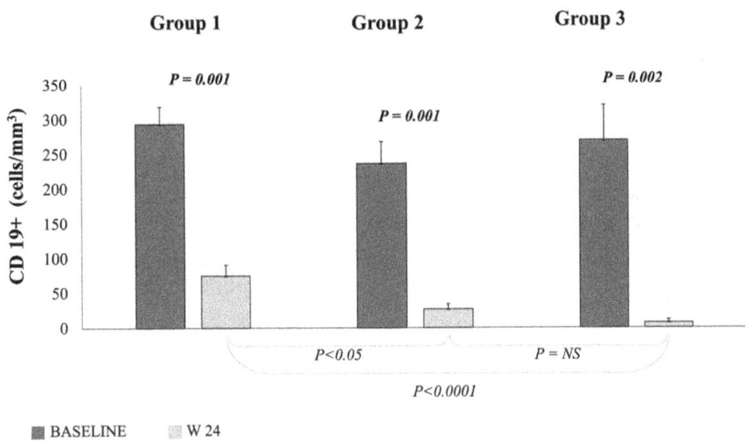

FIGURE 5 | Peripheral B cell count measured at baseline (dark grey) and 24 weeks (light grey) after treatment with different doses of RTX. Group 1 = 100 mg; Group 2 = 500 mg; Group 3 = 1000 mg x 2. Paired T test.

The QoL questionnaire used in the study has been validated and is specific for assessing quality of life changes in GO patients (18). It is divided into two sections, the first one assessing the impact of the aesthetic changes (appearance) on patients, the second one that of the eye dysfunction. The perception of self-appearance was found to improve at 24 weeks only in patients treated with 100 mg RTX in a single administration, while improvement of function was reported by those treated with a single larger dose of 500 mg. Improvement of inflammatory signs were in fact more rapidly observed after treatment with the low dose (>90% of patients inactivated at 12 weeks), whereas the impact of RTX on diplopia was found to be associated to the use of larger doses. This suggests that high doses of RTX might be preferable in patients with significant extraocular muscle involvement, as it would reduce the need of rehabilitative surgery. Unfortunately, we could not assess QoL outcome in Group 3 because of the small number of questionnaires returned, and this is a limitation of this study. Differences in the quality of life assessment were not associated to differences in the number of rehabilitative surgeries required, whichever dose of RTX was employed.

In two patients treated with the low dose, RTX therapy failed to inactivate GO and to prevent progression to DON. These patients may have had a subclinical form of DON at the time of treatment which might have been further exacerbated by the increase of intraorbital edema induced by an acute release of cytokines mediated by RTX as previously reported (9). In other studies RTX has been used in patients with DON (10) resulting in improvement of vision. In addition, the observation of the syndrome cytokine release in two patients receiving only 100 mg RTX, suggests that this adverse event is not related to the dose employed and can be prevented only by pretreating patients with fairly high intravenous methylprednisolone doses (up to 500 mg) (22). Caution is therefore suggested for the use of RTX in patients with suspected subclinical DON (1).

Restoration of euthyroidism after RTX may be due to either its effect on antibodies stimulating the TSH receptor (23) or to remission of hyperthyroidism after prolonged antithyroid treatment (24). While some authors have hypothesized that RTX does induce a decrease of serum TRAb in patients with GD (25, 26), others have shown that the levels of antibodies stimulating the TSH receptor (TSAb) are not modified in GO patients (23). RTX causes depletion of B lymphocytes in the peripheral blood but also in the thyroid (27) and in the orbit (9) and histological analysis of orbital tissues of patients who received RTX showed absence of both B and T lymphocytes (8). This observation supports the hypothesis that RTX blocks B cell function as antigen presenting cells and interaction with helper T cells, required for the initiation of the autoimmune process (28). Interestingly, we observed that the number of NK cells increased following RTX infusion in Group 1 and 2, compared to baseline values. Previous studies on rheumatoid arthritis and idiopathic membranous nephropathy have shown a rise in the NK number, associated with an altered NK cell function. Although, the clinical significance of this observation needs to be established, it has been associated with a better response to RTX treatment (29, 30).

This may explain why after CD19+ cells repopulation, inflammation does not relapse and the CAS continues to decrease until stable disease inactivation (31). We in fact did observe that although CD19+ cells return earlier (<24 weeks) in patients treated with the 100 mg dose, when compared to Groups 2 and 3, this does not result in GO reactivation.

In analyzing the use of RTX in GO, we also looked at the cost of therapy in relation to the administered dose. When compared to first line treatment with intravenous steroids, the cost of a full cycle of treatment with RTX in Europe is about 4.8, 24 and 61 times more expensive for the 100, 500 and 1000 x 2 mg dose, respectively. Given the more favorable response/relapse rate and the clinical evidence shown by this study, we believe that a single RTX 500 mg dose is best indicated as second line treatment for the majority of GO patients.

The results of this study have to be seen in light of some limitations: in first instance the retrospective study design, the small sample size and its heterogeneity. Indeed, cases had a different duration of GO (which was longer in patients belonging to Group 3 compared to Group 1 and 2) and were enrolled among Graves'disease, Hashimoto's thyroiditis and euthyroid GO patients. Furthermore, some patients received previous corticosteroid treatment that may have had influenced the final outcome.

In this study, in conclusion, we sought to understand, from the limited available evidence, which dose of RTX is optimal as second line therapy of active moderate-to-severe GO. In this analysis we considered, both the effectiveness of the drug in inactivating the disease, the possibility of changing its natural course, the effect on disease severity and the impact on the patients' quality of life. Prospective randomized studies specifically addressing RTX dosing in GO are warranted.

AUTHOR CONTRIBUTIONS

Data of each trial were collected by IC, DC, GV, MS, EL, LF, NC, LP and CG, BM and MD performed some serological assays and collected biochemical and cytofluorimetric data, the final database was produced by IM and EL, results were analyzed by IC and EL, the draft of the manuscript was written by IM and MS, the final manuscript was reviewed and revised by MS and MA. All authors contributed to the article and approved the submitted version.

SUPPLEMENTARY MATERIAL

Supplementary Figure 1 | Peripheral T cell, CD4+ (light gray) and CD8+ (white) and NK (dark grey) count measured at baseline and at different time-points after treatment with different doses of RTX. Test: Repeated measure ANOVA.

REFERENCES

1. Bartalena L, Baldeschi L, Boboridis K, Eckstein A, Kahaly GJ, Marcocci C, et al. The 2016 European Thyroid Association/European Group on Graves' Orbitopathy Guidelines for the Management of Graves' Orbitopathy. *Eur Thyroid J* (2016) 5:9–26. doi: 10.1159/000443828
2. Bartalena L, Kahaly GJ, Baldeschi L, Dayan CM, Eckstein A, Marcocci C, et al. EUGOGO †. The 2021 European Group on Graves' Orbitopathy (EUGOGO) Clinical Practice Guidelines for the Medical Management of Graves' Orbitopathy. *Eur J Endocrinol* (2021) 185:G43–67. doi: 10.1530/EJE-21-0479
3. Bartley GB. Rundle and His Curve. *Arch Ophthalmol* (2011) 129:356–8. doi: 10.1001/archophthalmol.2011.29
4. Bartalena L, Krassas GE, Wiersinga W, Marcocci C, Salvi M, Daumerie C, et al. Efficacy and Safety of Three Different Cumulative Doses of Intravenous Methylprednisolone for Moderate to Severe and Active Graves' Orbitopathy. *J Clin Endocrinol Metab* (2012) 97:4454–63. doi: 10.1210/jc.2012-2389
5. Dorner T, Lipsky PE. Beyond Pan-B-Cell-Directed Therapy – New Avenues and Insights Into the Pathogenesis of SLE. *Nat Rev Rheumatol* (2016) 12:645–57. doi: 10.1038/nrrheum.2016.158
6. Salvi M, Vannucchi G, Currò N, Campi I, Covelli D, Dazzi D, et al. Efficacy of B-Cell Targeted Therapy With Rituximab in Patients With Active Moderate to Severe Graves' Orbitopathy: A Randomized Controlled Study. *J Clin Endocrinol Metab* (2015) 100:422–3. doi: 10.1210/jc.2014-3014
7. Stan MN, Salvi M. Management of Endocrine Disease: Rituximab Therapy for Graves' Orbitopathy - Lessons From Randomized Control Trials. *Eur J Endocrinol* (2017) 176:R101–109. doi: 10.1530/EJE-16-0552
8. Salvi M, Vannucchi G, Campi I, Rossi S, Bonara P, Sbrozzi F, et al. Efficacy of Rituximab Treatment for Thyroid-Associated Ophthalmopathy as a Result of Intraorbital B-Cell Depletion in One Patient Unresponsive to Steroid Immunosuppression. *Eur J Endocrinol* (2006) 154:511–7. doi: 10.1530/eje.1.02119
9. Salvi M, Vannucchi G, Currò N, Introna M, Rossi S, Bonara P, et al. Small Dose of Rituximab for Graves' Orbitopathy: New Insights Into the Mechanism of Action. *Arch Ophthalmol* (2012) 130:122–4. doi: 10.1001/archopthalmol.2011.1215
10. Khanna D, Chong KK, Afifiyan NF, Hwang CJ, Lee DK, Garneau HC, et al. Rituximab Treatment of Patients With Severe, Corticosteroid-Resistant Thyroid-Associated Ophthalmopathy. *Ophthalmology* (2010) 117:133–9. doi: 10.1016/j.ophtha.2009.05.029

11. Descotes J. Immunotoxicity of Monoclonal Antibodies. *MAbs* (2009) 1:104–11. doi: 10.4161/mabs.1.2.7909
12. van Vollenhoven RF, Emery P, Bingham CO III, Keystone EC, Fleischmann RM, Furst DE, et al. Long-Term Safety of Rituximab in Rheumatoid Arthritis: 9.5- Year Follow-Up of the Global Clinical Trial Programme With a Focus on Adverse Events of Interest in RA Patients. *Ann Rheum Dis* (2013) 72:1496–502. doi: 10.1136/annrheumdis-2012-201956
13. Winkler U, Jensen M, Manzke O, Schulz H, Diehl V, Engert A. Cytokine-Release Syndrome in Patients With B-Cell Chronic Lymphocytic Leukemia and High Lymphocyte Counts After Treatment With an Anti-CD20 Monoclonal Antibody (Rituximab, IDEC-C2b8). *Blood* (1999) 94:2217–24. doi: 10.1182/blood.V94.7.2217.419k02_2217_2224
14. Vannucchi G, Campi I, Covelli D, Currò N, Lazzaroni E, Palomba A, et al. Efficacy Profile and Safety of Very Low-Dose Rituximab in Patients With Graves' Orbitopathy. *Thyroid* (2021) 31:821–8. doi: 10.1089/thy.2020.0269
15. Salvi M, Vannucchi G, Campi I, Currò N, Dazzi D, Simonetta S, et al. Treatment of Graves' Disease and Associated Ophthalmopathy With the Anti-CD20 Monoclonal Antibody Rituximab: An Open Study. *Eur J Endocrinol* (2007) 156:33–40. doi: 10.1530/eje.1.02325
16. Bredemeier M, Campos GG, de Oliveira FK. Updated Systematic Review and Meta-Analysis of Randomized Controlled Trials Comparing Low- Versus High-Dose Rituximab for Rheumatoid Arthritis. *Clin Rheumatol* (2015) 34:1801–5. doi: 10.1007/s10067-015-2977-z
17. Stan MN, Garrity JA, Carranza Leon BG, Prabin T, Bradley EA, Bahn RS. Randomized Controlled Trial of Rituximab in Patients With Graves' Orbitopathy. *J Clin Endocrinol Metab* (2015) 100:432–41. doi: 10.1210/jc.2014-2572
18. Bahn RS, Gorman CA. Choice of Therapy and Criteria for Assessing Treatment Outcome in Thyroid-Associated Ophthalmopathy. *Endocrinol Metab Clin North Am* (1987) 16:391–407. doi: 10.1016/S0889-8529(18)30485-7
19. Terwee CB, Gerding MN, Dekker FW, Prummel MF, Wiersinga WM. Development of a Disease Specific Quality of Life Questionnaire for Patients With Graves' Ophthalmopathy: The GO-QOL. *Br J Ophthalmol* (1998) 82:773–9. doi: 10.1136/bjo.82.7.773
20. Erdei A, Paragh G, Kovacs P, Karanyi Z, Berenyi E, Galuska L, et al. Rapid Response to and Long-Term Effectiveness of Anti-CD20 Antibody in Conventional Therapy Resistant Graves' Orbitopathy: A Five-Year Follow-Up Study. *Autoimmunity* (2014) 47:548–53. doi: 10.3109/08916934.2014.939266
21. El Fassi D, Nielsen CH, Kjeldsen J, Clemmensen O, Hegedüs L. Ulcerative Colitis Following B Lymphocyte Depletion With Rituximab in a Patient With Graves' Disease. *Gut* (2008) 57:714–5. doi: 10.1136/gut.2007.138305
22. Deltour JB, d'Assigny Flamen M, Ladsous M, Giovansili L, Cariou B, Caron P, et al. Efficacy of Rituximab in Patients With Graves' Orbitopathy: A Retrospective Multicenter Nationwide Study. *Graefes Arch Clin Exp Ophthalmol* (2020) 258:2013–21. doi: 10.1007/s00417-020-04651-6
23. El Fassi D, Banga JP, Gilbert JA, Padoa C, Hegedüs L, Nielsen CH. Treatment of Graves' Disease With Rituximab Specifically Reduces the Production of Thyroid Stimulating Autoantibodies. *Clin Immuno* (2009) 130:252–8. doi: 10.1016/j.clim.2008.09.007
24. Vannucchi G, Campi I, Bonomi M, Covelli D, Dazzi D, Currò N, et al. Rituximab Treatment in Patients With Active Graves' Orbitopathy: Effects on Proinflammatory and Humoral Immune Reactions. *Clin Exp Immunol* (2010) 161:436–43. doi: 10.1111/j.1365-2249.2010.04191.x
25. El Fassi D, Nielsen CH, Bonnema SJ, Hasselbalch HC, Hegedüs L. B Lymphocyte Depletion With the Monoclonal Antibody Rituximab in Graves' Disease: A Controlled Pilot Study. *J Clin Endocrinol Metab* (2007) 92:1769–72. doi: 10.1210/jc.2006-2388
26. Mitchell AL, Gan EH, Morris M, Johnson K, Neoh C, Dickinson AJ, et al. The Effect of B Cell Depletion Therapy on Anti-TSH Receptor Antibodies and Clinical Outcome in Glucocorticoid-Refractory Graves' Orbitopathy. *Clin Endocrinol* (2013) 79:437–42. doi: 10.1111/cen.12141
27. El Fassi D, Clemmensen O, Nielsen CH, Silkiss RZ, Hegedüs L. Evidence of Intrathyroidal B-Lymphocyte Depletion After Rituximab Therapy in a Patient With Graves' Disease. *J Clin Endocrinol Metab* (2007) 92:3762–3. doi: 10.1210/jc.2007-1238
28. Salvi M, Covelli D. B Cells in Graves' Orbitopathy: More Than Just a Source of Antibodies? *Eye* (2019) 33:230–4. doi: 10.1038/s41433-018-0285-y
29. Giollo A, Viapiana O, Carletto A, Ortolani R, Biasi D, Gatti D, et al. Rituximab Increases Peripheral Natural Killer Cells in Patients With Rheumatoid Arthritis. *Clin Exp Rheumatol* (2017) 35:241–6.

5

Epidemiology, Natural History, Risk Factors and Prevention of Graves' Orbitopathy

Luigi Bartalena, Eliana Piantanida, Daniela Gallo, Adriana Lai and Maria Laura Tanda*

Endocrine Unit, Department of Medicine and Surgery, University of Insubria, ASST dei Sette Laghi, Varese, Italy

***Correspondence:**
Luigi Bartalena
luigi.bartalena@uninsubria.it
orcid.org/0000000184475449

GO is the most frequent extrathyroidal manifestation of Graves' disease, although it may rarely occur in euthyroid/hypothyroid patients with chronic autoimmune thyroiditis. It is a relatively infrequent disorder, and men tend to have more severe ocular involvement at an older age. The prevalence of GO is lower than in the past among patients with recent onset Graves' hyperthyroidism, and moderate-to-severe forms requiring aggressive treatments are no more than 5–6% of all cases of GO. After an initial inflammatory (active) phase and a phase of stabilization (plateau phase), GO tends to improve and eventually inactivates (inactive or burnt-out phase). Minimal-to-mild GO often remits spontaneously, but complete *restitutio ad integrum* almost never occurs when GO is more than mild. Several risk factors contribute to its development on a yet undefined genetic background. Cigarette smoking is the most important of them. Early diagnosis, control and removal of modifiable risk factors, early treatment of mild forms of GO may effectively limit the risk of progression to more severe forms, which have a profound and dramatic impact on the quality of life of affected individuals, and remain a therapeutic challenge, often requiring long-lasting and multiple medical and surgical therapies.

Keywords: Graves' orbitopathy, Graves' disease, smoking, radioiodine (131I) treatment, TSH receptor antibodies, hyperthyroidism, hypothyroidism

INTRODUCTION

Graves' orbitopathy (GO), also named Graves' ophthalmopathy, Thyroid-eye disease, or Thyroid-associated ophthalmopathy, is a relatively rare, but disabling and disfiguring disease of the orbit, in most cases associated with hyperthyroidism due to Graves' disease (1). GO is a disorder of autoimmune origin, the pathogenic mechanisms of which remain to be fully elucidated (2). The close link of GO with thyroid autoimmune disorders, mainly Graves' disease, underpin the hypothesis that GO is triggered by immune reactions against one or more antigens shared by thyroid and orbit. The thyrotropin (TSH) receptor is the most likely culprit, supporting an important role of TSH receptor antibodies (TRAbs) in the pathogenesis and course not only of thyroid disease, but also of orbital disease (3, 4). The insulin-like growth factor-1 (IGF-1) receptor seems also to be involved, which may explain the recent promising results obtained by treating patients with active, moderate-to-severe GO with an IGF-1 receptor antagonist monoclonal antibody, teprotumumab (5, 6). This would also be in keeping with a putative, but yet to be proven, protective role of antibodies to the IGF-1 receptor found in serum of patients with GO (7).

The histopathologic changes underpinning orbital remodeling (expansion of the fibroadipose tissue, swelling of the extraocular muscles), as well the increased production of hydrophilic glycosaminoglycans by orbital fibroblasts provide a mechanical basis for understanding most of the clinical features of GO (soft tissue changes/inflammation, exophthalmos, diplopia, compressive dysthyroid optic neuropathy) (8).

EPIDEMIOLOGY

Incidence

Information on the incidence of GO is scant. In a study of residents in the Olmsted County, Minnesota, through a 15-year interval (1976–1990), 120 incident cases of GO were found, with an age-adjusted incidence of all-degree GO of 16/100,000 population/year for women and 2.9/100,000 population/year for men (9) (**Table 1**). In a more recent prospective multicenter study from Sweden, covering a population of more than 3,500,000 individuals, newly diagnosed cases of Graves' hyperthyroidism from 2003 to 2005 were 2,200, with an incidence of 21/100,000 population/year; of these, 20.1% had eye involvement of all degrees (4.9% moderate-to-severe), with an overall incidence of GO of 4.2/100,000 population/year (10). Because a 3.9:1 female to male ratio for Graves' hyperthyroidism was reported in that study, an approximate incidence of 3.3/100,000 population/year in women and 0.9/100,000 population/year in men can be derived for GO of all degrees (**Table 1**). Moderate-to-severe cases of GO would then have an incidence as low as 0.05/100,000 population/year, but classification criteria were not indicated in details (10). In a prospective registry-based study of patients with incident moderate-to-severe GO seen in Denmark during the period 1992–2009, 143 new cases of moderate-to-severe GO, classified following standardized criteria, were registered, with an incidence rate of 1.61/100,000 population/year (2.67/100,000 population/year for women, 0.54/100,000 population/year for men) (11). Figures were similar before and after iodine fortification of salt (11).The Danish study did not consider patients with mild GO (11). However, because about two thirds of Graves' patients have no or mild GO (13, 14), it was calculated that the incidence of GO of all degrees derived from the Danish study (11) might approximately be 4.83/100,000 population/year (8.01/100,000 population/year in women, 1.62/100,000 population/year in men) (12) (**Table 1**). The considerable differences among the various studies underscore the difficulties in establishing the true incidence of GO. Calculated figures derived from the two more recent studies (10, 11) appear to be lower than those reported in the older and pivotal study from USA (9). These differences might be apparent, due to difficulties in identifying patients with mild GO in registry-based studies (10, 11), or to persistent low referral rate of mild cases of GO, leading to an underestimation of all incident cases. On the other hand, this trend might be real and reflect a true decrease in the incidence of GO in recent years related to several factors, including changes in referral, improved interaction among general practitioners, endocrinologists and ophthalmologists, better control of risk factors, particularly smoking.

Prevalence

A recent study from the European Group on Graves' Orbitopathy (EUGOGO) used reported data on the incidence of GO (10, 11, 15) to estimate the prevalence of GO in the general population in Europe (12). By these calculations, it would appear that the prevalence of GO of all degrees in Europe might be between 90 and 155/100,000 population (12). Although this calculation is based on only three studies, these are large, epidemiological investigations and likely provide sound estimates of the overall prevalence of GO. Previous approximate calculations yielded an estimate of GO prevalence in Europe ranging from 100 to 305/100,000 population (16). The estimated prevalence derived from the Olmsted County, USA study was about 250/100,000 population (9). Other studies [reviewed in Ref. (17)] have led to an estimated prevalence of 100–300/100,000 population in Asia. Thus, although limitations inherent to the way of calculating prevalence from incidence data must be taken into account, it is reasonable to state that prevalence of GO does not substantially differ in different ethnic groups and is comprised between 90 and 300/100,000 population. GO, although relatively infrequent, does not fulfill the main criterion for being defined as a rare disease, i.e., a prevalence <50/100,000 population. However, several variants of the disease, namely, euthyroid GO, GO associated with thyroid dermopathy or acropachy are far below this threshold and can be considered as rare diseases, provided that distinct pathophysiological mechanisms can be identified (12).

Many patients with Graves' disease have no ocular involvement when first diagnosed with hyperthyroidism. A review of clinical records of the first 100 consecutive patients seen at a tertiary referral center in UK in 1960 and 1990 demonstrated that 57 and 35%, respectively, had clinically relevant GO with a parallel decrease in the proportion of severe forms in the two decades (**Figure 1**) (18) In a large and

TABLE 1 | Estimated incidence of Graves' orbitopathy (GO).

Author (year)	Years of observation	Estimated Incidence in Women	Estimated Incidence in Men	Ref.
Bradley (1994)	1976-1990	16/100,000/year	2.9/100,000/year	(9)
Abraham-Nordling (2011)	2003-2005	3.3/100,000/year	0.9/100,000/year	(10)
Laurberg (2012)	1992-2009	2.67/100,000/year* 8.01/100,000/year**	0.54/100,000/year* 1.62/100.000/year**	(11)

Moderate-to-severe forms of GO.
***All degrees of GO estimated by assuming that moderate-to-severe forms of GO represent 1/3 of cases (12).*

more recent series of 346 patients with newly diagnosed and recent onset Graves' hyperthyroidism seen at a single center in Italy, almost three quarters had no ocular involvement, and only 6% had moderate-to-severe GO (including 0.3% with sight-threatening GO) (**Figure 2**) (13). A recent meta-analysis and systematic review of 57 studies including 26,804 patients reported an overall prevalence of 40% (19). It should be noted that included papers likely comprised patients with early onset GO and patients with GO of longer duration. Thus, it can be concluded that the overall prevalence of GO of all grades among patients with Graves' hyperthyroidism is comprised between 25 and 40%. It is possible that early diagnosis and treatment of hyperthyroidism, as well as use of preventive measures, including removal of modifiable risk factors (see a subsequent section of this manuscript), may reduce the prevalence of clinically significant GO to the lower end of the above spectrum, or even lower. In addition, in those patients who have GO at onset, early referral and management may be associated with a change in the clinical manifestations of GO. In the PREGO (Presentation of Graves' Orbitopathy) study, patients referred to EUGOGO centers in the year 2012 were compared to patients referred to EUGOGO centers in the year 2000: the 2012 cohort had a shorter referral time and showed a much higher prevalence of mild forms (60.5 *vs.* 41.2%) and inactive forms (63.2 *vs.* 39.9%) of GO when compared with the 2000 cohort (14). Nowadays, moderate-to-severe forms of GO, which remain a major therapeutic challenge, represent 5–6% of cases (11, 13). Although it is difficult to draw definitive conclusions, it seems that the proportion of Graves' patients with GO of all grades and, particularly, with severe forms of the disease is possibly declining over time (20).

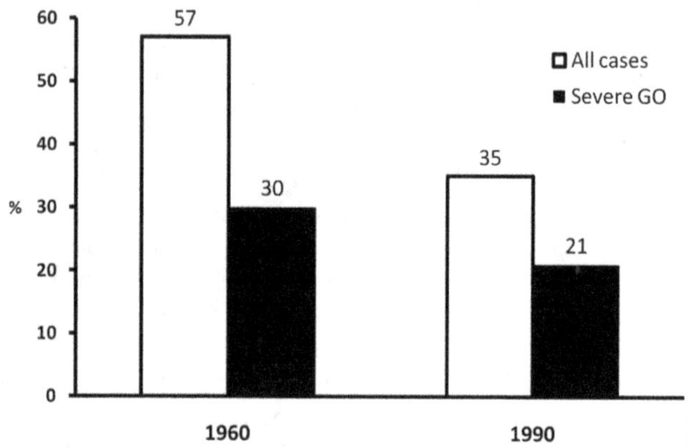

FIGURE 1 | Prevalence and severity of Graves' orbitopathy (GO) in the first 100 consecutive patients seen in a combined thyroid-eye clinic in UK in 1960 and 1990. Derived from Perros and Kendall-Taylor (18).

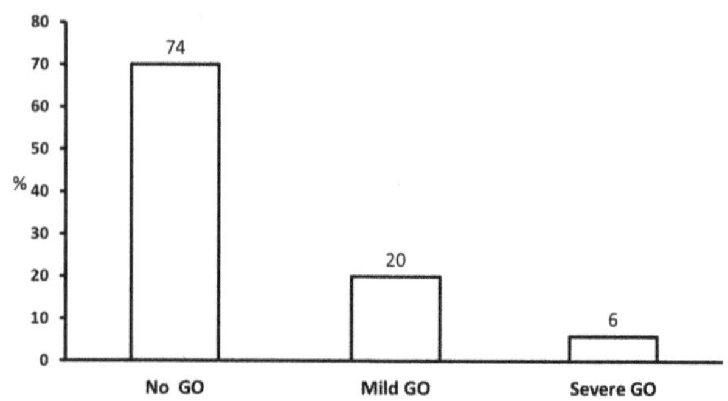

FIGURE 2 | Prevalence and severity of Graves' orbitopathy (GO) in 346 patients with recent onset and untreated Graves' hyperthyroidism. Severe GO: moderate-to-severe and sight-threatening GO. Derived from Tanda et al. (13).

Age, Gender, and Ethnicity

In the Olmsted County study, GO of all degrees showed a bimodal peak, 40–44 years and 60–64 years in women, 45–49 years and 65–69 years in men (9). In an observational Japanese study of 10,931 consecutive patients, the mean age of GO occurrence was 39 years in women and 43 years in men (21). In a study of 101 consecutive patients referred to a combined thyroid-eye clinic, the mean age was lower in patients without GO (40 years) than in those with GO (46 years) (22). In an Italian study mean age did not differ in Graves' patients without GO and in those with mild GO (46 and 44 years, respectively), but was significantly higher in patients with moderate-to-severe GO (54 years) (13). Likewise, in a Danish study of patients with moderate-to-severe GO, the median age was 50 and 56 years before and after salt iodization, respectively, and the risk of developing moderate-to-severe GO was lower in patients aged <40 years (11).Thus, age is a relevant factor affecting severity of GO, and the disease tends to be more severe in older patients (22). Although a questionnaire-based survey among European thyroidologists reported the presence of GO of all degrees in approximately one third of juvenile Graves' disease (23), clinically relevant GO in childhood is in general rarer than in adults and usually mild (24).

GO is more frequent in women than in men, although the female-to-male (F/M) ratio varies in different studies. In a study of 202 consecutive Graves' patients, the F/M ratio was 3.4 in patients without GO, 2.1 in patients with GO, and 0.7 in euthyroid GO (25). Other studies reported F/M ratios of 3.9 (21) and 4.2 (10). Gender affects also severity of GO, the F/M ratio progressively decreasing with increasing severity of GO (22). Likewise, in a cohort study of 2045 Graves' patients, although the proportion of patients with clinically relevant GO (NOSPECS class ≥2) was similar in women and men (51.5 and 52.7%, respectively), patients with more severe GO (NOSPECS class 4–6) were more frequently men (30.4 *vs.* 21.3%, $p < 0.001$), and their median age was also higher than in women with similar severity of GO (52 years *vs.* 40 years, $p < 0.05$) (27). Although a registry-based Danish study failed to show any significantly different risk of developing moderate-to-severe GO in men and women (11), it seems reasonable to conclude that GO tends to be relatively more frequent and severe in men, in whom it occurs at a more advanced age.

Relevance of ethnic factors in the occurrence of GO is controversial. In a study of 155 patients with newly diagnosed Graves' disease (116 Caucasians and 39 of Asian origin), the prevalence of GO was significantly higher in Caucasians than in

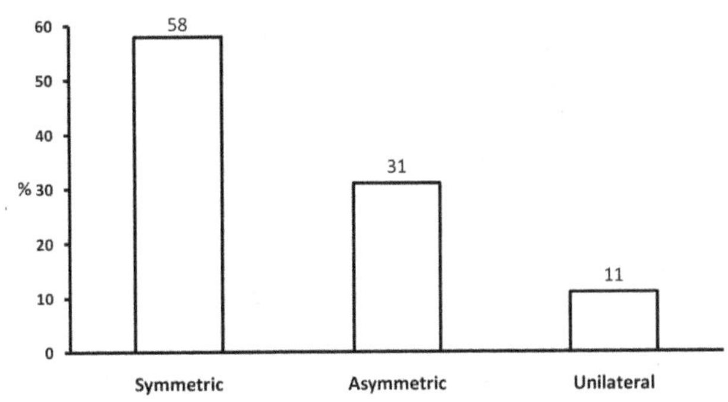

FIGURE 3 | Presentation of Graves' orbitopathy in a series of 269 patients referred to EUGOGO tertiary centers. Derived from Perros et al. (26).

Asians (42 *vs.* 7.7%, p = 0.0002), with a risk of developing GO 6.4-fold higher in Caucasians, possibly in relation to the high prevalence of smokers (>60%) among Caucasians (28). Conversely, a recent meta-analysis and systematic review showed a slightly lower prevalence of GO among Caucasians (37%) compared with Asians (45%) (19). A study from Australia reported that Caucasians have an increased risk (2.08, 95% CI, 1.56–2.76) of developing GO compared with non-Caucasian ethnicities (29). Conversely, other studies failed to link ethnic origin (including Caucasians, African Americans, Asian Americans, Asians, Latinos) to an increased for the occurrence of GO (30, 31). In summary, the role of ethnic factors, if any, remains, for the time being, unclear.

Phenotype

The majority of patients affected with GO have bilateral disease, but asymmetric or even unilateral GO may also develop (1). Asymmetric forms have been described in 4–14% of cases, unilateral forms in 9–34% of cases (9, 32–34). In a recent multicenter study of 269 patients referred to EUGOGO centers, although the majority (157 patients, 58%) had symmetric GO, many patients had either asymmetric or unilateral GO (26) (**Figure 3**). Interestingly, patients in the asymmetric group were older, were more frequently men, and tended to have more severe and active GO than the other groups (26). The reasons for asymmetric presentation of GO are unknown, but they might include differences in the anatomy of bony orbit or its vascularization. One study showed that patients with euthyroid/hypothyroid GO tend to have milder and more asymmetric forms of the disease (35). On the other hand, unilateral or asymmetric GO may sometimes progress to bilateral disease (34, 36). Asymmetric and unilateral forms of GO require an accurate diagnostic assessment to exclude other orbital diseases mimicking GO, reviewed in Ref. (37). Graves' disease may be an isolated disease or associated with other autoimmune disorders in the context of Autoimmune Polyglandular Syndromes: prevalence and severity of GO in these two different settings do not differ (38).

Relation With Thyroid Dysfunction

Most patients affected with GO are hyperthyroid (1), but a substantial proportion, ranging from 0.2 to 11% in different studies (35, 39–41), are euthyroid or subclinical/overt hypothyroid. TSH-receptor antibodies (TRAbs) are the ultimate responsible for hyperthyroidism due to Graves' disease (42), but they also strongly correlate with the clinical activity and severity of GO (3, 4, 43). But, in a series of 700 unselected patients with chronic autoimmune thyroiditis, overt GO was present in 44 (6%): among them TRAb bioassay for stimulating activities tested positive in 30/44 (68%) patients with GO *vs.* 36/656 (5.5%, p <0.001) patients without GO (44). Thus, it is conceivable that TRAbs can explain the rare occurrence of GO in patients without hyperthyroidism. A note of caution should be added by mentioning that cases of so-called euthyroid/hypothyroid GO might indeed be a manifestation of another emerging disease, IgG4 ophthalmic disease, which has clinical features similar to GO (45). This underscores again the need for a careful differential diagnosis in doubtful cases.

A close relationship exists between the onset of Graves' hyperthyroidism and the onset of GO, because in about 85% of cases GO develops within 18 months before or after the onset of hyperthyroidism (25, 46). Therefore, a normal thyroid status does not exclude the diagnosis of GO, because hyperthyroidism may occur long after the development of GO. On the other hand, when GO follows hyperthyroidism, a relevant question is whether treatment for hyperthyroidism can affect the development and course of GO (47). Hyperthyroidism *per se* negatively influences the course of GO, and restoration of euthyroidism is often associated with a stabilization/improvement of GO (48). But hypothyroidism can have a negative impact on the occurrence/progression of GO as well (45, 46). Thus, restoration and maintenance of euthyroidism is fundamental. While antithyroid drug treatment and thyroidectomy are apparently neutral to the course of GO, radioactive iodine (RAI) treatment is associated with a small, but definite risk of progression or *de novo* occurrence of GO, especially in smokers (49) (see a subsequent section).

Natural History

Following the initial description by Rundle and Wilson (50), it is widely accepted that overt GO clinically goes through an initial phase of inflammatory changes corresponding to ongoing activation of the pathogenic cascade of events occurring in the orbit (active phase); the disease then stabilizes when inflammation starts to subside (plateau or static phase), and then progressively improves in association with burning out of inflammation (inactive phase), without going back to normal (51). It is unknown how long it takes for GO to become inactive, but it is generally believed this occurs within 18–24 months. It should be mentioned that, although rarely, late reactivation of GO may occur (52). In a computer tomography-based study, the increase in the extraocular muscle volume appeared to be an early phenomenon, while the increase in the orbital fat volume occurred later (53). A precise definition of the natural course of GO of all degrees is, however, hampered by the fact that patients with moderate-to-severe and active GO cannot be left untreated and are, therefore, given disease-modifying treatments, namely intravenous glucocorticoids, orbital radiotherapy (54) or, more recently, biological agents (2).

In a series of 59 patients with untreated GO referred to a combined thyroid-eye clinic in UK, 13 patients (22%) improved substantially, 25 patients (42%) manifested only slight amelioration, 13 patients (22%) were stable, and 8 patients (14%) had a progression of GO over a median period of 12 months (55). In series of 196 Graves' patients, 81 (41%) developed GO, 53 of whom (65%) received no treatment, except for local measures: 25/53 (47%) improved substantially, 26/53 (49%) had unchanged GO at follow-up, 2/53 had a progression of GO (56). In a large series of 346 recent onset and untreated Graves' patients, 237 then completed a course of antithyroid drugs; 194 had no GO at baseline, and progression to moderate-to-severe GO occurred in <3% of cases; among the 43 patients with mild and inactive GO at baseline, progression to moderate-to-severe GO occurred in only 1 patient, while the majority of patients had a complete remission of ocular manifestations (13) (**Figure 4**). In another series of 65 patients, the large majority of whom had mild, minimally active GO and were followed without treatment for a median of 40 months, 51% improved spontaneously, 34% remained stable, 15% had some progression of GO (57). In summary, it would appear that mild/minimal GO rarely progresses to severe forms, particularly if hyperthyroidism is adequately managed and controlled, while stabilization and remission is frequent in mild forms of GO (20). This favorable course of mild GO is favored by control of modifiable risk factors (see a subsequent section). No conclusion can be drawn on the natural history of moderate-to-severe GO, because the latter is promptly treated by disease-modifying therapies. However, in a retrospective study of 226 patients with initially moderate-to-severe and active GO reexamined after a median of about 4 years after GO onset and various non-surgical and surgical treatments for GO, further amelioration was observed in 60% of responders to treatments at the last visit (58). This suggests that time (i.e., the natural history) is a key factor affecting also the long-term outcome of GO after treatment (58). In addition, in the placebo group of the second teprotumumab study, at the end of 6 months of observation a reduction in exophthalmos ≥2 mm was observed in 10% patients, an amelioration in diplopia in 29%, and a CAS 0-1 (inactive GO) in 21% (6). This suggests that the Rundle's curve description applies also to patients with moderate-to-severe GO. Obviously, this by no means implies that in this category of patients therapies should be postponed, because early immunosuppressive treatments improve and inactivate GO, thereby affecting substantially the natural history of GO, and reduce the time interval required to proceed to rehabilitative surgery, if needed.

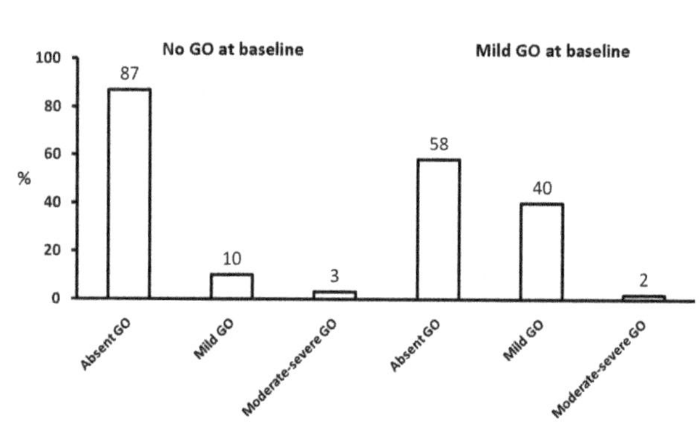

FIGURE 4 | Natural history of Graves' orbitopathy (GO) at the end of antithyroid drug treatment according the absence (n = 194) or presence (n = 43) of mild GO at baseline. Derived from Tanda et al. (13).

RISK FACTORS AND PREVENTION

GO results from a complex interaction of endogenous (unmodifiable) and exogenous/environmental (modifiable) risk factors. The former include age, gender, and genetic factors. As described in a previous section of this manuscript, GO tends to be more severe in men, in whom it occurs at an older age than in women. A search for genetic factors did not provide unequivocal information, with particular regard to differentiation between Graves' patients with or without GO (59–61). Likewise, results are conflicting as to the association between GO and Major Histocompatibility Complex (MHC), cytotoxic T-lymphocyte-associated antigen-4 (CTLA-4), protein tyrosine phosphatase or non-receptor type 22 (PTPN22), interleukins, intercellular adhesion molecule 1 gene polymorphisms, adipogenesis-related genes, TSH receptor or thyroglobulin (17, 62, 63).

Several modifiable risk factors for the occurrence/progression of GO have been identified. This is a very important issue, because controlling them may positively affect the course of GO (64) (**Table 2**).

Smoking

Smoking habit is probably the most important modifiable risk factor for GO (65, 66) (**Table 2**). The negative impact of smoking on GO is based on the following evidence: i) Graves' patients with GO are more frequently smokers (and heavy smokers) than those without GO, or patients with other thyroid disorders, including chronic autoimmune thyroiditis (67); ii) Among Graves' patients, smokers have a higher risk of developing GO than non-smokers (odds ratio, 7.7, 95% CI, 4.3–13.7, *vs.* 1.9, 95% CI, 1.1–3.2) (68); iii) Smokers are at high risk of developing severe forms of GO, with a dose-dependent relative risk of diplopia or exophthalmos (69) (**Figure 5**); iv) Response to treatments for GO is decreased and occurs later in smokers than in non-smokers (70, 71); v) *De novo* development or progression of GO after RAI treatment occurs more frequently in smokers (29, 49, 72); vi) Quit smoking decreases the risk of developing exophthalmos and diplopia, suggesting that current smoking is more important than lifetime tobacco consumption (69). Accordingly, refrain from smoking is a fundamental, general, preventive action strongly recommended by guidelines (54). It is possible, but yet unproven, that also passive smoking be relevant for the occurrence of GO (23). Whether e-cigarette may also concur to development/progression of GO remains for the time being unsettled. Mechanisms whereby cigarette smoking exerts a negative effect on GO are not fully understood, but they might involve oxygen free radical generation, hypoxia in the orbit, enhanced production of cytokines, stimulation of adipogenesis (64).

TABLE 2 | Risk factors for the occurrence/progression Graves' orbitopathy (GO) and preventive actions.

Risk Factor	Evidence (Ref.)	Preventive Action
Smoking Habit	• Patients with GO are more frequently smokers than those without GO (67) • Smokers have an increased risk of developing GO than non-smokers (68) • Smokers have a dose-dependent increased relative risk of developing severe GO (69) • Smokers have a lower and slower response to immunesuppressive treatments (70, 71), • Refrain from smoking reduces the risk of developing exophthalmos and diplopia (69) • Radioiodine associated progression og GO is more frequent in smokers (70, 72),	Urge patients to refrain from smoking
Thyroid Dysfunction	• Hyperthyroidism negatively influences GO and amelioration is associated with restoration of euthyroidism (48) • GO may develop during uncontrolled hypothyroidism (73)	Restore and stably maintain euthyroidism by antithyroid drugs (hyperthyroidism) or levothyroxine replacement (hypothyroidism)
Radioiodine treatment for hyperthyroidism	• Radioiodine treatment may cause occurrence or progression of GO (49, 74), particularly in smokers (72)	Give a short course of oral prednisone (steroid prophylaxis) in at risk patients
Oxidative stress	• GO is associated with an increased oxidative stress (75)	Provide a 6-month selenium supplementation in patients with mild GO of short duration
TSH receptor antibodies (TRAbs)	• TRAb levels are higher in patients with GO than in those without GO (76) • TRAb levels correlate with GO activity and severity (4, 43, 76),	In patients with relevant GO, control hyperthyroidism with antithyroid drugs, because this is usually associated with a decline in TRAb levels
Hypercholesterolemia	• Serum total and LDL cholesterol levels correlate the presence and activity of GO (77) • Serum total and LDL cholesterol levels are higher in patients with GO than in those without GO (78) • The use of statins was associated with a decreased risk of developing GO (31)	Correct dyslipidemia in patients with newly diagnosed Graves' hyperthyroidism

Thyroid Dysfunction

We mentioned above that both hyperthyroidism and hypothyroidism represent risk factors for the occurrence of GO (46, 48). Accordingly, a rapid restoration of euthyroidism and its stable maintenance, avoiding thyroid status fluctuations, are strongly recommended by guidelines as an important preventive measure (54) (**Table 2**). Mechanisms whereby thyroid dysfunction may favor the occurrence or progression of GO are probably related to the activation of the TSH receptor by either TRAbs (hyperthyroidism) or TSH (hypothyroidism) (64).

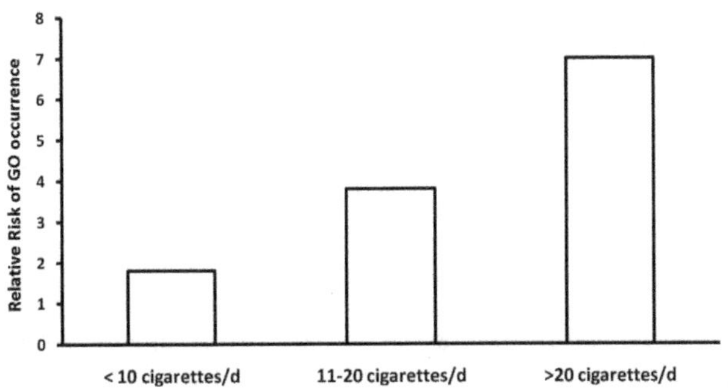

FIGURE 5 | Relative risk of developing exophthalmos and diplopia in relation to daily number of cigarettes. Derived from Pfeilschifter and Ziegler (67).

Radioiodine Treatment

RAI is a well-established and effective method of treatment for Graves' hyperthyroidism (79). RAI carries a small but definite risk of causing progression or *de novo* occurrence of GO, probably due to antigen release and related exacerbation of autoimmune reactions following RAI administration (1) (**Table 2**). In a randomized clinical trial of 168 patients, 114, aged 35 to 55 years, were randomized to either antithyroid drug treatment, RAI treatment, or subtotal thyroidectomy: GO developed or worsened in 4/38 patients (10%) treated with antithyroid drugs, 6/37 patients (16%) treated surgically, and 13/39 patients (33%) treated with RAI (74). In a randomized clinical trial of 443 patients, GO progressed in 23/150 patients (15%) treated with RAI, but in only 3/148 patients (3%) treated with antithyroid drugs (49). RAI-associated progression of GO was transient in some patients, but was permanent and required immunosuppressive treatments in 5% of patients (49). This untoward effect could be prevented in a third group of patients who received a concomitant short-term course of oral prednisone (steroid prophylaxis) (49), confirming a previous randomized clinical trial from the same group (80). This undue effect of RAI is more likely to occur in smokers (72), while it is unlikely in patients whose Graves' disease duration is >5 years (81) or whose GO is stably inactive (73). Relatively lower doses of oral prednisone (0.1–0.2 mg/bodyweight as starting dose, gradually tapered and withdrawn after 6 weeks) are equally effective as previously suggested highly doses (0.3–0.5 mg/bodyweight as starting dose, tapered and withdrawn after 3 months) (82) and safe (83). Based on the above studies, steroid prophylaxis is an important preventive measure in most Graves' patients undergoing RAI treatment for hyperthyroidism, and as such it is recommended in most patients by recent guidelines (54, 79). In particular, it should be given in patients who have mild and active GO and/or risk factors for its development/progression, especially smoking, while It can be avoided in patients with long-standing and inactive GO.

Oxidative Stress

Graves' orbitopathy is associated with an increased oxidative stress (75). Because of its antioxidant and immunoregulatory actions, selenium has been proposed as an adjuvant therapy in patients with mild GO. In a randomized clinical trial of 159 patients with mild and active GO, selenium administration for 6 months was associated with an improved quality of life and improved ocular involvement compared with placebo; in addition, it was more effective than placebo in preventing progression of GO from mild to moderate-to-severe (84). It is unclear whether selenium should be used only in patients who are selenium-deficient or also in patients with an adequate selenium intake. It is probably useless in patients with long-standing, inactive mild GO. Likewise, there is no evidence that a course of selenium may be beneficial also in patients with moderate-to-severe GO. With these limitations, current guidelines recommend a 6-month selenium supplementation in patients with recent onset, mild GO, because it improves ocular involvement and prevents progression to more severe forms of GO (54).

TSH-Receptor Antibody Levels

TRAbs are the only specific biomarker for Graves' disease and GO (3). TRAb levels correlate with the Clinical Activity Score (4, 43). TRAbs with stimulating activities in a recently developed bioassay tested positive in 150/155 patients with Graves' disease (97%) and 148/155 of those with GO (95%), their levels were 3-fold higher in patients with GO than in those without GO, and strongly correlated with GO activity and severity (76). TRAbs were shown to be an independent risk factor for GO and predictors of severity and outcome of the disease (85). In a study of 100 consecutive patients, the combination of high TRAb levels and absent thyroid peroxidase antibodies identified Graves' patients at high risk of developing GO (86). This finding was subsequently confirmed by a 3-year prospective study from the same group (87). In terms of prevention, for the time being, there is no treatment that blocks TRAb synthesis. However, while RAI treatment for hyperthyroidism is followed by a rise in TRAb levels (probably related to the cytolytic effect of RAI), which may last for several years, antithyroid drug treatment (either directly or through restoration of euthyroidism) and thyroidectomy are generally and gradually associated with a progressive reduction of serum TRAb concentration, which may be beneficial for GO (88).

Hypercholesterolemia

In a cross-sectional study of 250 patients with Graves' hyperthyroidism of recent onset, with (n = 133) or without GO (n = 117), a correlation between serum total and LDL cholesterol and the presence and activity of GO was reported (77). A second study, from the same group, of 86 consecutive patients with recent onset Graves' disease referred for RAI treatment, confirmed that serum total and LDL cholesterol were higher in patients than in those without GO, although there was no relationship between cholesterol and activity or severity of GO (78). The above reports might explain why the analysis of a large database from USA, including 8,404 patients with newly diagnosed Graves' disease, showed that the use of statins for at least two months in the year of observation was associated with a 40% decreased hazard ratio (HR) of developing GO (HR: 0.60, CI, 0.47–0.75) (31). Because the use of non-statin cholesterol lowering drugs was not associated with a decreased risk of GO occurrence (31), it is unsettled whether the purported protective/preventive effect of statins on GO is related to their anti-inflammatory action or to the cholesterol lowering effect. Clearly, further studies are needed to clarify this issue, but it is reasonable to state that correction of dyslipidemia in newly diagnosed Graves' patients may represent a useful preventive action against the occurrence of GO.

Prediction of GO Occurrence in Newly Diagnosed Graves' Patients

Because of the major role of exogenous factors in the development of GO, a prospective observational study was carried out in 10 EUGOGO centers to construct a predictive score (called PREDIGO, prediction of GO) for the development/progression of GO in 348 newly diagnosed and untreated Graves' patients without obvious GO (89). Four independent variables composed the PREDIGO score, i.e., the Clinical Activity Score, TRAbs (measured as TSH-binding inhibiting immunoglobulins, TBII), duration of hyperthyroidism, and smoking. Of the 348 patients, all submitted to antithyroid drug treatment, 53 (15%) developed GO, which was mild in 46 (13%) and moderate-to-severe in 7 (2%) (78). The PREDIGO score proved to be much better in identifying patients who will not develop GO (negative predictive value: 0.91, 95% CI, 0.87–0.94) than those who will (positive predictive value: 0.28, 95% CI, 0.20–0.37) (89). Although this represents an evident limitation and underpins the need for the improvement and refinement of this score with additional biomarkers, the PREDIGO score may represent a simple and useful tool to consider when discussing the general treatment plan of newly diagnosed Graves' patients with absent or very mild GO. Moreover, as mentioned earlier, early referral of patients with mild and active GO and/or effective control of modifiable risk factors for development/progression of the disease may substantially contribute to exacerbation of GO (54).

CONCLUDING REMARKS

GO is the most frequent extrathyroidal manifestation of Graves' disease, although it may rarely develop also in euthyroid/hypothyroid patients with chronic autoimmune thyroiditis. It is a relatively infrequent disorder, and men tend to have more severe ocular involvement at an older age. After an initial inflammatory (active) phase and a phase of stabilization (plateau phase), GO tends to improve and eventually inactivates (inactive or burnt-out phase). Mild GO tends spontaneously to remit spontaneously, but complete *restitutio ad integrum* almost never occurs when GO is more than minimal-to-mild. Several risk factors contribute to its development on a yet undefined genetic background. Cigarette smoking is the most important risk factor. Early diagnosis, control and removal of modifiable risk factors, early treatment of mild forms, stable control of thyroid dysfunction may effectively limit the risk of progression to more severe forms of GO, which have a profound and dramatic impact on the quality of life of affected individuals, and remain a therapeutic challenge, often requiring long-lasting and multiple medical and surgical therapies.

AUTHOR CONTRIBUTIONS

All the authors participated in searching literature, critically read the papers, critically revised the draft of the paper, checked illustrations, checked bibliography, and share responsibility for statements. All authors contributed to the article and approved the submitted version.

REFERENCES

1. Bartalena L, Tanda ML. Graves' ophthalmopathy. *N Engl J Med* (2009) 360:994–1001. doi: 10.1056/NEJMcp0806317
2. Taylor PN, Zhang L, Lee RWJ, Muller I, Ezra DG, Dayan CM, et al. New insights into the pathogenesis and nonsurgical management of Graves' orbitopathy. *Nat Rev Endocrinol* (2020) 16:104–16. doi: 10.1038/s41574-019-0305-4
3. Diana T, Ponto KA, Kahaly GJ. Thyrotropin receptor antibodies and Graves' orbitopathy. *J Endocrinol Invest* (2020). doi: 10.1007/s40618-020-01380-9
4. Nicolì F, Lanzolla G, Mantuano M, Ionni I, Mazzi B, Leo M, et al. Correlation between serum anti-TSH receptor autoantibodies (TRAbs) and the clinical feature of Graves' orbitopathy. *J Endocrinol Invest* (2020). doi: 10.1007/s40618-020-01353-y
5. Smith TJ, Kahaly GJ, Ezra DG, Fleming JC, Dailey RA, Tang RA, et al. Teprotumumab for thyroid-associated ophthalmopathy. *N Engl J Med* (2017) 376:1748–61. doi: 10.1056/NEJMoa1614949
6. Douglas RS, Kahaly GJ, Patel A, Sile S, Thompson EHZ, Perdok R, et al. Teprotumumab for the treatment of active thyroid eye disease. *N Engl J Med* (2020) 382:341–52. doi: 10.1056/NEJMoa1910434
7. Lanzolla G, Ricci D, Nicolì F, Sabini E, Sframeli A, Brancatella A, et al. Putative protective role of autoantibodies against the insulin-like growth factor-1 receptor in Graves' disease: results of a pilot study. *J Endocrinol Invest* (2020) 43:1759–68. doi: 10.1007/s40618-020-01341-2
8. Bahn RS. Graves' ophthalmopathy. *N Engl J Med* (2010) 362:726–38. doi: 10.1056/NEJMra0905750
9. Bartley GB. The epidemiologic characteristics and clinical course of ophthalmopathy associated with autoimmune thyroid disease in Olmsted County, Minnesota. *Trans Am Ophthalmol Soc* (1994) 92:477–588.
10. Abraham-Nordling M, Bystrom K, Torring O, Lantz M, Berg G, Calissendorf J, et al. Incidence of hyperthyroidism in Sweden. *Eur J Endocrinol* (2011) 165:899–905. doi: 10.1530/EJE-11-0548
11. Laurberg P, Berman DC, Bulow Pedersen I, Andersen S, Carlé A. Incidence and clinical presentation of moderate to severe Graves' orbitopathy in a Danish population before and after iodine fortification of salt. *J Clin Endocrinol Metab* (2012) 97:2325–32. doi: 10.1210/jc.2012-1275
12. Perros P, Hegedus L, Bartalena L, Marcocci C, Kahaly GJ, Baldeschi L, et al. Graves' orbitopathy as a rare disease in Europe: a European Group on Graves' Orbitopathy (EUGOGO) position statement. *Orphanet J Rare Dis* (2017) 12:72. doi: 10.1186/s13023-017-0625-1
13. Tanda ML, Piantanida E, Liparulo L, Veronesi G, Lai A, Sassi L, et al. Prevalence and natural history of Graves' orbitopathy in a large series of patients with newly diagnosed Graves' hyperthyroidism seen at a single center. *J Clin Endocrinol Metab* (2013) 98:1443–9. doi: 10.1210/jc.2012-3873
14. Perros P, Zarkovic M, Azzolini C, Ayvaz G, Baldeschi L, Bartalena L, et al. PREGO (presentation of Graves' orbitopathy) study: changes in referral patterns to European Group on Graves' Orbitopathy (EUGOGO) centres over the period from 2000 to 2012. *Br J Ophthalmol* (2015) 99:1531–5. doi: 10.1136/bjophthalmol-2015-306733
15. Zaletel K, Gaberscek S, Pirnat E. Ten-year follow-up of thyroid epidemiology in Slovenia after increase in salt iodization. *Croat Med J* (2011) 52:615–21. doi: 10.3325/cmj.2011.52.615
16. Lazarus JH. Epidemiology of Graves' orbitopathy (GO) and relationship with thyroid disease. *Best Pract Res Clin Endocrinol Metab* (2012) 26:273–9. doi: 10.1016/j.beem.2011.10.05
17. Hiromatsu Y, Eguchi H, Tani J, Kasaoka M, Teshima Y. Graves' ophthalmopathy: epidemiology and natural history. *Intern Med* (2014) 53:353–60. doi: 10.2169/internalmedicine.53.1518
18. Perros P, Kendall-Taylor P. Natural history of thyroid associated ophthalmopathy. *Thyroid* (1998) 8:423–5. doi: 10.1089/thy.1998.8.423
19. Chin YH, Ng CH, Lee MH, Koh JWH, Kiew J, Yang SP, et al. Prevalence of thyroid eye disease in Graves' disease: a meta-analysis and systematic review. *Clin Endocrinol (Oxf)* (2020). doi: 10.1111/cen.14296
20. Piantanida E, Tanda ML, Lai A, Sassi L, Bartalena L. Prevalence and natural history of Graves' orbitopathy in the XXI century. *J Endocrinol Invest* (2013) 36:444–9. doi: 10.3275/8937
21. Kozaki A, Inoue R, Komoto N, Maeda T, Inoue Y, Inoue T, et al. Proptosis in dysthyroid ophthalmopathy: a case series of 10,931 Japanese cases. *Optom Vis Sci* (2010) 87:200–4. doi: 10.1097/OPX.0b013e3181ce5702
22. Perros P, Crombie AL, Matthews JN, Kendall-Taylor P. Age and gender influence the severity of thyroid-associated ophthalmopathy: a study of 101 patients attending a combined thyroid-eye clinic. *Clin Endocrinol (Oxf)* (1993) 38:367–72. doi: 10.1111/j.1365-2265.1993.tb00516.x
23. Krassas GE, Segni M, Wiersinga WM. Childhood Graves' ophthalmopathy: results of a European questionnaire study. *Eur J Endocrinol* (2005) 53:515–21. doi: 10.1530/eje.1.01991
24. Bartalena L. Childhood Graves' orbitopathy. In: WM Wiersinga, GJ Kahaly, editors. *Graves' orbitopathy. A multisciplinary approach – questions and anwers, 3rd.* Basel: Karger (2017). 53:301–8. doi: 10.1159/000475968
25. Marcocci C, Bartalena L, Bogazzi F, Panicucci M, Pinchera A. Studies on the occurrence of ophthalmopathy in Graves' disease. *Acta Endocrinol (Copenh)* (1989) 120:473–8. doi: 10.1530/acta.0.1200473
26. Perros P, Zarkovic MP, Panagiotou GC, Azzolini C, Ayvaz G, Baldeschi L, et al. Asymmetry indicates more severe and active disease in Graves' orbitopathy: results from a prospective cross-sectional multicentre study. *J Endocrinol Invest* (2020) 43:1717–22. doi: 10.1007/s40618-020-01258-w
27. Manji N, Carr-Smith JD, Boelaert K, Allahabadia A, Armitage M, Chatterjee VK, et al. Influences of age, gender, smoking, and family history on autoimmune thyroid disease phenotype. *J Clin Endocrinol Metab* (2006) 91:4873–80. doi: 10.1210/jc.2006-1402
28. Tellez M, Cooper J, Edmonds C. Graves' ophthalmopathy in relation to cigarette smoking and ethnic origin. *Clin Endocrinol (Oxf)* (1992) 36:291–4. doi: 10.1111/j.1365-2265.1992.tb01445.x
29. Khong JJ, Finch S, De Silva C, Rylander S, Craig JE, Selva D, et al. Risk factors for Graves' orbitopathy; the Australian Thyroid-Associated Orbitopathy (ATOR) study. *J Clin Endocrinol Metab* (2016) 101:2716–20. doi: 10.1210/jc.2015-4294

30. Takakura A, Kirkeby K, Earle K, Silkiss RZ. Predicting the development of orbitopathy in Graves thyroidopathy patients: the potential role of TSI testing. *Ophthalm Plast Reconstr Surg* (2015) 31:369–72. doi: 10.1097/iop.0000000000000350
31. Stein JD, Childers D, Gupta S, Talwar N, Nan B, Lee BJ, et al. Risk factors for developing thyroid-associated ophthalmopathy among individuals with Graves disease. *JAMA Ophthalmol* (2015) 133:290–6. doi: 10.1001/jamaophthalmol.2014.5103
32. Prummel MF, Bakker A, Wiersinga WM, Baldeschi L, Mourits MP, Kendall-Taylor P, et al. Multi-center study on the characteristics and treatment strategies of patients with Graves' orbitopathy: the first European Group on Graves' Orbitopathy experience. *Eur J Endocrinol* (2003) 148:491–5. doi: 10.1530/eje.0.148049
33. Soroudi AE, Goldberg RA, McCann JD. Prevalence of asymmetric exophthalmos in Graves orbitopathy. *Ophthal Plast Reconstr Surg* (2004) 20:224–5. doi: 10.1097/01.iop.0000124675.80763.5
34. Daumerie C, Duprez T, Boschi A. Long-term multidisciplinary follow-up of unilateral thyroid-associatedorbitopathy. *Eur J Intern Med* (2008) 19:531–6. doi: 10.1016/j.ejim.2008.01.013
35. Eckstein AK, Losch C, Glowacka D, Schott M, Mann K, Esser J, et al. Euthyroid and primarily hypothyroid patients develop milder and significantly more asymmetrical Graves ophthalmopathy. *Br J Ophthalmol* (2009) 93:1052–6. doi: 10.1136/bjo.2007.137265
36. Strianese D, Piscopo R, Elefante A, Napoli M, Comune C, Baronissi I, et al. Unilateral proptosis in thyroid disease with subsequent contralateral involvement: retrospective follow-up study. *BMC Ophthalmol* (2013) 13:21. doi: 10.1186/1471-2415-13-21
37. Marinò M, Ionni I, Lanzolla G, Sframeli A, Latrofa F, Rocchi R, et al. Orbital diseases mimicking Graves' orbitopathy: a long-standing challenge in differential diagnosis. *J Endocrinol Invest* (2020) 43:401–11. doi: 10.1007/s40618-019-01141-3
38. Rotondi M, Virili C, Pinto S, Coperchini F, Croce L, Brusca N, et al. The clinical phenotype of Graves' disease occurring as an isolated condition or in association with other autoimmune diseases. *J Endocrinol Invest* (2020) 43:157–62. doi: 10.1007/s40618-019-01094-7
39. Khoo DH, Eng PH, Ho SC, Morgenthaler NG, Seah LL, Chee SP, et al. Graves' ophthalmopathy in the absence of elevated free thyroxine and triiodothyronine levels: prevalence, natural history, and thyrotropin receptor antibody levels. *Thyroid* (2000) 10:1093–100. doi: 10.1089/thy.2000.10.1093
40. Li Y, Kim J, Diana T, Olivo PD, Kahaly GJ. A novel bioassay for anti-thyrotrophin autoantibodies detects both thyroid-blocking and stimulating activities. *Clin Exp Immunol* (2013) 173:390–7. doi: 10.1111/cei.12129
41. Ponto KA, Binder H, Diana T, Matheis N, Otto AF, Pitz S, et al. Prevalence, phenotype, and psychological well-being in euthyroid/hypothyroid thyroid-associated orbitopathy. *Thyroid* (2015) 25:942–8. doi: 10.1089/thy.2015.0031
42. Smith TJ, Hegedus L. Graves' disease. *N Engl J Med* (2016) 375:1552–65. doi: 10.1056/NEJMra1510030
43. Gerding MN, van der Meer JW, Broenink M, Bakker O, Wiersinga WM, Prummel MF. Association of thyrotrophin receptor antibodies with the clinical features of Graves' ophthalmopathy. *Clin Endocrinol (Oxf)* (2000) 52:267–71. doi: 10.1046/j.1365-2265.2000.00959.x
44. Kahaly GJ, Diana T, Glang J, Kanitz M, Pitz S, Konig J. Thyroid stimulating antibodies are highly prevalent in Hashimoto's thyroiditis and associated orbitopathy. *J Clin Endocrinol Metab* (2016) 101:1998–2004. doi: 10.1210/jc.2016-1220
45. Bartalena L, Chiovato L. Graves'-like orbitopathy: do not forget IgG4-related disease. *J Endocrinol Invest* (2014) 37:1233–5. doi: 10.1007/s40618-014-0171-9
46. Wiersinga WM, Bartalena L. Epidemiology and prevention of Graves' ophthalmopathy. *Thyroid* (2002) 12:855–60. doi: 10.1089/105072502761016476
47. Marcocci C, Bartalena L, Bogazzi F, Bruno-Bossio G, Pinchera A. Relationship between Graves' ophthalmopathy and type of treatment of Graves' hyperthyroidism. *Thyroid* (1992) 2:171–8. doi: 10.1089/thy.1992.2.171
48. Prummel MF, Wiersinga WM, Mourits MP, Koornneef L, Berghout A, van der Gaag R. Effect of abnormal thyroid function on the severity of Graves' ophthalmopathy. *Arch Intern Med* (1990) 150:1098–101. doi: 10.1001/archinte.150.5.1098
49. Bartalena L, Marcocci C, Bogazzi F, Manetti L, Tanda ML, Dell'Unto E, et al. Relation between therapy for hyperthyroidism and the course of Graves' ophthalmopathy. *N Engl J Med* (1998) 338:73–8. doi: 10.1007/s40618-014-0171-9
50. Rundle FF, Wilson CW. Development and course of exophthalmos and ophthalmoplegia in Graves' disease with special reference to the effect of thyroidectomy. *Clin Sci* (1945) 5:177–94.
51. Bartalena L, Pinchera A, Marcocci C. Management of Graves' ophthalmopathy: reality and perspectives. *Endocr Rev* (2000) 21:168–99. doi: 10.1210/edrv.21.2.0393
52. Selva D, Chen C, King G. Late reactivation of thyroid orbitopathy. *Clin Exp Ophthalmol* (2004) 32:46–50. doi: 10.1046/j.1442-9071.2004.00756.x
53. Potgieser PW, Wiersinga WM, Regensburg NI, Mourits MP. Some studies on the natural history of Graves' orbitopathy: increase in orbital fat is a rather late phenomenon. *Eur J Endocrinol* (2015) 173:149–53. doi: 10.1530/EJE-14-1140
54. Bartalena L, Baldeschi L, Boboridis K, Eckstein A, Kahaly GJ, Marcocci C, et al. The 2016 European Thyroid Association /European Group on Graves' Orbitopathy guidelines for the management of Graves' orbitopathy. *Eur Thyroid J* (2016) 5:9–26. doi: 10.1159/000443828
55. Perros P, Crombie AL, Kendall-Taylor P. Natural history of thyroid associated ophthalmopathy. *Clin Endocrinol (Oxf)* (1995) 42:45–50. doi: 10.1111/j.1365-2265.1995.tb02597.x
56. Noth D, Gebauer M, Muller B, Burgi U, Diem P. Graves' ophthalmopathy: natural history and treatment outcomes. *Swiss Med Wkly* (2001) 131:603–9.
57. Menconi F, Profilo MA, Leo M, Sisti E, Altea MA, Rocchi R, et al. Spontaneous improvement of untreated mild Graves' ophthalmopathy: Rundle's curve revisited. *Thyroid* (2014) 24:60–6. doi: 10.1089/thy.2013.0240
58. Menconi F, Leo M, Sabini E, Mautone T, Nardi M, Sainato A, et al. Natural history of Graves' orbitopathy after treatment. *Endocrine* (2017) 57:226–33. doi: 10.1007/s12020-016-1136-x
59. Brix TH, Hegedus L. Twin studies as a model for exploring the aetiology of autoimmune thyroid disease. *Clin Endocrinol (Oxf)* (2012) 76:457–64. doi: 10.1111/j.1365-2265.2011.04318.x
60. Tomer Y. Mechanisms of autoimmune thyroid diseases: from genetics to epigenetics. *Annu Rev Pathol* (2014) 9:147–56. doi: 10.1146/annurev-pathol-012513-104713
61. Marinò M, Latrofa F, Menconi F, Chiovato L, Vitti P. Role of genetic and non-genetic factors in the etiology of Graves' disease. *J Endocrinol Invest* (2015) 38:283–94. doi: 10.1007/s40618-014-0214-2
62. Yin X, Latif R, Bahn R, Davies TF. Genetic profiling in Graves' disease: further evidence for lack of a distinct genetic contribution to Graves' orbitopathy. *Thyroid* (2012) 22:730–5. doi: 10.1089/thy.2012.0007
63. Jurecka-Lubieniecka B, Ploski R, Kula D, Szymanski K, Bednarczuk T, Ambroziak U, et al. Association between polymorphisms in the TSHR gene and Graves' orbitopathy. *PLoS One* (2014) 9:e102653. doi: 10.1371/journal.pone.0102653
64. Bartalena L. Prevention of Graves' orbitopathy. *Best Pract Res Clin Endocrinol Metab* (2012) 26:371–9. doi: 10.1016/j.beem.2011.09.004
65. Wiersinga WM. Smoking and thyroid. *Clin Endocrinol (Oxf)* (2013) 79:145–51. doi: 10.1111/cen.12222
66. Bartalena L, Piantanida E. Cigarette smoking: number one enemy for Graves' ophthalmopathy. *Pol Arch Med Wewn* (2016) 126:725–6. doi: 10.20452/pamw.3592
67. Bartalena L, Martino E, Marcocci C, Bogazzi F, Panicucci M, Velluzzi F, et al. More on smoking habits and Graves' ophthalmopathy. *J Endocrinol Invest* (1989) 12:733–7. doi: 10.1007/BF03350047
68. Prummel MF, Wiersinga WM. Smoking and risk of Graves' disease. *JAMA* (1993) 269:479–82. doi: 10.1001/jama.269.4.479
69. Pfeilschifter J, Ziegler R. Smoking and endocrine ophthalmopathy: impact of smoking severity and current versus lifetime tobacco consumption. *Clin Endocrinol (Oxf)* (1996) 45:477–81. doi: 10.1046/j.1365-2265.1996.8220832.x
70. Bartalena L, Marcocci C, Tanda ML, Manetti L, Dell'Unto E, Bartolomei MP, et al. Cigarette smoking and treatment outcomes in Graves' ophthalmopathy. *Ann Intern Med* (1998) 129:632–5. doi: 10.7326/0003-4819-129-8-199810150-00010
71. Eckstein AK, Quadbeck B, Mueller G, Rettemeier AW, Hoermann R, Mann K, et al. Impact of smoking on the response to treatment of thyroid associated ophthalmopathy. *Br J Ophthalmol* (2003) 73:773–6. doi: 10.1136/bjo.87.6.773
72. Traisk F, Tallstedt F, Abraham-Nordling M, Andersson T, Berg G, Calissendorff J, et al. Thyroid-associated ohthalmopathy after treatment for

Graves' hyperthyroidism with antithyroid drugs or iodine-131. *J Clin Endocrinol Metab* (2009) 94:3700–7. doi: 10.1136/bjo.87.6.773

73. Perros P, Kendall-Taylor P, Neoh C, Frewin S, Dickinson J. A prospective study of the effects of radioiodine therapy for hyperthyroidism in patients with minimally active Graves' ophthalmopathy. *J Clin Endocrinol Metab* (2005) 90:5321–3. doi: 10.1210/jc.2005-0507
74. Tallstedt L, Lundell G, Torring O, Wallin G, Ljunggren JG, Blomgren H, et al. Occurrence of ophthalmopathy after treatment for Graves' hyperthyroidism. *N Engl J Med* (1992) 326:1733–8. doi: 10.1056/NEJM199206253262603
75. Bartalena L, Tanda ML, Piantanida E, Lai A. Oxidative stress and Graves' ophthalmopathy: in vitro studies and therapeutic implications. *Biofactors* (2003) 19:155–63. doi: 10.1002/biof.5520190308
76. Lytton SD, Ponto KA, Kanitz M, Matheis N, Kohn LD, Kahaly GJ. A novel thyroid stimulating immunoglobulin bioassay is a functional indicator of activity and severity of Graves' orbitopathy. *J Clin Endocrinol Metab* (2010) 95:2123–31. doi: 10.1210/jc.2009-2470
77. Sabini E, Mazzi B, Profilo MA, Mautone T, Casini G, Rocchi R, et al. High serum cholesterol is a novel risk factor for Graves' orbitopathy: results of a cross-sectional study. *Thyroid* (2018) 28:386–94. doi: 10.1089/thy.2017.0430
78. Lanzolla G, Sabini E, Profilo MA, Mazzi B, Sframeli A, Rocchi R, et al. Relationship between serum cholesterol and Graves' orbitopathy (GO): a confirmatory study. *J Endocrinol Invest* (2018) 41:1417–23. doi: 10.1007/s40618-018-0915-z
79. Kahaly GJ, Bartalena L, Hegedus L, Leenhardt L, Poppe K, Pearce SH. European Thyroid Association Guideline for the management of Graves? Hyperthyroidism. *Eur Thyroid J* (2018) 7:167–86. doi: 10.1159/000490384
80. Bartalena L, Marcocci C, Bogazzi F, Panicucci M, Lepri A, Pinchera A. Use of corticosteroids to prevent progression of Graves' ophthalmopathy after radioiodine treatment for hyperthyroidism. *N Engl J Med* (1989) 321:1349–52. doi: 10.1056/NEJM198911163212001
81. Vannucchi G, Covelli D, Campi I, Currò N, Dazzi D, Rodari M, et al. Prevention of orbitopathy by oral or intravenous steroid prophylaxis in short duration Graves' disease undergoing radioiodine ablation: a prospective randomized control trial study. *Thyroid* (2019) 29:1828–33. doi: 10.1089/thy.2019.0150
82. Lai A, Sassi L, Compri E, Marino F, Sivelli P, Piantanida E, et al. Lower dose prednisone prevents radioiodine-associated exacerbation of initially mild or absent Graves' orbitopathy: a retrospective cohort study. *J Clin Endocrinol Metab* (2010) 95:1333–7. doi: 10.1210/jc.2009-213
83. Rosetti S, Tanda ML, Veronesi G, Masiello E, Premoli P, Gallo D, et al. Oral steroid prophylaxis for Graves' orbitopathy after radioactive iodine treatment for Graves' disease is not only effective, but also safe. *J Endocrinol Invest* (2020) 43:381–3. doi: 10.1007/s40618-019-01126-2
84. Marcocci C, Kahaly GJ, Krassas GE, Bartalena L, Prummel M, Stahl M, et al. Selenium and the course of mild Graves' ophthalmopathy. *N Engl J Med* (2011) 364:1920–31. doi: 10.1056/nejmoa1012985
85. Eckstein AK, Plicht M, Lax H, Neuhauser M, Mann K, Lederbogen S, et al. Thyrotropin receptor autoantibodies are independent risk factors for Graves' ophthalmopathy and help to predict severity and outcome of the disease. *J Clin Endocrinol Metab* (2006) 91:3464–70. doi: 10.1210/jc.-2005-2813
86. Khoo DHC, Ho SC, Seah LL, Fong KS, Tal ES, Chee SP, et al. The combination of absent thyroid peroxidase antibodies and high thyroid-stimulating immunoglobulin levels in Graves' disease identifies a group at markedly increased risk of ophthalmopathy. *Thyroid* (1999) 9:1175–80. doi: 10.1089/thy.1999.9.1175
87. Goh SH, Ho SC, Seah LL, Fong KS, Khoo DHC. Thyroid autoantibody profile in ophthalmic dominant and thyroid dominant Graves' disease differ and suggest ophthalmopathy is a multiantigenic disease. *Clin Endocrinol (Oxf)* (2004) 60:607. doi: 10.1111/j.1365-2265.2004.02033.x
88. Laurberg P, Wallin G, Tallstedt L, Abraham-Nordling M, Lundell G, Torring O. TSH-receptor autoimmunity in Graves' disease after therapy with anti-thyroid drugs, surgery, or radioiodine: a 5-year prospective randomized study. *Eur J Endocrinol* (2008) 158:69–75. doi: 10.1530/EJE-07-0450
89. Wiersinga WM, Zarkovic M, Bartalena L, Donati S, Perros P, Okosieme O, et al. Predictive score for the development or progression of Graves' orbitopathy in patients with newly diagnosed Graves' hyperthyroidism. *Eur J Endocrinol* (2018) 178:635–43. doi: 10.1530/EJE-18-0039

6

Simvastatin and ROCK Inhibitor Y-27632 Inhibit Myofibroblast Differentiation of Graves' Ophthalmopathy-Derived Orbital Fibroblasts *via* RhoA-Mediated ERK and p38 Signaling Pathways

Yi-Hsuan Wei[1,2], *Shu-Lang Liao*[1,3], *Sen-Hsu Wang*[1], *Chia-Chun Wang*[1] *and Chang-Hao Yang*[1,3]*

[1] *Department of Ophthalmology, National Taiwan University Hospital, Taipei, Taiwan,* [2] *Graduate Institute of Clinical Medicine, College of Medicine, National Taiwan University, Taipei, Taiwan,* [3] *Department of Ophthalmology, College of Medicine, National Taiwan University, Taipei, Taiwan*

***Correspondence:**
Chang-Hao Yang
chyangoph@ntu.edu.tw

Transforming growth factor-β (TGF-β)-induced differentiation of orbital fibroblasts into myofibroblasts is an important pathogenesis of Graves' ophthalmopathy (GO) and leads to orbital tissue fibrosis. In the present study, we explored the antifibrotic effects of simvastatin and ROCK inhibitor Y-27632 in primary cultured GO orbital fibroblasts and tried to explain the molecular mechanisms behind these effects. Both simvastatin and Y-27632 inhibited TGF-β-induced α-smooth muscle actin (α-SMA) expression, which serves as a marker of fibrosis. The inhibitory effect of simvastatin on TGF-β-induced RhoA, ROCK1, and α-SMA expression could be reversed by geranylgeranyl pyrophosphate, an intermediate in the biosynthesis of cholesterol. This suggested that the mechanism of simvastatin-mediated antifibrotic effects may involve RhoA/ROCK signaling. Furthermore, simvastatin and Y-27632 suppressed TGF-β-induced phosphorylation of ERK and p38. The TGF-β-mediated α-SMA expression was suppressed by pharmacological inhibitors of p38 and ERK. These results suggested that simvastatin inhibits TGF-β-induced myofibroblast differentiation *via* suppression of the RhoA/ROCK/ERK and p38 MAPK signaling pathways. Thus, our study provides evidence that simvastatin and ROCK inhibitors may be potential therapeutic drugs for the prevention and treatment of orbital fibrosis in GO.

Keywords: simvastatin, Y-27632, Ras homolog family member A (RhoA), Rho-associated protein kinase (ROCK), myofibroblast, Graves' ophthalmopathy, ERK, p38

INTRODUCTION

Graves' ophthalmopathy (GO) is the ocular manifestation of Graves' disease (GD) and occurs in 25–50% of GD patients (1). It is characterized by inflammation and fibrosis of the orbital tissue, including the retrobulbar fat, connective tissue, and extraocular muscles (2). The expansion of the orbital tissue displaces the orbital globe by pushing it forward and results in clinical signs such as proptosis, lagophthalmos, and even sight-threatening exposure keratopathy or compressive optic neuropathy (1). Fibrosis of orbital tissue and enlargement of extraocular muscles may lead to strabismus and diplopia, which strongly affect the quality of life of patients suffering from GO (3). Orbital fibroblasts appear to play a central role in the pathogenesis of GO. The thyroid-stimulating hormone receptor and the insulin-like growth factor receptor on orbital fibroblasts are the major autoantigens responsible for GO (4). Once activated, orbital fibroblasts may generate numerous inflammatory molecules and differentiate into adipocytes or myofibroblasts, leading to tissue remolding in GO (5).

Orbital fibrosis is an important pathological change that occurs in GO (6). Transforming growth factor-β (TGF-β) plays a pivotal role in the pathophysiology of many fibrotic disorders, including GO (7). In previous studies, TGF-β has been used to induce extracellular matrix production and myofibroblast differentiation in GO orbital fibroblasts. The expression of fibrotic markers, including that of α-smooth muscle actin (α-SMA), connective tissue growth factor (CTGF), fibronectin, and collagen, was increased after the stimulation of TGF-β in GO orbital fibroblasts (7).

Statins are a class of drugs that are commonly used to lower serum cholesterol and prevent the development of cardiovascular diseases by inhibiting the enzyme hydroxymethylglutaryl-coenzyme A (HMG-CoA) reductase, which plays a crucial role in cholesterol synthesis. Statins also show pleiotropic effects e.g., anti-inflammatory, antifibrotic, and immune-modulatory (8, 9). In a recent database study among GD patients, the use of statins was associated with a reduced chance of developing GO (10). However, the precise molecular mechanism for it has not been fully established. Statins exert their antifibrotic effects on several organs, such as heart, lungs, and intestines (9, 11–13). In this study, we aimed to explore the antifibrotic effect of statins in GO to explain the possible molecular mechanisms through which statins reduce/inhibit GO development.

Ras homolog family member A (RhoA) plays an essential role in cell adhesion, migration, and transformation by organizing the actin cytoskeleton (14) and the Rho-associated protein kinase (ROCK) is an important downstream effector of RhoA. There are two ROCK isoforms, ROCK1 and ROCK2, that are widely distributed in whole body tissues (15). The RhoA/ROCK signaling may play an important role in TGF-β signaling to control myofibroblast differentiation (16). Inhibition of the RhoA/ROCK pathway could reduce the TGF-β-induced expression of α-SMA, CTGF, and collagen I, as well as the myofibroblast differentiation of fibroblasts (17–19). Statins inhibit the synthesis of intermediates of cholesterol biosynthesis such as farnesyl pyrophosphate (FPP) and geranylgeranyl pyrophosphate (GGPP), which are essential for the post-translational modification of the Rho family proteins (8). Therefore, statins have a potential therapeutic role in fibrotic diseases owing to their inhibitory effects on RhoA/ROCK signaling (20, 21). Simvastatin, a type of statin, can suppress TGF-β-induced myofibroblast transformation of fibroblasts through RhoA/ROCK inhibition (20, 21).

In this study, we investigated the effects of simvastatin and ROCK inhibitor Y-27632 on TGF-β1-induced α-SMA production in cultured GO orbital fibroblasts. We also explored the possible pathways through which simvastatin and ROCK inhibitor Y-27632 affect TGF-β1 signaling. We hypothesized that simvastatin and ROCK inhibitor Y-27632 could inhibit the myofibroblast differentiation of GO orbital fibroblasts, as well as the process of fibrosis in GO.

MATERIALS AND METHODS

Orbital Tissue Collection

Orbital tissue specimens were collected from the surgical waste produced during the orbital decompression surgeries of six GO patients. The clinical characteristics of the patients are listed in **Table 1**. All patients were euthyroid, with a clinical activity score of less than three for more than 6 months prior to the surgery. None of them had received radiotherapy or steroid pulse therapy in the past. Patient recruitment for the study was carried out at the Department of Ophthalmology, National Taiwan University Hospital, Taiwan. The protocol was approved by the Institutional Review Board of National Taiwan University Hospital, Taiwan (201908011RINA). Informed consent was obtained from all participants in accordance with the Declaration of Helsinki and Good Clinical Practice.

Orbital Fibroblast Culture and Stimulation

Orbital fibroblasts were cultivated as previously reported (22). Orbital tissues were minced and placed in plastic culture

TABLE 1 | Clinical characteristics of the patients included in this study.

Age, years	Sex	Duration of GO, months	CAS	fT4 (ng/dL)	TSH (mU/L)	TBII (%)	Previous treatment for GO
34	F	12	2	1.36	0.48	61.2	None
38	M	10	1	1.14	1.17	19.7	None
41	F	28	1	1.01	1.96	24.3	None
47	F	22	2	0.82	2.07	38.3	Oral steroids
57	F	20	1	1.09	1.39	54.2	None
58	M	36	2	0.91	0.57	44.5	Oral steroids

CAS, clinical activity score; fT4, free thyroxine; TSH, thyroid stimulating hormone; TBII, thyrotropin binding inhibitory immunoglobulin.

dishes with Dulbecco's modified Eagle's medium (DMEM) supplemented with 20% fetal bovine serum (FBS) and 50 IU/mL penicillin-streptomycin (Gibco®; Thermo Fisher Scientific, Waltham, MA, USA), allowing orbital fibroblasts to grow out. Monolayers were covered with DMEM supplemented with 10% FBS and serially passaged with gentle trypsin/ethylenediaminetetraacetic acid (EDTA) (Gibco®; Thermo Fisher Scientific, Waltham, MA, USA) treatment. These were incubated in a humidified incubator at 37°C and 5% carbon dioxide (CO_2).

The orbital fibroblasts were seeded into six-well plates at a density of 2×10^5 cells per well and stimulated at 90% confluence with 3 ng/mL of recombinant human TGF-β1 (Cat. No. 580701; BioLegend, San Diego, CA, USA) with or without pretreatment with simvastatin (TargetMol, Boston, MA, USA) or ROCK inhibitor Y-27632 (Sigma-Aldrich, St. Louis, MO, USA). In some experiments, fibroblasts were pretreated with PD98059 (ERK inhibitor) and SB203580 (p38 inhibitor) obtained from Cell Signaling Technology (Beverly, MA, USA) before stimulation with TGF-β1. We purchased FPP ammonium salt (F6892), GGPP ammonium salt (G6025), and mevalonate (90469) from Sigma (St. Louis, MO, USA) for cell stimulation in some experiments. GGTI-298 (Cat. No. 2430) and FTI-277 (Cat. No. 2407) were purchased from Tocris Bioscience (Bristol, United Kingdom). All experiments were performed with fibroblasts between the third and eighth passages from culture initiation. Six independent strains from different donors were used for the repeated experiments.

Immunofluorescence Staining

The orbital fibroblasts were cultured on six-well plates containing glass coverslips, and the cells were fixed and blocked for the immunofluorescence assay. The coverslips were incubated with anti-α-SMA primary antibody ab5694 (Abcam, Cambridge, MA, USA) overnight at 4°C. After three washes, the coverslips were processed with VectaFluor Excel Amplified Anti-Rabbit IgG Kit, DyLight® 488 Antibody Kit (DK-1488; Vector Laboratories, Burlingame, CA, USA). The nuclei were counterstained using H-1500 DAPI (Vector Laboratories, Burlingame, CA, USA). The glass slides were then observed with a fluorescence microscope coupled to a CCD camera (EVOS FLc; Life Technologies, Carlsbad, CA, USA). The fluorescence intensity quantification was performed using ImageJ.

Real-Time Polymerase Chain Reaction

Total RNA was extracted from cultured orbital fibroblasts using the TRIzol reagent (Invitrogen; Carlsbad, CA, USA). Complementary DNA (cDNA) was synthesized using 1 μg of RNA according to the manufacturer's instructions for the iScript cDNA Synthesis Kit (Bio-Rad, Hercules, CA, USA). Real-time PCR was performed on a thermocycler (StepOne Real-Time PCR System; Applied Biosystems, Foster City, CA, USA) using SYBR Green Master Mix (Applied Biosystems, Foster City, CA, USA). All PCRs were performed in triplicate. The sequences of the primers used were as follows: α-SMA forward: 5′-CTC CCA GGG CTG TTT TCC CA-3′, reverse: 5′-CCA TGT CGT CCC AGT TGG TG-3'; CTGF forward: 5′-TGT GTG ACG AGC CCA AGG A-3′, reverse: 5′-TCT GGG CCA AAC GTG TCT TC-3'; and Fibronectin 1 (FN1) forward: 5'-CCA AGA AGG GCT CGT GTG A-3′, reverse: 5′-TGG CTG GAA CGG CAT CA-3′. The primers for glyceraldehyde 3-phosphate dehydrogenase (GAPDH) were obtained from Sino Biological, Inc. (Cat no. HP100003; Wayne, PA, USA). The messenger RNA (mRNA) levels of each target gene were normalized to GAPDH and represented as fold changes.

Western Blot Analysis

Proteins were extracted from tissue homogenates and cell lysates. After collecting the protein samples, equal amounts of protein (50 μg) were boiled in a sample buffer. The protein samples were separated in a 10% sodium dodecyl sulfate-polyacrylamide gel and transferred to a nitrocellulose membrane. The blots were blocked with 4% bovine serum albumin for 1 h at room temperature and then probed with primary antibodies at 4°C overnight. The ab5694 antibody for α-SMA (1:1000 dilution) was purchased from Abcam (Cambridge, MA, USA). The antibodies for RhoA (1:1000 dilution, no. 2117), ROCK1 (1:1000 dilution, no. 4035), Smad2/3 (1:1000 dilution, no. 5678), phospho-Smad2 (Ser465/467)/Smad3 (Ser423/425) (1:1000 dilution, no. 8828), ERK1/2 (1:1000 dilution, no. 9102), phospho-ERK1/2 (Thr202/Tyr204) (1:2000 dilution, no. 4370), p38 MAPK (1:1000 dilution, no. 8212), phospho-p38 MAPK (Thr180/Tyr182) (1:1000 dilution, no. 9211), JNK (1:1000 dilution, no. 9252), and phospho-JNK (Thr183/Tyr185) (1:1000 dilution, no. 4668) were purchased from Cell Signaling Technology (Beverly, MA, USA). Immunoreactive bands were detected with horseradish peroxidase-conjugated secondary antibodies and developed using enhanced chemiluminescence detection (MilliporeSigma, Burlington, MA, USA) and exposure to X-ray film. The relative amount of each immunoreactive band was quantified using the ImageJ software and normalized to the levels of the reference molecules.

Statistical Analyses

At least three cell strains from different individuals were used in all experiments, and all sample assays were carried out in triplicate. The experimental results are shown as the mean ± SD calculated from normalized measurements. Analysis of variance or the Student's t-test were used to determine statistical significance ($p < 0.05$) using GraphPad Prism 8.4.2 (GraphPad Software, San Diego, CA, USA).

RESULTS

Simvastatin and ROCK Inhibitor Y-27632 Inhibited TGF-β-Induced α-SMA Expression in GO Orbital Fibroblasts

To determine the effect of simvastatin and ROCK inhibitor Y-27632 on TGF-β-induced myofibroblast differentiation, immunofluorescence staining for α-SMA (marker for myofibroblast) was performed in cultured GO orbital fibroblasts. The expression of α-SMA and actin filament formation were markedly increased after TGF-β1 (3 ng/mL) stimulation for 48 h (**Figure 1**). However, pretreatment of the cells with different concentrations of simvastatin (1, 5, 10 μM) (**Figure 1A**) or ROCK inhibitor Y-27632 (1, 10, 30 μM) (**Figure 1B**) diminished TGF-β-induced α-SMA expression in orbital fibroblasts.

To further confirm the results, we used real-time PCR and western blot analysis to assess the mRNA and protein expression levels of α-SMA, respectively. As shown in **Figure 2**, TGF-β1 significantly induced an increase in mRNA and protein expression levels of α-SMA in GO orbital fibroblasts. Pretreatment with different concentrations of simvastatin (1, 5, 10 μM) (**Figures 2A, C**) or ROCK inhibitor Y-27632 (1, 10, 30 μM) (**Figures 2B, D**) significantly inhibited TGF-β-induced α-SMA mRNA expression and protein production. The inhibitory effect of simvastatin and Y-27632 appeared to be dose-dependent. Therefore, 10 and 30 μM concentrations of simvastatin and Y-27632, respectively, were used in the subsequent experiments to achieve a more prominent effect. As α-SMA is the most common marker for fibroblast-to-myofibroblast differentiation, these results suggested that simvastatin and ROCK-inhibitor Y-27632 have an inhibitory effect on the TGF-β-induced differentiation of orbital fibroblasts into myofibroblasts.

Inhibitory Effect of Simvastatin on TGF-β-Induced RhoA, ROCK1, and α-SMA Expression Was Reversed by GGPP

Simvastatin, an HMG-CoA reductase, inhibits the synthesis of mevalonate and other precursors of cholesterol such as FPP and GGPP, which are important for farnesylation and geranylgeranylation of Rho proteins. To investigate the mechanism of simvastatin-mediated inhibition of myofibroblast differentiation, we studied the effects of the HMG-CoA downstream intermediates, mevalonate, FPP, and GGPP, on the expressions of RhoA, ROCK1, and α-SMA. As shown in **Figures 3A–D**, simvastatin inhibited TGF-β1-induced expression of RhoA, ROCK1, and α-SMA in GO orbital fibroblasts. The addition of 10 μM of GGPP reversed the inhibitory effects of simvastatin on RhoA, ROCK1, and α-SMA expression. However, the addition of FPP or mevalonate failed to prevent the suppressive effects of simvastatin. Moreover, the geranylgeranyl transferase inhibitor (GGTI-298), not the farnesyl transferase inhibitor (FTI-227), showed simvastatin-like inhibition of TGF-β1-induced α-SMA (**Figure 3E**). Based on these results, we propose that the mechanism of simvastatin-mediated inhibition of myofibroblast differentiation may involve RhoA/ROCK signaling. Simvastatin may inhibit the TGF-β1-induced RhoA/ROCK signaling by blocking Rho geranylgeranylation, but not Rho farnesylation.

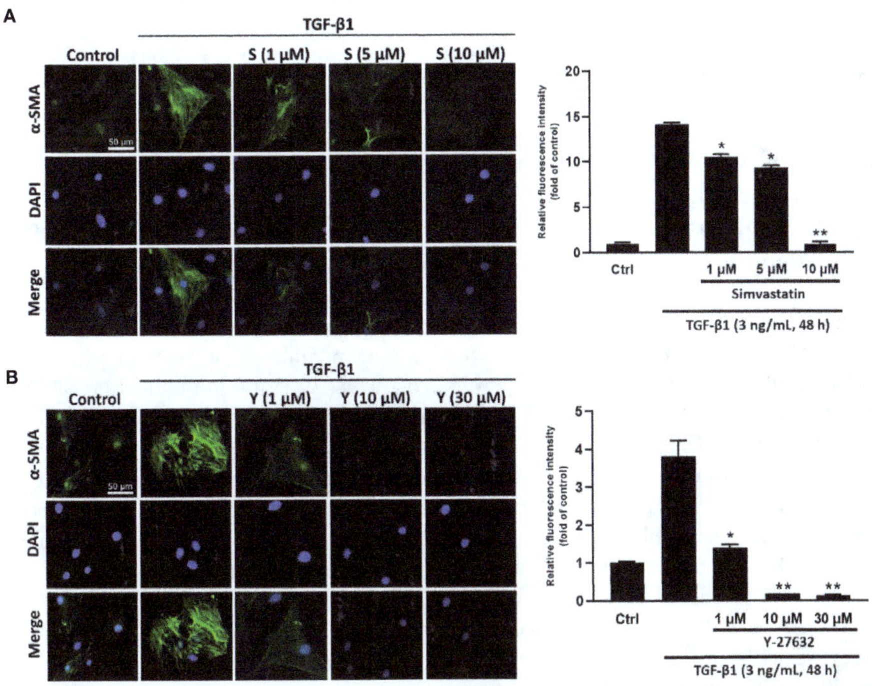

FIGURE 1 | Immunocytochemical characterization of transforming growth factor-β (TGF-β)-induced α-smooth muscle actin (α-SMA) expression in Graves' ophthalmopathy (GO) orbital fibroblasts. Primary cultured GO orbital fibroblasts were stimulated with 3 ng/mL TGF-β1 for 48 h with or without a 1-h pretreatment with different concentrations of simvastatin (1, 5, 10 μM) **(A)** or ROCK inhibitor Y-27632 (1, 10, 30 μM) **(B)**. α-SMA expression was detected using immunofluorescence staining (green). The bar charts show mean data of relative fluorescence intensity of α-SMA presented as the fold of control. *$p < 0.05$, **$p < 0.01$ compared to cells treated with TGF-β1 alone. S = simvastatin; Y = Y-27632.

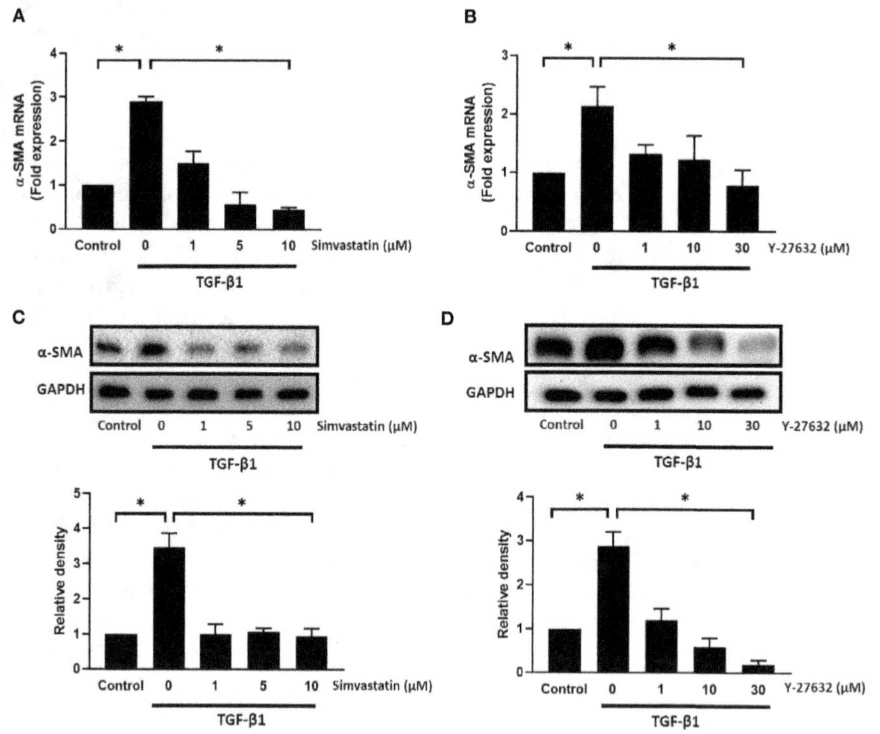

FIGURE 2 | Effect of simvastatin and ROCK inhibitor Y-27632 on transforming growth factor-β (TGF-β)-induced α-smooth muscle actin (α-SMA) messenger RNA (mRNA) and protein expression in Graves' ophthalmopathy (GO) orbital fibroblasts. Primary cultured GO orbital fibroblasts were stimulated with TGF-β1 (3 ng/mL) for 48 h with or without a 1-h pretreatment with different concentrations of simvastatin (1, 5, 10 μM) **(A, C)** or ROCK inhibitor Y-27632 (1, 10, 30 μM) **(B, D)**. The α-SMA mRNA expression was examined using real-time PCR **(A, B)**. The α-SMA protein production was determined using western blot analysis **(C, D)**. Data are presented as mean ± SD from at least three independent experiments. *p < 0.05.

Simvastatin and ROCK Inhibitor Y-27632 Inhibited TGF-β-Induced Phosphorylation of ERK and p38, But Not That of Smad

The signaling pathways implicated in TGF-β-induced myofibroblast differentiation include the Smad and non-Smad pathways, which incorporate the different branches of MAPK signaling (16). To explore the effects of simvastatin and ROCK inhibitor Y-27632 on TGF-β signaling in GO orbital fibroblasts, we investigated whether simvastatin and Y-27632 could inhibit TGF-β-induced phosphorylation of Smad2/3, ERK1/2, p38, and JNK. As shown in **Figures 4A–C**, 48 h of 3 ng/mL TGF-β treatment induced phosphorylation of Smad2/3, ERK1/2, and p38 in GO orbital fibroblasts. Simvastatin and Y-27632 successfully abrogated TGF-β-induced phosphorylation of ERK1/2 and p38. In contrast, they had no significant impact on TGF-β-induced phosphorylation of Smad2/3. Since the Smad and MAPK pathway could usually be activated in several minutes, we also assessed their phosphorylated states at early time-points (30, 60, 120 min) after TGF-β stimulation (**Figure 4D**). The results consistently demonstrated that simvastatin and Y-27632 inhibited TGF-β-induced phosphorylation of ERK1/2 and p38, but not Smad2/3. Our data suggested that simvastatin and Y-27632 could both inhibit the early- and late-phase activation of TGF-β-induced ERK and p38 signaling, but not Smad pathway in GO orbital fibroblasts.

Simvastatin and ROCK Inhibitor Y-27632 Inhibited TGF-β-Induced α-SMA Expression by Blocking ERK and p38 Signaling

To determine the potential involvement of ERK and p38 signaling in the mechanism by which simvastatin and Y-27632 inhibit myofibroblast differentiation, we investigated the effects of PD98059 (ERK inhibitor) and SB203580 (p38 inhibitor) on TGF-β-induced α-SMA expression. The results of western blot analysis showed that TGF-β-induced α-SMA expression in GO orbital fibroblasts was suppressed by PD98059 (**Figures 5A, C**) and SB203580 (**Figures 5B, D**). Based on previous data, simvastatin and Y-27632 have similar effects of ERK inhibitor and p38 inhibitor to block TGF-β-induced ERK and p38 signaling. These results suggested that simvastatin and Y-27632 inhibited TGF-β-induced α-SMA expression by blocking ERK and p38 signaling as well.

DISCUSSION

Orbital connective tissue remodeling and fibrosis are characteristic processes that appear relatively late in the clinical course of GO. The TGF-β produced by GO orbital fibroblasts may stimulate

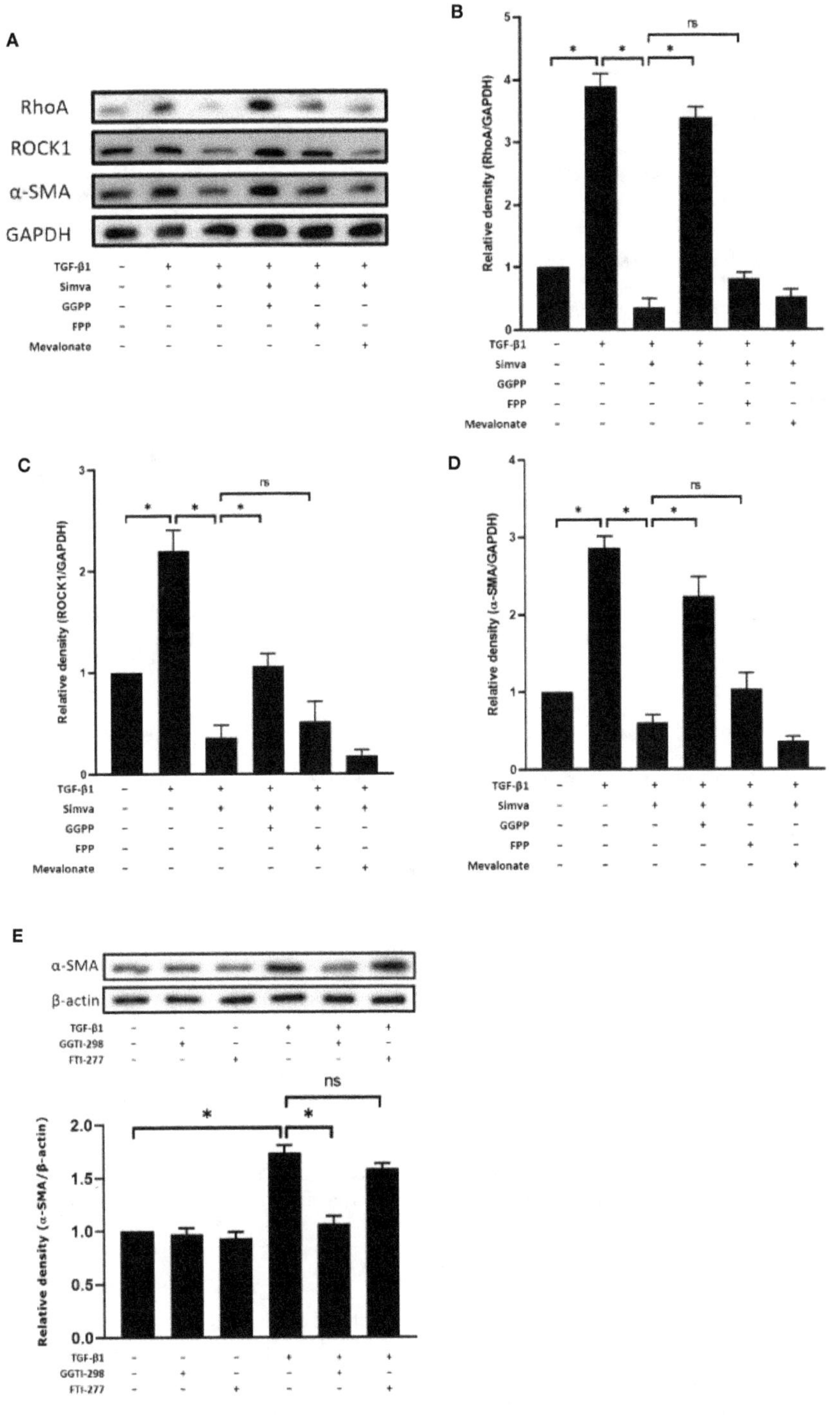

FIGURE 3 | Effects of hydroxymethylglutaryl-coenzyme A (HMG-CoA) downstream intermediates on simvastatin-mediated inhibition of transforming growth factor-β (TGF-β)-induced RhoA, Rho-associated protein kinase 1 (ROCK1), and α-smooth muscle actin (α-SMA) expression. **(A)** Graves' ophthalmopathy (GO) orbital fibroblasts were stimulated with TGF-β1 (3 ng/mL) for 48 h with or without a 1-h pretreatment with simvastatin (10 μM) and addition of geranylgeranyl pyrophosphate (GGPP) (10 μM), farnesyl pyrophosphate (FPP) (10 μM), or mevalonate (200 μM). The protein levels of RhoA, ROCK1, and α-SMA were determined using western blot analysis. **(B–D)** The densities of RhoA **(B)**, ROCK1 **(C)**, and α-SMA **(D)** protein bands were quantified and normalized to GAPDH. **(E)** GO orbital fibroblasts were stimulated with TGF-β1 (3 ng/mL) for 48 h with or without a 1-h pretreatment with geranylgeranyl transferase inhibitor (GGTI-298) (10 μM) or farnesyl transferase inhibitor (FTI-227) (10 μM). The α-SMA protein production was determined using western blot analysis. Data are presented as mean ± SD of at least three independent experiments. $^{*}p < 0.05$.

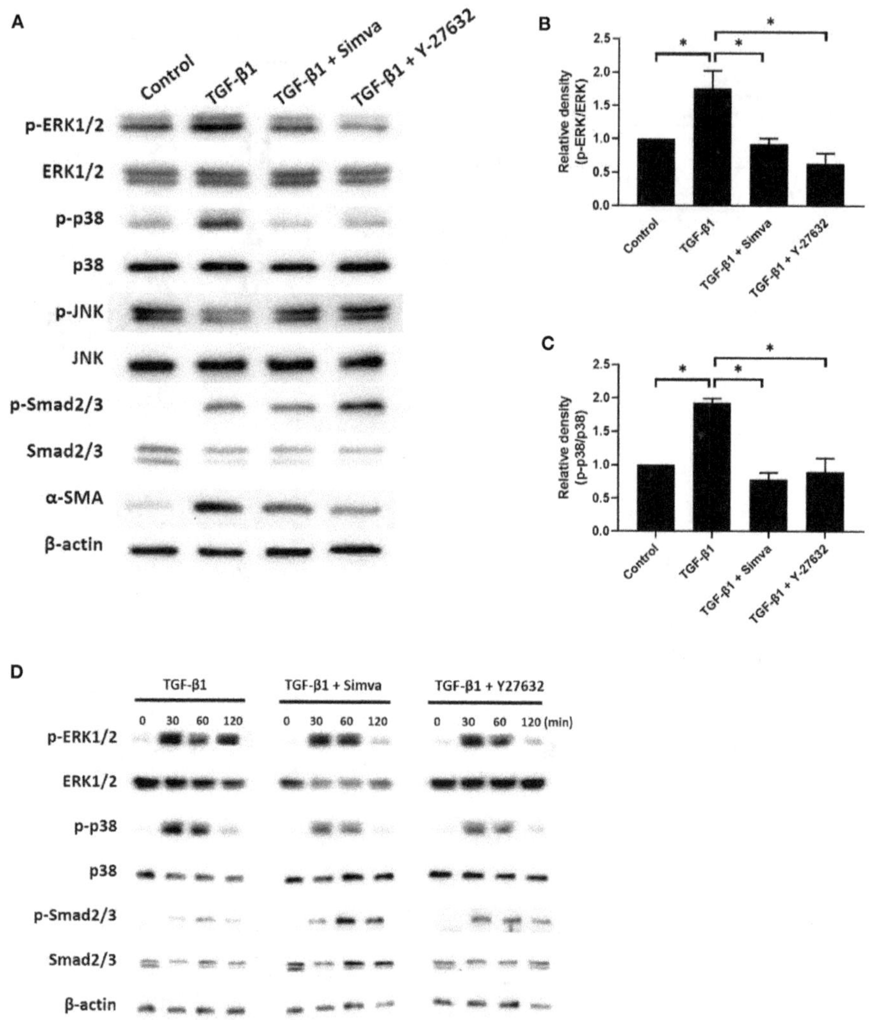

FIGURE 4 | Effects of simvastatin and ROCK inhibitor Y-27632 on transforming growth factor-β (TGF-β)-induced signaling. **(A)** Primary cultured Graves' ophthalmopathy (GO) orbital fibroblasts were stimulated with TGF-β1 (3 ng/mL) for 48 h with or without a 1-h pretreatment with simvastatin (10 μM) or ROCK inhibitor Y-27632 (30 μM). The expression and phosphorylation levels of Smad2/3, ERK1/2, p38, and JNK were determined using western blot analysis. **(B, C)** The densities of ERK1/2 **(B)** and p38 **(C)** protein bands were quantified and normalized to β-actin. **(D)** GO orbital fibroblasts were stimulated with TGF-β1 (3 ng/mL) for 30, 60, 120 min with or without a 1-h pretreatment with simvastatin (10 μM) or ROCK inhibitor Y-27632 (30 μM). The expression and phosphorylation levels of Smad2/3, ERK1/2, and p38 were determined using western blot analysis. Data are presented as mean ± SD of at least three independent experiments. *$p < 0.05$.

excessive production of extracellular matrix and differentiation of Thy-1-positive orbital fibroblasts into myofibroblasts, which express strong α-SMA immunoreactivity (22, 23). In this study, we showed that simvastatin and ROCK inhibitor Y-27632 inhibited the expression of TGF-β-induced α-SMA, which serves as a marker for fibrosis and indicates myofibroblast differentiation.

Some studies have demonstrated the inhibitory effects of simvastatin and Y-27632 on TGF-β-induced myofibroblast differentiation from fibroblasts derived from different disease specimens, such as nasal polyps (24), keloids (20), and penile tunica albuginea from Peyronie's disease (21). To the best of our knowledge, this is the first study to investigate the antifibrotic effects of simvastatin and Y-27632 in GO-derived fibroblasts. Further investigations on any synergistic effects of these two components will be helpful to understand their antifibrotic properties and potential therapeutic roles in GO.

Statins are commonly used to prevent coronary artery disease and stroke by reducing low-density lipoprotein cholesterol levels. Recently, the pleiotropic antifibrotic effects of statins have been proposed in various organ systems, such as heart (9, 11), liver (25, 26), and lungs (27, 28). Also, the possible protective role of statins in GO has been proposed (29). Statin usage is believed to be associated with a reduced risk of developing GO among patients with GD in a large cohort study (10). They found that

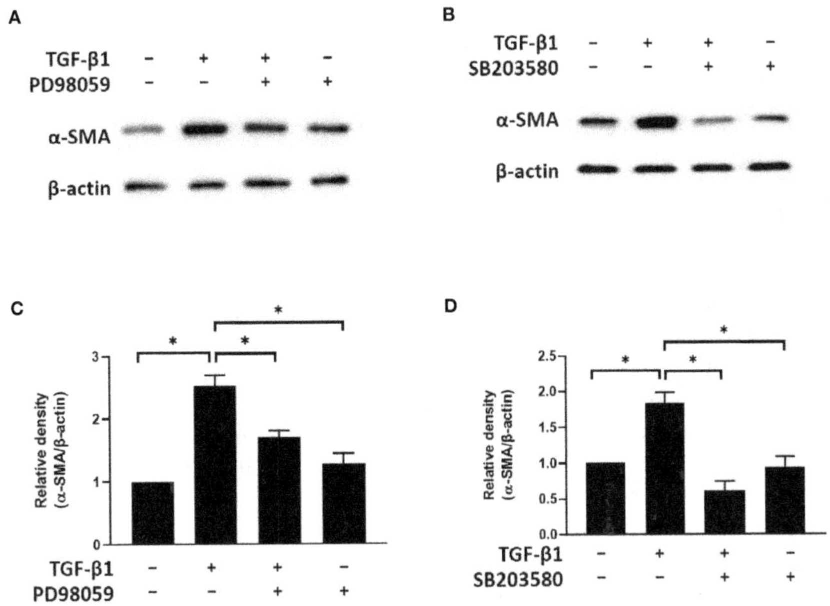

FIGURE 5 | Effects of ERK and p38 inhibitors on TGF-β-induced α-SMA expression in Graves's ophthalmopathy (GO) orbital fibroblasts. Primary cultured GO orbital fibroblasts were stimulated with transforming growth factor-β (TGF-β1) (3 ng/mL) for 48 h with or without a 1-h pretreatment with 10 μM of PD98059 (ERK inhibitor) **(A, C)** and 10 μM of SB203580 (p38 inhibitor) **(B, D)**. The protein levels of α-SMA were determined using western blot analysis. The densities of α-SMA protein bands were quantified and normalized to β-actin. Data are presented as mean ± SD of at least three independent experiments. *$p < 0.05$.

patients who used statins for at least 60 d during the period of observation had a 40% lower risk of developing GO. The precise molecular mechanisms by which statins reduce GO risk are not fully established. Some evidence suggests that statins may modulate both apoptosis and autophagic activities in patients with GD (29). This elucidation was based on the involvement of cellular apoptosis and autophagy in the pathogenesis of GO (30, 31). In addition, a recent study revealed that simvastatin may inhibit adipogenesis, as well as the expression of early and late adipogenic genes in human orbital fibroblasts (32). Our results provided *in vitro* evidence of simvastatin-mediated antifibrotic effects in GO that may also explain the possible protective effect of simvastatin against the development of GO.

The possible mechanism underlying statin-mediated antifibrotic effects is the inhibition of geranylgeranylated Rho protein, which in turn inhibits the Rho/ROCK signaling pathway (33, 34). Statins inhibit HMG-CoA reductase, the catalyst for the synthesis of mevalonate from HMG-CoA. This inhibition leads to a reduction of downstream intermediate compounds, including the isoprenoid GGPP and FPP. These molecules are necessary for the posttranslational modification of the Rho proteins, which is crucial for the Rho proteins to play their proper functions. In human keloid fibroblasts, simvastatin inhibited TGF-β-induced RhoA activation and RhoA/ROCK signaling by interfering with posttranslational geranylgeranylation of RhoA (20). In human airway fibroblasts, the inhibitory effects of simvastatin on TGF-β-induced fibronectin could be reversed by the addition of either GGPP or FPP (28). The study of human tenon fibroblasts suggested that the inhibition of Rho-geranylgeranylation, not Rho-farnesylation, was the mechanism for lovastatin to inhibit myofibroblast differentiation (35). In our study, we found that only GGPP, and not FPP, could reverse the simvastatin-mediated inhibition of TGF-β-induced α-SMA.

Consistently, only the geranylgeranyl transferase inhibitor (GGTI-298), not the farnesyl transferase inhibitor (FTI-227), showed simvastatin-like inhibition of TGF-β1-induced α-SMA. These findings suggested that geranylgeranylation rather than farnesylation of RhoA is crucial for TGF-β-induced α-SMA expression in GO orbital fibroblasts. And simvastatin may inhibit the TGF-β1-induced RhoA/ROCK signaling by blocking Rho geranylgeranylation, but not Rho farnesylation.

The RhoA/ROCK signaling pathway is known to regulate numerous cellular functions, including cell proliferation, migration, contraction, and adhesion (36). The profound involvement of the RhoA/ROCK pathway in various disease processes has made ROCK a potential therapeutic target in many kinds of diseases, e.g., cardiovascular (37), neoplastic (38), and neurologic (39). Moreover, ROCK inhibitors have been used as potential therapeutic drugs for several ophthalmic diseases, including glaucoma, corneal endothelial diseases, age-related macular degeneration, and diabetic retinopathy (40, 41). However, there are few studies that have investigated the role of Rho/ROCK signaling or that of ROCK inhibitors in GO. Using an *in vitro* model of GO, our study demonstrated the involvement of RhoA/ROCK signaling in TGF-β-induced myofibroblast differentiation and the antifibrotic effects of the ROCK inhibitor Y-27632. In many studies Y-27632 is a commonly used ROCK inhibitor that inhibits both ROCK1 and ROCK2 (42). Further investigations are necessary to explore the possible applications of ROCK inhibitors in the treatment of GO.

Transforming growth factor-β is the most potent inducer of myofibroblast differentiation and acts by activating the canonical Smad pathway or the non-Smad pathways, including Rho/ROCK signaling and different branches of the MAPK pathway (16, 43). The ROCK inhibitors were reported to inhibit TGF-β-induced myofibroblast differentiation by regulating the Smad or MAPK signaling pathways (19, 44). For example, Y-27632 suppressed TGF-β-induced phosphorylation of Smad3, but not that of Smad2, in ocular Tenon's capsule fibroblasts (44). It also inhibited TGF-β-induced phosphorylation of ERK and JNK, but not that of p38, in renal mesangial cells (19). In our study, Y-27632 abrogated TGF-β-induced phosphorylation of ERK and p38, but not that of JNK or Smad2/3. These results indicate that ROCK mediates MAPK signaling, but each MAPK signaling is regulated distinctively in different cells or by different stimuli. In our study, simvastatin showed an effect similar to that of Y-27632 in TGF-β-induced myofibroblast differentiation. These results suggest that, although simvastatin does not regulate the TGF-β-mediated Smad pathway in GO orbital fibroblasts, it regulates the TGF-β-mediated ERK/p38 MAPK pathways, probably in a ROCK-dependent manner. In summary, we propose that simvastatin can inhibit TGF-β-induced myofibroblast differentiation *via* suppression of the RhoA/ROCK/ERK and p38 MAPK signaling pathways (**Figure 6**).

Contrary to our findings, previous studies showed that simvastatin could inhibit TGF-β-mediated Smad phosphorylation in human ventricular (11) and intestinal fibroblasts (45). We believe that the cellular mechanisms of simvastatin's antifibrotic effect are diverse and complex in different cell types. Our data could not elucidate whether RhoA/ROCK/ERK and p38 MAPK signaling has any interaction with Smad2/3 signaling. Recently, Fang *et al.* reported that interleukin-17A can activate the JNK signaling in $CD90^+$ orbital fibroblasts to promote GO fibrosis initiated by TGF-β-mediated Smad transcription (46). Further investigation is needed to understand the possible interactions between the TGF-β-induced RhoA, MAPK, and Smad pathways in GO orbital fibroblasts.

Our study also had some limitations. First, the GO orbital fibroblasts were obtained from patients with inactive GO because of the surgical indication. Further studies must be conducted using specimens from patients with active GO to compare the results between different disease stages. Second, we only managed to obtain orbital tissues from a small cohort of

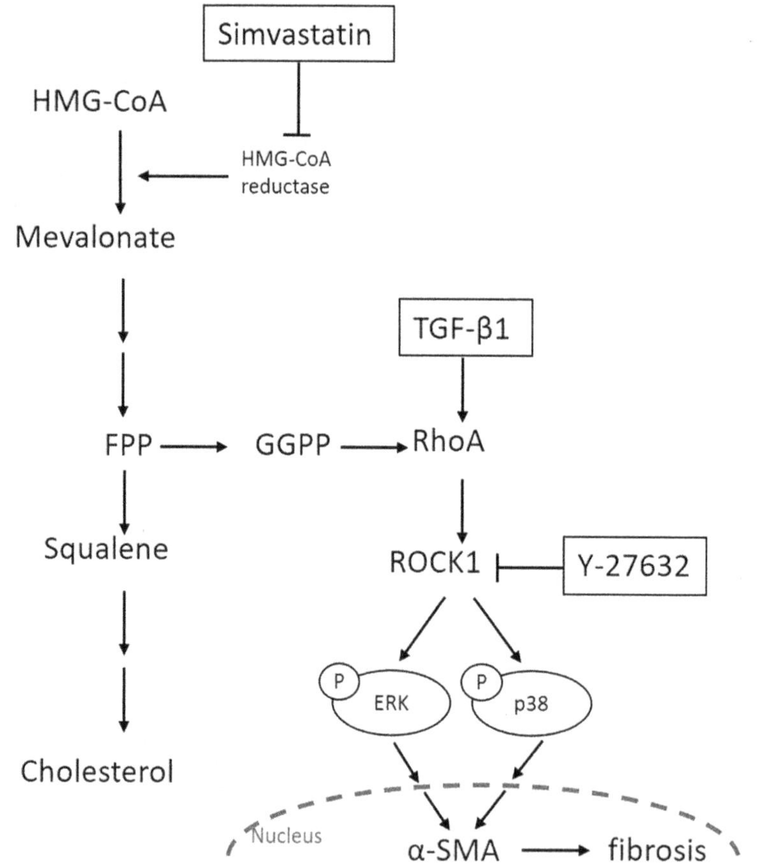

FIGURE 6 | Schematic diagram of the possible signaling mechanisms underlying simvastatin- and Y-27632-mediated inhibition of transforming growth factor-β (TGF-β1)-induced orbital tissue fibrosis in Graves' ophthalmopathy.

patients. We may need a larger sample size to validate our results in the future.

In conclusion, our results provide preliminary evidence that simvastatin and ROCK inhibitor Y-27632 inhibit TGF-β-induced differentiation of GO-derived fibroblasts into myofibroblasts. We propose that simvastatin and ROCK inhibitors may be potential candidates for the prevention and treatment of orbital tissue fibrosis in GO.

AUTHOR CONTRIBUTIONS

Y-HW, S-LL and C-CW conceptualized the experiments, designed the study, and secured funding. S-LL provided the surgical specimens. S-HW and C-CW performed the experiments and helped analyze the data. Y-HW interpreted the data and wrote the manuscript. C-HY supervised the research activity and revised the manuscript. All authors contributed to the article and approved the submitted version.

REFERENCES

1. Bahn RS. Graves' ophthalmopathy. *N Engl J Med* (2010) 362(8):726–38. doi: 10.1056/NEJMra0905750
2. Smith TJ. Pathogenesis of Graves' orbitopathy: a 2010 update. *J Endocrinol Invest* (2010) 33(6):414–21. doi: 10.1007/BF03346614
3. Lin IC, Lee CC, Liao SL. Assessing quality of life in Taiwanese patients with Graves' ophthalmopathy. *J Formos Med Assoc* (2015) 114(11):1047–54. doi: 10.1016/j.jfma.2013.12.002
4. Wang Y, Smith TJ. Current concepts in the molecular pathogenesis of thyroid-associated ophthalmopathy. *Invest Ophthalmol Vis Sci* (2014) 55 (3):1735–48. doi: 10.1167/iovs.14-14002
5. Dik WA, Virakul S, van Steensel L. Current perspectives on the role of orbital fibroblasts in the pathogenesis of Graves' ophthalmopathy. *Exp Eye Res* (2016) 142:83–91. doi: 10.1016/j.exer.2015.02.007
6. Shu DY, Lovicu FJ. Myofibroblast transdifferentiation: The dark force in ocular wound healing and fibrosis. *Prog Retin Eye Res* (2017) 60:44–65. doi: 10.1016/j.preteyeres.2017.08.001
7. Tsai CC, Wu SB, Kau HC, Wei YH. Essential role of connective tissue growth factor (CTGF) in transforming growth factor-beta1 (TGF-beta1)-induced myofibroblast transdifferentiation from Graves' orbital fibroblasts. *Sci Rep* (2018) 8(1):7276. doi: 10.1038/s41598-018-25370-3
8. Greenwood J, Steinman L, Zamvil SS. Statin therapy and autoimmune disease: from protein prenylation to immunomodulation. *Nat Rev Immunol* (2006) 6 (5):358–70. doi: 10.1038/nri1839
9. Oesterle A, Laufs U, Liao JK. Pleiotropic Effects of Statins on the Cardiovascular System. *Circ Res* (2017) 120(1):229–43. doi: 10.1161/ CIRCRESAHA.116.308537
10. Stein JD, Childers D, Gupta S, Talwar N, Nan B, Lee BJ, et al. Risk factors for developing thyroid-associated ophthalmopathy among individuals with Graves disease. *JAMA Ophthalmol* (2015) 133(3):290–96. doi: 10.1001/ jamaophthalmol.2014.5103
11. Rizvi F, Siddiqui R, DeFranco A, Homar P, Emelyanova L, Holmuhamedov E, et al. Simvastatin reduces TGF-beta1-induced SMAD2/3-dependent human ventricular fibroblasts differentiation: Role of protein phosphatase activation. *Int J Cardiol* (2018) 270:228–36. doi: 10.1016/j.ijcard.2018.06.061
12. Watts KL, Sampson EM, Schultz GS, Spiteri MA. Simvastatin inhibits growth factor expression and modulates profibrogenic markers in lung fibroblasts. *Am J Respir Cell Mol Biol* (2005) 32(4):290–300. doi: 10.1165/rcmb.2004-0127OC
13. Abe Y, Murano M, Murano N, Morita E, Inoue T, Kawakami K, et al. Simvastatin attenuates intestinal fibrosis independent of the anti-inflammatory effect by promoting fibroblast/myofibroblast apoptosis in the regeneration/healing process from TNBS-induced colitis. *Dig Dis Sci* (2012) 57(2):335–44. doi: 10.1007/s10620-011-1879-4
14. Heasman SJ, Ridley AJ. Mammalian Rho GTPases: new insights into their functions from in vivo studies. *Nat Rev Mol Cell Biol* (2008) 9(9):690–701. doi: 10.1038/nrm2476
15. Julian L, Olson MF. Rho-associated coiled-coil containing kinases (ROCK): structure, regulation, and functions. *Small GTPases* (2014) 5:e29846. doi: 10.4161/sgtp.29846
16. Carthy JM. TGFbeta signaling and the control of myofibroblast differentiation: Implications for chronic inflammatory disorders. *J Cell Physiol* (2018) 233(1):98–106. doi: 10.1002/jcp.25879
17. Itoh Y, Kimoto K, Imaizumi M, Nakatsuka K. Inhibition of RhoA/Rho-kinase pathway suppresses the expression of type I collagen induced by TGF-beta2 in human retinal pigment epithelial cells. *Exp Eye Res* (2007) 84(3):464–72. doi: 10.1016/j.exer.2006.10.017
18. Kita T, Hata Y, Kano K, Miura M, Nakao S, Noda Y, et al. Transforming growth factor-beta2 and connective tissue growth factor in proliferative vitreoretinal diseases: possible involvement of hyalocytes and therapeutic potential of Rho kinase inhibitor. *Diabetes* (2007) 56(1):231–38. doi: 10.2337/db06-0581
19. Nagai Y, Matoba K, Kawanami D, Takeda Y, Akamine T, Ishizawa S, et al. ROCK2 regulates TGF-beta-induced expression of CTGF and profibrotic genes via NF-kappaB and cytoskeleton dynamics in mesangial cells. *Am J Physiol Renal Physiol* (2019) 317(4):F839–51. doi: 10.1152/ajprenal.00596. 2018
20. Mun JH, Kim YM, Kim BS, Kim JH, Kim MB, Ko HC. Simvastatin inhibits transforming growth factor-beta1-induced expression of type I collagen, CTGF, and alpha-SMA in keloid fibroblasts. *Wound Repair Regener* (2014) 22(1):125–33. doi: 10.1111/wrr.12136
21. Milenkovic U, Ilg MM, Zuccato C, Ramazani Y, De Ridder D, Albersen M. Simvastatin and the Rho-kinase inhibitor Y-27632 prevent myofibroblast transformation in Peyronie's disease-derived fibroblasts via inhibition of YAP/TAZ nuclear translocation. *BJU Int* (2019) 123(4):703–15. doi: 10.1111/bju.14638
22. Smith TJ, Sempowski GD, Wang HS, Del Vecchio PJ, Lippe SD, Phipps RP. Evidence for cellular heterogeneity in primary cultures of human orbital fibroblasts. *J Clin Endocrinol Metab* (1995) 80(9):2620–25. doi: 10.1210/ jcem.80.9.7673404
23. Koumas L, Smith TJ, Feldon S, Blumberg N, Phipps RP. Thy-1 expression in human fibroblast subsets defines myofibroblastic or lipofibroblastic phenotypes. *Am J Pathol* (2003) 163(4):1291–300. doi: 10.1016/S0002-9440(10)63488-8
24. Park IH, Park SJ, Cho JS, Moon YM, Moon JH, Kim TH, et al. Effect of simvastatin on transforming growth factor beta-1-induced myofibroblast differentiation and collagen production in nasal polyp-derived fibroblasts. *Am J Rhinol Allergy* (2012) 26(1):7–11. doi: 10.2500/ajra.2012.26.3679
25. Trebicka J, Schierwagen R. Statins, Rho GTPases and KLF2: new mechanistic insight into liver fibrosis and portal hypertension. *Gut* (2015) 64(9):1349–50. doi: 10.1136/gutjnl-2014-308800
26. Janicko M, Drazilova S, Pella D, Fedacko J, Jarcuska P. Pleiotropic effects of statins in the diseases of the liver. *World J Gastroenterol* (2016) 22(27):6201–13. doi: 10.3748/wjg.v22.i27.6201
27. Zhu B, Ma AQ, Yang L, Dang XM. Atorvastatin attenuates bleomycin-induced pulmonary fibrosis via suppressing iNOS expression and the CTGF (CCN2)/ERK signaling pathway. *Int J Mol Sci* (2013) 14(12):24476–91. doi: 10.3390/ijms141224476
28. Schaafsma D, McNeill KD, Mutawe MM, Ghavami S, Unruh H, Jacques E, et al. Simvastatin inhibits TGFbeta1-induced fibronectin in human airway fibroblasts. *Respir Res* (2011) 12:113. doi: 10.1186/1465-9921-12-113
29. Bifulco M, Ciaglia E. Statin reduces orbitopathy risk in patients with Graves' disease by modulating apoptosis and autophagy activities. *Endocrine* (2016) 53(3):649–50. doi: 10.1007/s12020-015-0762-z
30. Yoon JS, Lee HJ, Chae MK, Lee EJ. Autophagy is involved in the initiation and progression of Graves' orbitopathy. *Thyroid* (2015) 25(4):445–54. doi: 10.1089/thy.2014.0300

31. Konuk O, Hondur A, Akyurek N, Unal M. Apoptosis in orbital fibroadipose tissue and its association with clinical features in Graves' ophthalmopathy. *Ocul Immunol Inflammation* (2007) 15(2):105–11. doi: 10.1080/09273940601186735
32. Shahida B, Johnson PS, Jain R, Brorson H, Asman P, Lantz M, et al. Simvastatin downregulates adipogenesis in 3T3-L1 preadipocytes and orbital fibroblasts from Graves' ophthalmopathy patients. *Endocr Connect* (2019) 8(9):1230–39. doi: 10.1530/EC-19-0319
33. Essig M, Nguyen G, Prie D, Escoubet B, Sraer JD, Friedlander G. 3-Hydroxy-3-methylglutaryl coenzyme A reductase inhibitors increase fibrinolytic activity in rat aortic endothelial cells. Role of geranylgeranylation and Rho proteins. *Circ Res* (1998) 83(7):683–90. doi: 10.1161/01.res.83.7.683
34. Mohammadalipour A, Hashemnia M, Goudarzi F, Ravan AP. Increasing the effectiveness of tyrosine kinase inhibitor (TKI) in combination with a statin in reducing liver fibrosis. *Clin Exp Pharmacol Physiol* (2019) 46(12):1183–93. doi: 10.1111/1440-1681.13157
35. Meyer-Ter-Vehn T, Katzenberger B, Han H, Grehn F, Schlunck G. Lovastatin inhibits TGF-beta-induced myofibroblast transdifferentiation in human tenon fibroblasts. *Invest Ophthalmol Vis Sci* (2008) 49(9):3955–60. doi: 10.1167/iovs.07-1610
36. Amano M, Nakayama M, Kaibuchi K. Rho-kinase/ROCK: A key regulator of the cytoskeleton and cell polarity. *Cytoskeleton (Hoboken)* (2010) 67(9):545–54. doi: 10.1002/cm.20472
37. Satoh K, Fukumoto Y, Shimokawa H. Rho-kinase: important new therapeutic target in cardiovascular diseases. *Am J Physiol Heart Circ Physiol* (2011) 301 (2):H287–96. doi: 10.1152/ajpheart.00327.2011
38. Wei L, Surma M, Shi S, Lambert-Cheatham N, Shi J. Novel Insights into the Roles of Rho Kinase in Cancer. *Arch Immunol Ther Exp (Warsz)* (2016) 64 (4):259–78. doi: 10.1007/s00005-015-0382-6
39. Mueller BK, Mack H, Teusch N. Rho kinase, a promising drug target for neurological disorders. *Nat Rev Drug Discovery* (2005) 4(5):387–98. doi: 10.1038/nrd1719
40. Moshirfar M, Parker L, Birdsong OC, Ronquillo YC, Hofstedt D, Shah TJ, et al. Use of Rho kinase Inhibitors in Ophthalmology: A Review of the Literature. *Med Hypothesis Discovery Innov Ophthalmol* (2018) 7(3):101–11.
41. Moura-Coelho N, Tavares Ferreira J, Bruxelas CP, Dutra-Medeiros M, Cunha JP, Pinto Proenca R. Rho kinase inhibitors-a review on the physiology and clinical use in Ophthalmology. *Graefes Arch Clin Exp Ophthalmol* (2019) 257 (6):1101–17. doi: 10.1007/s00417-019-04283-5
42. Liao JK, Seto M, Noma K. Rho kinase (ROCK) inhibitors. *J Cardiovasc Pharmacol* (2007) 50(1):17–24. doi: 10.1097/FJC.0b013e318070d1bd
43. Zhang YE. Non-Smad Signaling Pathways of the TGF-beta Family. *Cold Spring Harb Perspect Biol* (2017) 9(2). doi: 10.1101/cshperspect.a022129
44. Feng ZH, Zhang XH, Zhao JQ, Ma JZ. Involvement of Rho-associated coiled-coil kinase signaling inhibition in TGF-beta1/Smad2, 3 signal transduction in vitro. *Int J Ophthalmol* (2017) 10(12):1805–11. doi: 10.18240/ijo.2017.12.03
45. Burke JP, Watson RW, Murphy M, Docherty NG, Coffey JC, O'Connell PR. Simvastatin impairs smad-3 phosphorylation and modulates transforming growth factor beta1-mediated activation of intestinal fibroblasts. *Br J Surg* (2009) 96(5):541–51. doi: 10.1002/bjs.6577
46. Fang S, Huang Y, Zhong S, Li Y, Zhang Y, Li Y, et al. Regulation of Orbital Fibrosis and Adipogenesis by Pathogenic Th17 Cells in Graves Orbitopathy. *J Clin Endocrinol Metab* (2017) 102(11):4273–83. doi: 10.1210/jc.2017-01349

7

Integrative Analysis of Proteomics and DNA Methylation in Orbital Fibroblasts from Graves' Ophthalmopathy

Sita Virakul[1], *Poorichaya Somparn*[2,3], *Trairak Pisitkun*[2], *Peter J. van der Spek*[4], *Virgil A. S. H. Dalm*[5,6], *Dion Paridaens*[7,8], *P. Martin van Hagen*[5,6,7], *Nattiya Hirankarn*[9], *Tanapat Palaga*[1] *and Willem A. Dik*[5*]

[1] Department of Microbiology, Faculty of Science, Chulalongkorn University, Bangkok, Thailand, [2] Center of Excellence in Systems Biology, Research affairs, Faculty of Medicine, Chulalongkorn University, Bangkok, Thailand, [3] Translational Research in Inflammation and Immunology Research Unit (TRIRU), Department of Microbiology, Faculty of Medicine, Chulalongkorn University, Bangkok, Thailand, [4] Department of Bioinformatics, Erasmus University Medical Center, Rotterdam, Netherlands, [5] Department of Immunology, Laboratory Medical Immunology, Erasmus University Medical Center, Rotterdam, Netherlands, [6] Department of Internal Medicine, Division of Clinical Immunology, Erasmus University Medical Center, Rotterdam, Netherlands, [7] Rotterdam Eye Hospital, Rotterdam, Netherlands, [8] Department of Ophthalmology, Erasmus Medical Center, Rotterdam, Netherlands, [9] Center of Excellence in Immunology and Immune Mediated Diseases, Department of Microbiology, Faculty of Medicine, Chulalongkorn University, Bangkok, Thailand

***Correspondence:**
Willem A. Dik
w.dik@erasmusmc.nl

Background: Graves' ophthalmopathy (GO) is a frequent extrathyroidal complication of Graves' hyperthyroidism. Orbital fibroblasts contribute to both orbital tissue inflammation and remodeling in GO, and as such are crucial cellular elements in active GO and inactive GO. However, so far it is largely unknown whether GO disease progression is associated with functional reprogramming of the orbital fibroblast effector function. Therefore, the aim of this study was to compare both the proteome and global DNA methylation patterns between orbital fibroblasts isolated from active GO, inactive GO and healthy controls.

Methods: Orbital fibroblasts from inactive GO (n=5), active GO (n=4) and controls (n=5) were cultured and total protein and DNA was isolated. Labelled and fractionated proteins were analyzed with a liquid chromatography tandem-mass spectrometer (LC-MS/MS). Data are available *via* ProteomeXchange with identifier PXD022257. Furthermore, bisulphite-treated DNA was analyzed for methylation pattern with the Illumina Infinium Human Methylation 450K beadchip. In addition, RNA was isolated from the orbital fibroblasts for real-time quantitative (RQ)-PCR. Network and pathway analyses were performed.

Results: Orbital fibroblasts from active GO displayed overexpression of proteins that are typically involved in inflammation, cellular proliferation, hyaluronan synthesis and adipogenesis, while various proteins associated with extracellular matrix (ECM) biology and fibrotic disease, were typically overexpressed in orbital fibroblasts from inactive GO. Moreover, orbital fibroblasts from active GO displayed hypermethylation of genes that linked to inflammation and hypomethylated genes that linked to adipogenesis and autoimmunity. Further analysis revealed networks that contained molecules to which both hypermethylated and hypomethylated genes were linked, including NF-κB, ERK1/2, Alp, RNA polymerase II, Akt and IFNα. In addition, NF-κB, Akt and IFNα were also identified in networks that were derived from the differentially expressed proteins. Generally, poor correlation between protein expression, DNA methylation and mRNA expression was observed.

Conclusions: Both the proteomics and DNA methylation data support that orbital fibroblasts from active GO are involved in inflammation, adipogenesis, and glycosaminoglycan production, while orbital fibroblasts from inactive disease are more skewed towards an active role in extracellular matrix remodeling. This switch in orbital fibroblast effector function may have therapeutic implications and further studies into the underlying mechanism are thus warranted.

Keywords: graves' ophthalmopathy, orbital fibroblast, proteomics, DNA methylation, epigenetics

INTRODUCTION

Fibroblasts are crucial for maintaining tissue homeostasis, and are major producers of important cellular mediators for inflammatory and tissue remodeling processes during normal healing responses, but also under pathological conditions, including chronic inflammatory and fibrotic diseases (1). Chronic tissue inflammation and fibrosis are characterized by excessive fibroblast accumulation in affected tissues (1). Fibroblast accumulation occurs through different mechanisms, including enhanced proliferation by tissue resident CD34^{-} fibroblasts, recruitment of fibrocytes (a population of circulating cells with fibroblast-like properties that express CD34^{+} and extracellular matrix (ECM) molecules) and diminished apoptosis/prolonged survival (2–4). These fibroblasts can alter their phenotype and effector functions, as evidenced by their differentiation into myofibroblasts (5, 6). Myofibroblasts are considered to represent the end-effector cells in fibrotic reactions. Myofibroblasts express α-smooth muscle actin that facilitates cellular contraction and tissue distortion and actively produce high amounts of ECM molecules, such as collagen and hyaluronan (1).

Graves' ophthalmopathy (GO) is a disease of the orbital soft-tissues surrounding the eyes, and affects up to 50% of patients with Graves' disease (GD) (7). In general, GO patients first suffer from an initial phase of progressive disease (the 'active' phase) that is characterized by active inflammation (8). This active phase may last for months after which the activity subsides and progresses to a phase of slow spontaneous recovery. This 'chronic' phase may take months to years and is associated with pathological tissue alterations, including adipose tissue expansion, excessive hyaluronan accumulation and fibrosis (8). The orbital tissue alterations are largely responsible for several morbidities such as proptosis, chronic eye movement dysfunction, and eventually determines the 'severity' of GO (7). Previously, protein expression profiles of orbital tissues from GO with different disease activity and smoking status revealed differences in several proteins involved in inflammation and adipogenesis (9, 10). However, those proteins could not be specifically linked to their pathogenic cellular source.

Orbital fibroblasts represent the main effector cells in GO as they are crucially involved in regulation of both the local inflammatory and tissue remodeling responses. The effector functions of the orbital fibroblasts are in turn affected by several mediators, including the thyrotropin receptor (TSHR) stimulatory autoantibodies, cytokines, growth factors and physical cellular interactions (8). Importantly, orbital fibroblasts from GO patients may react in a different way to such stimuli than orbital fibroblasts isolated from healthy orbital tissue. For instance a stronger upregulation of CD40, Thy1, IGF1R and BAFF by GO orbital fibroblasts was reported (11–14). Moreover, orbital fibroblasts isolated from active GO display enhanced secretion of certain pro-inflammatory mediators in comparison to orbital fibroblasts from control tissue, even in the absence of further *in vitro* stimulation (15, 16). Furthermore, differentiation of orbital fibroblasts into adipocytes and pro-fibrotic myofibroblasts appears to be more restricted to the late inactive stage of disease and is associated with increased TSHR expression by these cells (17, 18).

Gradually, epigenetic regulation (e.g. histone modification, DNA methylation and non-coding RNA) has become the subject of studies in primary fibroblasts isolated from different fibroproliferative diseases, including idiopathic pulmonary fibrosis (IPF) and systemic sclerosis (SSc) (4, 19–22). Fibroblasts from IPF and SSc have altered DNA methylation profiles, which contribute to the regulation of gene transcription in these cells (19, 20). In GO, differential gene expression has been demonstrated in orbital tissue, suggesting a role for epigenetics in the pathogenesis of GO (23). However, data on DNA methylation in orbital fibroblasts from GO is lacking to date. Insight in this could help to develop novel therapeutic options that target aberrant epigenetic modifications in GO. Here we conducted a study to compare the proteome of orbital fibroblasts isolated from active GO, inactive GO and control orbital tissue and integrated these data with global DNA methylation analysis performed on the same orbital fibroblasts.

MATERIAL AND METHODS

Orbital Fibroblast Isolation From Orbital Tissue

Orbital fibroblasts were cultured from four patients with GO in an active stage (clinical activity score (CAS) ≥ 3/7) and five patients with GO in an inactive stage of disease (CAS < 3/7) (24), who underwent orbital decompression surgery. In addition, orbital fibroblasts were cultured from five controls without thyroid or inflammatory disease that underwent orbital surgery for other reasons, as described previously (25). GO patients were euthyroid and had not received immunosuppressive treatment for at least three months prior to orbital decompression surgery. Further patient characteristics are given in **Table 1**. All orbital tissues were obtained at the Rotterdam Eye Hospital (Rotterdam, the Netherlands), after informed consent and in accordance with the principles of the Declaration of Helsinki. Approval was given by the local medical ethics committee (protocol ID-2007-01). Orbital fibroblasts were cultured in Dulbecco's modified Eagle's medium (DMEM) supplemented with 10% fetal calf serum (FCS) and antibiotics (penicillin and streptomycin; Cambrex BioWhittaker, Verviers, Belgium) (25). Orbital fibroblasts were serially passaged with gentle treatment of trypsin/EDTA and used for experiments between the 2nd and 6th passage.

Proteome Analysis

Protein Extraction, Peptide Preparation and Labeling

Orbital fibroblasts from four patients with GO at an active stage and five GO patients at an inactive stage of disease, and five controls were included in this experiment. Orbital fibroblasts (5 x 10^6 cells) were obtained and pelleted after which Halt^{TM} Protease Inhibitor Cocktail and Phosphatase Inhibitor Cocktail (Thermo Fisher Scientific, Rockford, IL) was added before digestion and homogenization in 5% sodium deoxycholate with a sonicator. Protein concentration was determined with Pierce^{TM} BCA Protein Assay Kit (Thermo Fisher Scientific, Rockford, IL). For peptide preparation, 100 μg of protein was digested with 2 μg trypsin and labelled with 10-plex tandem mass tag (TMT) reagent according to the manufacturer's protocol (Thermo Fisher Scientific, Rockford, IL). Afterwards, the peptide mixture was passed through the Pierce High pH Reversed-Phase Peptide Fractionation Kit (Thermo Fisher Scientific, Rockford, IL).

TABLE 1 | Patients and controls data.

Participants	Cell ID	Age	Gender
Healthy control	**COF-3**	48	Female
	COF-4	82	Female
	COF-7	80	Female
	COF-9	59	Female
	COF-10	37	Female
Inactive GO	**GO-11**	43	Female
	GO-27	69	Female
	GO-31	46	Female
	GO-56	51	Female
	GO-89	32	Female
Active GO	**GO-19**	31	Female
	GO-37	62	Female
	GO-88	77	Male
	GO-90	84	Female

Peptide Analysis

The labelled fractionated peptides were analyzed with a liquid chromatography tandem-mass spectrometer (LC-MS/MS) (Q Exactive Plus mass spectrometer; Thermo Scientific, San Jose, CA). The LC-MS/MS methods included a full MS scan at a resolution of 70,000 followed by 10 data-dependent MS2 scans at a resolution of 37,500. The normalized collision energy of higher-energy collisional dissociation (HCD) fragmentation was set at 28%. MS scan range of 400 to 1,600 m/z was selected and precursor ions with unassigned charge states, a charge state of +1 and a charge state of greater than +8 were excluded. Proteome discoverer 2.1 software (Thermo Scientific, San Jose, CA) was used to analyze the MS raw data files with database containing forward and reverse peptide sequences from the human Uniprot Database. The search parameters were set for the fix modifications of carbamidomethylation of cysteine (+57.02146 Da) and TMT modifications (+229.2634 Da) at N-terminal and lysine, while oxidation of methionine (+15.99491 Da) was set for the variable modification. A maximum of four modifications and two missed cleavages per peptide were allowed. Parent and fragment monoisotopic mass errors were set at 10 ppm and 0.2 Da, respectively. A target–decoy approach was used to limit the false discovery rate (FDR) of the identified peptides to less than 1%. Differential protein expression was compared between orbital fibroblasts isolated from active and inactive GO by Student's t-test. The mass spectrometry proteomics data have been deposited to the ProteomeXchange Consortium *via* the PRIDE [1] partner repository with the dataset identifier PXD022257. Network, pathway and functional analysis were further performed on these differential expressed proteins using Ingenuity (Qiagen) filtering only for those networks and pathways that are based on experimentally obtained information.

DNA Methylation Analysis

Total DNA was extracted from orbital fibroblasts of active GO (n = 4), inactive GO (n = 4) and controls (n = 4). Global DNA methylation was measured using the Illumina Infinium Human Methylation 450K beadchip on bisulphite-treated DNA. DNA methylation analysis was performed by GenomeStudio methylation analysis package. Methylation level ranges from 0 (unmethylated) to 1 (fully methylated). Differential DNA methylation levels/patterns were analyzed by two approaches; 1) genes with differential DNA methylation using FDR < 0.05, and 2) differences in DNA methylation level of at least 2-fold between active and inactive GO. This was followed by network, pathway and functional analysis using Ingenuity (Qiagen) filtering only for those networks and pathways that are based on experimentally obtained information.

mRNA Expression by Orbital Fibroblasts

Messenger RNA was isolated (GenElute Mammalian Total RNA Miniprep Kit; Sigma-Aldrich, St. Louis, MO, USA) from orbital fibroblasts from the same culture experiment as used for the proteome and DNA methylation studies. The isolated mRNA was converted into cDNA and gene expression was determined by real-time quantitative (RQ)-PCR (QuantStudio 5 Real-Time PCR System; Applied Biosystems, Waltham, MA) and normalized to the control gene *ABL*, as described previously (25). Primer-probe combinations (*ABL*) and TaqMan gene expression assays (Life technologies, Foster, CA) used are listed in **Supplementary Table 1**. Data from mRNA expression was analyzed using ANOVA and subsequently analyzed with the Mann Whitney U test. A P-value < 0.05 was considered statistically significant.

RESULTS

Proteome Analysis in Orbital Fibroblasts

Twenty-five proteins differed significantly in their expression level between orbital fibroblasts from patients with active GO versus inactive GO (**Supplementary Table 2**). Cluster analysis revealed that the differentially expressed proteins clustered into three main groups (**Figure 1A**, indicated as cluster 1, cluster 2 and cluster 3). Proteins (n=6) in cluster 2 displayed higher expression in orbital fibroblasts from inactive GO compared to orbital fibroblasts from active GO and controls (**Figure 1B**). The proteins (n=16) in cluster 3 were higher expressed in orbital fibroblasts from active GO compared to inactive GO and controls (**Figure 1C**). The proteins (n=3) in cluster 1 were expressed at slightly higher level in orbital fibroblasts from active GO than orbital fibroblasts from inactive GO and controls.

Validation of Differential Protein Expression by RQ-PCR

For eleven of the proteins found to be differentially expressed (4 up-regulated and 7 down-regulated in inactive GO orbital fibroblasts compared to active GO) the expression levels of the corresponding mRNA molecules were determined by RQ-PCR (**Figures 1B, C**). From the 4 proteins (PSMB4, FBN2, COL6A1 and NCAM2) upregulated, only *NCAM2* mRNA was significantly higher expressed (P<0.05) in orbital fibroblasts from inactive GO compared to active GO (**Figure 1B**), while the mRNA levels of *PSMB4*, *FBN2* and *COL6A1* only showed a trend to higher expression in inactive GO orbital fibroblasts compared with active GO orbital fibroblasts (**Figure 1B**). Of the 7 proteins (PACSIN3, NFKB1, SMC3, GFER, GSDMD, UGDH and MT1X) that were expressed at significantly lower levels in orbital fibroblasts from inactive GO, none of the corresponding mRNAs was significantly decreased in inactive GO (**Figure 1C**). Unexpectedly, *NFKB1* mRNA expression was significantly up-regulated in inactive GO orbital fibroblasts compared to active GO (**Figure 1C**).

Orbital Fibroblast Expressed Proteins in Active GO Relate to Inflammation, Hyaluronan and Adipogenesis

Proteins overexpressed by orbital fibroblasts from active GO related to inflammation, hyaluronan synthesis and adipogenesis. One of the inflammation related proteins highly expressed in active GO orbital fibroblasts was NFKB1 (**Figure 1C**). The NFKB1 105 kD protein can be processed by the 26S proteasome into the DNA binding p50 subunit of the transcription factor NF-κB (26). NF-κB stimulates expression of genes involved in inflammation in many different cell types, including orbital fibroblasts (27, 28). The NFKB1 subunit exerts a protective role by dampening inflammation (29). Therefore, upregulation of NFKB1 may represent a counter regulatory mechanism to control the inflammatory response in orbital fibroblasts from active GO (8, 11).

ECM and fibrosis related proteins that were overexpressed in orbital fibroblasts from active GO included structural maintenance of chromosomes 3 (SMC3), growth factor, augmenter of liver regeneration (GFER) and uridine diphosphate-glucose dehydrogenase (UGDH) (**Figure 1C**). UGDH is involved in the biosynthesis of glycosaminoglycans (GAG), such as hyaluronan, chondroitin sulfate and heparan sulfate and was previously found elevated in urine from patients with active GO (30). Moreover, UGDH was found to be expressed at higher levels in orbital fibroblasts than in fibroblasts from other anatomical regions (31). This indicates that orbital fibroblasts in active GO acquire a phenotype very well equipped for GAG synthesis (32). Orbital fibroblasts from active GO also produced more protein kinase c and casein kinase substrate in neurons (PACSIN) 3, a protein involved in clathrin-mediated endocytosis that regulates glucose uptake by adipocytes (33, 34). The up-regulation of PACSIN3 in the active orbital fibroblasts may therefore relate to formation of adipocytes that finally accumulate in the inactive phase of GO (35).

Orbital Fibroblast Expressed Proteins in Inactive GO Relate to Extracellular Matrix Biology

Orbital fibroblasts from inactive GO overexpressed several proteins linked to ECM biology and fibrotic diseases. This included fibrillin-2 (FBN2), collagen type VI alpha 1 chain (COL6A1) and the neural adhesion molecule 2 (NCAM2) (**Figure 1B**) (36–39). FBN2 is involved in elastic fiber formation and is abundantly present in embryonic tissues, but is also elevated along with elastin in fibrotic tissue, for instance in systemic sclerosis (36, 40). Yet, data on elastin accumulation in orbital tissue from GO patients is lacking so far. The non-fibrillar collagen type VI is involved in structural organization of the ECM, for instance by interacting with a multitude of other key ECM components, including the fibrillary type-1 and type 3 collagens and hyaluronan (39, 41, 42). Increased COL6A1 tissue levels are present in lung fibrosis, liver fibrosis and keloid scarring (37–39). Furthermore, collagen type VI can bind a variety of different growth factors implicated in fibrosis, and as such serves as a reservoir that can regulate growth factor activity in the vicinity of fibroblasts and contribute to fibrosis (39, 42, 43). Although data on collagen type VI in GO orbital tissue is lacking so far, several growth factors that bind collagen type VI, including PDGF-AB, PDGF-

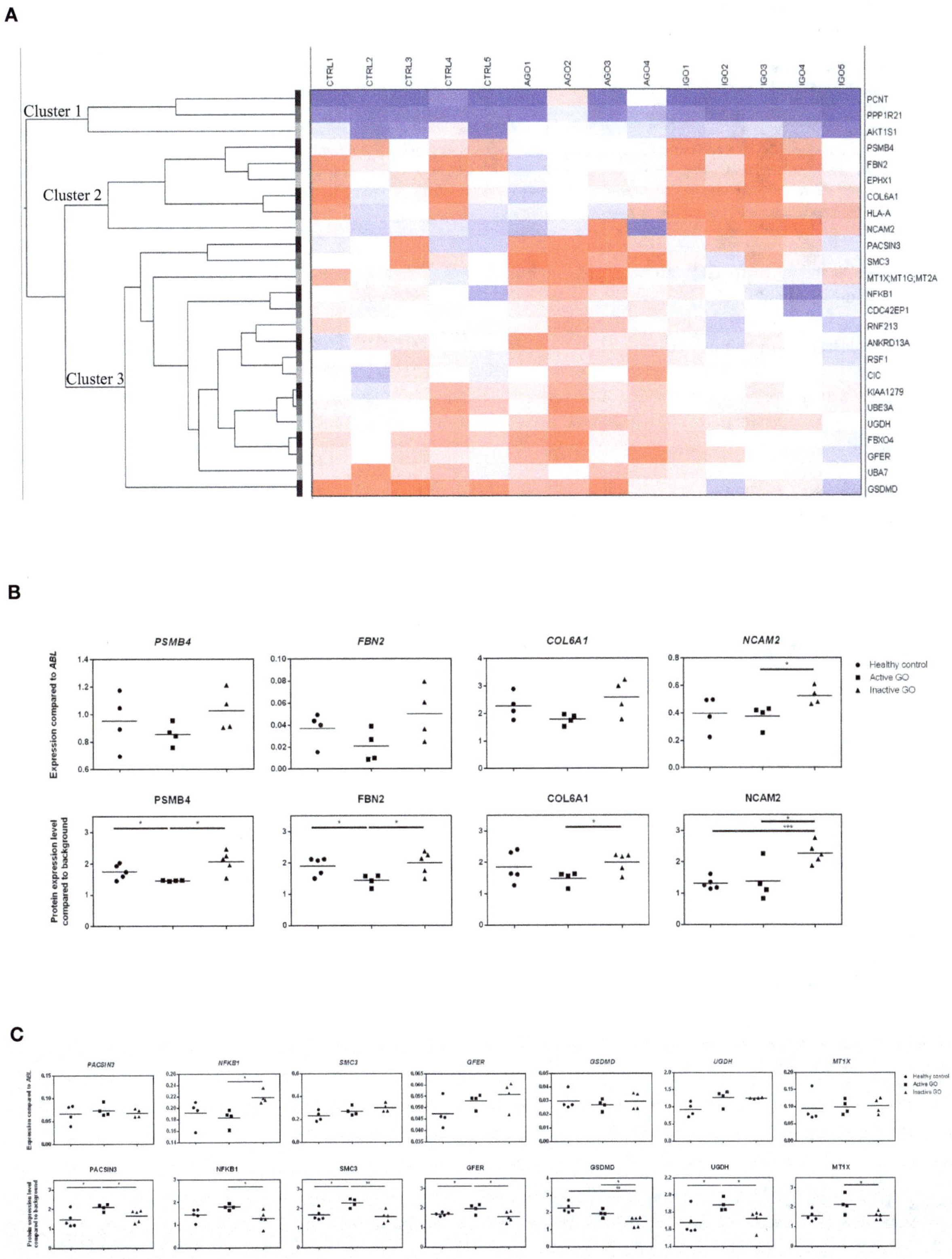

FIGURE 1 | Continued

FIGURE 1 | Proteomic profiles of orbital fibroblasts from inactive GO, active GO and healthy controls. **(A)** Cluster analysis of the differential protein expression between orbital fibroblasts from patients with inactive GO (n = 5), active GO (n = 4) and healthy controls (n = 5). Differentially expressed proteins grouped in three main clusters. Proteins within cluster 1 proteins were expressed at slightly higher level in orbital fibroblasts from active GO compared with orbital fibroblasts from inactive GO and controls. Proteins within cluster 2 displayed higher expression in orbital fibroblasts from inactive GO compared with orbital fibroblasts from active GO and controls. Proteins within cluster 3 were expressed at a higher level in orbital fibroblasts from active GO compared to inactive GO and controls. **(B)** Gene and protein expression level from proteins within cluster 2. Protein expression levels were compared to high abundant protein expression level. Four proteins (PSMB4, FBN2, COL6A1 and NCAM2) up-regulated in inactive GO orbital fibroblasts compared to active GO were related to extracellular matrix biology and further determined by RQ-PCR. * and *** indicate p-value < 0.05 and < 0.001, respectively. Individual symbols represent orbital fibroblast cultures from individual patients. Horizontal bar depicts the median. **(C)** Gene and protein expression level from proteins within cluster 3. Protein expression levels were compared to high abundant protein expression level. Seven proteins (PACSIN3, NFKB1, SMC3, GFER, GSDMD, UGDH and MT1X) down-regulated in inactive GO orbital fibroblasts compared to active GO related to inflammation, hyaluronan and adipogenesis were determined by RQ-PCR. * and ** indicate p-value < 0.05 and < 0.01, respectively. Individual symbols represent orbital fibroblast cultures from individual patients. Horizontal bar depicts the median.

BB, and HGF have been linked to GO pathogenesis (44–46). Neural adhesion molecule 2 (NCAM2) was also higher expressed by orbital fibroblasts from inactive GO. NCAM2 can activate fibroblast growth factor receptor (FGFR), and recent studies demonstrated that FGFR activation in orbital fibroblasts stimulates hyaluronan synthesis and adipogenesis (47–49). Therefore, it can be postulated that in late inactive GO, orbital fibroblast-derived NCAM2 might be involved in adipogenesis and hyaluronan synthesis through FGFR activation. Clearly further detailed study on the role of the molecules we here found to be expressed at higher levels in orbital fibroblasts from inactive GO is required. Yet, our data strongly suggest that in the inactive stage of GO the orbital fibroblasts acquire effector functions that are strongly related to ECM remodeling.

Proteome Pathway, Network and Functional Analysis

The proteins differentially expressed between orbital fibroblasts from active GO and inactive GO were fed into Ingenuity with the aim to link these proteins to networks and pathways of interest to GO pathogenesis. The top two identified canonical pathways were UDP-D-xylose and UDP-D-glucuronate biosynthesis (p-value = 0.00217) and protein ubiquitination pathway (p-value = 0.00305) (**Table 2**). Moreover, all these proteins, except MT1X, were linked to 2 networks (**Figure 2**). The first network is associated with

TABLE 2 | Top 5 canonical pathways and diseases and bio-functions from the differentially expressed proteins.

Top Canonical Pathways

Name	p-value	Overlap
UDP-D-xylose and UDP-D-glucuronate Biosynthesis	0.00217	50.0%
Protein Ubiquitination Pathway	0.00305	1.1%
Crosstalk between Dendritic Cells and Natural Killer Cells	0.00418	2.2%
Altered T Cell and B Cell Signaling in Rheumatoid Arthritis	0.00427	2.2%
OX40 Signaling Pathway	0.00427	2.2%

Top Diseases and Bio Functions
Diseases and Disorders

Name	p-value	#Molecules
Cancer	0.00000287 – 0.049	24
Endocrine System Disorders	0.00000287 – 0.0436	24
Organismal Injury and Abnormalities	0.00000087 – 0.0498	24
Reproductive System Disease	0.0000428 – 0.0436	19
Respiratory Disease	0.0000551 – 0.0394	13

Molecular and Cellular Functions

Name	p-value	Proteins (listing from the lowest p-value)
Cell-To-Cell Signaling and Interaction	0.000469 - 0.0434	HLA-A, NFKB1, UBE3A, CDC42EP1, NCAM2, SMC3
Carbohydrate Metabolism	0.00111 - 0.0445	UGDH, EPHX1, HLA-A, NFKB1
Cell Death and Survival	0.00111 - 0.0487	HLA-A, NFKB1, FBN2, PSMB4, GSDMD, SMC3, COL6A1, GFER, RSF1, AKT1S1, EPHX1, UBA7, UBE3A
Cell Morphology	0.00111 - 0.0434	NFKB1, PCNT, UBE3A, NCAM2, GFER, GSDMD, HLA-A, CDC42EP1
Cellular Assembly and Organization	0.00111 - 0.0424	KIF1BP, ANKRD13A, CDC42EP1, NCAM2, NFKB1, UBE3A, GFER, PCNT, RSF1, FBXO4, HLA-A

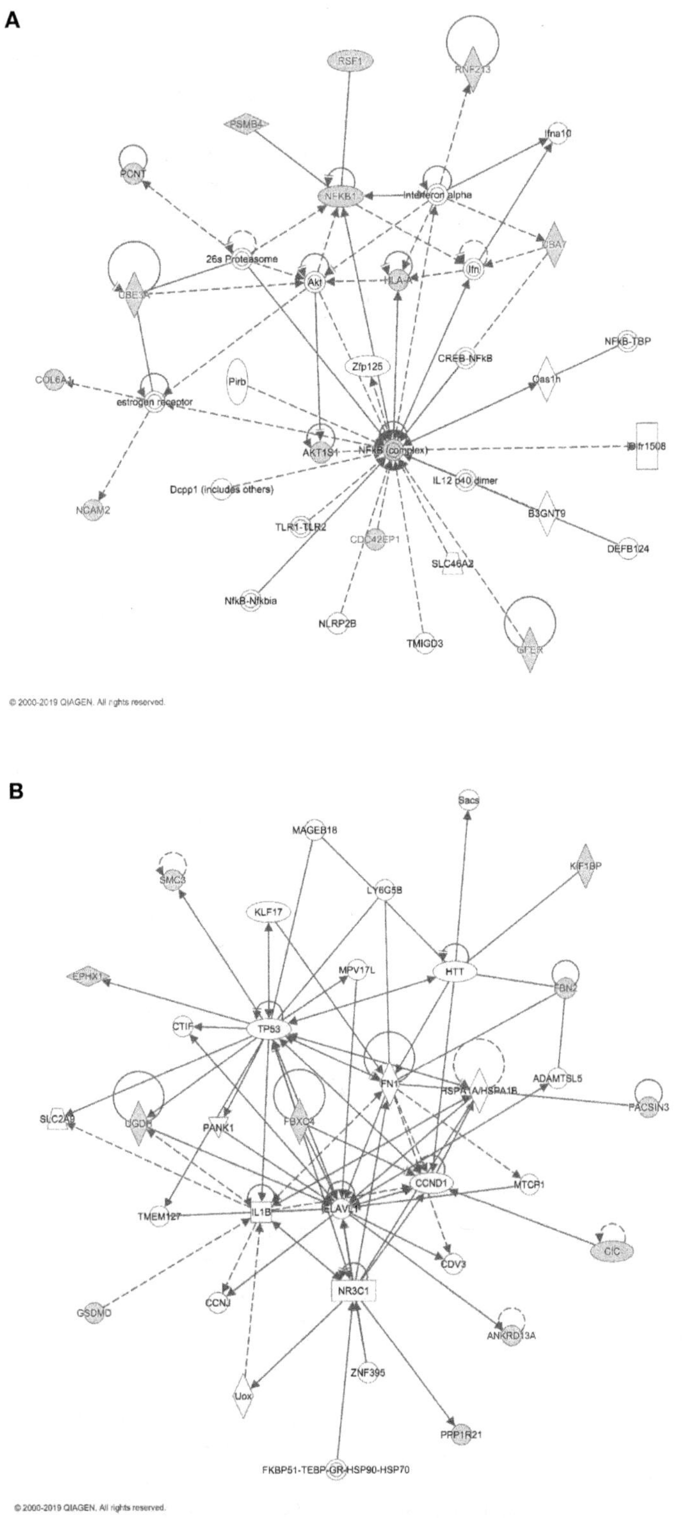

FIGURE 2 | Proteome based network analysis. **(A)** Network 1: linked to cellular development and connective tissue disorders. Differentially expressed proteins are highlighted in grey. The differentially expressed proteins labelled in red were the up-regulated while differentially expressed proteins labelled in blue were down-regulated in inactive GO comparing to active GO orbital fibroblasts. **(B)** Network 2: linked to free radical scavenging, DNA replication, recombination and repair and cellular assembly and organization. Differentially expressed proteins are highlighted in grey. The differentially expressed proteins labelled in red were up-regulated while differentially expressed proteins labelled in blue were down-regulated in inactive GO comparing to active GO orbital fibroblasts.

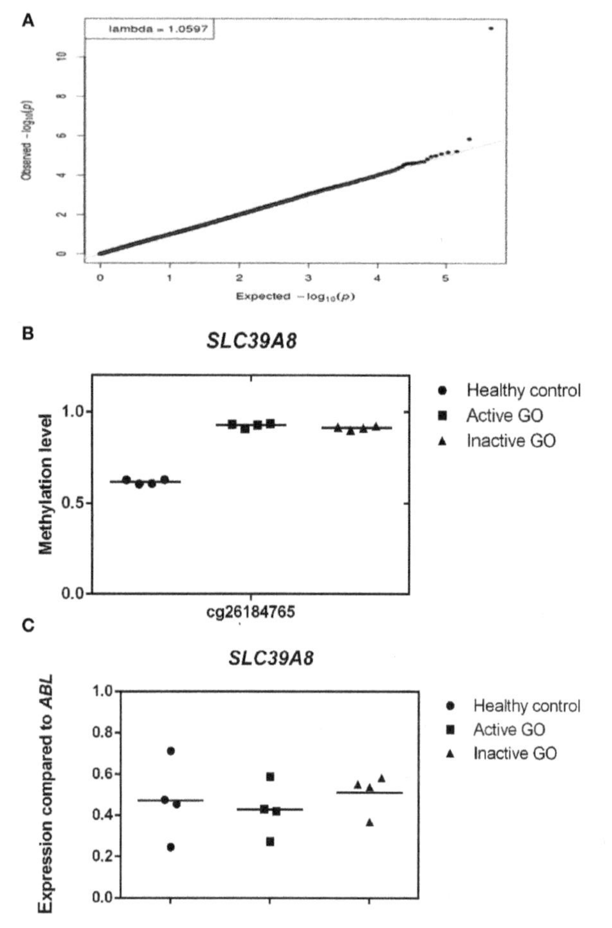

FIGURE 3 | Comparison of orbital fibroblast global DNA methylation profiles with FDR <0.05. **(A)** DNA methylation in active GO orbital fibroblasts (n = 4), inactive GO orbital fibroblasts (n = 4) and healthy control orbital fibroblasts (n = 4) were compared. Global DNA methylation was measured using the Illumina Infinium Human Methylation 450K beadchip on bisulphite-treated DNA and analyzed by GenomeStudio methylation analysis package. Genes with differential DNA methylation were further corrected for multiple testing using FDR < 0.05. **(B)** Methylation level of *SLC39A8*. Methylation level ranges from 0 (unmethylated) to 1 (fully methylated). Individual symbols represent orbital fibroblast cultures from individual patients. Horizontal bar depicts the median. **(C)** *SLC39A8* expression was determined by real-time quantitative (RQ)-PCR and normalized to the control gene *ABL*. Data from mRNA expression was analyzed using ANOVA and subsequently analyzed with the Mann Whitney U test. Individual symbols represent orbital fibroblast cultures from individual patients. Horizontal bar depicts the median.

cellular development and connective tissue disorders (**Figure 2A**), while the second network is linked to free radical scavenging, DNA replication, recombination and repair and cellular assembly and organization (**Figure 2B**). In network 1, the differentially expressed proteins were linked with NF-κB, Akt, 26s proteasome, interferon alpha and estrogen receptor (**Figure 2A**). On the other hand, the differentially expressed proteins in network 2 were linked to several transcriptional regulators, such as cellular tumor antigen p53 (TP53), huntingtin (HTT), cyclin D1 (CCND1), and also other (pathogenic) proteins including fibronectin 1 (FN1) and Hsp70-binding protein 1 (HSPA) (**Figure 2B**).

Global DNA Methylation Profile in Orbital Fibroblasts

After adjustment for multiple testing using false discovery rate (FDR < 0.05), none of the genes were differentially methylated when comparing the orbital fibroblasts isolated from active GO (n = 4) and inactive GO patients (n = 4), although hypermethylated *GNAS* (cg09885502) showed a trend to reach statistical significance (FDR = 0.0774) in inactive GO (**Supplementary Figure 1**). However, GNAS was not found differentially expressed at the protein level with the current technique used (**Supplementary Figure 1**). *SLC39A8* was the only gene that showed statistically significant difference when comparing control orbital fibroblasts (n = 4) with all GO patients (active and inactive GO; n = 8) (FDR = 1.404×10^{-6}) (**Figure 3A**), being hypermethylated in the 3'UTR region in the orbital fibroblasts from GO patients comparing to healthy control (**Figure 3B**). Although this could potentially be associated with decreased *SLC39A8* gene expression on GO orbital fibroblasts, no difference in mRNA expression was detected between the orbital fibroblast from inactive GO, active GO and controls (**Figure 3C**). Neither was SLC39A8 protein detected by our current proteomics approach. Gene expression level of enzymes regulating DNA methylation, the writers, DNA methyltransferases (DNMTs), and the erasers, ten eleven translocation (TET), were further examined; however, the expression level of all *DNMT* and *TET* were not significantly different in orbital fibroblasts from GO and healthy controls (**Supplementary Figure 2**).

Hypermethylated Genes in Orbital Fibroblasts From Active GO Patients

We further analyzed differences in methylation level in a less stringent manner by applying a cut-off difference of more than 2-fold between active and inactive GO patients. This resulted in a total of 142 hits, corresponding to 115 coding genes, that were hypermethylated in the orbital fibroblasts from active GO patients (**Figure 4** and **Supplementary Table 3**). Among the top 10 genes (with the fold differences ranging approximately from 3.1 to 6.9-fold), the highest fold difference was detected by a single probe located in the gene body of *WDR8* (**Supplementary Figure 3** and **Supplementary Table 3**). Several other genes were detected by more than one probe including *Mir548F5, MAB21L1, HTATIP2, TTC12, NIPAL2, TRIM2, PAQR5, OR2L13, RPH3AL, GPR6, MYOM2, DGKQ, ZNF234* and *SPAG1* (**Supplementary Figure 3**).

Hypomethylated Genes in Orbital Fibroblasts From Active GO Patients

Applying the cut-off difference of more than 2-fold between active and inactive GO patients yielded 66 hits, corresponding for 63 genes, that were hypomethylated in the orbital fibroblasts from active GO compared with orbital fibroblasts from inactive GO patients (**Figure 5** and **Supplementary Table 4**). The gene set hypomethylated in active GO orbital fibroblasts comprised a.o.: *RNF168* (with the highest fold change of 5.08-fold, as

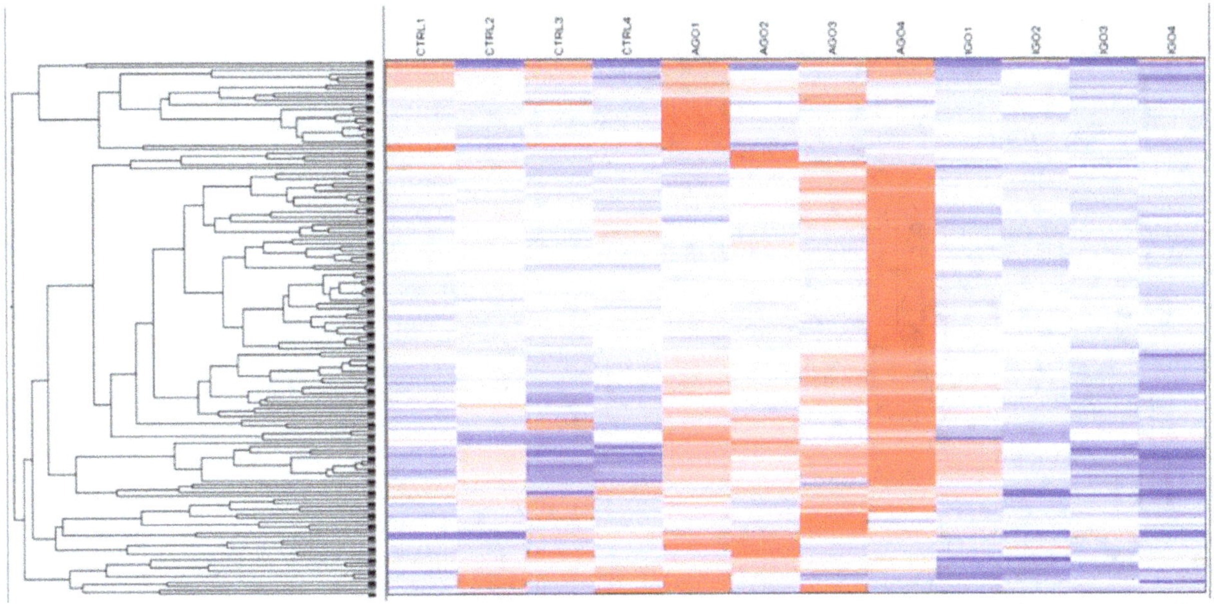

FIGURE 4 | Hypermethylated genes in orbital fibroblasts from active GO in comparison to orbital fibroblasts from inactive GO and healthy controls with a fold difference ≥ 2. DNA methylation in active GO orbital fibroblasts (n = 4) was compared with inactive GO orbital fibroblasts (n = 4). Global DNA methylation was measured using the Illumina Infinium Human Methylation 450K beadchip on bisulphite-treated DNA and analyzed by GenomeStudio methylation analysis package. Hypermethylated genes with differences in DNA methylation level of at least 2-fold in active GO orbital fibroblasts were clustered as shown in the heatmap.

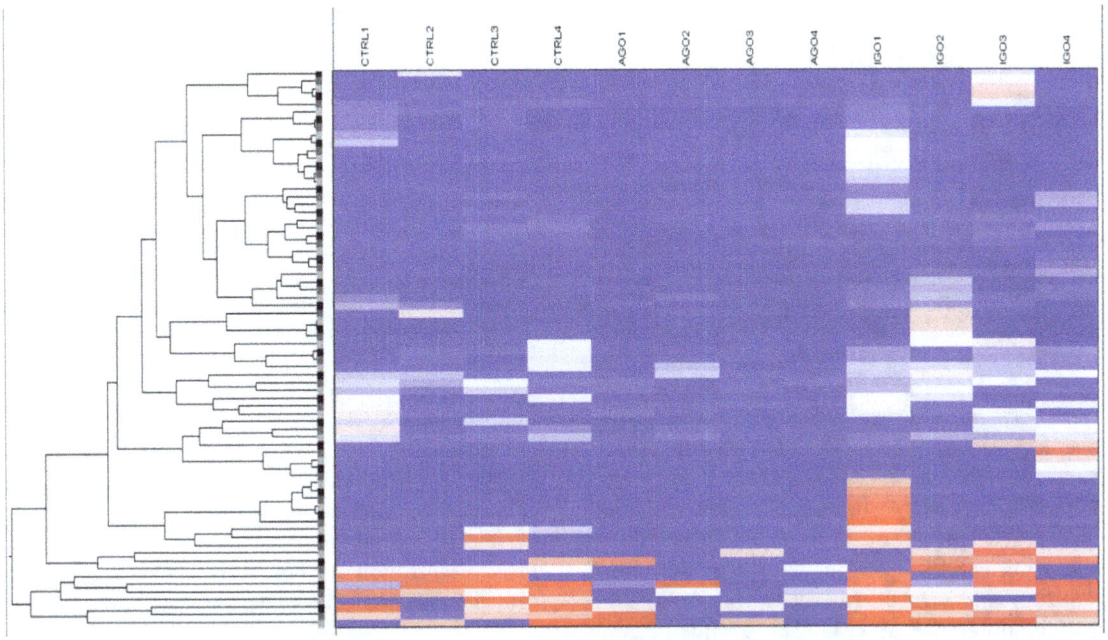

FIGURE 5 | Hypomethylated genes in orbital fibroblasts from active GO in comparison to orbital fibroblasts from inactive GO and healthy controls with a fold difference ≥ 2. DNA methylation in active GO orbital fibroblasts (n = 4) were compared with inactive GO orbital fibroblasts (n = 4). Global DNA methylation was measured using the Illumina Infinium Human Methylation 450K beadchip on bisulphite-treated DNA and analyzed by GenomeStudio methylation analysis package. Hypomethylated genes with differences in DNA methylation level of at least 2-fold in active GO orbital fibroblasts were clustered as shown in the heatmap.

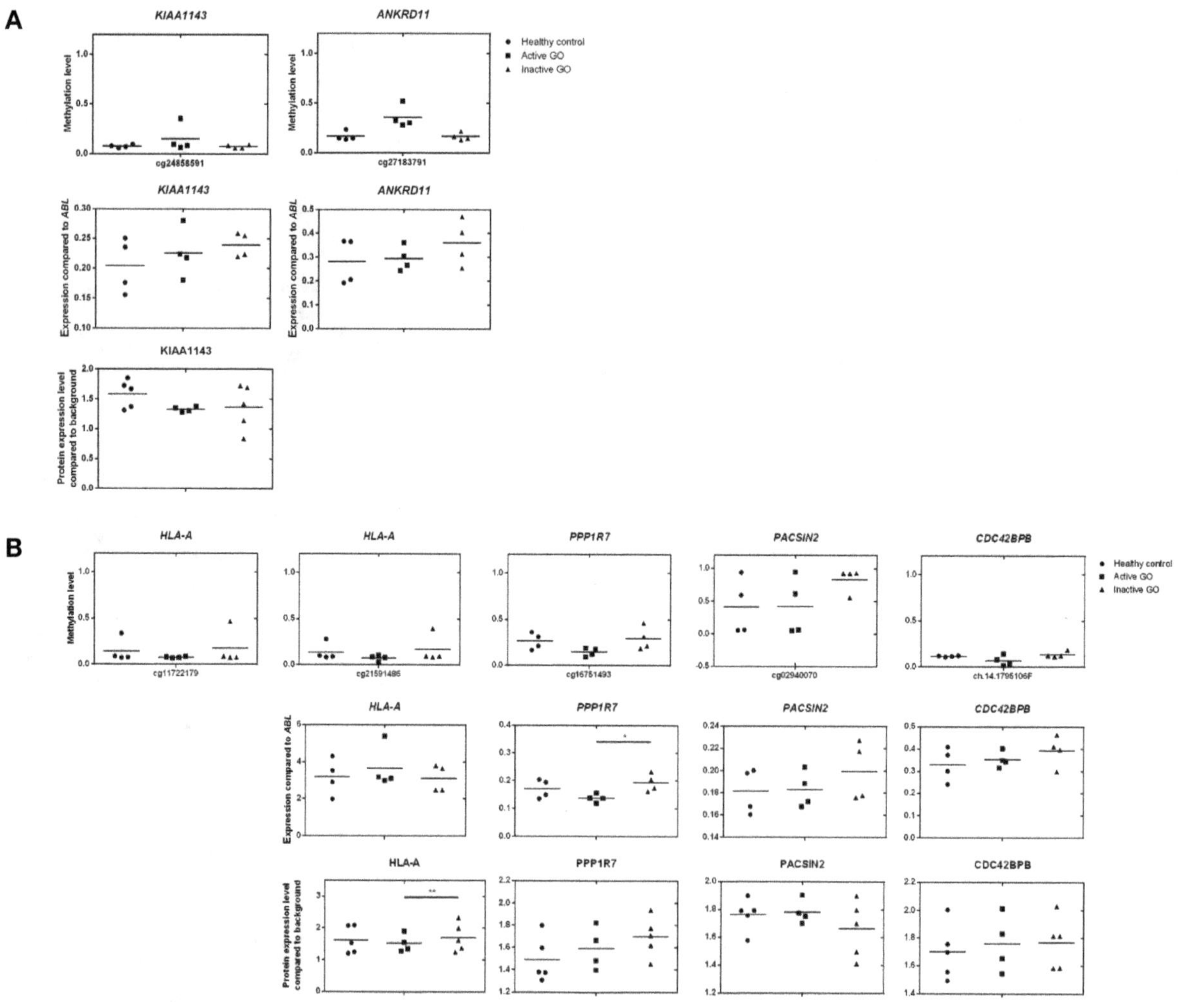

FIGURE 6 | Comparison of DNA methylation, mRNA expression and proteomic data. **(A)** Comparison of hypermethylated genes, mRNA expression and proteomic data. Gene expression was determined by real-time quantitative (RQ)-PCR and normalized to the control gene *ABL*. Data from mRNA expression was analyzed using ANOVA and subsequently analyzed with the Mann Whitney U test. Individual symbols represent orbital fibroblast cultures from individual patients. Horizontal bar depicts the median. **(B)** Comparison of hypomethylated genes, mRNA expression and proteomic data. Gene expression was determined by real-time quantitative (RQ)-PCR and normalized to the control gene *ABL*. Data from mRNA expression was analyzed using ANOVA and subsequently analyzed with the Mann Whitney U test. Individual symbols represent orbital fibroblast cultures from individual patients. Horizontal bar depicts the median.

detected by one probe in the gene body), *SIM2* (detected with 2 different probes located in the gene body: 2.19-fold differences at cg15316660 and 2.03-fold differences at cg23286646 in the gene body), *AIRE* (detected with 2 different probes: 2.35-fold difference at cg27251412 and 2.34-fold difference at cg09510531 200 nucleotides upstream of the transcriptional start site; TSS200) and *HLA-A* (detected with 2 different probes: 2.27-fold difference at cg11722179 and 2.22-fold difference at cg21591486 in the gene body) (**Figure 6B** and **Supplementary Figure 4**).

To investigate the effects of differential methylation at the TSS200 in *AIRE* and gene-body in *HLA-A*, mRNA expression levels were determined by RQ-PCR. *AIRE* gene expression was not detectable by RQ-PCR in any of the orbital fibroblasts (data not shown), while *HLA-A* was not differentially expressed at the mRNA level between fibroblasts from active GO and inactive GO (**Figure 6B**). AIRE protein expression was not detected by the current proteomics approach (data not shown), while HLA-A protein expression was significantly down-regulated in active GO orbital fibroblasts (**Figure 6B**).

Integrative Analysis of Proteomics and Gene Methylation in Orbital Fibroblasts From Active GO Patients

Upon integration of the DNA hypermethylation data with the proteome data, *KIAA* and the *ANKRD* gene family emerged from

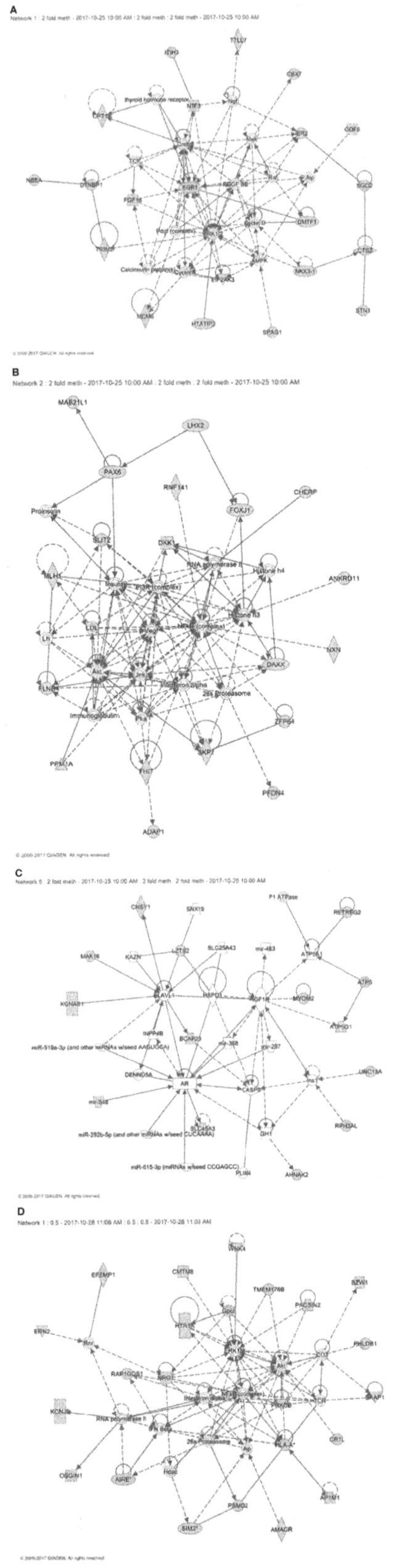

FIGURE 7 | Continued

FIGURE 7 | Methylation based network analysis. **(A)** Network 1 derived from hypermethylated genes in orbital fibroblasts from active GO: linked to neurological disease, organismal injury and abnormalities, and nervous system development and function Network analysis was further performed on these differentially hypermethylated genes (highlighted in grey) using Ingenuity (Qiagen) filtering only for those networks and pathways that are based on experimentally obtained information. **(B)** Network 2 derived from hypermethylated genes in orbital fibroblasts from active GO: linked to embryogenic development, nervous system development and function, and organ development. Network analysis was further performed on these differentially hypermethylated genes (highlighted in grey) using Ingenuity (Qiagen) filtering only for those networks and pathways that are based on experimentally obtained information. **(C)** Network 3 derived from hypermethylated genes in orbital fibroblasts from active GO: linked to cardiovascular system development and function, organismal development, and cellular assembly and organization. Network analysis was further performed on these differentially hypermethylated genes (highlighted in grey) using Ingenuity (Qiagen) filtering only for those networks and pathways that are based on experimentally obtained information. **(D)** Network 4 derived from hypomethylated genes in orbital fibroblasts from active GO: linked to cellular growth and proliferation, nervous system development and function, and cell-to-cell signaling and interaction. Network analysis was further performed on these differentially hypomethylated genes (highlighted in grey) using Ingenuity (Qiagen) filtering only for those networks and pathways that are based on experimentally obtained information.

both types of analyses and were therefore further examined by RQ-PCR. Although hypermethylation of *KIAA1143* and *ANKRD11* genes was more than 2-fold, neither *KIAA1143* nor *ANKRD11* mRNA expression reached statistically significant difference in expression when comparing active and inactive GO orbital fibroblasts (**Figure 6A**). In addition, ANKRD11 protein was not detected by the current proteomics approach (data not shown). Neither the difference on gene expression data and proteome data reached statistical significance nor corresponded to the DNA methylation data.

Integration of the DNA hypermethylation data with the proteome data revealed overlap for PPP1R, PACSIN, and the CDC42 family, which were subsequently further validated by RQ-PCR. Although trends towards elevated mRNA expression for *PACSIN2* and *CDC42BPB* were observed in inactive GO, no statistical significance existed among orbital fibroblast groups, while *PPP1R7* mRNA expression was significantly ($p < 0.05$) higher in inactive GO orbital fibroblasts than in active GO orbital fibroblasts ($P < 0.05$) (**Figure 6B**). However, neither the mRNA expression data nor the proteome data corresponded to the DNA methylation data.

Network Analysis From Methylated Genes in Orbital Fibroblasts From GO Patients

Next, all the genes that displayed differential DNA methylation between orbital fibroblasts from active GO and inactive GO were fed into Ingenuity pathway analysis to identify potential critical molecular networks involved in GO pathogenesis. The top network with the highest score obtained for hypermethylated genes in active GO orbital fibroblasts genes included TSHR signaling, PDGF-BB signaling and the ERK1/2 signal transduction pathway, as depicted in network 1 (**Figure 7A**). Ingenuity linked this network mainly to neurological disease, organismal injury and abnormalities, and nervous system development and function. *EGR1*, one of the top 10 genes with the highest fold methylation difference, was also found in this network. The second network with the second highest score (designated as network 2) contained genes that were associated with the PI3K, NF-κB, JNK and Akt signaling pathways (**Figure 7B**). Ingenuity linked this network mainly to embryogenic development, nervous system development and function, and organ development. Clearly, these signaling cascades exert several important roles in immune activation as well as fibrosis (27, 44, 50, 51). In addition, *Mir548F5* was found in another network (network 3) together with *MYOM2* and *RPH3AL* and were connected to IGF-1R, androgen receptor and various non-coding RNAs (**Figure 7C**). Ingenuity linked this network mainly to cardiovascular system development and function, organismal development, and cellular assembly and organization. Moreover, *LZTS2* and *MYOM2* found in this network are among the top 10 genes with the highest fold difference in methylation status (**Figure 7C**).

For hypomethylated genes in active GO orbital fibroblasts, 6 of the top 10 genes with the highest fold difference were found in network 4, including *ERN2, CMTM8, BZW1, PRKCB, PSMD2* and *AP1M1* (**Figure 7D**). Of the genes that were found hypomethylated in orbital fibroblasts from active GO, *AIRE* and *SIM2* linked to network (network 4) that also contained NF-κB, ERK1/2 and Akt signaling pathways (**Figure 7D**). *HLA-A* and *PSMD2* (proteasome 26S subunit, non-ATPase 2), that are associated with peptide degradation, antigen presentation and TCR signaling processes, also linked to network 4 (**Figure 7D**). Ingenuity associated network 4 mainly with cellular growth and proliferation, nervous system development and function, and cell-to-cell signaling and interaction.

Pathway and Functional Analysis From Methylated Genes in the Orbital Fibroblasts From GO Patients

The top 5 canonical pathways obtained from genes hypermethylated in orbital fibroblasts from active GO are shown in **Table 3**, while for genes hypomethylated in orbital fibroblasts form active GO the top 5 canonical pathways are given in **Table 4**. When all the functions from genes hypermethylated and hypomethylated in active GO (**Tables 3** and **4**) were integrated, overlapping bio-functions and diseases became apparent. The top disease/disorder identified to be shared between the hypo- and hypermethylated genes was organismal injury and abnormalities, containing ninety-seven hypermethylated genes (p-value = $1x10^{-6}$ – 0.0145) and sixty-two hypomethylated genes (p-value = $9.88x10^{-5}$ – 0.0498). For the molecular and cellular functions, cellular development and cellular growth and proliferation were among the top molecular and cellular functions that were shared between the hypo- and hypermethylated genes. Cellular development linked to 28 hypermethylated genes (p-value = $7.02x10^{-5}$ – 0.0145) (**Table 3**) and nineteen hypomethylated genes (p-value = 0.00132 – 0.0469) (**Table 4**), while cellular growth and proliferation linked to twenty-five hypermethylated genes (p-value = $7.02x10^{-5}$ – 0.0145) (**Table 3**) and seventeen hypomethylated genes (p-value = $1.32x10^{-4}$ – 0.0498) (**Table 4**).

TABLE 3 | Top 5 canonical pathways and diseases and bio-functions from the hypermethylated genes with the cut-off at more than 2-fold difference in the active GO orbital fibroblasts.

Top Canonical Pathways

Name	p-value	Overlap
Tyrosine Biosynthesis IV	0.0145	33.3%
Phenylalanine Degradation I (Aerobic)	0.0193	25.0%
Chondroitin and Dermatan Biosynthesis	0.0289	16.7%
Glutamate Receptor Signaling	0.0315	3.5%
NAD Biosynthesis from 2-amino-3-carboxymuconate Semialdehyde	0.0336	14.3%

Top Diseases and Bio Functions
Diseases and Disorders

Name	p-value	#Molecules
Cancer	$1x10^{-6}$ – 0.0145	95
Gastrointestinal Disease	$1x10^{-6}$ – 0.0145	90
Organismal Injury and Abnormalities	$1x10^{-6}$ – 0.0145	97
Developmental Disorder	$2.22x10^{-5}$ – 0.0145	26
Ophthalmic Disease	$2.22x10^{-5}$ – 0.0145	9

Molecular and Cellular Functions

Name	p-value	#Molecules
Gene Expression	$7.0x10^{-5}$ – 0.00209	30
Cellular Development	$7.0x10^{-5}$ – 0.0145	28
Cellular Growth and Proliferation	$7.0x10^{-5}$ – 0.0145	25
Cell Cycle	$4.85x10^{-4}$ – 0.0145	18
Cell Morphology	$4.85x10^{-4}$ – 0.0145	14

TABLE 4 | Top 5 canonical pathways and diseases and bio-functions from the hypomethylated genes with the cut-off at more than 2-fold difference in the active GO orbital fibroblasts.

Top Canonical Pathways

Name	p-value	Overlap
Lipoate Salvage and Modification	0.003	100.0%
Lipoate Biosynthesis and Incorporation II	0.00598	50.0%
Dopamine-DARPP32 Feedback in cAMP Signaling	0.0132	1.8%
Nur77 Signaling in T Lymphocytes	0.0136	3.4%
Wnt/Ca^{2+} pathway	0.0154	3.2%

Top Diseases and Bio Functions
Diseases and Disorders

Name	p-value	#Molecules
Cancer	$9.88x10^{-5}$ – 0.0498	61
Organismal Injury and Abnormalities	$9.88x10^{-5}$ – 0.0498	62
Dermatological Diseases and Conditions	$4.73x10^{-4}$ – 0.0496	43
Gastrointestinal Disease	0.00106 – 0.044	55
Metabolic Disease	0.00172 – 0.0498	8

Molecular and Cellular Functions

Name	p-value	#Molecules
Cellular Growth and Proliferation	$1.32x10^{-4}$ – 0.0498	17
Cellular Movement	0.00117 – 0.0498	12
Cell-To-Cell Signaling and Interaction	0.00132 – 0.0498	13
Cellular Development	0.00132 – 0.0469	19
Drug Metabolism	0.00132 – 0.0452	4

DISCUSSION

Disease activity and characteristics of GO alter with disease progression. Early active GO is characterized by active inflammation that progresses into a late inactive phase without apparent inflammation but characterized by extensive orbital tissue remodeling (increased adipose tissue formation, excessive hyaluronan deposition and fibrosis). Orbital fibroblasts represent the main effector cells in GO and contribute to both the early active and late inactive phases of disease (8). Here, we performed extensive proteomics and global DNA methylation analysis of orbital fibroblasts from active and inactive GO as well as control individuals. Our data clearly demonstrate distinctive proteome and DNA methylation profiles between orbital fibroblasts from patients with active and inactive GO. These profiles can be linked to pathologically relevant molecular networks specifically associated with active/inactive disease stage, including inflammation, cellular development, growth, proliferation and tissue remodeling. Therefore, this data clearly illustrates that with GO disease progression orbital fibroblasts exhibit specific characteristics linked to disease stage specific pathology, and that epigenetic regulation is involved in controlling this.

Orbital fibroblasts from active GO displayed overexpression of proteins typically involved in inflammation, cellular proliferation, hyaluronan synthesis and adipogenesis (**Figure 1C**). In contrast, various proteins linked to ECM biology and fibrotic disease were overexpressed in orbital fibroblasts from inactive GO (**Figure 1B**). These findings corroborated with the different types of networks identified, which included cellular development and connective tissue disorders, DNA replication, recombination and repair and cellular assembly and organization (**Figure 2**). Although our current protein findings fit the pathophysiological model of GO, further studies to unravel the exact function of these proteins in orbital fibroblasts as well as their contribution to the different stages of GO are required.

To our knowledge, our study is the first that explored DNA methylation in orbital fibroblasts from GO patients. Comparison of DNA methylation with stringent analysis using FDR between healthy controls and all the GO orbital fibroblasts included in our study resulted in a significant difference in methylation only for *SLC39A8* (hypermethylation in 3'UTR region in case of the GO orbital fibroblasts; **Figure 3**). SLC39A8 is a member of the major zinc transporter SLC39 (ZIP) family, and cellular zinc import by SLC39A8 is crucial in the control of immune activation and function (52, 53). SLC39A8 methylation status did not correlate with mRNA expression, while SLC39A8 protein was not detected at all. However, the SLC93A8 hypermethylation in GO orbital fibroblasts located to the 3'UTR region, a region in which hypermethylation does not necessarily relate to transcriptional repression as commonly reported in promoter regions (54–56). We can, however, not exclude that SLC39A8 expression is also controlled by other regulatory mechanism such as small non-coding RNAs. SLC39A8 is also thought to be the primary transporter of the toxic cation cadmium, which is found in cigarette smoke. In this study we did not detect SLC93A8 protein, which might be related to the sensitivity of the technique we applied. Yet, we propose that additional studies to understand the role of the SLC39A8 and other SLC39 family of solute carriers in the pathogenesis of GO are potentially of great interest considering that smoking is a major environmental risk factor for GO (57).

Additional analysis of global DNA methylation using a 2-fold difference cut-off was conducted with the intend to lower the stringency from FDR analysis. A drawback of this approach is however that individual outliers have a relatively large effect on the final outcome, which either may mask potential important

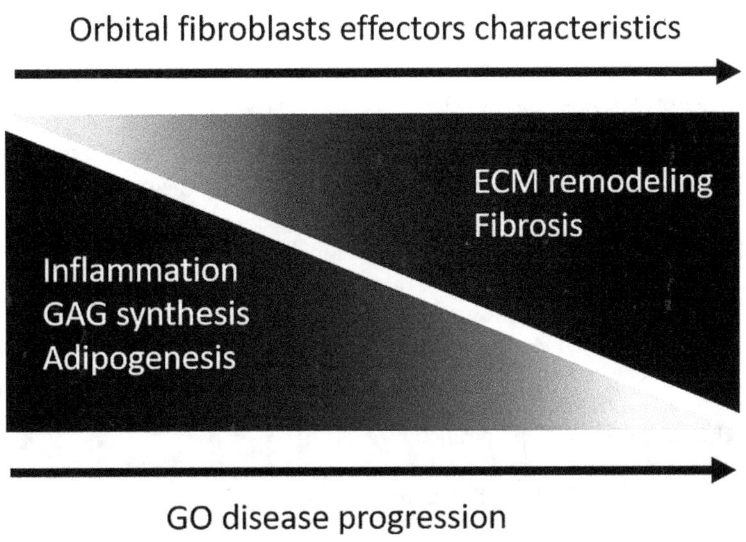

FIGURE 8 | Model depicting orbital fibroblast effector characteristics upon GO disease progression. During active disease orbital fibroblasts are skewed towards a functional phenotype involved in in inflammation, glycosaminoglycan synthesis and adipogenesis. With disease progression the orbital fibroblasts undergo a switch from this "inflammatory/pro-adipogenic primed" effector cell towards a "remodelling/pro-fibrotic" type of effector cell.

differences in methylation or identify false positive methylation differences, especially with the small groups (n = 4 per group) used in this study. Nonetheless, the overall DNA methylation patterns we observed suggest that orbital fibroblasts from inactive GO are more comparable to control orbital fibroblasts than to orbital fibroblasts from active GO (**Figures 4** and **5**). The global DNA methylation patterns and associated networks we found corroborate with the networks generated from the proteomics analysis, including NF-κB, Akt and IFNα (**Figures 2** and **7**), as well as previous reports that linked these pathways to GO pathogenesis (58–60). Other genes hypermethylated in inactive GO orbital fibroblasts also linked to other pathogenic pathways previously reported in GO, including PDGF (44), thyroid hormone receptor (61), NGF (62), AMPK (63) and ERK1/2 signaling pathways (64, 65) (**Figure 7**). In orbital fibroblasts from active GO hypermethylated genes clearly linked to inflammation, while hypomethylated genes linked to adipogenesis and autoimmune-related genes. This is in line with the association to inflammation and adipogenesis that we observed for the proteome of active GO orbital fibroblasts.

Genes hypomethylated in active GO orbital fibroblasts included *AIRE* and *HLA-A* (**Figure 6B** and **Supplementary Figure 4**). *AIRE* controls tissue specific antigen expression by medullary thymic epithelial cells to control thymic T-cell selection, and AIRE deficiency is associated with autoimmune disease (66, 67). CpG methylation in the promoter of the *AIRE* gene has previously been reported to control its tissue-specific expression pattern (68). Although hypomethylation of *AIRE* promoter was found in orbital fibroblasts from active GO (**Supplementary Figure 4**), *AIRE* expression was undetectable at mRNA and protein level (data not shown). Several studies showed *AIRE* expression in fibrocytes that typically infiltrate the orbital tissue form GO patients (69, 70). Potentially, fibrocyte numbers in our heterogeneous orbital fibroblast populations were low, which did however still allow detection of differences in *AIRE* methylation but not in AIRE mRNA or protein. *HLA-A* hypomethylation was detected in the gene body in orbital fibroblasts from active GO (**Figure 6B**). While *HLA-A* mRNA expression level did not differ between active and inactive GO, HLA-A protein expression was significantly down-regulated in active GO orbital fibroblasts (**Figure 6B**). Decreased HLA-A protein expression as observed in the orbital fibroblasts from active GO might regulate antigen presentation by these cells.

Fibroblasts isolated from fibrotic tissue display phenotypes that remain stable in *in vitro* culture for prolonged periods of time (71, 72). This allows investigation of epigenetic alterations and regulation, including histone modification, DNA methylation and non-coding RNA (71, 73). In general, we observed a poor correlation between protein expression, DNA methylation and mRNA expression. Poor correlations between DNA promotor methylation level and gene expression, as well as both positive and negative correlations between DNA gene body methylation and gene expression, have been reported (74–76). Our study thus clearly indicates that the proteome alterations we observed in orbital fibroblasts in relation to the specific GO disease stage are controlled by regulatory layers additional to DNA methylation (e.g. histone modifications and small regulatory RNA molecules) that remain so-far hardly studied in GO. For example, several microRNAs, including miR-322, miR-508-3p, miR-9 and miR-16 have been described to target *NFKB1* mRNA (77–80). miR-16 was previously found to be upregulated in orbital tissue from inactive GO patients and might thus be involved in downregulating NFKB1 and resolving inflammation that occurs during this disease stage (81). Altogether, the current data support the role of NF-κB signaling in regulating inflammation in GO orbital fibroblasts. Moreover, the data point towards existence of a complex epigenetic regulation machinery that controls NFKB1 expression and activity with GO disease progression.

There are several limitations associated with our study. First, the sample size is small, and it cannot be excluded that the extended orbital fibroblast isolation protocol and culture procedure altered the *in vivo* phenotypic/effector cell character of the orbital fibroblasts, although long term (epigenetic)stability of fibroblasts in culture is previously described (71, 72). Second, orbital fibroblasts are heterogeneous (8). Therefore, use of purified fibroblast subpopulations on the basis of cell surface marker expression, for instance Thy-1, CD34 and TSHR, could generate more in-depth insight into epigenetic regulation and fibroblast-subtype specific proteomes in GO. Despite these limitations, our proteomic and DNA methylation analysis identified known as well as novel molecules and molecular networks in relation to the pathogenesis of GO. In addition, both the proteomics and DNA methylation support that, with GO disease progression, orbital fibroblasts undergo a switch from an "inflammatory/pro-adipogenic primed" effector cell to a "remodeling/pro-fibrotic" type of effector cell, as depicted in **Figure 8**. We propose that detailed molecular understanding of this "inflammatory/pro-angiogenic-to-remodeling/pro-fibrotic switch" should be an active field of future research as it can contribute to improvement of treatment protocols.

AUTHOR CONTRIBUTIONS

SV designed research, performed research, analyzed and interpreted data, wrote the paper. PS performed research, analyzed data, wrote the paper. TPi designed research, analyzed data, contributed analytic tools, prepared manuscript. PS analyzed data, contributed analytic tools. DP contributed patient materials. VD, PH, NH, and TPa analyzed data, prepared manuscript. WD designed research, analyzed and interpreted data, prepared manuscript. All authors contributed to the article and approved the submitted version.

SUPPLEMENTARY MATERIAL

Supplementary Figure 1 | Comparison of GNAS DNA methylation and protein expression data.

Supplementary Figure 2 | Expression of *DNMT* and *TET* genes were determined by real-time quantitative (RQ)-PCR and normalized to the control gene *ABL*. Individual symbols represent orbital fibroblast cultures from individual patients. Horizontal bar depicts the median.

Supplementary Figure 3 | Methylation level of hypermethylated genes in orbital fibroblasts from active GO. Methylation level ranges from 0 (unmethylated) to 1 (fully methylated). Genes that were detected with the highest fold difference between active and inactive GO orbital fibroblasts, *WDR8*, and genes that were detected by more than one probe, *Mir548F5* and *MAB21L1*, are shown in this figure. Individual symbols represent orbital fibroblast cultures from individual patients. Horizontal bar depicts the median.

Supplementary Figure 4 | Methylation level of hypomethylated genes in orbital fibroblasts from active GO. Methylation level ranges from 0 (unmethylated) to 1 (fully methylated). Genes that were detected with the highest fold difference between active and inactive GO orbital fibroblasts, *RNF168*, and genes that were detected by more than one probe, *AIRE* and *SIM2*, are shown in this figure. Individual symbols represent orbital fibroblast cultures from individual patients. Horizontal bar depicts the median.

REFERENCES

1. Kendall RT, Feghali-Bostwick CA. Fibroblasts in fibrosis: novel roles and mediators. *Front Pharmacol* (2014) 5:123.
2. Reilkoff RA, Bucala R, Herzog EL. Fibrocytes: emerging effector cells in chronic inflammation. *Nat Rev Immunol* (2011) 11(6):427–35.
3. Kis K, Liu X, Hagood JS. Myofibroblast differentiation and survival in fibrotic disease. *Expert Rev Mol Med* (2011) 13:e27.
4. Korfei M, Skwarna S, Henneke I, MacKenzie B, Klymenko O, Saito S, et al. Aberrant expression and activity of histone deacetylases in sporadic idiopathic pulmonary fibrosis. *Thorax* (2015) 70(11):1022–32.
5. Wynn TA, Ramalingam TR. Mechanisms of fibrosis: therapeutic translation for fibrotic disease. *Nat Med* (2012) 18(7):1028–40.
6. Darby IA, Zakuan N, Billet F, Desmouliere A. The myofibroblast, a key cell in normal and pathological tissue repair. *Cell Mol Life Sci* (2016) 73 (6):1145–57.
7. Bahn RS. Graves' ophthalmopathy. *N Engl J Med* (2010) 362(8):726–38.
8. Dik WA, Virakul S, van Steensel L. Current perspectives on the role of orbital fibroblasts in the pathogenesis of Graves' ophthalmopathy. *Exp Eye Res* (2016) 142:83–91.
9. Matheis N, Lantz M, Grus FH, Ponto KA, Wolters D, Brorson H, et al. Proteomics of Orbital Tissue in Thyroid-Associated Orbitopathy. *J Clin Endocrinol Metab* (2015) 100(12):E1523–30.
10. Cheng KC, Huang HH, Hung CT, Chen CC, Wu WC, Suen JL, et al. Proteomic analysis of the differences in orbital protein expression in thyroid orbitopathy. *Graefes Arch Clin Exp Ophthalmol* (2013) 251(12):2777–87.
11. Hwang CJ, Afifiyan N, Sand D, Naik V, Said J, Pollock SJ, et al. Orbital fibroblasts from patients with thyroid-associated ophthalmopathy overexpress CD40: CD154 hyperinduces IL-6, IL-8, and MCP-1. *Invest Ophthalmol Vis Sci* (2009) 50(5):2262–8.
12. Pritchard J, Han R, Horst N, Cruikshank WW, Smith TJ. Immunoglobulin activation of T cell chemoattractant expression in fibroblasts from patients with Graves' disease is mediated through the insulin-like growth factor I receptor pathway. *J Immunol* (2003) 170(12):6348–54.
13. Khoo TK, Coenen MJ, Schiefer AR, Kumar S, Bahn RS. Evidence for enhanced Thy-1 (CD90) expression in orbital fibroblasts of patients with Graves' ophthalmopathy. *Thyroid* (2008) 18(12):1291–6.
14. Tang F, Chen X, Mao Y, Wan S, Ai S, Yang H, et al. Orbital fibroblasts of Graves' orbitopathy stimulated with proinflammatory cytokines promote B cell survival by secreting BAFF. *Mol Cell Endocrinol* (2017) 446:1–11.
15. Virakul S, Heutz JW, Dalm VA, Peeters RP, Paridaens D, van den Bosch WA, et al. Basic FGF and PDGF-BB synergistically stimulate hyaluronan and IL-6 production by orbital fibroblasts. *Mol Cell Endocrinol* (2016) 433:94–104.
16. Lee WM, Paik JS, Cho WK, Oh EH, Lee SB, Yang SW. Rapamycin enhances TNF-alpha-induced secretion of IL-6 and IL-8 through suppressing PDCD4 degradation in orbital fibroblasts. *Curr Eye Res* (2013) 38(6):699–706.
17. Mimura LY, Villares SM, Monteiro ML, Guazzelli IC, Bloise W. Peroxisome proliferator-activated receptor-gamma gene expression in orbital adipose/connective tissues is increased during the active stage of Graves' ophthalmopathy. *Thyroid* (2003) 13(9):845–50.
18. Wakelkamp IM, Bakker O, Baldeschi L, Wiersinga WM, Prummel MF. TSH-R expression and cytokine profile in orbital tissue of active vs. inactive Graves' ophthalmopathy patients. *Clin Endocrinol (Oxf)* (2003) 58(3):280–7.
19. Altorok N, Tsou PS, Coit P, Khanna D, Sawalha AH. Genome-wide DNA methylation analysis in dermal fibroblasts from patients with diffuse and limited systemic sclerosis reveals common and subset-specific DNA methylation aberrancies. *Ann Rheum Dis* (2015) 74(8):1612–20.
20. Huang SK, Scruggs AM, McEachin RC, White ES, Peters-Golden M. Lung fibroblasts from patients with idiopathic pulmonary fibrosis exhibit genome-wide differences in DNA methylation compared to fibroblasts from nonfibrotic lung. *PloS One* (2014) 9(9):e107055.
21. Hemmatazad H, Rodrigues HM, Maurer B, Brentano F, Pileckyte M, Distler JH, et al. Histone deacetylase 7, a potential target for the antifibrotic treatment of systemic sclerosis. *Arthritis Rheum* (2009) 60(5):1519–29.
22. Bagnato G, Roberts WN, Roman J, Gangemi S. A systematic review of overlapping microRNA patterns in systemic sclerosis and idiopathic pulmonary fibrosis. *Eur Respir Rev* (2017) 26(144).
23. Khong JJ, Wang LY, Smyth GK, McNab AA, Hardy TG, Selva D, et al. Differential Gene Expression Profiling of Orbital Adipose Tissue in Thyroid Orbitopathy. *Invest Ophthalmol Vis Sci* (2015) 56(11):6438–47.
24. Bartalena L, Baldeschi L, Dickinson AJ, Eckstein A, Kendall-Taylor P, Marcocci C, et al. Consensus statement of the European group on Graves' orbitopathy (EUGOGO) on management of Graves' orbitopathy. *Thyroid* (2008) 18(3):333–46.
25. van Steensel L, Paridaens D, Schrijver B, Dingjan GM, van Daele PL, van Hagen PM, et al. Imatinib mesylate and AMN107 inhibit PDGF-signaling in orbital fibroblasts: a potential treatment for Graves' ophthalmopathy. *Invest Ophthalmol Vis Sci* (2009) 50(7):3091–8.
26. Concetti J, Wilson CL. NFKB1 and Cancer: Friend or Foe? *Cells* (2018) 7(9).
27. Mussbacher M, Salzmann M, Brostjan C, Hoesel B, Schoergenhofer C, Datler H, et al. Cell Type-Specific Roles of NF-kappaB Linking Inflammation and Thrombosis. *Front Immunol* (2019) 10:85.
28. van Steensel L, Paridaens D, Dingjan GM, van Daele PL, van Hagen PM, Kuijpers RW, et al. Platelet-derived growth factor-BB: a stimulus for cytokine production by orbital fibroblasts in Graves' ophthalmopathy. *Invest Ophthalmol Vis Sci* (2010) 51(2):1002–7.
29. Oakley F, Mann J, Nailard S, Smart DE, Mungalsingh N, Constandinou C, et al. Nuclear factor-kappaB1 (p50) limits the inflammatory and fibrogenic responses to chronic injury. *Am J Pathol* (2005) 166(3):695–708.
30. Kahaly G, Forster G, Hansen C. Glycosaminoglycans in thyroid eye disease. *Thyroid* (1998) 8(5):429–32.
31. Smith TJ, Tsai CC, Shih MJ, Tsui S, Chen B, Han R, et al. Unique attributes of orbital fibroblasts and global alterations in IGF-1 receptor signaling could explain thyroid-associated ophthalmopathy. *Thyroid* (2008) 18(9):983–8.
32. Vigetti D, Viola M, Karousou E, De Luca G, Passi A. Metabolic control of hyaluronan synthases. *Matrix Biol* (2014) 35:8–13.
33. Roach W, Plomann M. PACSIN3 overexpression increases adipocyte glucose transport through GLUT1. *Biochem Biophys Res Commun* (2007) 355(3):745–50.
34. Aoh QL, Graves LM, Duncan MC. Glucose regulates clathrin adaptors at the trans-Golgi network and endosomes. *Mol Biol Cell* (2011) 22(19):3671–83.
35. Meyer zu Horste M, Stroher E, Berchner-Pfannschmidt U, Schmitz-Spanke S, Pink M, Gothert JR, et al. A novel mechanism involved in the pathogenesis of Graves ophthalmopathy (GO): clathrin is a possible targeting molecule for inhibiting local immune response in the orbit. *J Clin Endocrinol Metab* (2011) 96(11):E1727–36.
36. Brinckmann J, Hunzelmann N, Kahle B, Rohwedel J, Kramer J, Gibson MA, et al. Enhanced fibrillin-2 expression is a general feature of wound healing and sclerosis: potential alteration of cell attachment and storage of TGF-beta. *Lab Invest* (2010) 90(5):739–52.
37. Chen W, Zhao W, Yang A, Xu A, Wang H, Cong M, et al. Integrated analysis of microRNA and gene expression profiles reveals a functional regulatory module associated with liver fibrosis. *Gene* (2017) 636:87–95.

38. Specks U, Nerlich A, Colby TV, Wiest I, Timpl R. Increased expression of type VI collagen in lung fibrosis. *Am J Respir Crit Care Med* (1995) 151 (6):1956–64.
39. Theocharidis G, Drymoussi Z, Kao AP, Barber AH, Lee DA, Braun KM, et al. Type VI Collagen Regulates Dermal Matrix Assembly and Fibroblast Motility. *J Invest Dermatol* (2016) 136(1):74–83.
40. Fleischmajer R, Jacobs L, Schwartz E, Sakai LY. Extracellular microfibrils are increased in localized and systemic scleroderma skin. *Lab Invest* (1991) 64 (6):791–8.
41. Specks U, Mayer U, Nischt R, Spissinger T, Mann K, Timpl R, et al. Structure of recombinant N-terminal globule of type VI collagen alpha 3 chain and its binding to heparin and hyaluronan. *EMBO J* (1992) 11(12):4281–90.
42. Somasundaram R, Schuppan D. Type I, II, III, IV, V, and VI collagens serve as extracellular ligands for the isoforms of platelet-derived growth factor (AA, BB, and AB). *J Biol Chem* (1996) 271(43):26884–91.
43. Schuppan D, Schmid M, Somasundaram R, Ackermann R, Ruehl M, Nakamura T, et al. Collagens in the liver extracellular matrix bind hepatocyte growth factor. *Gastroenterology* (1998) 114(1):139–52.
44. Virakul S, van Steensel L, Dalm VA, Paridaens D, van Hagen PM, Dik WA. Platelet-derived growth factor: a key factor in the pathogenesis of graves' ophthalmopathy and potential target for treatment. *Eur Thyroid J* (2014) 3 (4):217–26.
45. Yamane K, Mazaki T, Shiozaki Y, Yoshida A, Shinohara K, Nakamura M, et al. Collagen-Binding Hepatocyte Growth Factor (HGF) alone or with a Gelatin-furfurylamine Hydrogel Enhances Functional Recovery in Mice after Spinal Cord Injury. *Sci Rep* (2018) 8(1):917.
46. Nowak M, Sieminska L, Karpe J, Marek B, Kos-Kudla B, Kajdaniuk D. Serum concentrations of HGF and IL-8 in patients with active Graves' orbitopathy before and after methylprednisolone therapy. *J Endocrinol Invest* (2016) 39 (1):63–72.
47. Virakul S, Dalm VA, Paridaens D, van den Bosch WA, Mulder MT, Hirankarn N, et al. Platelet-Derived Growth Factor-BB Enhances Adipogenesis in Orbital Fibroblasts. *Invest Ophthalmol Vis Sci* (2015) 56(9):5457–64.
48. Rasmussen KK, Falkesgaard MH, Winther M, Roed NK, Quistgaard CL, Teisen MN, et al. NCAM2 Fibronectin type-III domains form a rigid structure that binds and activates the Fibroblast Growth Factor Receptor. *Sci Rep* (2018) 8(1):8957.
49. Schrijver B, Kooiman MA, Kasteleijn E, van Holten-Neelen C, Virakul S, Paridaens D, et al. Basic Fibroblast Growth Factor Induces Adipogenesis in Orbital Fibroblasts: Implications for the Pathogenesis of Graves' Orbitopathy. *Thyroid* (2019) 29(3):395–404.
50. Foglia B, Cannito S, Bocca C, Parola M, Novo E. ERK Pathway in Activated, Myofibroblast-Like, Hepatic Stellate Cells: A Critical Signaling Crossroad Sustaining Liver Fibrosis. *Int J Mol Sci* (2019) 20(11).
51. Fruman DA, Chiu H, Hopkins BD, Bagrodia S, Cantley LC, Abraham RT. The PI3K Pathway in Human Disease. *Cell* (2017) 170(4):605–35.
52. Fraker PJ, King LE. Reprogramming of the immune system during zinc deficiency. *Annu Rev Nutr* (2004) 24:277–98.
53. Liu MJ, Bao S, Galvez-Peralta M, Pyle CJ, Rudawsky AC, Pavlovicz RE, et al. ZIP8 regulates host defense through zinc-mediated inhibition of NF-kappaB. *Cell Rep* (2013) 3(2):386–400.
54. Malumbres M, Perez de Castro I, Santos J, Fernandez Piqueras J, Pellicer A. Hypermethylation of the cell cycle inhibitor p15INK4b 3'-untranslated region interferes with its transcriptional regulation in primary lymphomas. *Oncogene* (1999) 18(2):385–96.
55. Maussion G, Yang J, Suderman M, Diallo A, Nagy C, Arnovitz M, et al. Functional DNA methylation in a transcript specific 3'UTR region of TrkB associates with suicide. *Epigenetics* (2014) 9(8):1061–70.
56. Shen Z, Zhu L, Zhang C, Cui X, Lu J. Overexpression of BHLHE41, correlated with DNA hypomethylation in 3'UTR region, promotes the growth of human clear cell renal cell carcinoma. *Oncol Rep* (2019) 41(4):2137–47.
57. Hegedius L, Brix TH, Vestergaard P. Relationship between cigarette smoking and Graves' ophthalmopathy. *J Endocrinol Invest* (2004) 27(3):265–71.
58. Romero-Kusabara IL, Filho JV, Scalissi NM, Melo KC, Demartino G, Longui CA, et al. Distinct inflammatory gene expression in extraocular muscle and fat from patients with Graves' orbitopathy. *Eur J Endocrinol* (2017) 176(4):481–8.
59. Li B, Smith TJ. PI3K/AKT pathway mediates induction of IL-1RA by TSH in fibrocytes: modulation by PTEN. *J Clin Endocrinol Metab* (2014) 99 (9):3363–72.
60. Gillespie EF, Raychaudhuri N, Papageorgiou KI, Atkins SJ, Lu Y, Charara LK, et al. Interleukin-6 production in CD40-engaged fibrocytes in thyroid-associated ophthalmopathy: involvement of Akt and NF-kappaB. *Invest Ophthalmol Vis Sci* (2012) 53(12):7746–53.
61. Iyer S, Bahn R. Immunopathogenesis of Graves' ophthalmopathy: the role of the TSH receptor. *Best Pract Res Clin Endocrinol Metab* (2012) 26(3):281–9.
62. Molnar I, Bokk A. Decreased nerve growth factor levels in hyperthyroid Graves' ophthalmopathy highlighting the role of neuroprotective factor in autoimmune thyroid diseases. *Cytokine* (2006) 35(3-4):109–14.
63. Li H, Yuan Y, Zhang Y, Zhang X, Gao L, Xu R. Icariin Inhibits AMPK-Dependent Autophagy and Adipogenesis in Adipocytes In vitro and in a Model of Graves' Orbitopathy In vivo. *Front Physiol* (2017) 8:45.
64. Tsui S, Naik V, Hoa N, Hwang CJ, Afifiyan NF, Sinha Hikim A, et al. Evidence for an association between thyroid-stimulating hormone and insulin-like growth factor 1 receptors: a tale of two antigens implicated in Graves' disease. *J Immunol* (2008) 181(6):4397–405.
65. Krieger CC, Perry JD, Morgan SJ, Kahaly GJ, Gershengorn MC. TSH/IGF-1 Receptor Cross-Talk Rapidly Activates Extracellular Signal-Regulated Kinases in Multiple Cell Types. *Endocrinology* (2017) 158(10):3676–83.
66. Perniola R. Twenty Years of AIRE. *Front Immunol* (2018) 9:98.
67. Gough SC, Simmonds MJ. The HLA Region and Autoimmune Disease: Associations and Mechanisms of Action. *Curr Genomics* (2007) 8 (7):453–65.
68. Kont V, Murumagi A, Tykocinski LO, Kinkel SA, Webster KE, Kisand K, et al. DNA methylation signatures of the AIRE promoter in thymic epithelial cells, thymomas and normal tissues. *Mol Immunol* (2011) 49(3):518–26.
69. Fernando R, Lu Y, Atkins SJ, Mester T, Branham K, Smith TJ. Expression of thyrotropin receptor, thyroglobulin, sodium-iodide symporter, and thyroperoxidase by fibrocytes depends on AIRE. *J Clin Endocrinol Metab* (2014) 99(7):E1236–44.
70. Smith TJ. Potential Roles of CD34+ Fibrocytes Masquerading as Orbital Fibroblasts in Thyroid-Associated Ophthalmopathy. *J Clin Endocrinol Metab* (2019) 104(2):581–94.
71. O'Reilly S. Epigenetics in fibrosis. *Mol Aspects Med* (2017) 54:89–102.
72. Albrengues J, Bertero T, Grasset E, Bonan S, Maiel M, Bourget I, et al. Epigenetic switch drives the conversion of fibroblasts into proinvasive cancer-associated fibroblasts. *Nat Commun* (2015) 6:10204.
73. Lund AH, van Lohuizen M. Epigenetics and cancer. *Genes Dev* (2004) 18 (19):2315–35.
74. Yang X, Han H, De Carvalho DD, Lay FD, Jones PA, Liang G. Gene body methylation can alter gene expression and is a therapeutic target in cancer. *Cancer Cell* (2014) 26(4):577–90.
75. Kulis M, Heath S, Bibikova M, Queiros AC, Navarro A, Clot G, et al. Epigenomic analysis detects widespread gene-body DNA hypomethylation in chronic lymphocytic leukemia. *Nat Genet* (2012) 44(11):1236–42.
76. Deaton AM, Webb S, Kerr AR, Illingworth RS, Guy J, Andrews R, et al. Cell type-specific DNA methylation at intragenic CpG islands in the immune system. *Genome Res* (2011) 21(7):1074–86.
77. Yang TQ, Lu XJ, Wu TF, Ding DD, Zhao ZH, Chen GL, et al. MicroRNA-16 inhibits glioma cell growth and invasion through suppression of BCL2 and the nuclear factor-kappaB1/MMP9 signaling pathway. *Cancer Sci* (2014) 105 (3):265–71.
78. Guo LM, Pu Y, Han Z, Liu T, Li YX, Liu M, et al. MicroRNA-9 inhibits ovarian cancer cell growth through regulation of NF-kappaB1. *FEBS J* (2009) 276(19):5537–46.
79. Huang T, Kang W, Zhang B, Wu F, Dong Y, Tong JH, et al. miR-508-3p concordantly silences NFKB1 and RELA to inactivate canonical NF-kappaB signaling in gastric carcinogenesis. *Mol Cancer* (2016) 15:9.
80. Zhang K, Song F, Lu X, Chen W, Huang C, Li L, et al. MicroRNA-322 inhibits inflammatory cytokine expression and promotes cell proliferation in LPS-stimulated murine macrophages by targeting NF-kappaB1 (p50). *Biosci Rep* (2017) 37(1).

8

A 'Real Life' Service Evaluation Model for Multidisciplinary Thyroid Eye Services

Soma Farag[1,2], Claire Feeney[2,3], Vickie Lee[3,4], Sonali Nagendran[4], Rajni Jain[3], Ahmad Aziz[3,4], Rashmi Akishar[3], Vassiliki Bravis[2] and Karim Meeran[1,2]*

[1] Imperial College School of Medicine, Imperial College London, London, United Kingdom, [2] Department of Metabolism, Digestion and Reproduction, Imperial College London, London, United Kingdom, [3] Department of Ophthalmology, The Western Eye Hospital, Imperial College Healthcare National Health Service (NHS) Trust, London, United Kingdom, [4] Department of Ophthalmology, Central Middlesex Hospital, London North West Healthcare NHS Trust, London, United Kingdom

***Correspondence:**
Vickie Lee
vickie.lee@nhs.net*

Background/Aims: There is no universal consensus on the practical implementation and evaluation of the Amsterdam Declaration on Graves Orbitopathy in a Multidisciplinary Thyroid Eye Disease (MDTED) pathway. Recent recommendations from the UK TEAMeD-5 and BOPSS initiative highlight the importance of prevention, screening, and prompt referral of patients with moderate to severe and sight-threatening thyroid eye disease to multidisciplinary (MDTED) clinics and recommends annual auditing. We propose a practical service evaluation model with Key Performance Indicators (KPI) that are achievable and could be implemented across most TED pathways.

Material and Methods: We conducted a service evaluation from an integrated TED pathway in London with three MDTED clinics. Data was collected retrospectively from consecutive TED patients included: 1) Patient demographics, 2) Referral to first appointment time, 3) Documented smoking cessation and selenium supplementation advice, 4) Presenting disease activity and severity, 5) Investigations and treatments, including radio-iodine, 6) Time from decision to treatment initiation, 7) Initial and subsequent thyroid status.

Results: The median age was 49.0 yrs, 77.5% (183/236) were female and 49.5% (101/204) Afro-Caribbean or Asian. At their first clinic attendance, 47.6% (110/231) were biochemically euthyroid and 76.7% (79/103) at discharge. All 23.1% (52/225) current smokers received smoking cessation advice and 64.8% (153/236) received selenium supplementation advice. Intravenous methylprednisolone was given to 33.9% (80/236) patients and 12.7% (30/236) received second-line immunosuppression. All 7.2% (17/236) patients with sight-threatening disease received treatment within two weeks of diagnosis.

Conclusions: This study forms a waymark for other units using TEAMeD-5 and BOPSS audit criteria. Dedicated electronic patient records with ongoing data capture, including quality of life assessments, and diagnostic coding would significantly aid future auditing, improve patient care, and facilitate a national audit of TED management. A future survey when the TED standards have become embedded would be instructive to see whether this has improved TED care.

Keywords: thyroid-associated ophthalmopathy, Graves ophthalmopathy, optic neuropathy, Graves disease, Graves orbitopathy, thyroid eye disease

INTRODUCTION

Thyroid Eye Disease (TED) is a distressing and sometimes sight-threatening complication of Graves' Disease (GD) which affects up to 400,000 people in the UK and an estimated 9 per 10,000 population in Europe (1, 2). Women are more commonly affected than men (1, 3). There have been several European initiatives including Amsterdam Declaration of 2009 (3) and the 2016 European Group on Graves Orbitopathy (EUGOGO) recommendations for timely therapeutic interventions in order to optimise outcomes (4, 5).

In response TEAMeD-5 (Thyroid Eye Disease Amsterdam Declaration Implementation Group) was launched in 2017 (6) to raise awareness among endocrinologists and patients with GD about the importance of prevention, early detection and prompt referral of moderate to severe and sight-threatening TED to a specialist multidisciplinary thyroid eye disease (MDTED) clinic (4). TEAMeD-5 recommended mainly endocrinological Key Performance Indications (KPIs). In 2019, TEAMeD and the British Oculoplastic Surgery Society (BOPSS) published further recommendations based on a national survey of TED services and that were endorsed by all the UK TED stakeholder organizations. In our study, we aimed to carry out a service evaluation of a large multi-disciplinary TED network in a multi-ethnic metropolitan setting, as a waymark for implementation of the aforementioned recommendations.

MATERIAL AND METHODS

Patient Recruitment

We conducted a retrospective observational study of patient databases from three MDTED clinics led by consultant ophthalmic and oculoplastic surgeons (VL, RJ and AA), and endocrinology consultants (including KM VB and CF). The patients' care also included orthoptists who assessed for ocular motility disturbance and an immunosuppression specialist (RA), for patients requiring second-line immuno suppression. There is an integrated network of other specialists including head and neck radiologists, radiotherapists for orbital radiotherapy, thyroid surgeons for thyroidectomy and an elective rehabilitation pathway (including orbital decompression ocular muscle surgery for diplopia and eyelid surgery) for patients with quiescent residual disfiguring and debilitating disease.

We formulated the KPIs used in this study from the 2019 recommendations of the British Oculoplastic Surgery Society (BOPSS) and TEAMeD-5 (**Table 1**) (7).

Patients were identified from MDTED clinic databases at Imperial College Healthcare NHS Trust and Central Middlesex Hospital (CMH) (part of London North West University Healthcare NHS Trust). Data was collected at a contemporaneous post clinic 'board round' consensus of all the MDT consultants, who are also authors of this paper.

Additional clinical data was collected from the electronic record systems and included clinic letters, biochemical and radiology results. All patient data was collected from inception of the MDT clinic. The duration of the service evaluation started from the inception of the MDT clinics - CMH (Nov 2011), Imperial College sites at the Western Eye Hospital (WEH) Jan 2016) and Charing Cross Hospital (CXH) Jan 2017).

Database lock was on 31st January 2019, which was six months before the initiation of analysis.

This study was registered and approved by the Audit Department of the Trusts. This study adhered to the tenets of the Declaration of Helsinki.

Clinical Assessment

All TED patients had a Clinical Activity Score (CAS) assigned by a consultant ophthalmologist at each visit. A CAS of ≥ 3 defined clinically active TED, although other factors such as proptosis, ocular motility disturbance and optic nerve compromise were also taken into account. The severity of the disease was graded according to the EUGOGO categories of disease severity (mild, moderate to severe and sight-threatening) (4). All patients with a CAS of 3 or above were classified as having at least moderate disease severity. MRI was the imaging modality of choice as it offers superior soft tissue resolution making it an appropriate assessment of TED, which is a soft tissue disease. First-line immunosuppression was once weekly intravenous methylprednisolone (IVMP) infusions given over 12 weeks, as recommended by the EUGOGO consensus (4). All patients had at least one endocrine assessment, with optimisation of thyroid status, where appropriate. In the majority of patients with hyperthyroidism, the treatment was either antithyroid medication (Carbimazole first-line and Propylthiouracil second-line), thyroxine replacement, or both (i.e., 'block and replace'). Hypothyroid patients and post thyroidectomy patients were treated with thyroxine replacement guided by their thyroid function.

The following data was retrospectively collected for each patient:

1) Demographic data: age, gender, ethnicity, family history (in first or second-degree relatives) of thyroid disease, smoking status (current, ex-smoker, never smoked), diabetes mellitus (type 1 and 2)

TABLE 1 | The British Oculoplastic Surgery Society proposed audit criteria for the review of services managing thyroid eye disease (6) and the findings of this study.

i)	BOPSS audit criteria	Audit results
(1) Efficacy	Consideration of oral selenium supplements for patients with mild, active TED.	Out of the 135 new patients seen after the introduction of TEAMeD-5 in 2017, 60.0% (81/135) were advised to take oral selenium supplements.
	Smoking cessation advice for patients who are smokers.	The 23.1% (52/223) documented smokers in our cohort 100% received smoking cessation advise.
	Prompt correction of dysthyroidism and maintenance of euthyroidism.	Not formally audited. 76.7% (79/103) were biochemically euthyroid at discharge from MDTED clinic
	Where systemic steroid treatment is indicated, use of intravenous pulses of methylprednisolone in preference to oral steroids.	Departmental SOP is IVMP only for first line immunosuppression. No patients had oral prednisolone as first-line treatment. 80/236 (33.9%) of our patients received IVMP.
	Number receiving urgent treatment for sight-threatening orbitopathy including surgical decompression for patients who fail to respond to high dose intravenous steroids.	7.20% (17/236) received the EUGOGO protocol of 3-day high dose IVMP for sight-threatening orbitopathy followed by the standard 12 week course. 9 of these 17 patients also underwent emergency decompression surgery.
	Prevalence of patients treated orbital irradiation.	38/236 (16.1%) patients received orbital irradiation.
	Patients undergoing elective orbital decompression and rehabilitative surgery for patients with inactive or minimally active disease who are significantly impaired (socially or psychologically) as a result of TED.	16/236 (6.78%) patients underwent elective orbital decompression as part of rehabilitative surgery for TED.
(2) Safety	Patient education for recognising side-effects of steroids and other immunosuppressive treatments.	Our patients receive information leaflets provided by the local trust and leading TED patient charities on the side effects of steroid and immunosuppressive medication. 12.7% (30/236) of our patients received second-line immunosuppression under care of the MDTED immunosuppression specialist.
	Appropriate selection of patients with TED who are being considered for radioiodine for suitability of steroid cover.	There is a departmental SOP for RAI treatment, with recommendations for adjunctive oral steroid cover for at risk patients. 25% (2/8) patients under our MDTED clinic received steroid cover. The remainder were sent for RAI suitability screening.
	Safe use of immunosuppressive treatments (exclusion of those for whom there are contraindications, assessment, and monitoring of risks of serious adverse effects	100% (80/80) of those requiring intravenous steroids were given in the day unit of a large teaching hospital with acute services. 100% (30/30) of those requiring second-line immunosuppression received this under the care of an immunosuppression specialist who is part of the MDTED clinic.
	Timely assessment of response to high dose intravenous steroids and withdrawal of steroid treatment in favour of other therapies for those with inadequate response.	There is a SOP that patients are seen monthly in MDT clinic and their treatment response is assessed, with a personalised management plan formulated. Our departments compliance with SOP was not formally audited
(3) Patient-centred care	Availability of good quality information about GO, its usual course, likely outcomes, and potential treatments, complemented by high quality written information and access to patient-led organisations.	100% (236/236) given written information on TED.
	Formulation of personalised management plans following multidisciplinary discussion.	100% (236/236) of the patient management plans are discussed with consultant Endocrinologist and Ophthalmologists at every visit. A board round is conducted at the end of each clinic to ensure a consensual and personalised management plan for each patient.
	Good communication between the clinical team and the patient.	100% (236/236) patients have their management plans discussed with them and are sent copies of clinic letters.
	Patient engagement with the decision process about management of TED.	
	Use of validated tools to assess the impact of GO on their quality of life.	Our study found that there was no uniform QOL collection as a result of this finding the departmental SOP was changed to ensure MDTED patients have a GOQOL assessment at each clinic visit
(4) Timely	Patients with sight-threatening TED (dysthyroid optic neuropathy resulting in significant reduction in visual acuity, corneal breakdown with impending or established infection, globe subluxation) should be treated urgently within 2 weeks	100% (17/17) achieved this. Median (range) decision to treatment time was 1.6 (0-6) days.
	Patients with moderate-to-severe, active TED should be offered treatment within six weeks from presentation	96.3% (77/80) received treatment within six weeks from presentation.
	Multiple surgical treatments in patients requiring complex rehabilitative surgery, should follow the sequence: orbital decompression/eye muscle surgery/lid surgery	This sequence was not audited, however it is in the departmental SOP.
(5) Efficient	Referral pathways from primary to secondary and tertiary care, should be well-defined and seamless	75.2% (177/236) were seen in a MDTED clinic within three months of referral.

BOPSS, British Oculoplastic Surgery Society; IVMP, Intravenous methylprednisolone; MDTED, Multidisciplinary Thyroid Eye Disease Clinic; RAI, Radio-iodine; SOP, Standard operating protocol; TED, Thyroid Eye Disease.

2) Endocrine data:

i) Thyroid status at first MDTED clinic visit

ii) Management of thyroid disease - treatment (drugs, radioiodine (RAI), thyroidectomy), endocrine control and relapse of thyroid dysfunction

iii) Initial thyroid status of patients at referral and during period of treatment and at the last follow-up visit

iv) Number of patients who received RAI treatment

v) TSH-R antibody status

3) MDTED clinical metrics data:

i) Time between referral and a specialist review at first MDTED clinic

ii) Disease activity (determined by CAS at the first and last MDTED clinic). Patients with a CAS ≥3 were deemed to have active disease.

iii) Disease severity (determined by a clinical assessment) in line with EUGOGO classification

iv) Outcome of patients referred to MDTED clinic (with a confirmed diagnosis of TED), including investigations and treatment given

4) Management of TED:

i) Duration of treatment for TED: this was estimated from the patient reported date of TED onset, date of referral and of first MDTED clinic

ii) Number of patients receiving documented advice on smoking cessation and selenium supplementation

iii) Time from decision to treat to initiation of treatment for moderate to severe and sight-threatening active disease. Time from decision to treatment was recorded for: IVMP infusions, orbital decompression (urgent and elective) and orbital radiotherapy.

Inclusion and Exclusion Criteria

Inclusion criteria:

i) At least 18 years of age

ii) A diagnosis of TED (any severity, active or inactive)

Exclusion criteria:

i) Seen at MDTED, where a diagnosis of TED was excluded

ii) Where the patient's endocrinology care was not at Imperial or CMH and where it was not possible to access their blood results or advise on their endocrine care.

Statistical Analyses

Statistical analyses were performed using IBM SPSS statistics v.25 and GraphPad Prism v.8. The demographic data are presented as number and percentage. Descriptive statistics for non-normally distributed data used median and inter-quartile range.

RESULTS

Patient Demographics

There were 303 patients who attended the three MDTED clinics over the study period. After applying the exclusion criteria, 49 patients were excluded from the study as they did not have a diagnosis of TED; 15 patients had inadequate records and 3 were seen at other hospitals where we could not access their endocrine records. Consequently, 236 patients were included in this study; 106 were at CMH, 82 at the WEH, and 48 at CXH. The baseline patient demographic data are shown in **Table 2**. Out of the 13.6% (32/236) patients who were diabetic: 12.5% (4/32) were type 1, 84.4% (27/32) type 2 and one patient had diabetes secondary to thyroid hormone resistance syndrome with a G332E mutation.

TABLE 2 | Patient demographics across 3 multidisciplinary clinics.

	All TED group *n* = 236		Central Middlesex Hospital *n* = 106		Western Eye Hospital *n* = 82		Charing Cross Hospital *n* = 48	
	n		*n*		*n*		*n*	
Age at first TED clinic(yrs)	**236**		**106**		**82**		**48**	
Median (IQR)		49 (36-57)		43 (33-55		52 (43.8-60)		48 (34.5-54.8)
Range		18 - 82		18 - 82		23 - 82		23 - 77
No. (%) Female	**236**	183 (77.5)	**106**	83 (78.3)	**82**	63 (76.8)	**48**	37 (77.1)
Ethnicity	**204[a]**		**99[b]**		**69[c]**		**36[d]**	
No. (%) Caucasian		71 (34.8)		25 (25.3)		26 (37.7)		20 (55.6)
No. (%) Afro-Caribbean		55 (27.0)		36 (36.4)		12 (17.4)		7 (19.4)
No. (%) Asian		46 (22.5)		33 (33.3)		9 (13.0)		4 (11.1)
Smoking status	**223[e]**		**106**		**69[c]**		**48**	
No. (%) Current smokers		52 (23.1)		26 (24.5)		13 (18.8)		13 (27.1)
No. (%) Ex-smokers		41 (17.9)		12 (11.3)		18 (26.1)		11 (20.8)
No. (%) Positive family history	**236**	74 (31.4)	**106**	34 (32.1)	**82**	23 (28.0)	**48**	17 (35.4)
No. (%) Diabetes	**236**	32 (13.6)	**106**	11 (10.4)	**82**	14 (17.1)	**48**	7 (14.6)
Thyroid status at first clinic	**231[f]**		**102[g]**		**81[h]**		**48**	
No. (%) Euthyroid		110 (47.6)		57 (55.9)		29 (35.8)		24 (50.0)
No. (%) Hyperthyroid		96 (41.6)		36 (35.3)		39 (48.1)		21 (43.8)
No. (%) Hypothyroid		25 (10.8)		9 (8.8)		11 (13.6)		5 (10.4)

[a]Data unrecorded n=32, [b]data missing n=7, [c]data missing n=13, [d]data missing n=12, [e]data missing n=13, [f]data missing n=5, [g]data missing n=4, [h]data missing n=1.

Data recorded from inception of the clinic until January 2019; July 2012 to January 2019 for Central Middlesex Hospital, January 2016 to January 2019 for Western Eye Hospital and January 2017 to January 2019.

In bold: n refers to the number of patients (participants) which had the data available in their patient record notes for each demographic/endocrinology/ophthalmology characteristic.

Timing of Referral

After referral, 75.2% (177/236) patients were seen in a MDTED clinic within three months of referral. The median time from the patients reported first onset of symptoms and date of their first MDTED clinic was 135 days (**Figure 1**).

Management of Thyroid Dysfunction

The baseline thyroid status of the patients is shown in **Tables 3** and **4**. Patients who were euthyroid at their first MDTED appointment were the result of well controlled thyroid disease or euthyroid GD. Out of 166 patients who had TSH antibody titre measurement, 75.9% (126/166) had a positive titre status. In our cohort, 23.7% (56/236) patients had a recurrence (relapse) of hyperthyroidism; 66.7% (37/56) had this before and 33.3% (19/56) after their first attendance at the MDTED clinics. One hundred and three patients were discharged from the MDTED clinics during the study period and 76.7% (79/103) were biochemically euthyroid at discharge.

Radioiodine Treatment (RAI)

Twenty-nine patients received RAI treatment; 72.4% (21/29) had the treatment before the diagnosis of TED. Two of the eight patients with an established TED diagnosis had adjunctive oral steroid cover during their RAI treatment. The others were deemed to be low risk for eye disease progression by the MDT team, therefore were not prescribed oral steroid cover.

Smoking and Selenium

Baseline smoking status, where it was documented for patients is shown in **Table 2**. All current smokers received documented smoking cessation advice. Out of the 135 new patients seen after the introduction of TEAMeD-5 in 2017, 60.0% (81/135) received documented advice regarding the potential benefits of selenium supplementation.

Activity and Severity of TED

Two hundred and nineteen patients (91.5%) had a documented CAS at their first MDTED clinic attendance; 20.1% (44/219) were had a CAS of 3 or more. In our cohort, 7.2% (17/236) had sight-threatening disease (dysthyroid optic neuropathy and/or sight-threatening corneal exposure) (**Tables 3** and **4**).

Investigations and Treatment

Seventy percent (165/236) had one or more orbital Magnetic Resonance imaging (MRI) scans; 57.6% (95/165) were reported to have radiological evidence of orbital inflammation on their baseline scan (either qualitatively with STIR sequences or quantitatively with non-echo planar diffusion weighted imaging - DWI).

As first-line immunosuppression treatment, 33.9% (80/236) received intravenous methylprednisolone (IVMP), as recommended by the EUGOGO consensus (**Table 1**). The median time (range) from decision to treat and treatment initiation was 7 (1-90) days. In our cohort, 12.7% (30/236) received second-line immunosuppressant therapy usually with

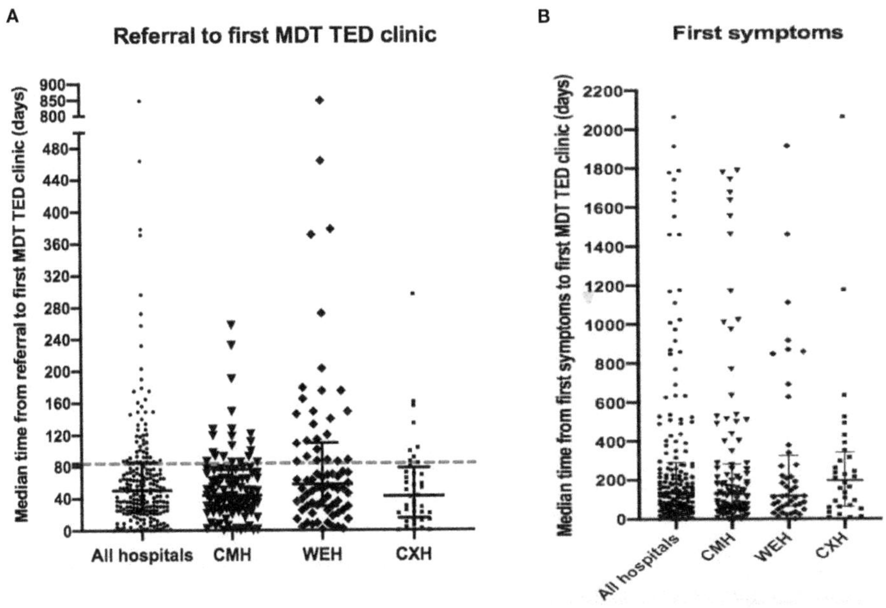

FIGURE 1 | **(A)** Time from referral to first MDTED clinic. The median (IQR) time (days) from referral to date of first MDTED clinic. All hospitals n=215, CMH n=101, WEH n=74, CXH: n=40. Horizontal line represents the target time by TEAMeD-5 (84 days or 3 months). **(B)** Time from first symptoms to first MDTED clinic. The median (IQR) time (months) from patient reported onset of first symptoms of Graves' Orbitopathy and the date of their first specialist multidisciplinary thyroid eye disease clinic. All hospitals n=177, CMH n= 101, WEH n= 44, CXH n= 32. Calculation from patient data available on symptom onset and referral time. CMH, Central Middlesex Hospital (part of London North West University Healthcare NHS Trust); WEH, Western Eye Hospital; CXH, Charing Cross Hospital.

TABLE 3 | Patient baseline characteristics by disease activity at presentation.

		Cohort 1 (CAS 0 - 1) *n* = 127		Cohort 2 (CAS 2) *n* = 31		Cohort 3 (CAS ≥ 3 and non-sight threatening) *n* = 44		Cohort 4 (DON) *n* = 17
	n		*n*		*n*		*n*	
Age (yrs)	**127**		**31**		**44**		**17**	
Median (IQR)		48 (35.0 - 57.0)		40(31.0 - 49.0)		49.0 (35.5 - 53.5)		57.0 (53.0 - 71.5)
Range		18 - 82		21 - 73		25 - 76		35 - 80
No. (%) Female	**127**	105 (82.7)	**31**	21 (67.7)	**44**	32 (72.7)	**17**	12 (70.6)
Ethnicity	**104**[a]		**28**[b]		**42**[c]		**15**[c]	
No. (%) Caucasian		36 (34.6)		7 (25.0)		16 (38.1)		6 (40.0)
No. (%) Afro-Caribbean		26 (25.0)		9 (32.1)		14 (33.3)		3 (20.0)
No. (%) Asian		25 (24.0)		10 (35.7)		7 (16.7)		2 (13.3)
Smoking status	**118**[d]		**30**[e]		**42**[c]		**17**	
No. (%) Current smokers		28 (23.7)		9 (30.0)		10 (23.8)		2 (11.8)
No. (%) Ex-smokers		23 (19.5)		3 (10.0)		9 (21.4)		2 (11.8)
No. (%) Positive family history	**127**	39 (30.7)	**31**	12 (38.7)	**44**	18 (40.9)	**17**	3 (17.6)

[a]Data missing n= 23, [b]data missing n= 3, [c]data missing n=2, [d]data missing n=9, [e]data missing n= 1.
Summary of 219 patients who had a recorded baseline clinical activity score (CAS) from July 2012 to January 2019.
DON, Dysthyroid Optic Neuropathy (sight-threatening disease).
In bold: n refers to the number of patients (participants) which had the data available in their patient record notes for each demographic/endocrinology/ophthalmology characteristic.

TABLE 4 | Endocrinological characteristics of the cohort by disease activity.

		Cohort 1 (CAS 0 - 1) *n* = 127		Cohort 2 (CAS 2) *n* = 31		Cohort 3 (CAS ≥ 3 and non-sight threatening) *n* = 44		Cohort 4 (DON) *n* = 17
	n		*n*		*n*		*n*	
Positive autoantibody								
No. (%) TSH	**90**[a]	59 (65.6)	**24**[b]	20 (83.3)	**30**[c]	28 (93.3)	**10**[d]	7 (70.0)
No. (%) TPO	**64**[e]	31 (48.4)	**20**[f]	8 (40.0)	**23**[g]	13 (56.5)	**7**[h]	3 (42.9)
TSH antibody titre (AU/mL)	**90**[a]							
Median (IQR)		4.2 (1.1 -13.7)	**24**[b]	12.3 (3.6 - 20.9)	**30**[c]	15.4 (5.0 - 29.7)	**8**[i]	4.0 (1.2 - 14.4)
Range		0.5 - 100.0		0.7 - 59.6		0.3 - 56.8		0.9 - 15.0
TPO antibody titre (AU/mL)								
Median (IQR)	**46**[j]	121.5 (12.7 - 357.2)	**20**[f]	152.0 (5.3 - 285.0)	**23**[g]	196.0 (20.0-491.2)	**7**[h]	56.5 (31.1 - 83.2)
Range		2.0 - 2379.0		1.0 - 617.0		1.0 - 879.0		25.8 - 88.9
Free T3 (pmol/L)								
Median (IQR)	**112**[k]	5.7 (3.8 - 12.7)	**30**[l]	7.8 (4.0- 15.5)	**43**[l]	7.3 (4.4 - 22.6)	**13**[m]	7.1 (4.8 - 14.9)
Range		0.4 - 46.2		1.6 - 46.1		0.9 - 47.1		0.9 - 46.1
Thyroid status at first clinic	**122**[o]							
No.(%) Hyperthyroid	36 (29.5)	**31**	18 (58.1)	**44**	26 (59.1)	**16**[l]	7 (43.8)	
No. (%) Hypothyroid	15 (12.3)		2 (6.5)		6 (13.6)		1 (6.3)	
No. (%) Euthyroid	71 (58.2)		11 (35.5)		12 (27.3)		8 (50.0)	
No. (%) Diabetes	**127**	15 (11.8)	**31**	3 (9.7)	**44**	7 (15.9)	**17**	4 (23.5)
HbA1c (mmol/l)	**72**[p]							
Median (IQR)		38.2 (36.0 - 42.0)	**20**[f]	38.0 (35.3 - 40.8)	**31**[q]	40.0 (36.0 - 45.0)	**14**[r]	42.0 (36.0 - 45.3)
Range		26.0 - 48.0		33.0 - 66.0		30.0 - 77.0		35.0 - 61.0
Thyroid medication	**87**[s]							
No. (%) Carbimazole (block and replace)		12 (13.8)		5 (23.8)		6 (16.2)		1 (7.7)
No. (%) Carbimazole (titration)		58 (67.7)	**21**[h]	12 (57.1)	**37**[d]	23 (62.2)	**13**[m]	9 (69.2)
No. (%) PTU		9 (10.3)		1 (4.8)		5 (13.5)		1 (7.7)
No. (%) Thyroxine		8 (9.2)		3 (14.3)		3 (8.1)		2 (15.4)
No. (%) Previous radioiodine	**127**	11 (8.7)	**31**	2 (6.5)	**44**	5 (11.4)	**17**	1 (5.9)
No. (%) Thyroidectomy	**127**	19 (16.8)	**31**	1 (3.2)	**44**	7 (14.3)	**17**	0 (0.0)

[a]Data unrecorded n=37, [b]data unrecorded n=7, [c]data unrecorded n=14, [d]data unrecorded n=7, [e]data unrecorded n=63, [f]data unrecorded n= 11, [g]data unrecorded n= 21, [h]data unrecorded n= 10, [i]data unrecorded n= 9, [j]data missing n= 81, [k]data missing n=15, [l]data missing n= 1, [m]data missing n= 4, [o]data missing n= 5, [p]data unrecorded n= 55, [q]data unrecorded n=13, [r]data unrecorded n= 3, [s]data missing n= 40.
Summary of the endocrinological characteristics stratified by disease activities as measured by clinical activity score (CAS).
DON; Dysthyroid Optic Neuropathy (sight-threatening disease), PTU; Propylthiouracil, TPO; Thyroid Peroxidase, TSH; Thyroid stimulating Hormone.
Normal ranges: TSH: <0.4AU/mL, TPO: <75 AU/mL, free T3: 2.5-5.7 pmol/L.
In bold: n refers to the number of patients (participants) which had the data available in their patient record notes for each demographic/endocrinology/ophthalmology characteristic.

mycophenolate mofetil (Cellcept). Further, 16.1% (38/236) patients required orbital radiotherapy (OR). Twenty-five of these patients' notes showed time of referral and date of treatment; the median time (range) from referral to OR was 30.5 (7-70) days. Twenty-five (10.6%) patients underwent orbital decompression surgery during the follow-up period, of these nine (36.0%) were emergency decompressions as adjunctive treatment for sight-threatening disease (median decision to treatment time: 1.6 days, range 0-6). All our 17 patients with sight-threatening disease started their sight preserving treatment within 2 weeks of diagnosis (**Table 1**).

DISCUSSION

The concept of combined multidisciplinary clinics has been well established in many disciplines to harness best available expertise to optimise patient management and outcomes. It has also been shown to improve the time to diagnosis and treatment in TED (5, 6, 8). Endocrinologists and ophthalmologists simultaneously seeing patients in these MDT clinics, ensures that a consistent and coherent management plan is clearly communicated and discussed with the patient and any concerns promptly addressed with readily available subspecialist expertise. The inception of two of our clinics at CMH (2011) and WEH (2015) predate the publication of TEAMeD-5 (2017) and the BOPSS audit criteria (December 2019). Data collection for this study predated the publication of the BOPSS criteria. Therefore, our multi-centre retrospective study of three MDTED clinics can be interpreted as a 'real world' snapshot of the MDT management of thyroid eye disease prior to introduction of established TED standards in a metropolitan multi-ethnic setting.

We had a similar age range and female:male ratio to other published multi-centre audits (9, 10). Our ethnically diverse cohort was comprised of 49.5% Afro-Caribbean or South Asian patients and this reflects the multi-ethnic London population. Previous audits of MDTED clinics have been less comprehensive in describing the ophthalmological and endocrinological profile of their patients (9, 10). Our prevalence of sight-threatening disease of 7.2% is higher compared to many other studies (11–13). We also had a higher number of patients requiring immunosuppression; 33.9% and 16.2% of our cohort received IVMP and orbital radiotherapy respectively compared to the PREGO study (23.0% and 6.0%), possibly reflecting a cohort with more severe disease (13). Only 75.9% of our cohort had a TSH-receptor positive titre, demonstrating that TED is primarily a clinical (and radiological) diagnosis, although serological testing is useful to identify Graves' Disease patients at risk (as per TEAMeD-5) (6). Most of our patients who received RAI did so prior to attending a MDTED clinic. There may be a very long gap between date of RAI treatment and onset of TED, so it is difficult to deduce whether RAI has contributed to the TED (14). However, out of those who received RAI after an established diagnosis of TED, only a quarter had prophylactic oral steroid cover. Oral steroids have a range of undesirable side effects for example weight gain, diabetes, and osteoporosis (15). These adverse effects must be considered before prescribing steroids, especially in patients deemed to be low risk for eye progression. There may also be a trend that with increasing awareness of TED, pre-RAI TED screening may account for increasing referrals to eye services. It is also encouraging that some of the key initiatives of TEAMeD-5 have already been implemented with 100% smoking cessation advice given to current smokers in our cohort. There is also increasing numbers (almost two-thirds of our cohort) who have received documented advice about selenium supplementation. In our experience, many patients have started selenium supplementation by the time of their first attendance at the MDTED clinic usually on the advice of their endocrinologists.

Limitations

This is a retrospective descriptive study at a single time point prior to the introduction of established TED standards. It would be interesting and informative to repeat this service evaluation in the future to evaluate for changes in practice after the TED standards have become embedded.

Data on every variable could not be recorded due to missing information from patients' notes. TSH-R measurement was less widespread prior to 2015, therefore only 70.3% of our patients had a recorded TSH antibody titre. In our cohort, there were some patients who had clinically active TED but a low CAS. CAS, having been developed in a predominantly white Dutch TED cohort, in our experience underestimates activity in patients with a high Fitzpatrick skin type due to its reliance on soft tissue appearance, such as erythema, and this is pertinent in a cohort of high ethnic diversity. The CAS scoring system places a greater weight on symptoms resulting from acute orbital congestion, as these comprise 5 of the total 7 points which can be allocated on the first visit. Ocular muscle involvement is not reflected in the scoring system, neither is posterior orbital pathology (16). Highly relevant signs such as diplopia at the first visit are also not included in the CAS scoring system (17). Therefore, changes in visual function are not scored for in the first visit where CAS is scored out of 7, so patients can have severe ocular motility restriction and decreased acuity that is not scored for in this setting (17). Recently, non-echo planar diffusion weighted imaging (DWI) MRI has been evaluated as a valuable tool, in adjunction with CAS, for investigating posterior orbital disease in TED and in providing higher resolution orbital images (16, 17). This imaging has been an invaluable adjunct for TED patient management in our clinics for the past eight years. Nevertheless, CAS also has a strong inter-specialty understanding and is used interchangeably by endocrinologists and ophthalmologists. Our aim with our ongoing collaboration alongside our radiological colleagues is to develop a Radiological Activity Score (RAS) to complement CAS to enable a more comprehensive assessment of disease activity and severity. It is well recognised that TED can significantly impact on Quality of Life (QoL) (18–21). QoL measurement with a validated instrument such as the GO-QOL, which is the gold standard in assessing the impact of TED, is recommended as part of the ongoing clinical assessment (19–21). However during the study period, the regular use of the validated GO-QOL questionnaire remained inconsistent in the aforementioned clinics.

Thyroid Eye Care in the Post Covid-19 Landscape

This service evaluation was carried out before the Covid-19 pandemic. In the height of the COVID pandemic, all routine face to face MDT clinic appointments were suspended. We stopped all our patients undergoing intravenous steroid treatment for non-sight-threatening disease and a significant proportion relapsed meaning we had to resume immunosuppression generally in the form of oral steroids during the lockdown period. In practice TEDmanagement is complex and relies on many face to face interactions such as orthoptic measurements, blood tests and ophthalmic and systemic assessments and we have found that a significant proportion of patients had significantly deteriorated despite reporting stability over a virtual consultation. The thyroid MDT clinic was one of the first, with the support of our management, to resume face to face activity for all patients once the height of the pandemic subsided and decisions regarding starting or resuming immunosuppression were made on the basis of these face to face consultations. With the investment of National Health Service (NHS) information technology in the UK, there may be a role for virtual MDT-lite clinics, which can enable more patients to have access to this modality, especially in parts of the country where there is significant geographical separation between endocrine and ophthalmic services. MDT clinics reduce duplication of appointments, avoids patients attending hospitals twice for the same condition and offers a consistent management strategy with a wholistic approach. We recognise however in a post COVID healthcare landscape, there will be significant fiscal constraints as regards service developments.

Implications for Future Work

There is consensus that TED management should be safe, timely, efficacious, equitable and patient-centred. In the UK, TEAMeD has worked closely with BOPSS to set up sustainable targets (7). Regular auditing of key performance indicators (KPIs) is of paramount importance. One of our recommendations is the set up of a dedicated electronic patient record platform to record this data prospectively in the clinic setting to avoid an onerous audit process, with a system to enable continuous and effortless GO-QOL evaluations at every consultation. The MDT service would also benefit from having dedicated co-ordinators as presently this administrative burden is mainly borne by clinical staff. This would be highly beneficial to provide more patient-centred care. We highlight the important of signposting patients to support organisations for additional support. In the UK, these include the British Thyroid Foundation and Thyroid Eye Disease Charitable Trust (TEDct). Ideally patients should have access to psychological counselling in view of the burden of significant disfigurement from TED. We believe that our approach, integrating TEAMeD-5 audit standards with the BOPSS recommendations forms a more complete service evaluation model for future MDTED services to implement the aims of the Amsterdam Declaration on Graves Orbitopathy. The clinical findings of our service evaluation in a multi-ethnic metropolitan population may not be widely applicable to all TED populations. Our main aim is to show the feasibility of producing key performance indicators for benchmarking TED care in a multi-disciplinary setting. We would look forward to other centres with a different cohort demographic to conduct a similar service evaluation to establish the range of TED presentations in an MDT setting designed to enable earlier diagnosis and treatment of TED.

AUTHOR CONTRIBUTIONS

VL conceived and designed the study. SF acquired, analysed, and interpreted the data. SF, CF, and VL drafted the manuscript. RA, RJ, AA, VB, and KM contributed to the manuscript. All authors contributed to the article and approved the submitted version.

ACKNOWLEDGMENTS

The authors would like to thank all of their colleagues working at the multidisciplinary thyroid eye disease pathways at the hospitals mentioned in this paper.

REFERENCES

1. Lazarus JH. Epidemiology of Graves' Orbitopathy (GO) and Relationship With Thyroid Disease. *Best Pract Res Clin Endocrinol Metab* (2012) 26:273–9. doi: 10.1016/j.beem.2011.10.005
2. Perros P, Hegedüs L, Bartalena L, Marcocci C, Kahaly GJ, Baldeschi L, et al. Graves' Orbitopathy as a Rare Disease in Europe: A European Group on Graves' Orbitopathy (Eugogo) Position Statement. *Orphanet J Rare Dis* (2017) 12(1):1–6. doi: 10.1186/s13023-017-0625-1
3. Perros P. The Amsterdam Declaration on Graves' Orbitopathy. *Graves' Orbitopathy Karger Publishers* (2017) 20:338–44. doi: 10.1159/000475973
4. Bartalena L, Baldeschi L, Boboridis K, Eckstein A, Kahaly GJ, Marcocci C, et al. The 2016 European Thyroid Association/European Group on Graves' Orbitopathy Guidelines for the Management of Graves' Orbitopathy. *Eur Thyroid J* (2016) 5:9–26. doi: 10.1159/000443828

5. Benzimra JD, Quinn AG, Kersey T, McGrane D, Goss L, Vaidya B. Management of Patients in a Combined Thyroid Eye Clinic in Secondary Care. *Int Ophthalmol* (2014) 34:1–6. doi: 10.1007/s10792-013-9768-9
6. Dayan C. Improving Outcomes in Thyroid Eye Disease-the Teamed 5 Programme. Society for Endocrinology Bes 2017. *BioScientifica* (2017) 131:18. doi: 10.1530/endoabs.50.CMW4.1
7. Lee V, Avari P, Williams B, Perros P, Dayan C. A Survey of Current Practices by the British Oculoplastic Surgery Society (BOPSS) and Recommendations for Delivering a Sustainable Multidisciplinary Approach to Thyroid Eye Disease in the United Kingdom. *Eye* (2019) 34:1–10. doi: 10.1038/s41433-019-0664-z
8. Avari C, Bravis V, Robinson S, Meeran K, Lee V. Sharing and Caring? Perspectives of Multidisciplinary Working Between Endocrinologists and Ophthalmologists in Thyroid Eye Disease. *Endocrinologist* (2018) 129:9.
9. Mellington FE, Dayan CM, Dickinson AJ, Hickey JL, MacEwen CJ, McLaren J, et al. Management of Thyroid Eye Disease in the United Kingdom: A Multi-Centre Thyroid Eye Disease Audit. *Orbit* (2017) 36:159–69. doi: 10.1080/01676830.2017.1280057
10. Babwah F, Viswanath A, Sandramouli S. Thyroid Eye Disease Audit-the Wolverhampton Experience. *Endocrine Abstracts* (2015) 38:abstract P456. doi: 10.1530/endoabs.38.P456
11. Tanda ML, Piantanida E, Liparulo L, Veronesi G, Lai A, Sassi L, et al. Prevalence and Natural History of Graves' Orbitopathy in a Large Series of Patients With Newly Diagnosed Graves' Hyperthyroidism Seen At a Single Center. *J Clin Endocrinol Metab* (2013) 98:1443–9. doi: 10.1210/jc.2012-3873
12. Laurberg P, Berman DC, Bülow Pedersen I, Andersen S, Carlé A. Incidence and Clinical Presentation of Moderate to Severe Graves' Orbitopathy in a Danish Population Before and After Iodine Fortification of Salt. *J Clin Endocrinol Metab* (2012) 97:2325–32. doi: 10.1210/jc.2012-1275
13. Perros P, Žarković M, Azzolini C, Ayvaz G, Baldeschi L, Bartalena L, et al. PREGO (Presentation of Graves' Orbitopathy) Study: Changes in Referral Patterns to European Group On Graves' Orbitopathy (Eugogo) Centres Over the Period From 2000 to 2012. *Br J Ophthalmol* (2015) 99:1531–5. doi: 10.1136/bjophthalmol-2015-306733
14. Acharya SH, Avenell A, Philip S, Burr J, Bevan JS, Abraham P. Radioiodine Therapy (RAI) for Graves' Disease (GD) and the Effect on Ophthalmopathy: A Systematic Review. *Clin Endocrinol* (2008) 69:943–50. doi: 10.1111/j.1365-2265.2008.03279.x
15. Hougardy DM, Peterson GM, Bleasel MD, Randall CT. Is Enough Attention Being Given to the Adverse Effects of Corticosteroid Therapy? *J Clin Pharm Ther* (2000) 25:227–34. doi: 10.1046/j.1365-2710.2000.00284.x
16. Lingam RK, Mundada P, Lee V. Novel Use of non-Echo-Planar Diffusion Weighted MRI in Monitoring Disease Activity and Treatment Response in Active Grave's Orbitopathy: An Initial Observational Cohort Study. *Orbit* (2018) 37:325–30. doi: 10.1080/01676830.2017.1423343
17. Feeney C, Lingam RK, Lee V, Rahman F, Nagendran S. Non-EPI-DWI for Detection, Disease Monitoring, and Clinical Decision-Making in Thyroid Eye Disease. *Am J Neuroradiol* (2020) 41(8):1466–72. doi: 10.3174/ajnr.A6664
18. Hiromatsu Y, Eguchi H, Tani J, Kasaoka M, Teshima Y. Graves' Ophthalmopathy: Epidemiology and Natural History. *Internal Med* (2014) 53:353–60. doi: 10.2169/internalmedicine.53.1518
19. Estcourt S, Quinn AG, Vaidya B. Quality of Life in Thyroid Eye Disease: Impact of Quality of Care. *Eur J Endocrinol* (2011) 164:649–55. doi: 10.1530/EJE-11-0055
20. Terwee CB, Gerding MN, Dekker FW, Prummel MF, Wiersinga WM. Development of a Disease Specific Quality of Life Questionnaire for Patients With Graves' Ophthalmopathy: The Go-Qol. *Br J Ophthalmol* (1998) 82:773–9. doi: 10.1136/bjo.82.7.773
21. Wickwar S, McBain HB, Ezra DG, Hirani SP, Rose GE, Newman SP. What are the Psychosocial Outcomes of Treatment for Thyroid Eye Disease? A Systematic Review. *Thyroid* (2014) 24:1407–18. doi: 10.1089/thy.2014.0037

9

Asymmetric Graves' Orbitopathy

Grigorios Panagiotou[1*] *and Petros Perros*[2]

[1] Department of Acute and Intensive Care Medicine, Northwick Park Hospital, London North West University Healthcare NHS Trust, Harrow, United Kingdom, [2] Department of Endocrinology, Royal Victoria Infirmary, Newcastle-upon-Tyne, United Kingdom

***Correspondence:**
Grigorios Panagiotou
gpanayio@gmail.com

Graves' Orbitopathy (GO) is an autoimmune orbital disorder usually presenting as a sequala of autoimmune thyroid disease. The presence of GO is associated with increased psychological burden and, in severe cases may cause blindness. While most patients with GO present with bilateral disease, asymmetric or unilateral GO may affect a significant proportion of patients diagnosed with GO. Older age, male sex, active and severe disease correlate with asymmetric disease. However, the exact mechanisms causing asymmetry remain elusive. Herein, we review the literature on asymmetric GO and highlight its differences compared with bilateral GO.

Keywords: asymmetry, Graves' disease, exophthalmos, unilateral, hyperthyroidism

INTRODUCTION

Graves' orbitopathy (GO) is the most common extrathyroidal feature of Graves' disease (1) with an estimated prevalence of 10/10,000 persons in European populations (2), while more recent data have shown variable prevalence between 25% and over 50% in Graves' hyperthyroidism cases (3) worldwide. GO is closely associated with thyroid autoimmunity, and although it is classically linked with hyperthyroidism, GO features have been described in hypothyroid or euthyroid individuals (4).

Autoimmune processes resulting in proliferation of orbital fibroblasts, increased adipogenesis, and extracellular matrix expansion are involved in its pathophysiology (5) and Thyroid Stimulating Hormone (TSH) Receptor Antibodies (TRAb) seem to be a key determinant. In fact, TRAb titer together with smoking, duration of thyroid dysfunction and clinical activity score (CAS) at baseline are regarded as main risk factors for developing GO (6).

The disease most often presents bilaterally and symmetrically with lid retraction, exophthalmos. and diplopia (3) being the most common features. In severe cases GO can be sight-threatening, thus requiring a prompt referral to specialist services (7) upon diagnosis. GO may also cause a psychological and financial burden (8), primarily but not exclusively due to cosmetic concerns, as well as increase the risk for suicide (9), and impairment of quality of life of patients (10).

However, some patients might exhibit asymmetric or unilateral symptoms, for yet unknown reasons. It has been suggested that unilateral GO may progress to bilateral disease (11) and we have also found that asymmetry was associated with more severe and active GO (12). Asymmetry and/or unilateral GO can impose diagnostic challenges (13) and it is therefore important that awareness for asymmetric GO be raised. Clinicians involved in the care of patients with GO need to be able to identify unilateral or asymmetric GO, as timely recognition of asymmetry may expedite referral to specialist services and facilitate further management. However, whether unilateral and/or asymmetric disease represent a distinct variant of GO remains unclear and a better understanding of their underlying mechanisms may provide useful insight on the pathogenesis of

GO, in general. Herein, we review the available literature on asymmetric GO and highlight differences compared with bilateral disease.

ASSESSMENT OF ASYMMETRIC AND/OR UNILATERAL GO

Asymmetry of the human face is well documented (14, 15), while asymmetry in the orbital anatomy of normal human skulls has been shown to be the norm. In a study of 127 human skulls (254 orbits) of individuals aged between newborn to 76 years, asymmetry in orbital anatomy (greater horizontal diameter, greater vertical diameter, orbital perimeter and orbital base area) was present in all cases except four, with variability between 2.47 and 4.47% between the right and left orbit (16). In the same study asymmetry was more prevalent in females and measurements from the right orbit were greater than the left (16). This is of importance, as facial asymmetry in itself can be a cause of significant distress (17).

On the other hand, orbital volume calculation using CT scanning has shown no differences between orbits or gender in a Taiwanese normal population (18). A large study of 653 normal Caucasians subjects aged 21–80 years found asymmetry to be rare (2%), minor (difference in exophthalmos readings <2mm), and unrelated to gender or age. Another study however showed a linear negative correlation between proptosis and age between the ages of 31 and 80 (19), which was also confirmed independently (20). In the latter study, recruiting a large sample (n = 1,063) of normal Iranian subjects including children, a significantly greater proptosis in the right eye compared with the left via exophthalmometry was shown, though the difference was never greater than 2 mm (21).

In the past, asymmetry has been variably defined as difference in proptosis between eyes by ≥2 mm (13), >2 mm (11, 22), or any one of the following criteria: retrobulbar pain or > or =1 grade in soft tissue involvement, and/or of > or =2 mm in exophthalmos, and/or > or =8 degrees in elevation (23), or repeatable asymmetry with regard to more than one symptom and more than one external or anterior segment finding for a duration of two or more visits at least 1 month apart at any time during the initial or follow-up period (23). Radiological criteria for asymmetry, such a right-to-left ratio of more than 1.4 in extraocular muscle diameter, as obtained by CT measurements based on normative data, have also been proposed (24). Unilateral GO is likewise variably defined as one or more features in one eye without any such manifestations in the other eye (20), proptosis >2 mm in one eye with normal examination of the other eye (25), or proptosis difference between eyes >4 mm, and/or if clinical signs and symptoms of GO found unilaterally (26). In our recently published study, asymmetry was defined as bilateral disease with one or more of the following features: difference between the two eyes in exophthalmos by ≥2 mm; difference in palpebral aperture by ≥2 mm; difference in eyelid swelling by ≥1 grades; difference in eyelid erythema by ≥1 grades; difference in conjunctival redness by ≥1 grades; presence of dysthyroid optic neuropathy in one eye only. Unilateral disease was defined as one or more clinical features of GO in one eye without any evidence of GO in the contralateral eye (12). Moreover, disease severity is assessed similarly to bilateral disease, using clinically evaluated standardized tools, such as CAS (27) and Vision, Inflammation, Strabismus, Appearance (VISA) (28). Clearly, there is a need for a consensus in the definitions of asymmetric and unilateral disease.

EPIDEMIOLOGY OF ASYMMETRIC AND/OR UNILATERAL GO

Different studies have estimated prevalence of unilateral disease between 4.5 and 14% (13, 25, 29–31), while asymmetry was evident in 9–34% of patients with GO (13, 26, 32). More recently, in our multi-center prospective cohort recruiting 269 newly diagnosed patients from 13 different centers across Europe, we have found a prevalence of 30.9% for asymmetric and 10.7% for unilateral GO (12). However, in a recently published retrospective hospital-based report from India, unilateral disease was much higher at 36% and significantly more common among silent presenters compared to the clinically active group (33). It is important to note that published studies have used different definitions of asymmetry and/or unilateral GO and this might explain the big variation in reported epidemiology among published data. Furthermore, less is known in regards to the epidemiology of unilateral or asymmetric GO in children.

Many risks factors have been associated with asymmetry. Shorter duration of symptoms (29) and thyroid status might be associated with asymmetry. In specific, small studies have suggested that euthyroid and primarily hypothyroid patients develop more asymmetrical GO (34, 35), which tends to present more mildly. In a larger study, Ponto et al. showed that a seven-fold higher risk for unilateral GO in hypothyroid or euthyroid subjects, compared with hyperthyroid GO (26). Moreover, previous studies have shown no difference in regards to race (13) and sex (29), but more recent data, including our recent multicenter study (12) and a cohort of 354 Chinese patients (36), have shown that male sex is associated with asymmetry. In another study, male subjects exhibited asymmetric disease (proptosis and overall asymmetry) three-fold more frequently compared with women, while women with hyperthyroidism demonstrated more symmetry compared with euthyroid and hypothyroid individuals of either sexes (23). With regards to correlation with older age, we have confirmed previous findings supporting higher prevalence and more severe asymmetry in older and especially men (12, 37), in keeping with previously described associations between age and male gender with severity of GO in patients with bilateral disease (38).

SPECIFIC CONSIDERATIONS IN ASYMMETRIC GO

It is important that unilateral GO be differentially diagnosed from orbital diseases affecting one eye, such as orbital tumors, such as lymphoma (39, 40). Other differentials affecting the orbit including other orbital tumors or pseudotumors, carotid cavernous fistulae, and dermoid and/or epidermoid cysts need to be excluded, too. Diagnosing unilateral or asymmetric GO without any other signs of GO and especially in the absence of hyperthyroidism or high TRAb titer suggestive of Graves' disease can be challenging (41) and requires increased clinical awareness and usually imaging of the orbits.

With regards to pathophysiology, the autoimmune processes in asymmetric and unilateral GO, causing expansion of orbital contents seem to be similarly to bilateral disease. However, mechanical, vascular, and inflammatory factors as well as anatomical variances may contribute to development of asymmetric disease.

More specifically, Soroudi et al. have speculated that asymmetric distribution of antigen or inflammatory processes may be the cause of asymmetrical expansion of orbital contents (13), though this was not explored in any studies so far. They have also postulated, that anatomical differences causing differential blood flow or lymphatic drainage may be present (13). Elasticity of orbital septae or other local factors, associated with unilateral triggers such as infections or difference in potential for adipogenesis have also been suggested (12). Others have examined the effect of sleeping position but found no significant correlation with asymmetric GO (32). However, despite previous postulations the exact mechanisms remain elusive. Therefore, more studies are needed to study asymmetric GO and shed light on the mechanisms leading to asymmetry. Such studies may provide further answers in regards to GO development and management.

TREATMENT OF UNILATERAL AND/OR ASYMMETRIC GO

Given that the pathophysiological mechanisms causing unilateral or asymmetric GO appear to be similar to the well-described bilateral GO, treatment of asymmetric GO is generally the same with bilateral disease and is usually dependent on disease severity. However, since asymmetric disease may progress to bilateral GO thereby increasing patients' anxiety and deteriorating their mental health status and quality of life as alluded to above, it is important that patients are managed promptly. Therefore, the goal in managing asymmetric or unilateral GO should be: a) to ensure symptoms are alleviated and sight is not threatened, similarly to bilateral GO; b) to take measures that may prevent progression to bilateral symptomatology; c) surgical rehabilitation when indicated.

Smoking cessation advice and restoring the euthyroid state are important pillars in the management of asymmetric GO. There is no contraindication in regards to any treatment modality including antithyroid drugs, radioactive iodine, and/or total thyroidectomy for mild asymmetric and/or unilateral GO, while in moderate to severe cases radioiodine should be avoided, similarly to bilateral symmetric disease (42).

In mild cases of asymmetric GO patients may still benefit from selenium supplementation (43). However, there are no prospective data evaluating whether early selenium supplementation in asymmetric GO cases may halt progression to bilateral symptoms. For more severe cases, methylprednisolone infusion (44) and/or administration of immune-modifying therapies, such as rituximab (45) and/or mycophenolate mofetil (46) may need to be considered. Targeted therapies such as teprotumumab, an anti-Insulin Growth Factor 1 (IGF-1) receptor monoclonal antibody, were shown to be effective in patients with active GO (47), but its role in asymmetric or unilateral GO is unexplored. Decompression surgery may be used in appropriate cases.

DISCUSSION AND CONCLUSIONS

Asymmetric and unilateral GO are recognized features of GO with variable prevalence among different studies; however, they do not seem to represent a distinct variant of classical GO, rather than the extreme of the spectrum, and thus focused studies are scarce. Therefore, prospective multicenter studies recruiting patients with different socioeconomic, demographic, ethnic, and anthropometric background are needed to better elucidate the epidemiology as well as other parameters of asymmetry and/or unilateral disease. Furthermore, previous studies have shown associations of asymmetric/unilateral GO with disease activity and severity and it is crucial that large cohorts include patients of different clinical status. There is a need for better documentation of the suggestions that asymmetric/unilateral GO might run a milder course or be a prelude to bilateral disease. The mechanisms leading to asymmetric disease discussed are speculative. Animal and mechanistic studies are needed to provide more in depth understanding of the mechanisms leading to disease progression and bilaterality and could identify possible novel therapeutic targets at a molecular level. Wide agreement and consensus among experts on the definition of asymmetry and unilaterality is paramount and will facilitate diagnosis, management, and research into this fascinating clinical entity.

In conclusion, although the available literature is limited, asymmetric and/or unilateral GO tend to be present in older age and male patients and is associated with more active and severe GO. Current evidence suggests that patient presenting with asymmetric or unilateral GO may progress to bilateral disease, which clinicians treating patients with GO need to be aware of. The present mini-review summarizes important information for both clinicians and researchers and also provides the impetus for further research. More specifically, in everyday clinical practice, unilateral disease needs to be differentiated from other pathologies affecting one eye. In the future, mechanistic studies are needed to explore the underlying pathological processes in asymmetric/unilateral GO. Most importantly, longitudinal studies evaluating individuals who are at higher risk for developing bilateral symptoms as well as the effect of various treatments in impeding progression of unilateral and/or asymmetric disease to bilateral GO are warranted.

AUTHOR CONTRIBUTIONS

GP: literature search, data acquisition, and writing of the manuscript. PP: conceptualization, literature search, and writing of the manuscript. All authors contributed to the article and approved the submitted version.

REFERENCES

1. Abraham-Nordling M, Bystrom K, Torring O, Lantz M, Berg G, Calissendorff J, et al. Incidence of hyperthyroidism in Sweden. *Eur J Endocrinol* (2011) 165:899–905. doi: 10.1530/EJE-11-0548
2. Perros P, Hegedus L, Bartalena L, Marcocci C, Kahaly GJ, Baldeschi L, et al. Graves' orbitopathy as a rare disease in Europe: a European Group on Graves' Orbitopathy (EUGOGO) position statement. *Orphanet J Rare Dis* (2017) 12:72. doi: 10.1186/s13023-017-0625-1
3. Chin YH, Ng CH, Lee MH, Koh JWH, Kiew J, Yang SP, et al. Prevalence of thyroid eye disease in Graves' disease: A meta-analysis and systematic review. *Clin Endocrinol* (2020). doi: 10.1111/cen.14296
4. Bahn RS. Graves' ophthalmopathy. *N Engl J Med* (2010) 362:726–38. doi: 10.1056/NEJMra0905750
5. Taylor PN, Zhang L, Lee RWJ, Muller I, Ezra DG, Dayan CM, et al. New insights into the pathogenesis and nonsurgical management of Graves orbitopathy. *Nat Rev Endocrinol* (2020) 16:104–16. doi: 10.1038/s41574-019-0305-4
6. Wiersinga W, Zarkovic M, Bartalena L, Donati S, Perros P, Okosieme O, et al. Predictive score for the development or progression of Graves' orbitopathy in patients with newly diagnosed Graves' hyperthyroidism. *Eur J Endocrinol* (2018) 178:635–43. doi: 10.1530/EJE-18-0039
7. Fox TJ, Anastasopoulou C. *Graves Orbitopathy*. Treasure Island (FL: StatPearls (2020).
8. Kahaly GJ, Petrak F, Hardt J, Pitz S, Egle UT. Psychosocial morbidity of Graves' orbitopathy. *Clin Endocrinol* (2005) 63:395–402. doi: 10.1111/j.1365-2265.2005.02352.x
9. Ferlov-Schwensen C, Brix TH, Hegedus L. Death by Suicide in Graves' Disease and Graves' Orbitopathy: A Nationwide Danish Register Study. *Thyroid* (2017) 27:1475–80. doi: 10.1089/thy.2017.0365
10. Ponto KA, Hommel G, Pitz S, Elflein H, Pfeiffer N, Kahaly GJ. Quality of life in a german graves orbitopathy population. *Am J Ophthalmol* (2011) 152:483–490 e1. doi: 10.1016/j.ajo.2011.02.018
11. Strianese D, Piscopo R, Elefante A, Napoli M, Comune C, Baronissi I, et al. Unilateral proptosis in thyroid eye disease with subsequent contralateral involvement: retrospective follow-up study. *BMC Ophthalmol* (2013) 13:21. doi: 10.1186/1471-2415-13-21
12. Perros P, Zarkovic MP, Panagiotou GC, Azzolini C, Ayvaz G, Baldeschi L, et al. Asymmetry indicates more severe and active disease in Graves' orbitopathy: results from a prospective cross-sectional multicentre study. *J Endocrinol Invest* (2020) 43:1717–22. doi: 10.1007/s40618-020-01258-w
13. Soroudi AE, Goldberg RA, McCann JD. Prevalence of asymmetric exophthalmos in Graves orbitopathy. *Ophthalmic Plast Reconstr Surg* (2004) 20:224–5. doi: 10.1097/01.IOP.0000124675.80763.5A
14. Chebib FS, Chamma AM. Indices of craniofacial asymmetry. *Angle Orthodontist* (1981) 51:214–26. doi: 10.1043/0003-3219(1981)051<0214:IOCA>2.0.CO;2
15. Shah SM, Joshi MR. An assessment of asymmetry in the normal craniofacial complex. *Angle Orthodontist* (1978) 48(2):141–8. doi: 10.1043/0003-3219(1978)048<0141:AAOAIT>2.0.CO;2
16. Seiji F, Moreira RS, De Angelis MA, Smith Chairman RL. Orbital asymmetry in development: an anatomical study. *Orbit* (2009) 28:342–6. doi: 10.3109/01676830903162841
17. Shackelford TK, Larsen RJ. Facial asymmetry as an indicator of psychological, emotional, and physiological distress. *J Pers Soc Psychol* (1997) 72:456–66. doi: 10.1037/0022-3514.72.2.456
18. Shyu VB, Hsu CE, Chen CH, Chen CT. 3D-assisted quantitative assessment of orbital volume using an open-source software platform in a Taiwanese population. *PloS One* (2015) 10:e0119589. doi: 10.1371/journal.pone.0119589
19. Ahmadi H, Shams PN, Davies NP, Joshi N, Kelly MH. Age-related changes in the normal sagittal relationship between globe and orbit. *J Plastic Reconstr Aesthet Surg* (2007) 60:246–50. doi: 10.1016/j.bjps.2006.07.001
20. Kashkouli MB, Kaghazkanani R, Heidari I, Ketabi N, Jam S, Azarnia S, et al. Bilateral versus unilateral thyroid eye disease. *Indian J Ophthalmol* (2011) 59:363–6. doi: 10.4103/0301-4738.83612
21. Kashkouli MB, Nojomi M, Parvaresh MM, Sanjari MS, Modarres M, Noorani MM. Normal values of hertel exophthalmometry in children, teenagers, and adults from Tehran, Iran. *Optom Vision Sci* (2008) 85:1012–7. doi: 10.1097/OPX.0b013e3181890dc7
22. Tsai CC, Kau HC, Kao SC, Hsu WM. Exophthalmos of patients with Graves' disease in Chinese of Taiwan. *Eye* (2006) 20:569–73. doi: 10.1038/sj.eye.6701925
23. Kavoussi SC, Giacometti JN, Servat JJ, Levin F. The relationship between sex and symmetry in thyroid eye disease. *Clin Ophthalmol* (2014) 8:1295–300. doi: 10.2147/OPTH.S61041
24. Sheikh M, Abalkhail S, Doi SA, Al-Shoumer KA. Normal measurement of orbital structures: implications for the assessment of Graves' ophthalmopathy. *Australas Radiol* (2007) 51:253–6. doi: 10.1111/j.1440-1673.2007.01721.x
25. Daumerie C, Duprez T, Boschi A. Long-term multidisciplinary follow-up of unilateral thyroid-associated orbitopathy. *Eur J Internal Med* (2008) 19:531–6. doi: 10.1016/j.ejim.2008.01.013
26. Ponto KA, Binder H, Diana T, Matheis N, Otto AF, Pitz S, et al. Prevalence, Phenotype, and Psychosocial Well-Being in Euthyroid/Hypothyroid Thyroid-Associated Orbitopathy. *Thyroid* (2015) 25:942–8. doi: 10.1089/thy.2015.0031
27. Mourits MP, Prummel MF, Wiersinga WM, Koornneef L. Clinical activity score as a guide in the management of patients with Graves' ophthalmopathy. *Clin Endocrinol* (1997) 47:9–14. doi: 10.1046/j.1365-2265.1997.2331047.x
28. Dolman PJ, Rootman J, Classification for Graves orbitopathy VISA. Ophthalmic plastic and reconstructive surgery. *Ophthalmic Plast Reconstr Surg* (2006) 22:319–24. doi: 10.1097/01.iop.0000235499.34867.85
29. Wiersinga WM, Smit T, van der Gaag R, Mourits M, Koornneef L. Clinical presentation of Graves' ophthalmopathy. *Ophthalmic Res* (1989) 21:73–82. doi: 10.1159/000266782
30. Bartley GB. The epidemiologic characteristics and clinical course of ophthalmopathy associated with autoimmune thyroid disease in Olmsted County, Minnesota. *Trans Am Ophthalmol Soc* (1994) 92:477–588.
31. Prummel MF, Bakker A, Wiersinga WM, Baldeschi L, Mourits MP, Kendall-Taylor P, et al. Multi-center study on the characteristics and treatment strategies of patients with Graves' orbitopathy: the first European Group on Graves' Orbitopathy experience. *Eur J Endocrinol* (2003) 148:491–5. doi: 10.1530/eje.0.1480491
32. Wiersinga WM, Bleumink M, Saeed P, Baldeschi L, Prummel MF. Is sleeping position related to asymmetry in bilateral Graves' ophthalmopathy? *Thyroid* (2008) 18:541–4. doi: 10.1089/thy.2007.0302
33. Naik MN, Vasanthapuram VH. Demographic and clinical profile of 1000 patients with thyroid eye disease presenting to a Tertiary Eye Care Institute in India. *Int Ophthalmol* (2020). doi: 10.1007/s10792-020-01571-6
34. Eckstein AK, Losch C, Glowacka D, Schott M, Mann K, Esser J, et al. Euthyroid and primarily hypothyroid patients develop milder and significantly more asymmetrical Graves ophthalmopathy. *Br J Ophthalmol* (2009) 93:1052–6. doi: 10.1136/bjo.2007.137265
35. Jang SY, Lee SY, Lee EJ, Yoon JS. Clinical features of thyroid-associated ophthalmopathy in clinically euthyroid Korean patients. *Eye* (2012) 26:1263–9. doi: 10.1038/eye.2012.132
36. Li Q, Ye H, Ding Y, Chen G, Liu Z, Xu J, et al. Clinical characteristics of moderate-to-severe thyroid associated ophthalmopathy in 354 Chinese cases. *PLoS One* (2017) 12:e0176064. doi: 10.1371/journal.pone.0176064

37. Kendler DL, Lippa J, Rootman J. The initial clinical characteristics of Graves' orbitopathy vary with age and sex. *Arch Ophthalmol* (1993) 111:197–201. doi: 10.1001/archopht.1993.01090020051022
38. Perros P, Crombie AL, Matthews JN, Kendall-Taylor P. Age and gender influence the severity of thyroid-associated ophthalmopathy: a study of 101 patients attending a combined thyroid-eye clinic. *Clin Endocrinol* (1993) 38:367–72. doi: 10.1111/j.1365-2265.1993.tb00516.x
39. Moura Neto A, Denardi FC, Delamain MT, Tambascia MA, Vassallo J, Caldato R, et al. Orbital lymphoma mimicking ophthalmopathy in a patient with Graves'. *Am J Med Sci* (2012) 344:418–21. doi: 10.1097/MAJ.0b013e3182582330
40. Buescu A, Teixeira P, Coelho S, Donangelo I, Vaisman M. Orbital lymphoma misdiagnosed as Graves' ophthalmopathy. *Endocr Pract* (2001) 7:110–2. doi: 10.4158/EP.7.2.110
41. Verma SK, Jain N, Saraf S, Singh SK. Asymmetric graves ophthalmopathy as a sole manifestation of autoimmune hypothyroidism. *BMJ Case Rep* (2013) 2013:bcr2012007485. doi: 10.1136/bcr-2012-007485
42. Laurberg P, Wallin G, Tallstedt L, Abraham-Nordling M, Lundell G, Torring O. TSH-receptor autoimmunity in Graves' disease after therapy with anti-thyroid drugs, surgery, or radioiodine: a 5-year prospective randomized study. *Eur J Endocrinol* (2008) 158:69–75. doi: 10.1530/EJE-07-0450
43. Marcocci C, Kahaly GJ, Krassas GE, Bartalena L, Prummel M, Stahl M, et al. Selenium and the course of mild Graves' orbitopathy. *N Engl J Med* (2011) 364:1920–31. doi: 10.1056/NEJMoa1012985
44. Tu X, Dong Y, Zhang H, Su Q. Corticosteroids for Graves' Ophthalmopathy: Systematic Review and Meta-Analysis. *BioMed Res Int* (2018) 2018:4845894. doi: 10.1155/2018/4845894
45. Salvi M, Vannucchi G, Campi I, Rossi S, Bonara P, Sbrozzi F, et al. Efficacy of rituximab treatment for thyroid-associated ophthalmopathy as a result of intraorbital B-cell depletion in one patient unresponsive to steroid immunosuppression. *Eur J Endocrinol* (2006) 154:511–7. doi: 10.1530/eje.1.02119
46. Ye X, Bo X, Hu X, Cui H, Lu B, Shao J, et al. Efficacy and safety of mycophenolate mofetil in patients with active moderate-to-severe Graves' orbitopathy. *Clin Endocrinol* (2017) 86:247–55. doi: 10.1111/cen.13170
47. Douglas RS, Kahaly GJ, Patel A, Sile S, Thompson EHZ, Perdok R, et al. Teprotumumab for the Treatment of Active Thyroid Eye Disease. *N Engl J Med* (2020) 382:341–52. doi: 10.1056/NEJMoa1910434

10

Association of Other Autoimmune Diseases with Thyroid Eye Disease

Mary Kelada[1,2], Parizad Avari[2], Soma Farag[1,2], Rashmi Akishar[3], Rajni Jain[3], Ahmad Aziz[3], Claire Feeney[2], Vassiliki Bravis[2], Karim Meeran[2] and Vickie Lee[2,3,4]*

[1] Imperial College School of Medicine, Imperial College London, London, United Kingdom, [2] Department of Metabolism, Digestion and Reproduction, Imperial College London, London, United Kingdom, [3] The Western Eye Hospital, Imperial College Healthcare NHS Trust, London, United Kingdom, [4] Department of Ophthalmology, Central Middlesex Hospital, London North West Healthcare NHS Trust, London, United Kingdom

Correspondence:
Vickie Lee
vickie.lee@nhs.net

Background: Thyroid eye disease (TED) is a potentially disfiguring and sight-threatening autoimmune (AI) orbitopathy, affecting up to 400,000 people in the UK. There are no accurate early predictors of TED severity. Although polyautoimmunity has been shown to affect AI disease severity, its influence on TED severity has never been investigated. The prevalence of polyautoimmunity among TED patients is also unclear, with discordant results reported in the literature. This study evaluates the prevalence of non-thyroid/ "other" AI (OAI) conditions in an ethnically diverse TED cohort and assesses how polyautoimmunity affects TED severity and activity.

Methods: A retrospective study of patients presenting to multidisciplinary TED clinics across three North-West London hospitals between 2011 and 2019. Data collected included: 1) demographics; 2) OAI conditions and management; 3) endocrine management of thyroid dysfunction; 4) details of TED and clinical activity score at presentation.

Results: Two hundred and sixty-seven patients with a median age of 46 (35–54) years were included, 79.4% were female and 55% were Black, Asian and minority ethnic (BAME). Thirty-seven patients (13.9%) had OAI conditions, with rheumatoid arthritis (3.7%), vitiligo (3.0%) and psoriasis (3.0%) among the most prevalent. Of patients with OAI conditions, 43.2% (16/37) required immunosuppression prior to TED onset. Non-immunosuppressed patients with OAI conditions had a significantly higher clinical activity score at presentation than TED-only and previously immunosuppressed patients ($p=0.02$). No significant differences were observed in thyroid receptor antibody titers between these groups.

Conclusions: This study finds a 13.9% prevalence of OAI conditions among TED patients. Patients with OAI conditions overall have a tendency for more severe and significantly more clinically active TED than those without OAI conditions. Larger, prospective studies are warranted to further evaluate polyautoimmunity as an early predictor of TED severity.

Keywords: thyroid eye disease, polyautoimmunity, disease severity, ethnically diverse, clinical activity score, immunosuppression, rheumatoid arthritis, psoriasis

INTRODUCTION

Thyroid eye disease (TED), also known as Graves' ophthalmopathy/ orbitopathy, is a distressing, disfiguring, and potentially sight threatening, autoimmune disease (1). TED affects an estimated 400,000 people in the UK (2) and is the most common extrathyroidal manifestation of Graves' Disease (GD) (3–5). TED can cause a significant disease burden, causing pain, discomfort, double vision and considerable psychosocial distress to its sufferers (1, 6, 7). Around 5% of TED cases are estimated to progress to sight-threatening disease (8); however, there are currently no accurate early predictors of disease severity.

There is a well-established tendency for distinct autoimmune (AI) conditions to co-exist in patients who have previously been diagnosed with an AI condition, such as autoimmune thyroiditis (i.e. polyautoimmunity) (9–11). Although polyautoimmunity has been shown to affect AI disease severity (12–15), its association with TED severity has never been investigated.

There is also a paucity of medical literature investigating the prevalence of polyautoimmunity among TED patients. Only two studies have investigated the prevalence of non-thyroid AI, or "other AI" (OAI), conditions among TED patients. They estimate the prevalence of OAI conditions to be 8%–19% among TED patients (16, 17). However, both studies were carried out in monoethnic cohorts of Graves' hyperthyroidism patients only. Given that around 3% of TED patients have autoimmune hypothyroidism (Hashimoto's thyroiditis) and a further 2% never experience thyroid dysfunction (18), these results may not be applicable to all TED patients.

This study aims to evaluate the presence of non-thyroid AI conditions in an ethnically diverse, metropolitan TED cohort and to assess whether there is an association between the presence of polyautoimmunity and TED severity or clinical activity.

METHODOLOGY

This was a retrospective multi-center patient-cohort study based on patients attending three multidisciplinary thyroid eye disease (MDTED) clinics based in North West London, UK, at Imperial College Healthcare NHS Trust (ICHNT; Charing Cross Hospital CXH, Western Eye Hospital WEH) and Central Middlesex Hospital CMH, London North West Healthcare NHS Trust (LNWH). The audit was registered and approved by the relevant Trust departments.

Clinical records of all patients added to the joint MDT-TED clinic databases at CHX, WEH and CMH hospital sites from January 2011 to November 2019 were evaluated for eligibility. Patients were excluded if they had less than 3 months of follow-up, no TED diagnosis according to clinical/radiological criteria or incomplete clinic notes (i.e. no past medical history stated/no letters available for subsequent visits). Patients who had received ophthalmic or endocrine care outside Imperial or LNWH Trusts were also excluded as their hospital records were not accessible.

Data were collected from the electronic hospital records of eligible patients. Demographic data included: age at first presentation at the MDT-TED clinic, gender, ethnicity, smoking status, and family history of thyroid disease (i.e. primary or secondary relative affected). Details of their endocrine care were collected to include: thyroid diagnosis (GD, Hashimoto's thyroiditis, Hashitoxicosis, hypothyroidism, euthyroid or other) at presentation, initial thyroid receptor antibody (TRAb) titer and thyroid dysfunction management [medication, thyroidectomy, and/or radioiodine (RAI) therapy].

Data collected on TED included: clinical activity score (CAS) at presentation; the patient's initial and most severe disease severity classification according to European Group on Graves' Orbitopathy (EUGOGO) criteria; management {selenium supplements, lubricating eyedrops, immunosuppression [first line treatment with intravenous methylprednisolone (IVMP) and/or second line immunosuppression, urgent or elective orbital decompression surgery, orbital radiotherapy (OR)]}.

Other autoimmune (OAI) conditions were only recorded for patients if the diagnosis had been confirmed by a specialist (for example, dermatologist, rheumatologist or gastroenterologist) following relevant clinical examinations and investigations. Steroid cover and immunomodulatory therapy for OAI were also recorded.

Statistical Analyses

All data were anonymized for statistical analyses using GraphPad Prism, version 8.0. The Shapiro-Wilks test was used to assess the normality of continuous data. Where data are not normally distributed, continuous variables have been expressed as medians (interquartile range). A Spearman rank correlation was used to evaluate the degree of association between two non-parametric variables (i.e. CAS score and TRAb titers). For groupwise analysis of non-parametric continuous data, a Kruskall-Wallis test was carried out, followed by Mann-Whitney *U* tests. Where more comparisons have been made than there are number of groups, alpha values have been adjusted using Bonferroni's correction to account for multiple comparisons. Chi squared tests were used to compare two categoric variables between groups.

RESULTS

Demographics

Two hundred and sixty-seven patients were included in the study. On average, patients were seen within 1.8 (0.8–2.9) months of referral from endocrine clinic to MDT-TED. Patients had a median age of 46 (35–54) years. Of these, 92.5% (247/267) had Graves hyperthyroidism, 3.7% (10/267) had Hashitoxicosis, 3.0% (8/267) had no thyroid hormonal dysfunction and 0.7% (2/267) had other thyroid pathologies, namely thyroid hormone resistance and follicular carcinoma of the thyroid. 79.4% were female and over half the participants (55%) were Black, Asian or minority ethnic (BAME). 13.9% (37/267) patients were noted to have OAI conditions, of whom 21.7% (8/37) had more than OAI condition. Nearly half [43% (16/37)] of patients with OAI conditions required immunosuppressive therapy prior to TED symptom onset. 42.6% (98/267) of patients were euthyroid at TED onset.

OAI Conditions

The most commonly observed AI condition was rheumatoid arthritis (RA) with the highest prevalence among Caucasian TED patients, (six compared to two BAME patients; **Table 1**). 3.0% (eight patients) had vitiligo and the same for psoriasis. Seven of the eight vitiligo patients were BAME, so this was the most prevalent OAI condition among BAME patients. 1.5% (4/267) had relapsing-remitting multiple sclerosis (RRMS). Overall, we did not detect statistically significant differences in the distribution of OAI conditions among Caucasian and BAME patients (p>0.05, post-hoc analysis not displayed).

In total, 6.0% patients (16/267) underwent immunosuppressive therapy for their OAI conditions before TED symptom onset with no statistically significant differences between the ethnic groups. On average, immunomodulatory therapy for OAI conditions was commenced 60 (2–120) months prior to TED symptom onset; only 18.8% (3/16) of patients were still receiving immunosuppressive therapy at the time of TED diagnosis. Treatment of TED included steroids, monoclonal antibodies and disease modifying drugs. 31.3% (5/16) of patients used prednisolone prior to TED symptom onset, 31.3% (5/16) had taken monoclonal antibodies, namely natalizumab, alemtuzumab or tocilizumab, and 50.0% (8/16) had commenced disease modifying therapies, such as methotrexate, prior to TED symptom onset.

Table 2 describes the characteristics of patients within three groups: those with TED only, those with TED + OAI conditions who had received immunosuppression for their AI conditions prior to TED symptom onset and those with OAI who had not been immunosuppressed. Significant differences were observed in the median age of presentation to MDT-TED clinic between the three groups. The median age of presentation to MDT-TED clinic of previously immunosuppressed patients was 52 (46.3–57.8) years, which was significantly higher than that of patients with TED only, 45 (33.8–54.0) years (p = 0.04). No differences were observed in the distribution of sex, ethnicity, or smoking status in TED-only patients compared to patients with OAI conditions, regardless of prior immunosuppression.

A similar proportion of TED-only patients (49.6%) and patients with OAI conditions (43.2%) presented to MDT-TED clinic with hyperthyroidism, regardless of prior use of immunosuppression. The proportion of patients that underwent radioiodine therapy for thyroid dysfunction was also comparable across the three groups of patients.

Patients with OAI who had not received prior immunosuppressive therapy had the highest median CAS score at presentation (2, IQR: 1–4), compared to TED-only patients (p = 0.02; **Figure 1**) and previously immunosuppressed patients (p = 0.02; **Figure 1**).

Similar proportions of OAI (no prior immunosuppression) patients and OAI (prior immunosuppression) patients required first-line immunosuppressive therapy (IVMP) for TED (9.5% *vs.* 12.5%). However, only 6.3% of OAI (prior immunosuppression) patients required further (second-line) immunosuppressive TED therapy in the form of OR and/or MMF, while 28.6% of OAI (no prior immunosuppression) required first line (IVMP) and second line (OR and/or MMF) treatment.

TABLE 1 | Prevalence of non-thyroid autoimmune conditions in patients grouped by ethnicity.

	Ethnicity			Total (n= 267)
	Caucasian (n = 74)	BAME (n = 147)	Not Stated (n = 46)	
Non-thyroid Autoimmune Conditions				
Rheumatoid Arthritis	6 (8.1%)	2 (1.4%)	2 (4.3%)	10 (3.7%)
Vitiligo	1 (1.3%)	7 (4.8%)	0 (0%)	8 (3.0%)
Psoriasis	2 (2.8%)	3 (2.0%)	3 (6.5%)	8 (3.0%)
Relapsing-Remitting Multiple Sclerosis	1 (1.3%)	2 (1.4%)	1 (2.2%)	4 (1.5%)
Systemic Lupus Erythematosus	0 (0%)	2 (1.4%)	0 (0%)	2 (0.7%)
Crohn's Disease	1 (1.3%)	1 (0.7%)	0 (0%)	2 (0.7%)
Type 1 Diabetes Mellitus	1 (1.3%)	1 (0.7%)	0 (0%)	2 (0.7%)
Juvenile Idiopathic Arthritis	0 (0%)	1 (0.7%)	0 (0%)	1 (0.4%)
Alopecia Areata	1 (1.3%)	0 (0%)	0 (0%)	1 (0.4%)
Giant Cell Arteritis	1 (1.3%)	0 (0%)	0 (0%)	1 (0.4%)
Polymyalgia Rheumatica	1 (1.3%)	0 (0%)	0 (0%)	1 (0.4%)
Sjogren's Disease	0 (0%)	2 (1.4%)	0 (0%)	2 (0.7%)
Sarcoidosis	1 (1.3%)	0 (0%)	0 (0%)	1 (0.4%)
AI Pancreatitis	0 (0%)	1 (0.7%)	0 (0%)	1 (0.4%)
AI Neutropenia	1 (1.3%)	0 (0%)	0 (0%)	1 (0.4%)
AI Pernicious Anemia	0 (0%)	1 (0.7%)	0 (0%)	1 (0.4%)
pANCA Vasculitis	0 (0%)	0 (0%)	1 (2.2%)	1 (0.4%)
Coeliac	0 (0%)	0 (0%)	1 (2.2%)	1 (0.4%)
Urticarial Vasculitis	0 (0%)	0 (0%)	1 (2.2%)	1 (0.4%)
Myasthenia Gravis	0 (0%)	1 (0.7%)	0 (0%)	1 (0.4%)
Patients with >1 non-thyroid AI condition	2 (2.8%)	5 (3.4%)	1 (2.2%)	8 (3.0%)
Patients with one non-thyroid AI condition	10 (13.6%)	12 (8.2%)	7 (15.2%)	29 (10.9%)
Use of immunosuppressive therapy prior to TED symptom onset	6 (8.1%)	7 (4.8%)	3 (6.5%)	16 (6.0%)

The presence of non-thyroid AI conditions was recorded if the condition had been diagnosed by a specialist following relevant examinations and investigations and reported in the patient's medical records. Data presented as "count (percentage of cohort)".

TABLE 2 | Summary of patient demographics, thyroid dysfunction and thyroid eye disease (TED) data categorized by the presence of non-thyroid autoimmune conditions and whether or not patients with non-thyroid autoimmune conditions had commenced immunosuppressive therapy prior to TED symptom onset.

		TED only (n = 230)	TED + OAI conditions		p-value
			No Previous Immunosuppression (n = 21)	Previous Immunosuppression (n = 16)	
Patient Demographics					
Sex	*Female*	182 (79.1%)	16 (76.2%)	14 (87.5%)	0.78
	Male	48 (20.7%)	5 (23.8%)	2 (12.5%)	
Age at first MDT-TED clinic		45 (34 - 54)	48 (43.5-61.5)	52 (44.8-57.8)	0.04*
Smoking status	*Current smoker*	54 (23.5%)	0 (0%)	2 (11.1%)	0.07
	Previous smoker	41 (17.8%)	3 (14.3%)	5 (27.8%)	
	Vapes	4 (1.7%)	1 (4.8%)	1 (5.5%)	
	Never Smoked	131 (57.0%)	17 (81.0%)	8 (50.0%)	
Ethnicity	*Caucasian*	62 (27.0%)	6 (28.6%)	6 (37.5%)	0.75
	BAME	127 (55.2%)	12 (57.1%)	9 (56.3%)	
	Not Stated	41 (17.8%)	3 (14.3%)	1 (6.2%)	
Thyroid Dysfunction					
Family history of thyroid dysfunction		61 (26.5%)	3 (14.3%)	5 (27.8%)	–
Diagnosed Thyroid Pathology	*Graves*	200 (87.0%)	17 (80.1%)	15 (93.8%)	0.23
	Hashimoto's	7 (3.0%)	2 (9.5%)	0 (0%)	
	None	4 (1.7%)	2 (9.5%)	1 (6.2%)	
	Other	2 (0.9%)	0 (0%)	0 (0%)	
Thyroid status at TED onset	*Hypothyroid*	18 (7.8%)	4 (19.0%)	0 (0%)	0.25
	Euthyroid	98 (42.6%)	8(38.1%)	9 (56.2%)	
	Hyperthyroid	114 (49.6%)	9 (42.9%)	7 (43.8%)	
Previous Radioiodine Therapy		32 (13.9%)	4 (19.0%)	1 (6.3%)	–
Thyroid Eye Disease					
CAS at presentation		1 (1-2)	2 (1-4)	1 (1-2)	0.04*
Selenium recommended		183 (79.6%)	20 (95.2%)	14 (87.5%)	–
Proportion of patients requiring further therapy	*IVMP only*	35 (15.2%)	2 (9.5%)	2 (12.5%)	–
	IVMP + MMF	25 (10.9%)	2 (9.5%)	0 (0%)	
	IVMP + Radio	18 (7.8%)	1 (4.8%)	1 (6.3%)	
	IVMP + MMF + Radio	9 (3.9%)	3 (14.3%)	0 (0%)	

Categoric data are presented as "count (percentage)"; all continuous variables are presented as "median (interquartile range)."
**represents statistical significance, where p < 0.05.*
OAI, other autoimmune; TED, thyroid eye disease; BAME, black and minority ethnic; CAS, clinical activity score; IVMP, intravenous methylprednisolone; MMF, mycophenolate mofetil; Radio, orbital radiotherapy.

Thyroid Receptor Antibody (TRAb) Titer

61.4% (164/267) of patients were tested for TRAb antibodies and 88.4% of these (145/164) were TRAb positive. There were no significant differences in the TRAb titers of patients with TED only compared to those with OAI, regardless of prior immunosuppression (p = 0.66; **Figure 2**). However, we note there was a tendency for OAI (no prior immunosuppression) patients conditions to have higher titers, 13.35 U/L (0.90–30.0), compared to OAI (prior immunosuppression) patients, 4.90 U/L (1.55–5.90), and those with TED only, 4.00 U/L (1.37–15.10; p>0.05).

Further sub-analysis found no correlation between TRAb titers and CAS of all included patients (r = 0.079, p = 0.32). There were also no correlations between TRAb and CAS within the three patient sub-groups.

We did not distinguish between stimulating and blocking TSH receptor antibodies as it was not possible to establish which assays had been used in the various laboratories across the three sites from 2011 to 2019.

DISCUSSION

This was the first study to evaluate the prevalence of non-thyroid OAI conditions in an ethnically diverse, metropolitan TED cohort and to assess potential associations between the presence of polyautoimmunity and TED severity or clinical activity.

The findings of this study, taken together with the results of the Cruz and Ferrari studies, suggest TED patients may have a higher prevalence of certain AI conditions compared to the general population. For example, RA and psoriasis was found to have a prevalence of 3.7% and 3% in our cohort, compared to a prevalence of 0.4%–1.2% and 1.3% in the general population (19). Our study also corroborates findings from the aforementioned studies that vitiligo and RA were among the most prevalent OAI conditions among TED patients. However, we also found a higher prevalence of psoriasis and MS in our cohort (16, 17).

A number of immune-related genes have been found in TED and OAI, presumably underpinning the inherited susceptibility to autoimmunity (20). There is evidence to suggest that

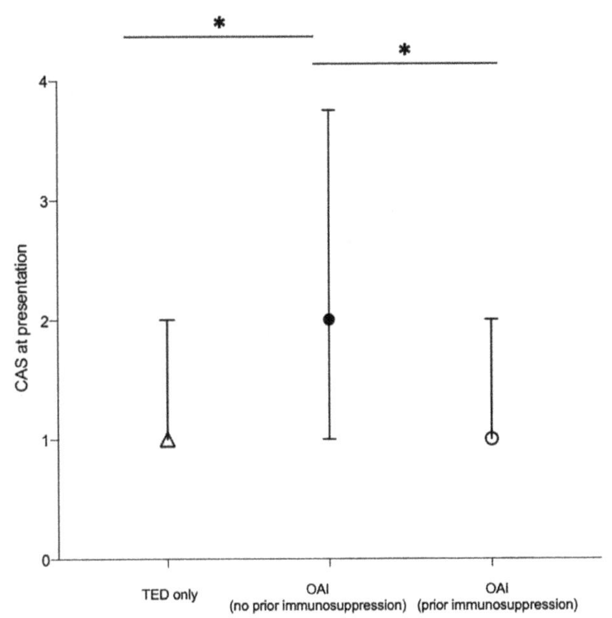

FIGURE 1 | Median clinical activity score (CAS) at presentation of patients categorized by the presence of non-thyroid autoimmune conditions and whether or not patients with non-thyroid autoimmune conditions had commenced immunosuppressive therapy prior to TED symptom onset. Median value of each cohort plotted. Error bars represent the interquartile range. *represents statistical significance, where $p < 0.0167$ by Bonferroni's correction. CAS, clinical activity score; OAI, other autoimmune; TED, thyroid eye disease.

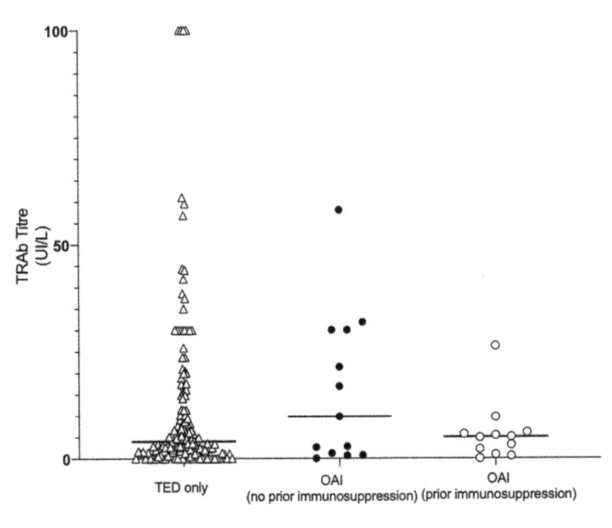

FIGURE 2 | Initial thyroid receptor antibody (TRAb) titer of patients categorized by the presence of non-thyroid autoimmune conditions and whether or not patients with non-thyroid autoimmune conditions had commenced immunosuppressive therapy prior to TED symptom onset. Data were collected from clinic notes and patient hospital records. Points represent the initial TRAb titer of each patient in the cohort; solid lines represent the median TRAb titer of each cohort. No significant differences were found in the TRAb titers of the three groups. OAI, other autoimmune; TED, thyroid eye disease.

mutations in the interleukin-23 receptor (IL23R) gene could confer increased susceptibility to AI conditions, such as RA, psoriasis and TED (21–23), which may explain the association of RA and psoriasis in our cohort. The link between IL23R gene mutations and TED pathophysiology is uncertain with only a few conflicting studies in the literature. For example, a study of Caucasian patients demonstrated the RA-associated single nucleotide polymorphisms of the IL23R gene to be associated with TED (24) while a similar study on Japanese patients did not identify such a trend (25). Further studies are needed to fully understand the role, if any, of the IL23R gene.

Vitiligo has previously been demonstrated to be associated with autoimmune thyroid diseases, such as Graves and Hashimoto's thyroiditis (26–28). Similarly, autoimmune thyroid diseases have been demonstrated to be the most common co-existing AI conditions in MS and RA patients (29). It would be interesting to compare the prevalence of each AI conditions in patients with AITD and no orbitopathy to patients with TED to establish whether there is an association between TED and these AI conditions, or rather if the presence of AITD in the studied population was a confounder. Further studies are required on the potential value of screening with thyroid antibodies in patients with OAI conditions that appear to be most prevalent in those eventually presenting with TED.

We found 13.9% of patients to have at least one non-thyroid OAI condition, of whom 48.6% had prior immunosuppression before their TED diagnosis. Patients in the TED only and OAI (no prior immunosuppression) subgroups presented with more active and severe disease compare to the subgroup with OAI (prior immunosuppression) and required more immunosuppression for their TED. It is possible this finding is a chance association and further studies are required to confirm this.

This study found a higher proportion of euthyroid patients at presentation to TED-MDT compared to figures previously published in the literature (30). The nature of the referral pathway to these TED-MDTs is such that the majority of patients are referred from an endocrine clinic where therapy such as radioiodine, which is known to have an adverse effect on TED (30), may have been used to establish a euthyroid state.

A limitation of this study is that the term "immunosuppression" included patients who had taken monoclonal antibodies, disease modifying drugs or steroids prior to TED symptom onset. It is therefore unclear if the different mechanisms of action of various immunosuppressive agents could have different effects on TED severity or activity. Although only one patient had taken alemtuzumab, a recent study has demonstrated this drug to trigger the onset of TED in "at risk" patients (31). Whether other monoclonal therapies can have a similar effect is unknown. Beyond this, the effects of alemtuzumab on TED severity remain unclear. It would therefore be interesting to further study the effects of steroids, monoclonal antibodies and other disease modifying drugs on TED severity and activity. A further limitation of this study reflects this being a single-center, retrospective study. While our findings are comparable to the ethnic diversity of London, UK (BAME population of 40.2% as per the Office of National Statistics 2011 Census), the findings may not be representative of other parts in the

UK (32). Furthermore, the study does not account for the effects of other medications, such as statins and metformin, among others, that could have an immunomodulatory properties (33).

Although the patients in this study were treated in the pre COVID-19 era, during the pandemic all first line intravenous steroid immunosuppression for non-sight threatening TED were stopped. We monitored and treated patients with severe relapse with oral steroids in line with best practice recommendations (34–36). All our second line immunosuppression patients continued treatment abiding with governmental shielding protocols. Careful consideration and constant evaluation has to be deployed regarding the choice and timing of immunosuppression in the post-COVID landscape.

In conclusion, the findings of this study were overall concordant with similar studies of monoethnic populations. Certain AI conditions, such as rheumatoid arthritis and vitiligo, appear to have an increased prevalence in TED patients. Whether or not this is due to a common pathway in their pathogeneses remains unclear.

This study was also the first to demonstrate that patients with polyautoimmunity receiving immunosuppression prior to TED diagnosis may have less severe and less clinically active TED than those who have received no prior immunosuppressive therapy. Larger, prospective studies are warranted to evaluate how polyautoimmunity affects TED severity and activity and whether the presence of polyautoimmunity could be used as an early predictor of TED severity.

AUTHOR CONTRIBUTIONS

VL conceived and designed the study. MK acquired the data, analyzed, and interpreted the data. MK, PA, and VL drafted the manuscript. SF, RA, RJ, AA, CF, VB, and KM contributed to the manuscript. All authors contributed to the article and approved the submitted version. VL and MK are the guarantors of this work and, as such, had full access to all the data in the study and take responsibility for the integrity of the data and the accuracy of the data analysis.

REFERENCES

1. Wiersinga WM, Kahaly G. *Graves" orbitopathy : a multidisciplinary approach.* Karger (2007) p. 1–22. S. Karger (Firm). doi: 10.1159/isbn.978-3-8055-8343-5
2. Lazarus JH. Epidemiology of Graves' orbitopathy (GO) and relationship with thyroid disease. *Best Pract Res Clin Endocrinol Metab* (2012) 26(3):273–9. doi: 10.1016/j.beem.2011.10.005
3. Vanderpump MPJ. The epidemiology of thyroid disease. *Br Med Bull* (2011) 99(1):39–51. doi: 10.1093/bmb/ldr030
4. Vangheluwe O, Ducasse A, Vaudrey C, Maes B, Delisle MJ. Prevalence de l'ophtalmopathie dans la maladie de basedow. Suivi des malades a un an apres la decouverte de leur hyperthyroidie. *J Fr Ophtalmol* (1994) 17(5):331–8.
5. Bartley GB, Fatourechi V, Kadrmas EF, Jacobsen SJ, Ilstrup DM, Garrity JA, et al. Long-term follow-up of Graves ophthalmopathy in an incidence cohort. *Ophthalmology* (1996) 103(6):958–62. doi: 10.1016/S0161-6420(96)30579-4
6. Park JJ, Sullivan TJ, Mortimer RH, Wagenaar M, Perry-Keene DA. Assessing quality of life in Australian patients with Graves' ophthalmopathy. *Br J Ophthalmol* (2004) 88(1):75–8. doi: 10.1136/bjo.88.1.75
7. Ponto KA, Merkesdal S, Hommel G, Pitz S, Pfeiffer N, Kahaly GJ. Public health relevance of graves' orbitopathy. *J Clin Endocrinol Metab* (2013) 98 (1):145–52. doi: 10.1210/jc.2012-3119
8. Mellington FE, Dayan CM, Dickinson AJ, Hickey JL, MacEwen CJ, McLaren J, et al. Management of thyroid eye disease in the United Kingdom: A multi-centre thyroid eye disease audit. *Orbit* (2017) 36(3):159–69. doi: 10.1080/01676830.2017.1280057
9. Bliddal S, Nielsen CH, Feldt-Rasmussen U. Recent advances in understanding autoimmune thyroid disease: The tallest tree in the forest of polyautoimmunity. *F1000Research* (2017) 6:1766. doi: 10.12688/f1000research.11535.1
10. Agnoli A, Ruggieri S, Denaro A, Bruno G. New Strategies in the Management of Parkinson's Disease: A Biological Approach Using a Phospholipid Precursor (CDP-Choline). *Neuropsychobiology* (1982) 8(6):289–96. doi: 10.1159/000117914
11. Cellini M, Santaguida MG, Stramazzo I, Capriello S, Brusca N, Antonelli A, et al. Recurrent Pregnancy Loss in Women with Hashimoto's Thyroiditis with Concurrent Non-Endocrine Autoimmune Disorders. *Thyroid* (2020) 30 (3):457–62. doi: 10.1089/thy.2019.0456
12. Ramos-Casals M, Nardi N, Lagrutta M, Brito-Zerón P, Bové A, Delgado G, et al. Vasculitis in Systemic Lupus Erythematosus. *Medicine (Baltimore)* (2006) 85(2):95–104. doi: 10.1097/01.md.0000216817.35937.70
13. Christensen PB, Jensen TS, Tsiropoulos I, SOrensen T, Kjaer M, Højer-Pedersen E, et al. Associated autoimmune diseases in myasthenia gravis A population-based study. *Acta Neurol Scand* (2009) 91(3):192–5. doi: 10.1111/j.1600-0404.1995.tb00432.x
14. Marinó M, Ricciardi R, Pinchera A, Barbesino G, Manetti L, Chiovato L, et al. Mild Clinical Expression of Myasthenia Gravis Associated with Autoimmune Thyroid Diseases*. *J Clin Endocrinol Metab* (1997) 82(2):438–43. doi: 10.1210/jcem.82.2.3749
15. Avouac J, Airò P, Dieude P, Caramaschi P, Tiev K, Diot E, et al. Associated autoimmune diseases in systemic sclerosis define a subset of patients with milder disease: Results from 2 large cohorts of European Caucasian patients. *J Rheumatol* (2010) 37(3):608–14. doi: 10.3899/jrheum.090815
16. Cruz AAV, Akaishi PMS, Vargas MA, de Paula SA. Association Between Thyroid Autoimmune Dysfunction and Non-Thyroid Autoimmune Diseases. *Ophthalmic Plast Reconstr Surg* (2007) 23(2):104–8. doi: 10.1097/IOP.0b013e318030b06b
17. Ferrari SM, Fallahi P, Ruffilli I, Elia G, Ragusa F, Benvenga S, et al. The association of other autoimmune diseases in patients with Graves' disease (with or without ophthalmopathy): Review of the literature and report of a large series. *Autoimmun Rev* (2019) 18:287–92. doi: 10.1016/j.autrev.2018.10.001
18. Leo M, Menconi F, Rocchi R, Latrofa F, Sisti E, Profilo MA, et al. Role of the underlying thyroid disease on the phenotype of graves' orbitopathy in a tertiary referral center. *Thyroid* (2015) 25(3):347–51. doi: 10.1089/thy.2014.0475
19. Symmons D, Turner G, Webb R, Asten P, Barrett E, Lunt M, et al. The prevalence of rheumatoid arthritis in the United Kingdom: new estimates for a new century. *Rheumatology* (2002) 41(7):793–800. doi: 10.1093/rheumatology/41.7.793
20. Franco J-S, Amaya-Amaya J, Anaya J-M. Thyroid disease and autoimmune diseases. (2013). https://www.ncbi.nlm.nih.gov/books/NBK459466/.

21. Faragó B, Magyari L, Sáfrány E, Csöngei V, Járomi L, Horvatovich K, et al. Functional variants of interleukin-23 receptor gene confer risk for rheumatoid arthritis but not for systemic sclerosis. *Ann Rheum Dis* (2008) 67(2):248–50. doi: 10.1136/ard.2007.072819
22. Cargill M, Schrodi SJ, Chang M, Garcia VE, Brandon R, Callis KP, et al. A large-scale genetic association study confirms IL12B and leads to the identification of IL23R as psoriasis-risk genes. *Am J Hum Genet* (2007) 80 (2):273–90. doi: 10.1086/511051
23. Duerr RH, Taylor KD, Brant SR, Rioux JD, Silverberg MS, Daly MJ, et al. A genome-wide association study identifies IL23R as an inflammatory bowel disease gene. *Science (80-)* (2006) 314(5804):1461–3. doi: 10.1126/science.1135245
24. Huber AK, Jacobson EM, Jazdzewski K, Concepcion ES, Tomer Y. Interleukin (IL)-23 Receptor Is a Major Susceptibility Gene for Graves' Ophthalmopathy: The IL-23/T-helper 17 Axis Extends to Thyroid Autoimmunity. *J Clin Endocrinol Metab* (2008) 93(3):1077–81. doi: 10.1210/jc.2007-2190
25. Ban Y, Tozaki T, Taniyama M, Nakano Y, Yoneyama KI, Ban Y, et al. Association studies of the IL-23R gene in autoimmune thyroid disease in the Japanese population. *Autoimmunity* (2009) 42(2):126–30. doi: 10.1080/08916930802422265
26. Gey A, Diallo A, Seneschal J, Léauté-Labrèze C, Boralevi F, Jouary T, et al. Autoimmune thyroid disease in vitiligo: multivariate analysis indicates intricate pathomechanisms. *Br J Dermatol* (2013) 168(4):756–61. doi: 10.1111/bjd.12166
27. Gill L, Zarbo A, Isedeh P, Jacobsen G, Lim HW, Hamzavi I. Comorbid autoimmune diseases in patients with vitiligo: A cross-sectional study. *J Am Acad Dermatol* (2016) 74(2):295–302. doi: 10.1016/j.jaad.2015.08.063
28. Sheth VM, Guo Y, Qureshi AA. Comorbidities associated with vitiligo: A ten-year retrospective study. *Dermatology* (2014) 4):311–5. doi: 10.1159/000354607
29. Rojas-Villarraga A, Amaya-Amaya J, Rodriguez-Rodriguez A, Mantilla RD, Anaya J-M, García-Carrasco M. Introducing Polyautoimmunity: Secondary Autoimmune Diseases No Longer Exist. *Autoimmune Dis* (2012) 2012. doi: 10.1155/2012/254319
30. McAlinden C. An overview of thyroid eye disease. *Eye Vis* (2014) 1(1):1–4. doi: 10.1186/s40662-014-0009-8
31. Roos JCP, Moran C, Chatterjee VK, Jones J, Coles A, Murthy R. Immune reconstitution after alemtuzumab therapy for multiple sclerosis triggering Graves' orbitopathy: a case series. *Eye* (2019) 33(2):223–9. doi: 10.1038/s41433-018-0282-1
32. Regional ethnic diversity. GOV.UK Ethnicity facts and figures. https://www.ethnicity-facts-figures.service.gov.uk/uk-population-by-ethnicity/national-and-regional-populations/regional-ethnic-diversity/latest.
33. Koch CA, Krabbe S, Hehmke B. Statins, metformin, proprotein-convertase-subtilisin-kexin type-9 (PCSK9) inhibitors and sex hormones: Immunomodulatory properties? *Rev Endocr Metab Disord* (2018) 19:363–95. doi: 10.1007/s11154-018-9478-8
34. Bartalena L, Chiovato L, Marcocci C, Vitti P, Piantanida E, Tanda ML. Management of Graves' hyperthyroidism and orbitopathy in time of COVID-19 pandemic. *J Endocrinol Invest* (2020) 43(8):1149–51. doi: 10.1007/s40618-020-01293-7
35. Schön MP, Berking C, Biedermann T, Buhl T, Erpenbeck L, Eyerich K, et al. COVID-19 and immunological regulations – from basic and translational aspects to clinical implications. *JDDG J der Dtsch Dermatologischen Gesellschaft* (2020) 18: (8):795–807. doi: 10.1111/ddg.14169
36. TED Immunosuppression advice during Covid-19 – BOPSS. Available at: https://www.bopss.co.uk/covid/ted-immunosuppression-advice-during-covid-19.

11

Emerging Insights into the Role of Epigenetics and Gut Microbiome in the Pathogenesis of Graves' Ophthalmopathy

Yan Wang[1], *Xiao-Min Ma*[1], *Xin Wang*[2], *Xin Sun*[2], *Ling-Jun Wang*[2], *Xin-Qi Li*[2], *Xiao-Yan Liu*[2] *and Hong-Song Yu*[1*]

[1] *Department of Immunology, Special Key Laboratory of Ocular Diseases of Guizhou Province, Zunyi Medical University, Zunyi, China,* [2] *School of Basic Medical Sciences, Special Key Laboratory of Gene Detection and Therapy of Guizhou Province, Zunyi Medical University, Zunyi, China*

***Correspondence:**
Hong-Song Yu
yuhongsong@163.com

Graves' Ophthalmopathy (GO) is an organ-specific autoimmune disease that is often characterized by infiltration of orbital tissues and is considered as the most common extra-thyroid manifestation of Graves' disease (GD). Although genetic susceptibility has been found to be critical for the phenotype of GO, the associated risk alleles in a single gene are generally insufficient to cause the disease. Accruing evidence has shown that epigenetic disorders can act as the potentially missing link between genetic risk and clinically significant disease development. Abnormal epigenetic modifications can lead to pro-inflammatory cascades and activation of orbital fibroblasts (OFs) by promoting the various inflammatory response pathways and regulating the diverse signaling molecules that are involved in the fibrogenesis and adipogenesis, thereby leading to the significant expansion of orbital tissues, fibrosis and inflammation infiltration. Additionally, emerging evidence has shown that the gut microbiome can possibly drive the pathogenesis of GO by influencing the secretion of Thyrotropin receptor antibody (TRAb) and T-helper 17 (Th17)/regulatory T cells (Treg) imbalance. This paper describes the latest epigenetic research evidence and progress made in comprehending the mechanisms of GO development, such as DNA methylation, histone modification, non-coding RNAs, and the gut microbiome.

Keywords: Graves' ophthalmopathy, epigenetics, DNA methylation, histone modification, noncoding RNAs, gut microbiome

INTRODUCTION

Graves' ophthalmopathy (GO), also known as thyroid-related ophthalmopathy, is an autoimmune disease associated with Graves' disease (GD) that involves orbital tissues. It has been found that about 25% of GD patients develop GO during their disease course (1, 2). Approximately 90% of GO develop in hyperthyroidism caused by GD, whereas GO sometimes occurs in patients with euthyroid or hypothyroid chronic autoimmune thyroiditis (3, 4). Although the ratio of female to male (F/M) has been found to vary based on the different studies, the incidence of GO is significantly higher in women than in men (5). The common clinical characteristics of GO are eyelid retraction, swelling, exophthalmos, retrobulbar pain, and even vision impairment resulting from optic neuropathy (6). Similar to GD, the autoreactive inflammatory process of orbital tissue plays a major role in the pathogenesis of GO. The extraocular muscles and connective tissue of GO patients are infiltrated by activated monocytes (such as T cells), as well as a small number of plasma cells, macrophages and mast cells (7). Activated T cells, mainly $CD4^{+}$T cells, produce a large number of cytokines to amplify and maintain orbital inflammation and stimulate the proliferation of orbital fibroblasts (OFs) and the synthesis of glycosaminoglycans (GAG) (8). OFs are heterogeneous cells, and when activated, fibroblasts with a high level of thymocyte differentiation antigen 1(Thy1) surface expression (Thy1+) are more likely to form myofibroblasts, on the contrary, fibroblasts with little or no Thy1 (Thy1 -) are more likely to form adipocytes (9, 10). Accumulation of GAG leads to edema of extraocular muscles (11) and eventually leads to orbital swelling, tissue expansion and fibrosis development.

As mentioned above, cytokines and immune mechanisms play an important role in the pathogenesis of GO. $CD4^{+}$T cells can be divided into auxiliary T helper 1(Th1), Th2, Th17, regulatory T (Treg) cells and other subtypes, which are considered to be related to the occurrence and development of GO (8). Studies have shown that Th1 cytokines are not only related to the progression of GO, but may play a dominant role in the orbital involvement in the early stage of GO. On the contrary, Th2 cytokines have no direct correlation with disease progression, but may play a greater role in the later stage of the disease (12–14). IL-17A secreted by Th17 cells has pro-inflammatory and pro-fibrosis effects, which further drives the clinical manifestation of GO (15). Treg cells are a subgroup of T cells with immune regulatory function, and impaired Th17/Treg balance may also be an important cause of GO (16). Furthermore, activated T cells activate the differentiation of B cells into plasma cells and the production of antibodies by secreting IL-4 (8). GD related hyperthyroidism is primarily caused by binding of TRAb to the thyrotropin receptor (TSHR) on the thyroid follicular endothelial cells, thereby stimulating the excessive secretion of the thyroid hormones. Furthermore, recent studies have reported that TRAb can effectively stimulate the proliferation of OFs, which is positively correlated with the clinical features of GO and can adversely affect the prognosis (17). Another crucial autoantigen involved in the pathogenesis of GO is insulin-like growth factor I receptor (IGF-IR), which forms a physical and functional complex with TSHR in OFs from GO patients (18). Antibodies of the IgG class generated by GD patients are able to bind to IGF-1R and initiate the signaling from the TSHR/IGF-IR protein complex. Furthermore, Teprotumumab, an IGF-IR blocking monoclonal antibody, has been approved in the US FDA for the treatment of GO and works by attenuating signaling from TSHR or IGF-IR (19). Currently, substantial progress has been made in treating GO, but the moderate-to-severe GO patients usually do not completely respond to available medical treatments, and complete *restitutio ad integrum* almost never occurs (5, 20). Therefore, more extensive studies are needed to explore the pathogenesis of GO and develop prompt prediction, timely referral and novel therapeutic strategies for GO.

In the past decade, increasing evidence has shown that genetic susceptibility plays a crucial role in the pathogenesis of GD and GO (21–24), but the associated risk alleles in a single gene are generally insufficient to cause disease. Moreover, several studies have performed Human leukocyte antigen *(HLA)*, cytotoxic T lymphocyte antigen-4 *(CTLA4)*, Interleukin (IL) - 23 receptor *(IL23R)*, and *TSHR* genotyping on GO and non-GO patients in GD patients. The results show no statistical differences in allele and genotype frequency between the two groups, thereby plausibly suggesting that GO might not have significant genetic susceptibility in GD patients (25). These results suggested that epigenetics and/or environmental influences could possibly also play an important role in the pathogenesis of GO. Epigenetics as a research hotspot in recent years, researchers have found that the decreased level of *ICAM1* methylation is significantly associated with exophthalmos in patients with GD (26). Similarly, micro RNAs (miRNAs) have been correlated with the level of autoimmune antibodies such as TPOAb, TgAb and TRAb (27). These findings provided us with vital background to explore the potential pathogenesis of GO. A number of previous epigenetics related studies have shown that different environmental factors can also functionally regulate gene expression and phenotypes in the disease development process without altering the DNA sequences, primarily through epigenetic mechanisms such as those of DNA methylation, histone modification, and non-coding RNAs (28). Epigenetic modifications have been found to be involved in the dysregulation of the different signaling molecules and receptors in a variety of autoimmune/inflammatory conditions, including GO (29–32). Thus, epigenetic studies could serve as interesting targets for elucidating the pathogenesis of GO. Interestingly, all environmental factors involved in the pathogenesis of GD and GO can effectively alter the balance of microorganisms located in the gut and influence the immune system, particularly the proportion of Treg and Th17 cells. A recent study demonstrated that gut dysbiosis can lead to the imbalance of Th17/Treg through the propionic acid regulated pathway, and promote the occurrence of GD (33). A number of studies in GD/GO mice model have also shown that the gut microbiome might induce the clinical manifestation of GO by influencing the levels of TRAb and Th17/Treg imbalance (34, 35). Therefore, this paper reviews the latest epigenetics landscape and progress made in deciphering the mechanisms of GO by encompassing the various aspects of DNA methylation, histone modification, noncoding RNAs and gut microbiome, with an aim to provide new effective potential therapeutic strategies for the management of GO.

ABNORMAL DNA METHYLATION AND GO

As one of the most common forms of epigenetic modification, DNA methylation is catalyzed by DNA methyltransferases (DNMTs) by using S-adenosyl-L-methionine (SAM) as a methyl donor, and forming 5-methylcytosine (5-MC) by the transfer of the methyl group to the five carbon atoms of the CpG dinucleotide cytosine base. Accumulating evidence has suggested that DNA methylation in the promoter regions of the CpG island is primarily linked to gene transcriptional inhibition; and the methylated CpG binding domain (MBD) family can effectively recognize and bind to methylated CpG to cause significant transcriptional inhibition (36).

In recent years, several studies have shown that DNA methylation exhibits important functions in the pathogenesis of GO by altering the gene expression profile. Xin et al. (37) have identified 841 differentially methylated sites by sequencing the whole wide genomic DNA methylation in 6 patients with GO. It was found that 148 different genes were located near or at the methylation sites. These genes include various genes mediating immune responses such as Cluster of Differentiation 14 *(CD14)*, interleukin 17 receptor E *(IL17RE)*, beclin1*(BECN1)*, cyclin dependent kinase 5 *(CDK5)*, oxidative stress regulation genes including ATP-Binding cassette transporter superfamily D1 *(ABCD1)*, homeobox B13 *(HOXB13)*, thyroid function regulating gene such as dopamine receptor D4 *(DRD4)*. The aforementioned genes *IL17RE* and *CDK5* have been positively associated with Clinical Activity Score (CAS) and TRAb, respectively. The authors also performed enrichment of genes associated with the diverse biological processes, cellular composition, and molecular functions. To further understand the pathogenesis of GO, pathway analysis of these identified genes was carried out, and four potentially important pathways, including toxoplasmosis pathway, axon guidance pathway, focal adhesion pathway, and proteoglycans in cancer pathway, were found to be closely associated to the occurrence and development of GO. Moreover, other important pathway genes such as *LDLR*, *CDK5*, and phosphatidylinositol-4,5-bisphosphate 3-kinase catalytic subunit beta *(PIK3CB)* that play an important role in regulating inflammatory have also been found to be significantly correlated with GO phenotypes (32). These observations further confirmed the potential relationship between the DNA methylation level and its functions in the regulation of specific genes involved in the pathogenesis of GO. In another study, Shi et al. (38) carried out genome scale screening of DNA methylation in the peripheral blood samples of patients with GO and healthy controls. They next screened the different candidate genes with a good topological performance by constructing a gene regulatory network of hypermethylated and hypomethylated genes. They further expanded the sample for verification by monomethylated sequencing, thus confirming that, the methylation level of boule homolog *(BOLL)* was lower, and the methylation level of myelin basic protein *(MBP)* and *CDK5* was markedly higher. *BOLL*, *MBP*, and *CDK5* genes were found to be associated with increased risk of GO. The possible mechanism can be described by the fact that *MBP* is related to the activation of *MBP* specific CD8 lymphocytes and *CDK5* could promote oxidative stress. Khong et al. (39) used microarray analysis to detect the gene expression profile of orbital adipose tissue obtained from GO patients. In combination with gene set enrichment analysis (GSEA), they found that compared with inactive GO, the gene enrichment of active GO showed significantly more prominent epigenetic characteristics of acute myeloid leukemia (AML). Moreover, the abnormal hypomethylation of epigenetic markers in AML was associated with immunodeficiency signaling, cytotoxic T cell-mediated apoptosis, and dysregulation of T cell receptor signaling (40). In summary, the pathogenesis of GO is driven by aberrant DNA methylation of specific genes such as ABCD1 and PIK3CB, which may cause oxidative stress and immune dysregulation leading to inflammation (**Figure 1**).

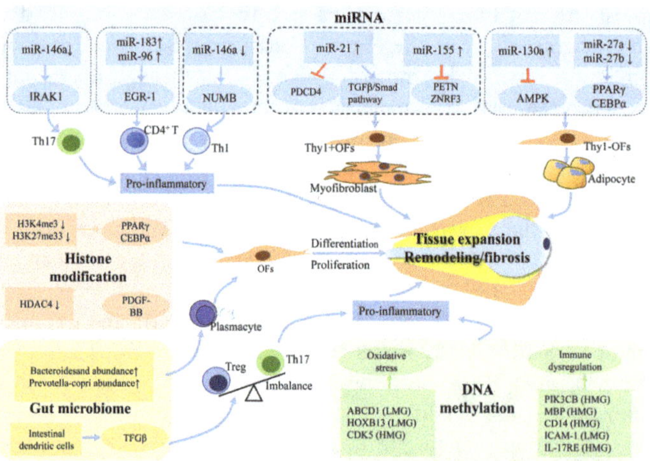

FIGURE 1 | Potential mechanism of epigenetics and gut microbiome in the pathogenesis of GO. Abnormal epigenetic modifications may promote pro-inflammatory cascades and disrupt the expression of signaling molecules that are involved in the fibrogenesis and adipogenesis of orbital fibroblasts. Gut microbiome possibly drives the pathogenesis of GO by influencing secretion of TRAb and Th17/Treg imbalance. The process of all these changes will lead to the hyaluronan production and the activation of orbital fibroblasts, which eventually develop into tissue expansion, fibrosis and inflammation. LMG, lowly methylated genes; HMG, highly methylated genes; TRAb, Thyrotropin receptor antibody; Treg, regulatory T; Th17, T-helper 17.

Furthermore, OFs play a crucial role in the initiation and maintenance of the inflammatory response as well as in orbital tissue expansion and remodeling. Hu et al. (41) performed DNA methylation sequencing and orbital computer tomography (CT) measurement on the peripheral blood samples from patients with GO and healthy controls. They found that the abnormal methylation of *MBP* gene was significantly correlated with the ratio of the total cross-sectional area of the orbital muscles (OM) to the total orbital area in GO patients. Virakul et al. (42) similarly carried out the detection of various OFs, and further reported that OFs in active versus inactive GO patients might have different proteomic and DNA methylation characteristics, thereby indicating that OFs can show specific pathological characteristics that might be related to the disease stage during the progression of GO. These observations highlighted the potential role of OFs as a future therapeutic target in GO. These findings also suggested that DNA methylation occurs in the fibroblasts and epigenetic understanding of the transition of OFs from "inflammatory/pre-lipogenic" to "remodeling/pre-fibrotic" effector cells should be a critical area of research in the future studies.

Genetic polymorphisms of a few selected DNA methylation regulatory genes can also lead to abnormal DNA methylation and dysfunction of these genes, which can further increase the susceptibility of the host (43). For example, methylenetetra-hydrofolate reductase *(MTHFR)* reduces 5, 10-methylenetra-hydrofolate to 5-methylenetrahydrofol -ate in the folic acid metabolic pathway, thus extending to the methyl transport pathway and indirectly facilitating methyl groups for the DNA methylation and protein methylation through the re-methylation of homocysteine residues. Lee et al. (44) reported that *MTHFR* polymorphism was closely associated with GO susceptibility and that *MTHFR 677 TT* can serve as an independent risk factor for GO. Moreover, SNPs *677C>T* of the *MTHFR* gene have been demonstrated to result in pronounced alteration of its enzymatic activity (45), providing indirect evidence for the important role of DNA methylation in GO pathogenesis.

Taken together, DNA methylation plays an important role in the occurrence and development of GO, but the related research is rather limited. Therefore, more studies are needed to explore the key role of DNA methylation in the pathogenesis of GO, to develop biomarkers for the rapid detection of early DNA methylation changes and establish effective GO treatment strategies.

HISTONE MODIFICATION AND GO

The nucleosome constitutes the basic structural unit of chromosomes. It consists of an octamer composed of four different pairs of core histones (H3, H4, H2A, and H2B) and a 147bp length of the double-stranded DNA surrounding the octamer. The core histones moieties are generally spherical, and the non-structural N-terminal amino acids extended by each histone can be modified after translation. The common histone modifications events include methylation, acetylation, phosphorylation, ubiquitination, adenosine diphosphate (ADP) ribosylation, etc. (46). Currently, histone modification studies have primarily focused on the methylation and acetylation, thereby providing some evidence for the possible role of histone modification in regulating immune tolerance and autoimmune thyroid diseases (47–49).

Histone methylation can be catalyzed by histone methyltransferase (HMT) and occurs mainly on the lysine and arginine residues of H3 and H4 histones, but the transcriptional output from histone methylation primarily depends on the nature of the specific residues involved. Histone H3 methylation is one of the most well characterized epigenetic modifications and actively involved in the adipogenesis of OFs. The differentiation of OFs into adipocytes is primarily a peroxisome proliferator-activated receptor gamma (*PPARγ*) and CCAAT/enhancer binding protein alpha (*CEBPα*) dependent process (50). Khong et al. (39) conducted GSEA on the expression profile of the various differentiated genes in the active phase of GO and found that the unmethylated histone H3 in the genes with high CpG density promoters (HCP) found in embryonic fibroblast was significantly downregulated compared with the normal controls. Methylation at K4 (H3K4me3) and K27 (H3K27me33) on histone 3, which is in bivalent status on HCP has been directly related to cell lineage commitment. *PPARγ* often remains in a bivalent state during embryonic fibroblast differentiation (51). Matsumura et al. (52) reported that the H3K4me3 and H3K27me3 bivalent state might change to H3K4/H3K9me3 during lineage specification. The characteristics of H3K4/H3K9me3 bivalent chromatin signature can possibly maintain *CEBPα* and *PPARγ* gene expression at a very low level in lineage-committed mesenchymal stem cells (MSCs) and preadipocytes by silencing or by maintaining developmental genes to poise for subsequent activation, and they may constitute a distinct pseudo heterochromatin/euchromatin boundary which is important for adipocyte differentiation. The above studies suggested that histone H3 methylation might play an important role in the pathogenesis of GO by targeting some genes that are related to adipogenesis. However, at present, there are only few related studies, and there are no reports to establish that abnormal histone methylation might be related to the occurrence of GO. Therefore, additional studies are needed to decipher the specific mechanisms underlying these observations.

Histone acetylation and deacetylation are important components of the gene regulatory machinery. Histone acetylation is usually catalyzed by histone acetyltransferase (HAT), and addition of acetyl groups to the target histones can activate the various transcription factors which can specifically bind to the different DNA binding sites and promote gene transcription. Histone deacetylase (HDAC) can also catalyze the deacetylation of histones to make DNA more tightly encapsulated around the nucleosomes, thus inhibiting gene expression (46). Histone acetylation and deacetylation can effectively maintain a dynamic balance in the nucleus. For example, loss of HDAC expression in the thyroid and immune cells of patients with autoimmune thyroid diseases has been confirmed (53). Recently, Ekronarongchai et al. (31) reported HDAC4 mRNA upregulation and protein expression in OFs by Platelet-Derived Growth Factor-BB (PDGF-BB). It was observed that the expression of HDAC4 mRNA in the OFs of GO patients was significantly higher as compared to the healthy control group, and the lysine 9 acetylation of histone H3 (H3K9ac) was markedly decreased under PDGF-BB stimulation. It was also found that the expression of hyaluronan synthase 2 (*HAS2*), collagen type I alpha 1 chain (*COL1A1*), proliferation marker Ki67 (*Ki67*), and α-smooth muscle actin (*α-SMA*) mRNA and the production of hyaluronic acid in PDGF-BB stimulated OFs were significantly decreased upon HDAC4 silencing. These data suggested that HDAC4-induced H3K9 deacetylation could potentially exacerbate GO OFs hyperproliferation and extracellular matrix production by functionally regulating PDGF-BB, thus suggesting that HDAC4 might serve as a new target for GO therapy.

Therefore, histone modification has been related to the occurrence and development of GO. Histone H3 methylation and HDAC may be potential targets for GO therapy, but the specific mechanisms are still not clear. More studies are needed to identify abnormal histone modifications associated with GO and to clarify their molecular mechanisms in GO.

NON-CODING RNAS AND GO

Non-coding RNAs are a class of RNA transcripts that lack the function of coding proteins. They can be classified into miRNAs, circular RNAs (circRNAs) and long noncoding RNAs (lncRNAs), which have been reported to play an important role in the pathogenesis of the various autoimmune thyroid diseases (54).

MiRNAs and GO

MiRNAs are endogenous small non-coding RNA molecules that contain 18 to 23 nucleotides in length, and that by binding to the untranslated 3' domain of the target gene mRNA, miRNAs can effectively mediate the degradation of mRNA or inhibit its translation, thus exerting a strong negative regulatory effect on the gene expression at the post-transcriptional level (55). MiRNAs can regulate more than 60% of protein- coding genes in the humans and have been implicated in the various biological processes such as the lineage commitment in the immune system, cell proliferation, differentiation, apoptosis, and maintenance of immune homeostasis (56, 57). An abnormal expression of miRNAs has been closely related to the pathogenesis of various autoimmune-mediated eye diseases such as GO (58). Circulating miRNAs can be detected in the peripheral blood and orbital tissues of GO patients, with different expression levels in the active disease stage of GO.

Circulating miRNAs and GO

A number of recent studies have shown that some circulating miRNAs might be directly involved in the development of GO, and have been found to be closely related to the regulation of differentiation or activation of immune cells and immune responses.

MiR-146a-5p is one of the most widely studied miRNAs and has an important role in regulating GO progression. MiR-146a is a typical multifunctional miRNA whose expression can be induced by toll-like receptor 4 (TLR4)/nuclear factor-kappa B (NF-κB) pathway, which acts as an important regulator of immune and inflammatory response pathways (59). By targeting tumor necrosis factor receptor-associated factor 6 (TRAF6) and IL-1 receptor-associated kinase 1 (IRAK1), miR-146a can negatively inhibit the feedback of NF-κB signaling cascade and modulate the signal transduction by the related receptors and subsequent cytokine release (60, 61). A few studies have shown that the peripheral blood level of miR-146a-5p in GO patients was significantly decreased as compared with their healthy counterparts as well as GD patients which lack GO phenotype (62–64). Additionally, reduced expression of miR-146a-5p has been negatively correlated with the CAS and IL-17 levels in GO patients. IL-17 levels have been positively correlated with CAS, and the downregulation of miR-146a can effectively lead to a paradoxical increase in IL-17 levels possibly due to their inability to inhibit IRAK1. This finding suggested that IRAK1 could play a key regulatory role in the differentiation of Th17 cell (62). The orbital tissues are infiltrated by activated mononuclear cell such as $CD4^+$ T cells, which exert a key role on GO activity (7). A number of recent studies have also suggested that the down-regulated expression of miR-146a in $CD4^+$T cells of GO patients might facilitate GO development by targeting NUMB genes, thus resulting in the development of inflammatory Th1 response, which can lead to orbital inflammation in GO patients (63, 64). In other words, the downregulation of circulating miR-146a may indirectly promote the development of GO by regulating the expression of various inflammatory mediators. Contrary to the downregulation of miR-146a, miR-155 levels have been reported to be increased in the peripheral venous blood in GO patients. In turn, both miR-155 and miR-146a have multiple target genes in the TLR4/NF-κB pathway, which can mutually regulate the immune response. The upregulation of miR-155 may also promote autoimmune inflammation through the targeted inhibition of cytokine signaling 1 (SOCS1) and SH2 domain-containing inositol-5-phosphatase 1 (SHIP1) (65). Other miRNAs such as miR-Let7d-5p, miR-96-5p and miR-301a-3p, were also found to be differentially expressed in the serum of GO patients versus control group, which might contribute to the regulated expression of the different inflammatory mediators *in vivo* and can lead to the occurrence as well as the development of GO (27). In addition, Thiel and colleagues (66) have reported an increased expression of miR-183 and miR-96 in $CD4^+$T cells of GO patients and in activated T cells of mice. It has been found that these two kinds of miRNAs promote the activation of $CD4^+$T cells by effectively regulating the expression of early growth response 1 (EGR-1), which can directly be related to the activation of PTEN/Akt signal axis, and thus participate in the occurrence as well as the development of GO. At present, based on the special characteristic of the differential expression of miRNAs, it will be of great significance to study the role of the various influencing factors involved in the pathogenesis and to decipher the mechanisms of the transition from an active stage to static stage, to facilitate early diagnosis and treatment possibilities of GO.

The clinical utility of miRNAs in GO has also been explored. For instance, Shen et al. (67) found that the low serum miR-224-

5p could be correlated with GO glucocorticoid (GC) insensitivity, and overexpression of miR-224-5p *in vitro* increased GC sensitivity and glucocorticoid receptor protein *via* targeting glycogen synthase kinase 3 beta. Moreover, the combination of baseline serum miR-224-5p and TRAb was an independent risk factor for GC insensitivity. Recently, a number of studies have analyzed the possible role of miRNAs in the assessment of GO severity and disease outcomes. One study by Martinez-Hernandez et al. (27) reported that miR-let7D-5P expression was markedly decreased in GO patients as compared with GD patients without GO and was also found to be negatively correlated with CAS. Meanwhile, Zhang et al. (68) performed miRNAs profiling of the thyroid tissues in GO patients using next-generation sequencing (NGS) and then identified their serum expression. They found that novel:19_15038 and hsa-miR-27a-3p were up-regulated in GO, while hsa-miR-22-3p was down-regulated in GO as compared to healthy controls. To sum up, the detection of the various differentially expressed miRNAs might be used as the potential biomarkers to predict the development and progression of GD into GO.

Orbital Tissue miRNAs and GO

OFs are both the target cell and effector cell in the pathogenesis process of GO. A number of recent studies have suggested that miRNA inhibitors or mimics can be used to up-regulate or down-regulate miRNAs expression in orbital tissues, thus regulating the corresponding biological behavior. Recent studies have also indicated that some miRNAs might be associated with orbital fibrosis, adipose tissue formation and inflammatory cell development.

For example, miR-146a acts as a key regulatory factor of GO orbital tissue fibrosis. To our knowledge, the level of miR-146a might be variable in the different types of tissues (63, 69). Unlike the downregulation of miR-146a in peripheral blood summarized previously, it is mostly up-regulated in orbital tissues. Wang et al. (69) reported that up-regulation of miR-146a in the orbital connective tissue of GO patients could significantly increase IL-6 level by inhibiting Notch2, thereby effectively promoting mitotic activity of fibroblasts in GO patients, inhibiting cellular apoptosis, and subsequently worsening the deterioration of GO. Woeller et al. (70) reported that TSHR signaling could induce the production of miR-146a and miR-155 on the OFs of GO patients. The expression of the different cell proliferation suppressor genes *ZNRF3* and *PTEN* were substantially decreased, thereby indirectly promoting the proliferation response of OFs, which could possibly explain the pathological mechanisms of partial fibroplasia observed in GO. However, a few studies have also shown that miR-146a can inhibit the fibrosis process. MiR-146a also plays an active role in the anti-inflammatory and anti-fibrotic processes of OFs. Jang et al. (71, 72) have reported that inflammatory stress can significantly up-regulate miR-146a expression in OFs, but inhibit the expression of IL-6, ICAM-1, and other inflammatory proteins. It can also negatively regulate levels of transforming growth factor beta (TGF-β) -induced fibrosis markers such as fibronectin (FN), collagen I α, and α -SMA. Type I collagen is considered to be a critical marker of fibrosis, and hyaluronic acid is a glycosaminoglycan. Liu et al. (73) recently reported that miR-146a expression was markedly down-regulated in the secretion of hyaluronic acid and type I collagen in GO OFs *in vitro*, which can reduce the aggregation of glycosaminoglycan and collagen deposition, and thereby delay the progression of the disease. Li et al. (65) hypothesized that miR-155, in contrast to miR-146a, can enhance the development of inflammatory T cells by promoting different autoimmune responses. In particular, the levels of miR146a in circulating and orbital tissues have been found to be inconsistent, which may be because the inflammation caused by miR-146 in peripheral blood may not fully reflect the inflammation in orbit. What is more, the contradictory functions about the relationship between miR-146a and differentiation of OFs can also be difficult to interpret, mainly due to the manifestation of the different targeting effects. Furthermore, miR-146a was found to play different functions in the regulation of the diverse signaling pathways or in interactions with the different target mRNAs. However, elucidation of the detailed mechanism of miR-146 in GO requires further investigation.

In addition to miR-146a, miR-21 has also been reported to play an important role in orbital muscle fibrogenesis. Lee et al. (74) found that in human OFs, PDGF-BB can significantly inhibit the expression of Programmed cell death factor 4 (PDCD4) by up-regulating miR-21, and thus promoting the proliferation of OFs. It is consistent with the study that the translation of PDCD4 was inhibited by miR-21 by Young et al. (75). Therefore, PDGF-BB/miRNA-21/PDCD4 pathway might form the basis of novel strategies for developing therapeutic interventions against GO. Tong et al. (76) reported that expression of miR-21-5p in GO eye fibroblasts was markedly higher than that of the control group and that it could enhance TGF-β 1-induced expression of total type I collagen and mRNA level of type I collagen. In addition, anti-miR-21 not only blocked decapentaplegic3 (Smad3) phosphorylation but can also mimic activated Smad3 phosphorylation. These results suggested that miR-21 could substantially enhance Smad3 phosphorylation and activate TGF-β/Smad signaling pathway to participate in orbital muscle fibrogenesis. In summary, these studies indicated that miR-21 may provide new targets for the treatment of GO.

Adipogenesis has been found to be closely related to the degree of ocular protruding (77). Therefore, efforts are being made to find effective ways to block the adipogenesis pathway as a new therapeutic option. Hammond et al. (78) reported that when Thy1- OFs were accumulated in GO, the miR-130a level was significantly increased, resulting in the decreased AMPK activity and promotion of the fat accumulation in orbit. Moreover, the expression level of miR-27a and miR-27b in the orbital adipose tissue of GO patients was significantly lower than that of the controls, which explains the inability to negatively regulate the mRNA expression of the various adipogenic genes such as *PPARγ* and *CEBPβ* in GO fibroblasts, thus indirectly causing the adipogenic differentiation of OFs (79). Therefore, blocking orbital muscle fibrogenesis and adipose generating pathways through modulating miRNA expression could provide novel therapeutic options.

In summary, multiple miRNAs can play an important role in the occurrence as well as the development of GO, and especially miR-146a may serve as an important target (**Table 1**). However,

TABLE 1 | Non-coding RNAs in the pathogenesis of GO.

Noncoding-RNAs	Samples/ cells	Expression change	Function	Effects in GO	References
miR-146a	Plasma	Downregulation	Promote the differentiation of Th17 cell	Pro-inflammatory	(62)
	CD4+ T	Downregulation	Increase Th1 response	Pro-inflammatory	(63, 64)
	Orbital tissue	Upregulation	Increase the IL-6 level	Exacerbate GO	(69)
	Orbital tissue	Upregulation	Decreases FN, collagen Iα, and α -SMA	Inhibit fibrosis process	(72, 73)
miR-183 and miR-96	CD4+ T	Upregulation	Contribute to the activation of CD4+ T cells	Pro-inflammatory	(66)
miR-21-5P	Orbital tissue	Upregulation	Promote collagen Iα and total collagen production	Promote fibrogenesis	(76)
miR-146a and miR-155	Orbital tissue	Upregulation	Reducing the expression of PTEN and ZNRF3	Promote proliferation	(70)
m iR-27a and miR-27b	Orbital tissue	Downregulation	Cause the adipogenic differentiation of OFs	Promote adipogenesis	(79)
m iR-130a	Orbital tissue	Upregulation	Enhance lipid accumulation	Fatty tissue accumulation	(78)
circRNA_14940	Orbital tissue	Upregulation	Regulate the Wnt signaling pathway, ECM receptor interaction and PIK3-AKT signaling pathway	Participate in the pathogenesis of GO	(80)

the therapeutic applications of miRNA have not been fully developed, and hence more studies are needed to clarify the possible effects of miRNAs on other target genes in GO or its pathogenesis. In the future, miRNAs are expected to aid significantly in the precise diagnosis and targeted therapy of GO.

Other Noncoding RNAs and GO

CircRNAs are endogenous entities formed by the covalent binding of 3' and 5' end reverse splicing, which can display important biological functions in acting as miRNA sponge adsorption, attaching to the different RNA-binding proteins, and participating in protein translation (81, 82). However, the role of circRNAs in GO development is still in its infancy. For example, Wu et al. identified (80) 163 differentially expressed circRNAs from the orbital fat/connective tissues of GO patients. Through circRNA-mRNA co-expression and circRNA-mRNA interaction analysis, possible crosstalk of circRNA_14940 with down-regulated mRNA tenascin XB *(TNXB)* and up-regulated mRNA cyclin D1(*CCND1)* was analyzed and it was observed that abnormal regulation of the Wnt signaling pathway, PI3K-Akt signaling cascade, and extracellular matrix (ECM) receptor might also be involved in the pathogenesis of GO. CircRNA_10135 can also interact with prostaglandin F receptor (PTGFR) through modulating the calcium signaling pathway and participating in the adipogenesis process of GO. Meanwhile, circRNA_14936 has been found to be correlated with up-regulated mRNA TNF receptor superfamily member 19 (TNFRSF19), and hsa-miR-10392-3p that may potentially affect the occurrence and development of GO by regulating the interactions between circRNA_14936 and TNFRSF19 which can influence B cell survival. Therefore, circRNAs might play an important role in the pathogenesis and progression of GO (**Table 1**). However, there are only few studies conducted to evaluate the role of circRNAs in the pathogenicity of GO, so the functions of most circRNAs are not clear and their molecular mechanism remains to be further elucidated.

LncRNAs are an important class of non-coding RNAs with a length of more than 200 nucleotides. LncRNAs can regulate the gene expression through affecting various mechanisms, including those related to epigenetics, transcriptional, post-transcriptional, and miRNAs regulation. A number of previous studies have reported that lncRNAs may play an important role in the pathogenesis of GD (83). For instance, Christensen et al. (84) reported the first lncRNA Heg to be associated with GD and showed that was negatively correlated with monocyte CD14 mRNA and serum TRAb level in GD patients. Moreover, anti-thyroid therapy could not change lncRNA Heg level in GD patients. The intimate temporal relationship between the onset of GD and GO also clearly suggests that these two diseases may have the same underlying etiology. Xia et al. (85) identified a novel lncRNA named Lnc-Smad3, which can maintain the tight chromatin structure of Smad3 promoter through direct interaction with HDAC1, thereby inhibiting Smad3 transcription and affecting inducible Treg (iTreg) cell polarization through modulating the TGFβ/Smad3 signaling pathway.

LncRNAs are also involved in the development of Treg cells, which provides a new direction to further study of the possible relationship between Lnc-Smad3 and GO. Although there are some difficulties in screening and studying lncRNAs, identifying their role and mechanism in GO may be a necessary direction for future research.

GUT MICROBIOME AND GO

The human gut microbiome consists of about 100 trillion different gut microbial cells and serves as the main entry point for bacteria. In a symbiotic manner, the human host primarily provides the gut microbiota with crucial nutrients for promoting growth. In contrast, the gut microbes play an important role in the food digestion, detoxification, protection from pathogens, and the regulation of the host immune system. In fact, the highest concentration of T cells in the human body is located in the intestinal mucosa, where lymphocytes are primed to respond to the various microorganisms. Furthermore, the intestinal microbiome can also effectively regulate the local intestinal immune system and the systemic immune response (86, 87).

Moreover, multiple human and animal studies have shown that gut microbiome have been closely related to a variety of autoimmune diseases, such as inflammatory colitis (IBD) (88), rheumatoid arthritis (RA) (89), type I diabetes (T1D) (90), and systemic lupus erythematosus (SLE) (91). For instance, Jiang et al. (92) sequenced the fecal samples of patients with GD and healthy controls, and found that the richness of intestinal microflora in patients with GD decreased significantly. This alteration was characterized by a significant increase in *Bacteroides*, which damaged intestinal barrier function, resulting in the release of a large number of pro-inflammatory factors outside the intestine, thus resulting in immune dysfunction. In addition, it was also found that changes in thyroid hormone levels can lead to an increase in the number of *Lactobacillus.* It may play a harmful role in GD by activating NF- κB signaling pathway and autoimmune response to thyroid gland. At present, there are only few studies on intestinal flora in GO. Several reports have suggested that there is a marked decrease in bacterial community diversity in GO. Shi et al. (93) sequenced the fecal samples of patients with GO and healthy controls and found that compared with the control group, the proportion of *Bacteroidetes* and *Prevotellaceae* in patients with GO at different levels increased significantly, while the proportion of *Blautia* and *Fusicatenibacter* decreased significantly. The proportion of the *Succinivibrionaceae* and *Subdoligranulum* was positively correlated with TRAb, and there was a negative correlation between *Parabacteroides_disasonis* and TRAb. Further analysis showed that *Prevotellaceae* could clearly distinguish GO patients from the control group. The level of *s_Prevotea_copri* was reported to be positively correlated with the level of serum TRAb, which may be related to active orbital inflammation (94). Thereafter, the researchers conducted a comparative analysis of GD, GO and healthy people for the first time. They found that the proportion of *Deinococcus-Thermus* and *Chloroflexi* in patients with GO was significantly lower than that in GD (95). Interestingly, after transplanting the normal human feces into type 2 diabetic mice, researchers found that the abundance of *Bacteroides* and some bacteria decreased and blood glucose levels recovered. This led to the speculation that it may be possibly increasing the diversity of intestinal microflora that can affect the different types of microorganisms in the intestines of mice to achieve the effect of treatment (96). Therefore, whether fecal microbiome transplantation can also have a therapeutic effect on GO can be an important direction for future research. Additional in-depth studies about the role of intestinal microorganisms in GO will possibly provide new methods and ideas for the treatment of GO. In addition, some studies have reported that Salmonella that can cause enteritis possesses an antigenic cluster similar to the thyroid stimulating hormone receptor protein, where antibodies against the thyrotropin receptor proteins might be produced after infection (96). These results laid a sound foundation for exploring the interaction between intestinal microorganisms and TRAb. However, the current findings may also be related to thyroid autoimmunity rather than GO, and might not be entirely specific for GO.

Masetti et al. (34) used intramuscular injection of eukaryotic expression plasmid (thyroid stimulating receptor) in two distinct experimental centers in two different countries (Center 1 and 2). The GD/GO disease model of BALB/C female mice was established by immunological method of TSHR. The results showed that only BALB/C mice from Center 2 displayed hyperthyroidism and apparent changes in orbital tissues. Interestingly, it was found that the abundance and species composition of intestinal flora were significantly different between BALB/C mice tested from the two centers by 16S rRNA gene sequencing and traditional microbial culture. In Center 2, the intestinal flora structure of different intervention groups (TSHR group, β Gal group) was analyzed by 16S rRNA gene sequencing and it was found that the intestinal flora of TSHR group changed significantly (increased relative abundance of *Lactobacillus*, decreased relative abundance of *bacteroides*, etc.). These alterations were also associated with some clinical features such as thyroxine levels (fT4), TRAb, orbital adipogenesis, and muscular atrophy. The same group constructed another GD/GO model by using BALB/c and C57BL/6J mice. The results indicated that the C57BL/6 mice had higher TRAb, but compared with BALB/c mice, the spleen T cells of C57BL/6 mice exhibited poor proliferation of TSHR response, and secreted mainly anti-inflammatory cytokines such as IL-10, without elevated thyroxine levels or any orbital lesions, while resembling immunized BALB/C mice showed orbital pathology. These observations suggested that there was a different pattern of correlation between the microbiomes and disease (endocrine and immune) characteristics between the two different mouse strains (97). In addition, Shi et al. (94) found that operational taxonomic units (OTUs) derived from the *bacteroidesstercoris* species were markedly associated with the thyroglobulin autoantibodies, whereas OTUs from the *bacteroides* genus were associated with CAS. Masetti et al. (98) deciphered that the effect of intestinal microorganisms on the immune system can be primarily revealed by maintaining a balance between the Tregs and pro-inflammatory Th17 cells and Th1 cells. When the microbiome might not be ideal, intestinal dendritic cells can secrete TGF-β, which can cause the Th17/Treg imbalance, thus leading to the loss of immune tolerance. In individuals with a particular genetic predisposition, the result can potentially lead to GD and GO. These results clearly suggested that the gut microbiome could play a critical role in shaping the immune response that might significantly influence the TRAb levels and immune tolerance, thereby influencing thyroid and eye disease phenotypes.

The above studies have provided a novel perspective research pathway to clarify the potential mechanisms of intestinal microbiome disorders observed in GO. Hence, understanding that how the composition of the gut bacterial microbiome and the abundance of specific bacterial strains might affect the autoimmune response in GD and GO remains the next important aspect.

CONCLUSION

With the emergence of novel bioinformatics tools and high-throughput gene sequencing technologies, the important role of epigenetics and gut microbiomes in GO has been gradually elucidated (**Figure 1**). Still, several crucial mechanisms especially from GD to GO remain unclear. At present, the study of GO epigenetics focuses primarily on only one kind of epigenetic modifications, but the role of its regulatory network in controlling molecular mechanisms of GO remains unknown. Therefore, there is an unmet need to conduct a combined analysis of the varying epigenetic modifications that can further explore the possible roles of various less explored epigenetic factors that have been implicated in the pathogenesis of GO.

Epigenetic inheritance can link environmental factors and diseases. How environmental factors can lead to the progression of GO by facilitating epigenetic inheritance and intestinal microbial dysregulation in GO remains to be elucidated. To date, GO is clinically diagnosed by an ophthalmologist with an adjunct imaging such as CT or magnetic resonance imaging (MRI). A few studies have shown that some epigenetic markers and intestinal microflora might be different in GD patients with or without GO. However, it is still difficult to predict which GD patients will develop into GO or severe GO, and which GD patients will be responsive or unresponsive to the different types of treatment. Further studies should focus on the current challenges in the future.

AUTHOR CONTRIBUTIONS

YW and H-SY participated in the conceptualization and writing. X-MM, XW, XS, L-JW, X-QL, and X-YL participated in the review and editing. All authors contributed to the article and approved the submitted version.

FUNDING

This work was supported by National Key R&D Program of China (grant number: 2018YFC1004300), National Natural Science Foundation Project of China (grant number: 82160154, 81670844), the Key Project of Guizhou Provincial Science and Technology Department (grant number: QKH-JC-2019-1464), the Excellent Talent Support Program of Guizhou Provincial Education Department (grant number: QJH-KY-2017-077), the Science and Technology Foundation of Guizhou Province (grant number: QKH-PTRC-2018-5772-042), the Science and Technology Project of Zunyi (grant number: ZSKH-HZ-2020-35), and the Program for Excellent Young Talents of Zunyi Medical University (grant number: 18-ZY-001).

REFERENCES

1. Edmunds MR, Boelaert K. Knowledge of Thyroid Eye Disease in Graves' Disease Patients With and Without Orbitopathy. *Thyroid* (2019) 29(4):557–62. doi: 10.1089/thy.2018.0665
2. Tanda ML, Piantanida E, Liparulo L, Veronesi G, Lai A, Sassi L, et al. Prevalence and Natural History of Graves' Orbitopathy in a Large Series of Patients With Newly Diagnosed Graves' Hyperthyroidism Seen at a Single Center. *J Clin Endocrinol Metab* (2013) 98(4):1443–9. doi: 10.1210/jc.2012-3873
3. Bahn RS. Graves' Ophthalmopathy. *N Engl J Med* (2010) 362(8):726–38. doi: 10.1056/NEJMra0905750
4. Bartley GB. The Epidemiologic Characteristics and Clinical Course of Ophthalmopathy Associated With Autoimmune Thyroid Disease in Olmsted County, Minnesota. *Trans Am Ophthalmol Soc* (1994) 92:477–588.
5. Bartalena L, Piantanida E, Gallo D, Lai A, Tanda ML. Epidemiology, Natural History, Risk Factors, and Prevention of Graves' Orbitopathy. *Front Endocrinol (Lausanne)* (2020) 11:615993. doi: 10.3389/fendo.2020.615993
6. Bartalena L, Baldeschi L, Boboridis K, Eckstein A, Kahaly GJ, Marcocci C, et al. The 2016 European Thyroid Association/European Group on Graves' Orbitopathy Guidelines for the Management of Graves' Orbitopathy. *Eur Thyroid J* (2016) 5(1):9–26. doi: 10.1159/000443828
7. Rotondo Dottore G, Torregrossa L, Lanzolla G, Mariotti S, Menconi F, Piaggi P, et al. Role of the Mononuclear Cell Infiltrate in Graves' Orbitopathy (GO): Results of a Large Cohort Study. *J Endocrinol Invest* (2021). doi: 10.1007/s40618-021-01692-4
8. Huang Y, Fang S, Li D, Zhou H, Li B, Fan X. The Involvement of T Cell Pathogenesis in Thyroid-Associated Ophthalmopathy. *Eye (Lond)* (2019) 33(2):176–82. doi: 10.1038/s41433-018-0279-9
9. Kuriyan AE, Woeller CF, O'Loughlin CW, Phipps RP, Feldon SE. Orbital Fibroblasts From Thyroid Eye Disease Patients Differ in Proliferative and Adipogenic Responses Depending on Disease Subtype. *Invest Ophthalmol Vis Sci* (2013) 54(12):7370–7. doi: 10.1167/iovs.13-12741
10. Koumas L, Smith TJ, Phipps RP. Fibroblast Subsets in the Human Orbit: Thy-1+ and Thy-1- Subpopulations Exhibit Distinct Phenotypes. *Eur J Immunol* (2002) 32(2):477–85. doi: 10.1002/1521-4141(200202)32:2<477::aid-immu477>3.0.co;2-u
11. Wiersinga WM, Prummel MF. Pathogenesis of Graves' Ophthalmopathy–Current Understanding. *J Clin Endocrinol Metab* (2001) 86(2):501–3. doi: 10.1210/jcem.86.2.7338
12. Wakelkamp IM, Bakker O, Baldeschi L, Wiersinga WM, Prummel MF. TSH-R Expression and Cytokine Profile in Orbital Tissue of Active vs. Inactive Graves' Ophthalmopathy Patients. *Clin Endocrinol (Oxf)* (2003) 58(3):280–7. doi: 10.1046/j.1365-2265.2003.01708.x
13. Aniszewski JP, Valyasevi RW, Bahn RS. Relationship Between Disease Duration and Predominant Orbital T Cell Subset in Graves' Ophthalmopathy. *J Clin Endocrinol Metab* (2000) 85(2):776–80. doi: 10.1210/jcem.85.2.6333
14. Xia N, Zhou S, Liang Y, Xiao C, Shen H, Pan H, et al. CD4+ T Cells and the Th1/Th2 Imbalance Are Implicated in the Pathogenesis of Graves' Ophthalmopathy. *Int J Mol Med* (2006) 17(5):911–6.
15. Fang S, Huang Y, Wang S, Zhang Y, Luo X, Liu L, et al. IL-17a Exacerbates Fibrosis by Promoting the Proinflammatory and Profibrotic Function of Orbital Fibroblasts in TAO. *J Clin Endocrinol Metab* (2016) 101(8):2955–65. doi: 10.1210/jc.2016-1882
16. Lv M, Shen J, Li Z, Zhao D, Chen Z, Wan H, et al. [Role of Treg/Th17 Cells and Related Cytokines in Graves' Ophthalmopathy]. *Nan Fang Yi Ke Da Xue Xue Bao = J South Med Univ* (2014) 34(12):1809–13.
17. Eckstein AK, Plicht M, Lax H, Neuhäuser M, Mann K, Lederbogen S, et al. Thyrotropin Receptor Autoantibodies Are Independent Risk Factors for Graves' Ophthalmopathy and Help to Predict Severity and Outcome of the Disease. *J Clin Endocrinol Metab* (2006) 91(9):3464–70. doi: 10.1210/jc.2005-2813

18. Tsui S, Naik V, Hoa N, Hwang CJ, Afifiyan NF, Sinha Hikim A, et al. Evidence for an Association Between Thyroid-Stimulating Hormone and Insulin-Like Growth Factor 1 Receptors: A Tale of Two Antigens Implicated in Graves' Disease. *J Immunol* (2008) 181(6):4397–405. doi: 10.4049/jimmunol.181.6.4397
19. Smith TJ. Insulin-Like Growth Factor Pathway and the Thyroid. *Front Endocrinol (Lausanne)* (2021) 12:653627. doi: 10.3389/fendo.2021.653627
20. Bartalena L, Kahaly G, Baldeschi L, Dayan C, Eckstein A, Marcocci C, et al. The 2021 European Group on Graves' Orbitopathy (EUGOGO) Clinical Practice Guidelines for the Medical Management of Graves' Orbitopathy. *Eur J Endocrinol* (2021) 185(4):G43–g67. doi: 10.1530/eje-21-0479
21. Hadj-Kacem H, Rebuffat S, Mnif-Feki M, Belguith-Maalej S, Ayadi H, Peraldi-Roux S. Autoimmune Thyroid Diseases: Genetic Susceptibility of Thyroid-Specific Genes and Thyroid Autoantigens Contributions. *Int J Immunogenet* (2009) 36(2):85–96. doi: 10.1111/j.1744-313X.2009.00830.x
22. Yin X, Latif R, Bahn R, Tomer Y, Davies TF. Influence of the TSH Receptor Gene on Susceptibility to Graves' Disease and Graves' Ophthalmopathy. *Thyroid* (2008) 18(11):1201–6. doi: 10.1089/thy.2008.0098
23. Du J, Wang X, Tan G, Wei W, Zhou F, Liang Z, et al. Predisposition to Graves' Disease and Graves' Ophthalmopathy by Genetic Variants of IL2RA. *J Mol Med (Berl)* (2021) 99(10):1487–95. doi: 10.1007/s00109-021-02111-0
24. Zhou F, Liang Z, Wang X, Tan G, Wei W, Zheng G, et al. The VDR Gene Confers a Genetic Predisposition to Graves' Disease and Graves' Ophthalmopathy in the Southwest Chinese Han Population. *Gene* (2021) 793:145750. doi: 10.1016/j.gene.2021.145750
25. Yin X, Latif R, Bahn R, Davies TF. Genetic Profiling in Graves' Disease: Further Evidence for Lack of a Distinct Genetic Contribution to Graves' Ophthalmopathy. *Thyroid* (2012) 22(7):730–6. doi: 10.1089/thy.2012.0007
26. Shalaby SM, Mackawy AMH, Atef DM, Atef RM, Saeed J. Promoter Methylation and Expression of Intercellular Adhesion Molecule 1 Gene in Blood of Autoimmune Thyroiditis Patients. *Mol Biol Rep* (2019) 46(5):5345–53. doi: 10.1007/s11033-019-04990-6
27. Martinez-Hernandez R, Sampedro-Nunez M, Serrano-Somavilla A, Ramos-Levi AM, de la Fuente H, Trivino JC, et al. A MicroRNA Signature for Evaluation of Risk and Severity of Autoimmune Thyroid Diseases. *J Clin Endocrinol Metab* (2018) 103(3):1139–50. doi: 10.1210/jc.2017-02318
28. Feil R, Fraga MF. Epigenetics and the Environment: Emerging Patterns and Implications. *Nat Rev Genet* (2012) 13(2):97–109. doi: 10.1038/nrg3142
29. Wang B, Shao X, Song R, Xu D, Zhang JA. The Emerging Role of Epigenetics in Autoimmune Thyroid Diseases. *Front Immunol* (2017) 8:396. doi: 10.3389/fimmu.2017.00396
30. Mazzone R, Zwergel C, Artico M, Taurone S, Ralli M, Greco A, et al. The Emerging Role of Epigenetics in Human Autoimmune Disorders. *Clin Epigenet* (2019) 11(1):34. doi: 10.1186/s13148-019-0632-2
31. Ekronarongchai S, Palaga T, Saonanon P, Pruksakorn V, Hirankarn N, van Hagen PM, et al. Histone Deacetylase 4 Controls Extracellular Matrix Production in Orbital Fibroblasts From Graves' Ophthalmopathy Patients. *Thyroid* (2021) 31(10):1566–76. doi: 10.1089/thy.2020.0948
32. Xin Z, Hua L, Yang YL, Shi TT, Liu W, Tuo X, et al. A Pathway Analysis Based on Genome-Wide DNA Methylation of Chinese Patients With Graves' Orbitopathy. *BioMed Res Int* (2019) 2019:9565794. doi: 10.1155/2019/9565794
33. Su X, Yin X, Liu Y, Yan X, Zhang S, Wang X, et al. Gut Dysbiosis Contributes to the Imbalance of Treg and Th17 Cells in Graves' Disease Patients by Propionic Acid. *J Clin Endocrinol Metab* (2020) 105(11):dgaa511. doi: 10.1210/clinem/dgaa511
34. Masetti G, Moshkelgosha S, Kohling HL, Covelli D, Banga JP, Berchner-Pfannschmidt U, et al. Gut Microbiota in Experimental Murine Model of Graves' Orbitopathy Established in Different Environments may Modulate Clinical Presentation of Disease. *Microbiome* (2018) 6(1):97. doi: 10.1186/s40168-018-0478-4
35. Moshkelgosha S, Verhasselt HL, Masetti G, Covelli D, Biscarini F, Horstmann M, et al. Modulating Gut Microbiota in a Mouse Model of Graves' Orbitopathy and Its Impact on Induced Disease. *Microbiome* (2021) 9 (1):45. doi: 10.1186/s40168-020-00952-4
36. Zhu H, Wang G, Qian J. Transcription Factors as Readers and Effectors of DNA Methylation. *Nat Rev Genet* (2016) 17(9):551–65. doi: 10.1038/nrg.2016.83
37. Xin Z, Hua L, Shi TT, Tuo X, Yang FY, Li Y, et al. A Genome-Wide DNA Methylation Analysis in Peripheral Blood From Patients Identifies Risk Loci Associated With Graves' Orbitopathy. *J Endocrinol Invest* (2018) 41(6):719–27. doi: 10.1007/s40618-017-0796-6
38. Shi TT, Hua L, Xin Z, Li Y, Liu W, Yang YL. Identifying and Validating Genes With DNA Methylation Data in the Context of Biological Network for Chinese Patients With Graves' Orbitopathy. *Int J Endocrinol* (2019) 2019:6212681. doi: 10.1155/2019/6212681
39. Khong JJ, Wang LY, Smyth GK, McNab AA, Hardy TG, Selva D, et al. Differential Gene Expression Profiling of Orbital Adipose Tissue in Thyroid Orbitopathy. *Invest Ophthalmol Vis Sci* (2015) 56(11):6438–47. doi: 10.1167/iovs.15-17185
40. Figueroa ME, Lugthart S, Li Y, Erpelinck-Verschueren C, Deng X, Christos PJ, et al. DNA Methylation Signatures Identify Biologically Distinct Subtypes in Acute Myeloid Leukemia. *Cancer Cell* (2010) 17(1):13–27. doi: 10.1016/j.ccr.2009.11.020
41. Hu YF, Hua L, Tuo X, Shi TT, Yang YL, Liu YF, et al. Preliminary Evidence of the Association Between DNAm and Orbital Volumetry in GO. *Endocr Connect* (2020) 9(7):617–26. doi: 10.1530/EC-20-0147
42. Virakul S, Somparn P, Pisitkun T, van der Spek PJ, Dalm V, Paridaens D, et al. Integrative Analysis of Proteomics and DNA Methylation in Orbital Fibroblasts From Graves' Ophthalmopathy. *Front Endocrinol (Lausanne)* (2020) 11:619989. doi: 10.3389/fendo.2020.619989
43. Kato N, Loh M, Takeuchi F, Verweij N, Wang X, Zhang W, et al. Trans-Ancestry Genome-Wide Association Study Identifies 12 Genetic Loci Influencing Blood Pressure and Implicates a Role for DNA Methylation. *Nat Genet* (2015) 47(11):1282–93. doi: 10.1038/ng.3405
44. Lee JY, Kim NK, Cho YW, Lew H. Association Between Methylenetetrahydrofolate Reductase (MTHFR) Polymorphisms and Susceptibility to Graves' Ophthalmopathy. *Mol Med Rep* (2016) 14 (3):2276–82. doi: 10.3892/mmr.2016.5458
45. Mao R, Fan Y, Zuo L, Geng D, Meng F, Zhu J, et al. Association Study Between Methylenetetrahydrofolate Reductase Gene Polymorphisms and Graves' Disease. *Cell Biochem Funct* (2010) 28(7):585–90. doi: 10.1002/cbf.1694
46. Kouzarides T. Chromatin Modifications and Their Function. *Cell* (2007) 128 (4):693–705. doi: 10.1016/j.cell.2007.02.005
47. Yan N, Zhou JZ, Zhang JA, Cai T, Zhang W, Wang Y, et al. Histone Hypoacetylation and Increased Histone Deacetylases in Peripheral Blood Mononuclear Cells From Patients With Graves' Disease. *Mol Cell Endocrinol* (2015) 414:143–7. doi: 10.1016/j.mce.2015.05.037
48. Stefan M, Wei C, Lombardi A, Li CW, Concepcion ES, Inabnet WB3rd, et al. Genetic-Epigenetic Dysregulation of Thymic TSH Receptor Gene Expression Triggers Thyroid Autoimmunity. *Proc Natl Acad Sci U S A* (2014) 111 (34):12562–7. doi: 10.1073/pnas.1408821111
49. Limbach M, Saare M, Tserel L, Kisand K, Eglit T, Sauer S, et al. Epigenetic Profiling in CD4+ and CD8+ T Cells From Graves' Disease Patients Reveals Changes in Genes Associated With T Cell Receptor Signaling. *J Autoimmun* (2016) 67:46–56. doi: 10.1016/j.jaut.2015.09.006
50. Jung SJ, Choi YJ, Park TK, Woo SE, Kim BY, Yoon JS, et al. Wnt Signalling Inhibits Adipogenesis in Orbital Fibroblasts From Patients With Graves' Orbitopathy. *Br J Ophthalmol* (2021). doi: 10.1136/bjophthalmol-2020-316898
51. Mikkelsen TS, Ku M, Jaffe DB, Issac B, Lieberman E, Giannoukos G, et al. Genome-Wide Maps of Chromatin State in Pluripotent and Lineage-Committed Cells. *Nature* (2007) 448(7153):553–60. doi: 10.1038/nature06008
52. Matsumura Y, Nakaki R, Inagaki T, Yoshida A, Kano Y, Kimura H, et al. H3K4/H3K9me3 Bivalent Chromatin Domains Targeted by Lineage-Specific DNA Methylation Pauses Adipocyte Differentiation. *Mol Cell* (2015) 60 (4):584–96. doi: 10.1016/j.molcel.2015.10.025
53. Sacristan P, Serrano-Somavilla A, Gonzalez-Amaro R, Martinez-Hernandez R, Marazuela M. Analysis of Expression of Different Histone Deacetylases in Autoimmune Thyroid Disease. *J Clin Endocrinol Metab* (2021) 106(11):3213–27. doi: 10.1210/clinem/dgab526
54. Yin L, Zeng C, Yao J, Shen J. Emerging Roles for Noncoding RNAs in Autoimmune Thyroid Disease. *Endocrinology* (2020) 161(8):bqaa053. doi: 10.1210/endocr/bqaa053

55. Mehta A, Baltimore D. MicroRNAs as Regulatory Elements in Immune System Logic. *Nat Rev Immunol* (2016) 16(5):279–94. doi: 10.1038/nri.2016.40
56. Friedman RC, Farh KK, Burge CB, Bartel DP. Most Mammalian mRNAs Are Conserved Targets of microRNAs. *Genome Res* (2009) 19(1):92–105. doi: 10.1101/gr.082701.108
57. Chen JQ, Papp G, Szodoray P, Zeher M. The Role of microRNAs in the Pathogenesis of Autoimmune Diseases. *Autoimmun Rev* (2016) 15(12):1171–80. doi: 10.1016/j.autrev.2016.09.003
58. Wei Y, Li N, Zhao L, Yang C, Ma B, Li X, et al. MicroRNAs and Autoimmune-Mediated Eye Diseases. *Front Cell Dev Biol* (2020) 8:818. doi: 10.3389/fcell.2020.00818
59. Ma X, Becker Buscaglia LE, Barker JR, Li Y. MicroRNAs in NF-kappaB Signaling. *J Mol Cell Biol* (2011) 3(3):159–66. doi: 10.1093/jmcb/mjr007
60. Jiang W, Kong L, Ni Q, Lu Y, Ding W, Liu G, et al. miR-146a Ameliorates Liver Ischemia/Reperfusion Injury by Suppressing IRAK1 and TRAF6. *PLoS One* (2014) 9(7):e101530. doi: 10.1371/journal.pone.0101530
61. Taganov KD, Boldin MP, Chang KJ, Baltimore D. NF-kappaB-Dependent Induction of microRNA miR-146, an Inhibitor Targeted to Signaling Proteins of Innate Immune Responses. *Proc Natl Acad Sci USA* (2006) 103(33):12481–6. doi: 10.1073/pnas.0605298103
62. Wei H, Guan M, Qin Y, Xie C, Fu X, Gao F, et al. Circulating Levels of miR-146a and IL-17 Are Significantly Correlated With the Clinical Activity of Graves' Ophthalmopathy. *Endocrine J* (2014) 61(11):1087–92. doi: 10.1507/endocrj.ej14-0246
63. Hu ZJ, He JF, Li KJ, Chen J, Xie XR. Decreased microRNA-146a in CD4+T Cells Promote Ocular Inflammation in Thyroid-Associated Ophthalmopathy by Targeting NUMB. *Eur Rev Med Pharmacol Sci* (2017) 21(8):1803–9.
64. Yang WJ, Ma PF, Li SP, Su H, Liu YJ. MicroRNA-146a Contributes to CD4(+) T Lymphocyte Differentiation in Patients With Thyroid Ophthalmopathy. *Am J Trans Res* (2017) 9(4):1801–9.
65. Li K, Du Y, Jiang BL, He JF. Increased microRNA-155 and Decreased microRNA-146a may Promote Ocular Inflammation and Proliferation in Graves' Ophthalmopathy. *Med Sci Monit* (2014) 20:639–43. doi: 10.12659/MSM.890686
66. Thiel J, Alter C, Luppus S, Eckstein A, Tan S, Fuhrer D, et al. MicroRNA-183 and microRNA-96 Are Associated With Autoimmune Responses by Regulating T Cell Activation. *J Autoimmun* (2019) 96:94–103. doi: 10.1016/j.jaut.2018.08.010
67. Shen L, Huang F, Ye L, Zhu W, Zhang X, Wang S, et al. Circulating microRNA Predicts Insensitivity to Glucocorticoid Therapy in Graves' Ophthalmopathy. *Endocrine* (2015) 49(2):445–56. doi: 10.1007/s12020-014-0487-4
68. Zhang L, Masetti G, Colucci G, Salvi M, Covelli D, Eckstein A, et al. Combining Micro-RNA and Protein Sequencing to Detect Robust Biomarkers for Graves' Disease and Orbitopathy. *Sci Rep* (2018) 8(1):8386. doi: 10.1038/s41598-018-26700-1
69. Wang N, Chen FE, Long ZW. Mechanism of MicroRNA-146a/Notch2 Signaling Regulating IL-6 in Graves Ophthalmopathy. *Cell Physiol Biochem* (2017) 41(4):1285–97. doi: 10.1159/000464430
70. Woeller CF, Roztocil E, Hammond C, Feldon SE. TSHR Signaling Stimulates Proliferation Through PI3K/Akt and Induction of miR-146a and miR-155 in Thyroid Eye Disease Orbital Fibroblasts. *Invest Ophthalmol Vis Sci* (2019) 60(13):4336–45. doi: 10.1167/iovs.19-27865
71. Jang SY, Chae MK, Lee JH, Lee EJ, Yoon JS. Role of miR-146a in the Regulation of Inflammation in an *In Vitro* Model of Graves' Orbitopathy. *Invest Ophthalmol Vis Sci* (2016) 57(10):4027–34. doi: 10.1167/iovs.16-19213
72. Jang SY, Park SJ, Chae MK, Lee JH, Lee EJ, Yoon JS. Role of microRNA-146a in Regulation of Fibrosis in Orbital Fibroblasts From Patients With Graves' Orbitopathy. *Br J Ophthalmol* (2018) 102(3):407–14. doi: 10.1136/bjophthalmol-2017-310723
73. Liu W, Ma C, Li HY, Chen L, Yuan SS, Li KJ. MicroRNA-146a Downregulates the Production of Hyaluronic Acid and Collagen I in Graves' Ophthalmopathy Orbital Fibroblasts. *Exp Ther Med* (2020) 20(5):38. doi: 10.3892/etm.2020.9165
74. Lee JY, Yun M, Paik JS, Lee SB, Yang SW. PDGF-BB Enhances the Proliferation of Cells in Human Orbital Fibroblasts by Suppressing PDCD4 Expression *Via* Up-Regulation of microRNA-21. *Invest Ophthalmol Vis Sci* (2016) 57(3):908–13. doi: 10.1167/iovs.15-18157
75. Young MR, Santhanam AN, Yoshikawa N, Colburn NH. Have Tumor Suppressor PDCD4 and Its Counteragent Oncogenic miR-21 Gone Rogue? *Mol Interventions* (2010) 10(2):76–9. doi: 10.1124/mi.10.2.5
76. Tong BD, Xiao MY, Zeng JX, Xiong W. MiRNA-21 Promotes Fibrosis in Orbital Fibroblasts From Thyroid-Associated Ophthalmopathy. *Mol Vision* (2015) 21:324–34.
77. Nishida Y, Tian S, Isberg B, Hayashi O, Tallstedt L, Lennerstrand G. Significance of Orbital Fatty Tissue for Exophthalmos in Thyroid-Associated Ophthalmopathy. *Graefes Arch Clin Exp Ophthalmol* (2002) 240(7):515–20. doi: 10.1007/s00417-002-0498-3
78. Hammond CL, Roztocil E, Gonzalez MO, Feldon SE, Woeller CF. MicroRNA-130a Is Elevated in Thyroid Eye Disease and Increases Lipid Accumulation in Fibroblasts Through the Suppression of AMPK. *Invest Ophthalmol Vis Sci* (2021) 62(1):29. doi: 10.1167/iovs.62.1.29
79. Jang SY, Chae MK, Lee JH, Lee EJ, Yoon JS. MicroRNA-27 Inhibits Adipogenic Differentiation in Orbital Fibroblasts From Patients With Graves' Orbitopathy. *PLoS One* (2019) 14(8):e0221077. doi: 10.1371/journal.pone.0221077
80. Wu L, Zhou R, Diao J, Chen X, Huang J, Xu K, et al. Differentially Expressed Circular RNAs in Orbital Adipose/Connective Tissue From Patients With Thyroid-Associated Ophthalmopathy. *Exp Eye Res* (2020) 196:108036. doi: 10.1016/j.exer.2020.108036
81. Hansen TB, Jensen TI, Clausen BH, Bramsen JB, Finsen B, Damgaard CK, et al. Natural RNA Circles Function as Efficient microRNA Sponges. *Nature* (2013) 495(7441):384–8. doi: 10.1038/nature11993
82. Bolisetty MT, Graveley BR. Circuitous Route to Transcription Regulation. *Mol Cell* (2013) 51(6):705–6. doi: 10.1016/j.molcel.2013.09.012
83. Wu GC, Pan HF, Leng RX, Wang DG, Li XP, Li XM, et al. Emerging Role of Long Noncoding RNAs in Autoimmune Diseases. *Autoimmun Rev* (2015) 14(9):798–805. doi: 10.1016/j.autrev.2015.05.004
84. Christensen NJ, Habekost G. Bratholm P. A RNA Transcript (Heg) in Mononuclear Cells is Negatively Correlated With CD14 mRNA and TSH Receptor Autoantibodies. *Clin Exp Immunol* (2008) 154(2):209–15. doi: 10.1111/j.1365-2249.2008.03744.x
85. Xia M, Liu J, Liu S, Chen K, Lin H, Jiang M, et al. Ash1l and lnc-Smad3 Coordinate Smad3 Locus Accessibility to Modulate Itreg Polarization and T Cell Autoimmunity. *Nat Commun* (2017) 8:15818. doi: 10.1038/ncomms15818
86. Covelli D, Ludgate M. The Thyroid, the Eyes and the Gut: A Possible Connection. *J Endocrinol Invest* (2017) 40(6):567–76. doi: 10.1007/s40618-016-0594-6
87. Kataoka K. The Intestinal Microbiota and Its Role in Human Health and Disease. *J Med Investigation: JMI* (2016) 63(1-2):27–37. doi: 10.2152/jmi.63.27
88. Conrad MA, Wu GD, Kelsen JR. The Gut Microbiota and Inflammatory Bowel Disease. *Pediatric Inflammatory Bowel Disease*. Springer International Publishing (2017) 45–54. doi: 10.1007/978-3-319-49215-5_4
89. Zhang X, Zhang D, Jia H, Feng Q, Wang D, Liang D, et al. The Oral and Gut Microbiomes Are Perturbed in Rheumatoid Arthritis and Partly Normalized After Treatment. *Nat Med* (2015) 21(8):895–905. doi: 10.1038/nm.3914
90. Kugelberg E. Microbiota: Diet can Protect Against Type 1 Diabetes. *Nat Rev Immunol* (2017) 17(5):279. doi: 10.1038/nri.2017.40
91. Edwards CJ, Costenbader KH. Epigenetics and the Microbiome: Developing Areas in the Understanding of the Aetiology of Lupus. *Lupus* (2014) 23(6):505–6. doi: 10.1177/0961203314531636
92. Jiang W, Yu X, Kosik RO, Song Y, Qiao T, Tong J, et al. Gut Microbiota May Play a Significant Role in the Pathogenesis of Graves' Disease. *Thyroid* (2021) 31(5):810–20. doi: 10.1089/thy.2020.0193
93. Shi TT, Xin Z, Hua L, Zhao RX, Yang YL, Wang H, et al. Alterations in the Intestinal Microbiota of Patients With Severe and Active Graves' Orbitopathy: A Cross-Sectional Study. *J Endocrinol Invest* (2019) 42(8):967–78. doi: 10.1007/s40618-019-1010-9
94. Shi TT, Hua L, Wang H, Xin Z. The Potential Link Between Gut Microbiota and Serum TRAb in Chinese Patients With Severe and Active Graves' Orbitopathy. *Int J Endocrinol* (2019) 2019:9736968. doi: 10.1155/2019/9736968
95. Shi TT, Xin Z, Hua L, Wang H, Zhao RX, Yang YL, et al. Comparative Assessment of Gut Microbial Composition and Function in Patients With Graves' Disease and Graves' Orbitopathy. *J Endocrinol Invest* (2021) 44(2):297–310. doi: 10.1007/s40618-020-01298-2
96. Han X, Wang Y, Zhang P, Zhu M, Li L, Mao X, et al. Kazak Faecal Microbiota Transplantation Induces Short-Chain Fatty Acids That Promote Glucagon-

Like Peptide-1 Secretion by Regulating Gut Microbiota in Db/Db Mice. *Pharm Biol* (2021) 59(1):1077–87. doi: 10.1080/13880209.2021.1954667

97. Moshkelgosha S, Masetti G, Berchner-Pfannschmidt U, Verhasselt HL, Horstmann M, Diaz-Cano S, et al. Gut Microbiome in BALB/c and C57BL/6J Mice Undergoing Experimental Thyroid Autoimmunity Associate With Differences in Immunological Responses and Thyroid Function. *Horm Metab Res* (2018) 50(12):932–41. doi: 10.1055/a-0653-3766
98. Masetti G, Ludgate M. Microbiome and Graves' Orbitopathy. *Eur Thyroid J* (2020) 9(Suppl 1):78–85. doi: 10.1159/000512255

12

Evidence that Baseline Levels of Low-Density Lipoproteins Cholesterol Affect the Clinical Response of Graves' Ophthalmopathy to Parenteral Corticosteroids

*Adriano Naselli, Diletta Moretti, Concetto Regalbuto, Maria Luisa Arpi, Fabrizio Lo Giudice, Francesco Frasca, Antonino Belfiore and Rosario Le Moli**

Endocrinology, Department of Clinical and Experimental Medicine, University of Catania, Garibaldi-Nesima Medical Center, Catania, Italy

Correspondence:
Rosario Le Moli
rlemoli@unict.it
orcid.org/0000-0002-1398-9271

Background: High dose intravenous glucocorticoid (ivGC) therapy is the first line treatment in moderate to severe Graves' ophthalmopathy (GO) and is associated with a clinical response rate ranging from 50% to 80%. Recently, a positive correlation between total cholesterol and low-density lipoproteins cholesterol (LDLc) with GO presentation and activity has been described.

Objective: We aimed at evaluating whether, in patients with moderate to severe active GO treated with ivGC therapy, cholesterol, and LDLc could represent valuable predictive factors of medium-term GO outcome.

Methods: This single center retrospective study was conducted in a consecutive series of 87 patients undergone ivGC therapy because affected by moderate to severe active GO. Clinical outcome of GO was evaluated at week 6 (W6) and 12 (W12) in respect to baseline conditions (week 0) by the seven points CAS according to EUGOGO recommendations. Univariate analysis and binary logistic regression were performed for the outcome variable W12CAS.

Results: In patients with active GO, an early positive clinical response to ivGC therapy (as evaluated by CAS at 6W) was a strong determinant (OR=13) of the clinical outcome at week 12. Moreover, high levels of LDLc at baseline were positively associated with a reduction in the likelihood of being classified as improved at 12W. Patients with LDLc >193.6 mg/dl were very likely to respond negatively to ivGC therapy independently from the response at 6W. Based on these results, we propose a predictive decision-making model to be tested in future prospective studies.

Discussion: We found that, in patients with active GO, both an early clinical response to ivGC therapy and baseline LDLc levels are significant determinants of GO outcome

(W12CAS). These data support the need of a cholesterol-lowering treatment before addressing these patients to ivGC therapy.

Keywords: cholesterol, low-density lipoprotein cholesterol, Graves' ophthalmopathy, parenteral corticosteroids, Graves' disease

INTRODUCTION

Graves' disease (GD) is an autoimmune disorder associated with the production of activating autoantibodies to the thyroid-stimulating hormone receptor (TSH-R) in the thyroid gland, leading to hyperthyroidism. A major extra-thyroidal complication of GD is Graves' ophthalmopathy (GO), an autoimmune and inflammatory condition characterized by orbital disfigurement, double vision, and decreased visual performance up to blindness (sight-threatening GO). All these factors are associated with proven decrease of quality of life and negative social impact (1, 2). Innate and adaptive immunity as well as a large number of inflammatory factors are implicated in GO pathogenesis (3). High dose ivGC therapy is the first choice in moderate to severe or severe active GO; other immunosuppressive drugs and/or retrobulbar irradiation are widely used in the treatment of GO. Surgical orbital decompression is, however, the best choice for treating patients with moderate to severe or severe inactive GO. Treatment with 131-iodine, severe hyperthyroidism and elevated anti TSH-R antibodies (TRAbs) are considered risks factors for GO presentation or exacerbation (4). Smoking is considered to be the most important risk factor for presentation, exacerbation of GO and resistance to corticosteroids (5). Low levels of miR-224-5p also appear to reduce the clinical efficacy of medium dose of ivGC therapy in patients with moderate to severe active GO (6). Recently a retrospective analysis of a large number of patients showed an independent effect of 3-hydrossi-3methylglutaryl CoA reductase inhibitors (statins) on the risk to develop GO (7). In patients with GD, statin use for approximately 60 days during a one-year observation period significantly reduced the risk of developing GO, an effect not obtained when patients were treated with cyclooxygenase-2 (COX-2) inhibitors alone (8). A significant correlation of GO presentation and activity with total cholesterol and LDLc has been described (9) revealing a role of cholesterol in the processes involved in GO pathogenesis. Those data suggest the possibility that cholesterol might not only increase the risk of GO but also its activity, corroborating previous data showing that chronically elevated cholesterol increases systemic inflammation and modulates innate and adaptive immunity (10). However, the possible impact of cholesterol levels on the clinical efficacy of ivGC therapy in patients with active GO is not known (8, 11, 12).

We aimed at evaluating whether serum cholesterol levels may serve as predictive factor of medium-term clinical activity GO outcome in patients with moderate to severe active GO treated with ivGC therapy.

Abbreviations: GD, Graves' Disease; GO, Graves' ophthalmopathy; ATD, anti-thyroid drugs; LDLc, low density lipoproteins cholesterol; PREDIGO, predictive score for the development or progression of Graves' orbitopathy;, ivGC, intravenous glucocorticoid; W6, week 6; W12, week 12; EuGoGo, The European Group on Graves' Orbitopathy; FT3, triiodothyronine; FT4, thyroxine or tetraiodothyronine; TSH, thyroid stimulating hormone; TRAbs, thyrotropin (TSH)-receptor autoantibodies; RAI, radioiodine; ROC, receiver operator characteristics. CTEC, combined thyroid eyes clinic.

PATIENTS AND METHODS

Patients

We retrospectively selected 87 consecutive patients with Graves' disease and GO referred to our out-patients thyroid clinic from January 2013 to July 2019 and treated with ivGC therapy because of moderate to severe active GO. Patients with a history of treatment with statins, corticosteroids, radioiodine (RAI) for Graves' hyperthyroidism, retrobulbar radiotherapy or with incomplete metabolic evaluation were excluded from the study. Six patients previously treated with thyroidectomy 11.1 (14.6) months earlier and stably euthyroid were included.

Graves' Ophthalmopathy Clinical Evaluation at Baseline

All patients were evaluated at the combined thyroid eye clinic (CTEC) of Endocrinology Unit at Garibaldi-Nesima Hospital, Catania, Italy. The same expert endocrinologist carried out the clinical examination of GO according to European Group of Graves' Ophthalmopathy (EuGoGo) criteria (4). The lid fissure width was evaluated in millimeters by a router, proptosis of each patient was evaluated by the same Hertel exophthalmometer. Diplopia was classified according to the Gorman score by four levels of severity: absent, intermittent, inconstant, or constant. A complete ophthalmological evaluation was carried out by the same expert ophthalmologist. The GO was defined as moderate to severe when eye disease had a sufficient impact on daily life with one or more of the following clinical signs, each part of a composite index (CI): lid retraction 2 mm or more, moderate or severe soft tissue involvement, exophthalmos 3 or more mm above 21, and inconstant or constant diplopia. GO activity was evaluated according to seven points CAS and was considered active when reaching a CAS ≥3.

Graves' Ophthalmopathy Clinical Outcome Evaluation

Clinical outcome of GO was evaluated at week 6 (W6) and 12 (W12) in respect to baseline conditions (week 0) by the seven points CAS and was defined clinically improved when CAS improved by almost 2 points in at least one eye. Deterioration was defined by CAS worsening of at least 2 points or when dysthyroid optic neuropathy (DON) or corneal breakdown occurred. No changes were defined as the condition in which changes less than those described above occurred. For each assessment, patients who improved were considered as group I, patients who did not improve or who worsened were defined as group NI. According to these groups and to the time of assessment we defined the following categories: week 6 CAS (I_{W6CAS} or NI_{W6CAS}), week 12 CAS (I_{W12CAS} or NI_{W12CAS}).

Pulse Therapy

Corticosteroid treatment for GO consisted of ivGC (Solumedrol; Pfizer, Karlsruhe, Germany) injections with a median cumulative dose of 52.3 mg/kg subdivided in 12 weekly infusions. Patients were asked to report to our endocrinology day hospital on the appointed day, an indwelling venous catheter was inserted into an antecubital vein between 8.30 and 9.30 and Solumedrol diluted in 250 ml of a 0.9 sodium chloride solution % was administered at an infusion rate of 120 ml/h in the post-absorption state and in a lying position. Blood pressure, blood glucose, lipid levels, thyroid, liver and kidney function were evaluated prior to initiating the corticosteroid infusion.

Analytical Methods

Serum hormones were measured by microparticle enzyme immunoassay (Abbot AxSYM-MEIA) with inter-assay coefficients of variation of less than 10% over the analytical ranges of 1.7–46.0 pmol/L for FT3, 5.15–77.0 pmol/L for FT4, and 0.03–10.0 mU/L for TSH. The within-run and between-run precisions for FT3, FT4, and TSH assays showed coefficients of variation <5%. Thyrotropin receptor antibodies (TRAbs) were measured by a III generation assay (SELco TRAbs Human, Dahlewitz/Berlino (Germany). Glycaemia, total cholesterol, high density lipoprotein (HDL) cholesterol and triglycerides were evaluated by standard methods. We calculated LDLc values by the formula of Martin/Hopkins that is reliable for a wide range of triglyceride values (13). The thyroid was evaluated by ultrasound and the volume of each lobe was calculated with the formula for ellipsoid volumes: Volume = length*width*depth*(π/6). The calculated thyroid volume was the sum of the volumes of the two lobes (14).

Statistical Methods

Statistical analyses were performed with the SPSS package (IBM SPSS Statistics for Windows, Version 26.0. Armonk, NY: IBM Corp). For the descriptive analysis, continuous variables were expressed as median (25th-75th percentile); categorical variables were expressed as numbers and percentages. We calculated that, to detect a moderate size effect (OR = 2) with a p value ≤ 0.05 and a statistical power of 0.8, a total of 84 patients would have needed (see supplementary data).

Univariate Analysis

Univariate analysis was performed to identify predictive variables significantly associated with the clinical outcome at W12CAS ("Improved" and "Not Improved"). Continuous variables were analyzed using the non-parametric Mann Whitney U test. The shapes of distribution of each variable were evaluated by visual inspection of the population pyramid charts; for distributions of similar shape we reported the medians, for distributions of different shapes we reported average ranks. The estimate of the effect size "r" was calculated when appropriate (15). Categorical variables were analyzed by the Chi-square test or, if cells with less than five expected cell numbers were found, by Fisher's exact test. The strength of the associations was quantified by calculating the Odds Ratio.

Binary Logistic Regression

A binary logistic regression was performed for the outcome variable (W12CAS). Covariates were selected on the basis of the results of univariate analysis and the final model was built using forced entry and a hierarchical method. Linearity of the continuous variables with respect to the logit of the dependent variable was assessed by the Box-Tidwell procedure (16) and a Bonferroni correction was applied using all terms in the model to assess its statistical significance (17). Multi-collinearity was excluded after checking tolerance (18) and variance inflation factor (VIF) (19) statistics and the proportion of the variance of each predictor's b value attributed to each eigenvalue.

The possible presence of outliers was verified by examining standardized residuals and values ≥1.96 or ≤-1.96 standard deviations were reported; cases whose standardized residuals exceeded such thresholds were inspected closely and the decision to eliminate or to keep them in the analysis was made after assessing if they exerted an undue influence on the model using the following influence statistics: Cook's distance, DFBeta, and Leverage statistics. The adequacy of the models was tested with the maximum likelihood method. The Wald test was used to verify that coefficients differed from 0. Odds ratios were calculated as the exponential of b values to give an indicator of the change in odds resulting from a unit change in the predictor. The proportion of variation in the dependent variable explained by each model was assessed by Nagelkerke pseudo-R^2 value (20). To predict the probability of improving at week 12 (W12CAS), we constructed our models on the basis of the theoretical model of the binary logistic regression, expressed by the following equation [Eq. 1]:

$$P(Y) = \frac{1}{1 + e - \left(b_0 + \sum_{i=1}^{n} b_i x_i\right)} \quad (1)$$

Where:

$P\ (Y)$: probability of Y occurring; in our study $Y = I_{W12CAS}$.

e: Euler's number

b_0: constant regression coefficient (interception at x axis)

b_i: regression coefficient of x_i

x_i: predictor variable

n: number of predictor variables

Logistic regression models assigned a predicted category on the basis of P (Y) values (predicted probability of improving). Using the standard cut-off P (Y) = 0.5 the models assigned a predicted category = Improved (I_{W12CAS}) when P (Y) ≥ 0.5; the remaining predicted category (NI_{W12CAS}) was assigned if P (Y) was < 0.5.

Receiver Operating Characteristic Curve Analysis and Youden's Test

These analyses were performed for the W12CAS binomial logistic regression model on the basis of the regression outputs.

The ability of the model to discriminate between outcome categories was investigated in more details by elaborating the ROC curve (21). The $P(I_{W12CAS})$ (predicted probability of improving at W12) provided by regression analysis was set as test variable, in order to study the model accuracy for different $P(I_{W12CAS})$ cut-offs. The cut-off with the best compromise between sensitivity and specificity was assessed using Youden's test (22).

All tests were considered statistically significant at a 2-tailed p value <0.05.

RESULTS

Patient characteristics at study entry are shown in **Table 1**. Eighty-seven patients completed the 12-week (12W) GO clinical assessment according to the seven-points CAS and 71.3% of them improved. Fifty-three patients who had a complete metabolic assessment were included in the analysis.

Univariate and Binomial Logistic Regression Analysis according to CAS Evaluation

On univariate analysis, the only two variables positively associated with GO improvement at 12W (I_{W12CAS}) were serum levels of LDLc (r= -0.25, p=0.045) and early improvement at W6 (I_{W6CAS}) (p<0.001) (**Figure 1**, **Table 2**). Notably, 90.6% patients classified as "improved" at W6 were also "improved" at W12. In contrast, 41.2% of patients 'not improved' at W6 (NI_{W6CAS}) were classified as 'improved' at W12 (OR=13.714, CI 95% 3.61–52.095, p<0.001, I_{W6CAS} vs NI_{W6CAS}).

We found a negative association between male gender and GO improvement at W12; however, this difference did not reach statistical significance (OR = 2.778, CI 95% 1.003–7.691, p=0.058).

TABLE 1 | Characteristics of patients at study entrance.

Variables	
Number of patients	87
ivGC treatment period	1/2013–7/2019
Sex: male/female (n, %)	22 (25.3)/ 65 (74.7)
Age (years)	45 (35–55)
BMI (Kg/mq)	24.1 (21.6–28)
Current smokers (n, %)	45 (51.7)
Previous Smokers (n, %)	29 (33.3)
Non Smokers (n, %)	13(14.9)
Thyroid volume (ml)	18.1 (13–24.3)
ivGC cumulative dose (mg/kg)	52.3 (40.2–68.2)
CAS	3 (3–4)
GO duration (months)	8 (3–12)
TSH (mU/L)	0.05 (0–0.9)
FT3 (pg/ml)	2.86 (2.53–3.64)
FT4 (ng/dl)	0.98 (0.86–1.29)
TRAbs (IU/l)	5.31 (2.44–18.15)
Total cholesterol (mg/dl)	200 (173–226)
HDL (mg/dl)	53 (47.8–61.3)
Triglycerides (mg/dl)	81.5 (60.8–115)
LDLc (mg/dl)	123.3 (104.1–151.9)
Glycaemia (mg/dl)	94 (87.8–102.3)

Data are reported as number and percentage or median and interquartile range.

Similarly, higher total cholesterol and older age showed some association with the lack in GO improvement at W12, without reaching statistical significance (p=0.094 and p=0.08, respectively) There was no association between smoking habit and W12 outcome and no association with any of the other continuous variables considered (**Table 2**). Prior thyroidectomy was not a contributing factor as at 12W three out of six patients were classified as improved and three as not improved.

Variables identified at univariate analysis (LDLc and W6CAS) were then evaluated by binomial logistic regression to further ascertain their effects on the likelihood to affect GO improvement at W12. The continuous independent variable was found to be linearly related to the logit of the dependent variable. There were two standardized residuals with a value of -5.986 and -4.706 standard deviations, which were kept in the analysis. The logistic regression model was statistically significant, $\chi2(2)$ = 15.985, p < 0.001. The model explained 41.1% (Nagelkerke R^2) (20) of the variance in W12CAS outcome and correctly classified 84.6% of cases. Sensitivity was 95.1%, specificity was 45.5%, positive predictive value was 86.7% and negative predictive value was 71.4%. Both predictor variables were statistically significant. I_{W6CAS} had 13 higher odds to be classified as I_{W12CAS} than NI_{W6CAS}. Increasing LDLc was associated with a reduction in the likelihood of being classified as I_{W12CAS}, since for each unit of LDLc reduction, the odds of improving at W12CAS increased by a factor of 1.03. **Table 3** reports the regression output of the final model. Based on the results of the binary logistic regression, the following model was constructed to predict the P(IW12CAS) (probability of improving at W12CAS) for individual patients [Eq. 2]:

$$P(I_{W12CAS}) = \frac{1}{1 + e^{-(2.95 - 0.025x_1 + 2.57x_2)}} \tag{2}$$

Where: x_1 = LDLc (mg/dl); x_2 = W6CAS outcome (x_2 = 1 for I_{W6CAS}; x_2 = 0 for NI_{W6CAS}). We tested the reliability of our model by performing several multivariate logistic regression analyses, with the aim of verifying that LDLc is an independent predictor for the W12CAS outcome. We also constructed an overfitted model constructed with 5 covariates (see supplementary data).

Receiver Operating Characteristic Curve Analysis

The ROC curve processed using the regression $P(I_{W12CAS})$ resulted in an excellent level of discrimination (0.805; 95% CI, 0.608–1.000) according to Hosmer et al. (23). (**Figure 2**). Youden's test identified a $P(I_{W12CAS})$ = 0.664 as best cut-off, with sensitivity 90.2%, specificity 81.8%, positive predictive value 94.9%, negative predictive value 69.2% and accuracy 88.5%. **Figure 3** highlights the impact that different $P(I_{W12CAS})$ cut-offs have on the prediction performance of the model.

W12CAS Binomial Logistic Regression Implementation

Almost every patient classified as "improved" at W6CAS had a $P(I_{W12CAS})$ between 0.8 and 1.0, allowing a correct diagnosis in

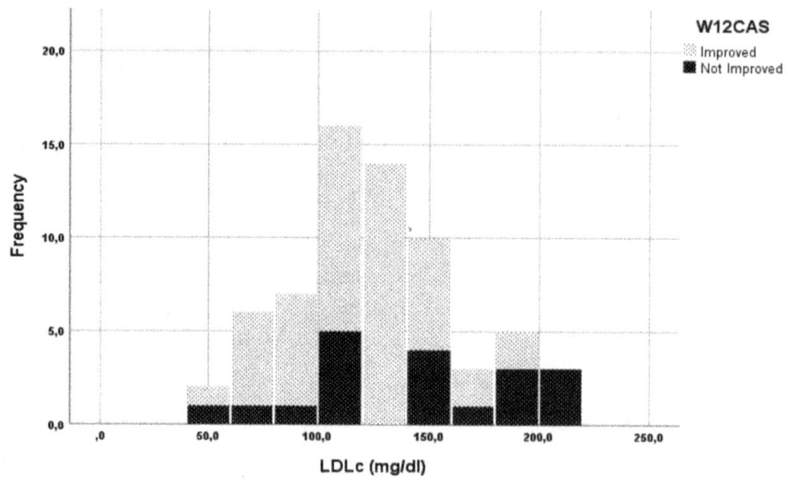

FIGURE 1 | Stacked histogram of low-density lipoproteins cholesterol (LDLc) levels grouped for W12CAS categories.

almost all of them. Within the I_{W6CAS} group the lower P (I_{W12CAS}) (ranging from 0.59 to 0.7) was assigned to the patients with a very high LDLc and the Youden's cut-off (unlike the standard cut-off $P(I_{W12CAS}) = 0.5$) allowed to correctly predict their W12CAS outcome. Considering that the two independent variables (LDLc and W6CAS outcome) are not available at the same time, since the first one is obtained at baseline and the second one after a 6 weeks pulse therapy, we aimed at identifying a LDLc cut-off that would give a $P(I_{W12CAS})$ <0.664 independently of W6CAS outcome; knowing this value may allow the physician to delay pulse therapy until this value is corrected. This LDLc cut-off was calculated using the binomial logistic regression model (Eq. 3) setting $P(I_{W12CAS}) < 0.664$ (as indicated by Youden's test):

$$P(I_{W12CAS}) = \frac{1}{1 + e^{-(2.95-0.025x_1+2.57x_2)}} < 0.664 \quad (3)$$

The resulting inequality was solved for both x_2 valid values (0 and 1) with the purpose to calculate which LDLc values (x_1) would certainly give a $P(I_{W12CAS})$ <0.664, independently from W6CAS outcome (x_2). Calculations resulted in x_1>193.6. According to this data, a patient showing a baseline LDLc >193.6 mg/dl can't reach a $P(I_{W12CAS})$ >0.664; in fact, in the best scenario ($x_2 = 1$), he would reach a $P(I_{W12CAS})$ value slightly lower than 0.664, while in the worst one ($x_2 = 0$) its $P(I_{W12CAS})$ should fall below 0.132. For W6CAS Improved patients, the outcome of the W6CAS itself is the most important predictor, with LDLc making a predominant contribution when it exceeds 190 mg/dL. Based on these results, a proposal for a decision algorithm was developed (**Figures 3** and **4**).

TABLE 2 | Univariate analysis for W12CAS outcome.

Variables	I_{W12CAS}	NI_{W12CAS}	p
Glycaemia (mg/dl)	93.5 (87.8–102)	95 (86.3–104.5)	0.885
Age*(years)	41.01	51.42	0.082
Females (%)	76.9	23.1	0.058
BMI (Kg/m^2)	24.1 (21.7–27.9)	25.6 (21.3–28.6)	0.929
Smokers (%)	68.9	31.1	0.643
ivGC CD (mg/Kg)	50.4 (40.2–67.2)	60 (50.6–73.2)	0.131
Thyroid (ml)	18.6 (11.9–24.3)	18.1 (14.5–39.9)	0.546
CAS	3 (3–4)	3 (3–4)	0.927
TSH (mU/L)	0.05 (0–0.9)	0.05 (0.01–1)	0.661
FT3 (pg/ml)	2.87 (2.56–3.43)	2.69 (2.39–3.76)	0.699
FT4 (ng/dl)	0.98 (0.84–1.25)	1.05 (0.89–1.3)	0.975
TRAbs (IU/l)	4.6 (2.2–16.5)	8.4 (3.3–28)	0.156
Cholesterol*	31.67	39.89	0.094
HDL*	35.06	29.63	0.298
Triglycerides (mg/dl)	76.0 (58–112)	89.0 (74–131)	0.315
LDLc*	30.49	40.95	0.045
I-W6CAS (n, %)	48 (90.6)	5 (9.4)	<0.001

Data are expressed as number or percentage percentage, median and interquartile range or mean ranks as indicated (*); CD, cumulative dose.

TABLE 3 | Outputs of the binary logistic regression for the outcome variable W12CAS.

	B	SE	Wald	df	p	Odds Ratio	95% CI of Odds Ratio	
							Lower	Upper
LDLc	-0.025	0.013	4.025	1	0.045	0.975	0.951	0.999
W6CAS	2.570	0.863	8.858	1	0.003	13.065	2.405	70.976
Constant	2.950	1.707	2.987	1	0.084	19.099		

Final model built with covariates LDLc and W6CAS.

DISCUSSION

Herein we found that in patients with active GO addressed to pulse therapy with corticosteroids, baseline serum levels of LDLc and early clinical response at week 6 (W6CAS) were the strongest determinants of the clinical outcome at week 12 according to CAS evaluation (W12CAS). A previous study correlated serum total cholesterol and LDLc levels with the onset and severity of GO, but their impact on the GO response to corticosteroids has not been determined (9). In our study, we modeled the predicted probability P (I_{W12CAS}) that each patient is classified as improved at W12CAS based on baseline serum levels of LDLc plus W6CAS outcome, showing that the LDLc level provides an independent contribution to the W6CAS data by overcoming the effect of W6CAS when it exceeds 190 mg/dl with a positive predictive value of 86.7% and a negative predictive value of 71.4%. Furthermore, the ROC curves indicated a sensitivity of 90.2% and a specificity of 81.8% in predicting a positive response of GO to corticosteroids at 12W.

Active GO is often an auto resolving condition, but several factors independently modulate its severity and ultimate clinical outcome. Although ivGC therapy is the most widely used medical treatment for active GO, its clinical efficacy is variable, and it is therefore important to have biomarkers that can predict its efficacy in the individual patient.

Few variables are known to influence the severity and outcome of GO. For example, smoking is a proven independent risk factor for the development and exacerbation of GO, and radioiodine (131-I) treatment of hyperthyroidism can also trigger GO and worsen its outcome. Furthermore, failure to achieve euthyroidism and persistence of high levels of TRAbs are negatively correlated with the clinical outcome of GO (24). Recently, a predictive risk score for the development of GO in patients with newly diagnosed Graves' hyperthyroidism has been proposed (25). This score (PREDIGO) aims to estimate the odds ratio of GO exacerbation according to CAS based on serum levels of TSH and TRAbs, duration of hyperthyroidism and smoking habits. In our study, GO was moderate to severe and active in patients with stable thyroid function and with similar TRAbs levels between responders and non-responders, therefore the risk of GO exacerbation was similar across the study population. In addition to the aforementioned risk factors, GO occurrence and severity have been positively associated with diabetes mellitus (DM) (12, 26) and serum levels of total cholesterol and LDLc (9). These data are of interest since both DM and hypercholesterolemia induce a chronic inflammatory

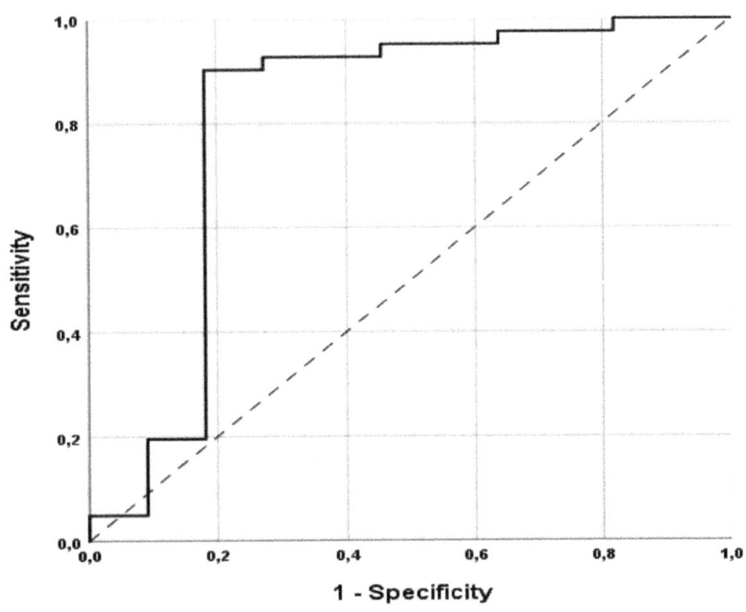

FIGURE 2 | Receiver operating characteristic (ROC) curve of the predicted probability of improvement at W12CAS calculated with binomial logistic regression.

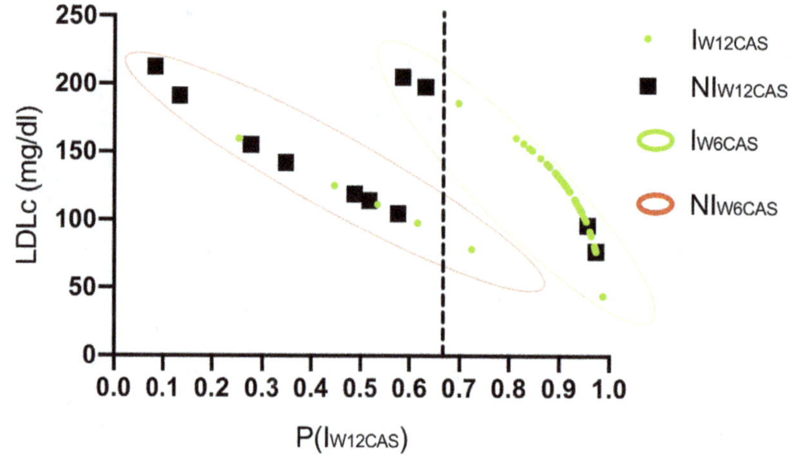

FIGURE 3 | Suggested decision-making algorithm. The graphs are constructed on the basis of binomial logistic regression prediction using the Youden's best cut-off $P(I_{W12CAS}) = 0.66$. Each dot refers to a single patient; green dots refer to patients classified as Improved at W12CAS, while black dots refer to Not Improved Patients. The predicted probability of improvement at W12CAS [$P(I_{W12CAS})$] provided by regression analysis is positioned on the x axis; cut-off = 0.664 (dotted line). The continuous predictive variable included in the model (LDLc) is positioned on the Y axis. The categories of the dichotomous predictive variable (W6CAS outcome) are highlighted in green (I_{W6CAS}) or red (NI_{W6CAS}) contour lines.

state that adds to GO immunological process and contributes to remodeling of the orbital tissues. Elevated LDLc levels have been hypothesized to increase the influx of free fatty acids into the liver causing the production of reactive oxygen radical species (ROS) and the secretion of interleukin-6 (IL-6). The increase in IL-6 activity within the orbital environment can promote greater secretion of insulin growth factor 1 (IGF-1) by orbital fibroblasts of GO patients and improve the proliferation of fibroblasts and the expansion of soft orbital tissues favoring IGF-1R - TSHR crosstalk (8, 27–29). These studies raise the need to investigate the impact of LDLc levels on the GO response to immunosuppressive therapy.

In our series of patients, none had previously received corticosteroids or retrobulbar radiation (30) and none had received radioiodine therapy to control hyperthyroidism. At week 6 after initiation of corticosteroid therapy, more than 90% of patients classified as responders maintained the same clinical rating at week 12. Corticosteroid responders at week 6

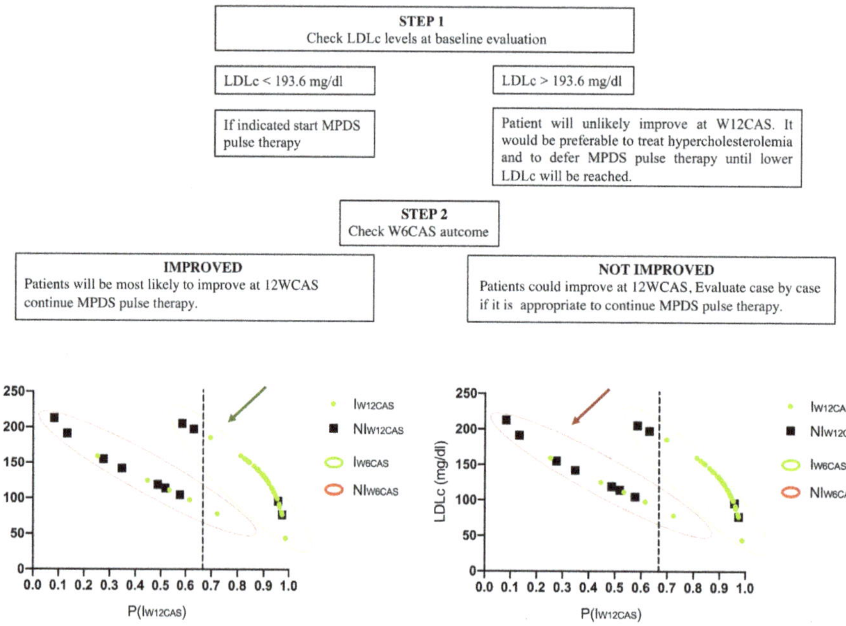

FIGURE 4 | Steps of the decision-making algorithm.

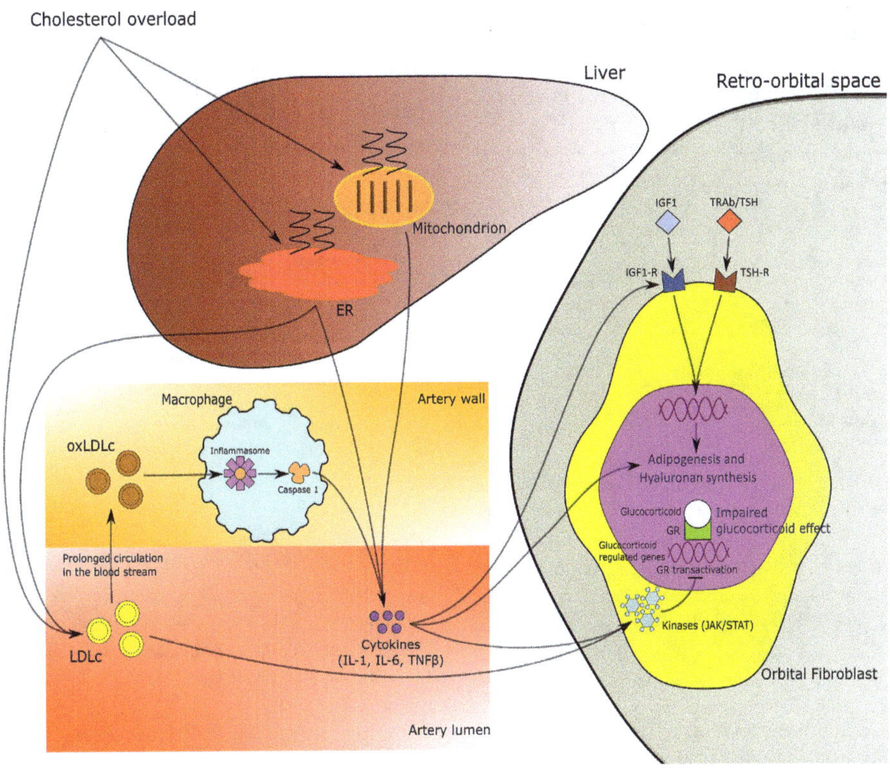

FIGURE 5 | Mechanistic hypothesis of relationship of hypercholesterolemia with chronic inflammation and resistance to corticosteroids effects in patients with Graves' ophthalmopathy (GO).

were significantly more likely than non-responders to have a positive outcome at week 12 (OR 13.7; p <0.001) confirming the previous observations (31). In our series, total cholesterol levels were higher in non-responders than in responders, but this difference did not reach statistical significance, while baseline LDLc levels were inversely related to GO clinical outcome at 12W. Other variables recognized as risk factor for GO presentation and/or exacerbation, such as cigarette smoking (24), male gender and age older than 60 yrs (32, 33) were not significantly predictive of GO response to ivGC at week 12. Although these findings may appear unexpected especially for smoking habit, the impact of smoking on the clinical response of GO to ivGC in a similar setting has not been previously investigated and deserves to be studied in prospective trials.

Our results are in agreement with the concept that hypercholesterolemia can promote chronic inflammation leading to resistance to the effects of corticosteroids characterized by inhibition of tissue macrophage functions, such as chemotaxis, phagocytosis, proliferation and antigen presentation (34). In particular, oxidized low-density lipoprotein (oxLDL) regulates the expression of dipeptidyl dipeptidase IV (DPP4) in macrophages leading to the increase of CD36 + cells which are representative of the inflammatory processes of atherosclerosis in obese and insulin resistant patients. Moreover, a direct effect of LDLc on transcriptional and translational activities of corticosteroids at the cellular levels has also been hypothesized (35, 36; **Figure 5**).

Our study has some limitations. Although all patients in our study were treated following a rigorous protocol, the study is retrospective, and the regression analysis was built on the basis of a small patient population. For these reasons, the reported algorithm is a suggestion that should be evaluated in a prospective context. However, our data indicate that patients with active GO may have a clinically limited response to ivGC therapy if LDLc levels are above 190 mg/dL.

CONCLUSIONS

Early clinical response to ivGC therapy in patients with active GO is a strong determinant of clinical outcome at week 12 when assessed by CAS. Additionally, baseline serum LDLc levels are also an independent predictor of response to ivGC therapy, and LDLc levels above 190 mg/dL greatly reduce the likelihood of a positive clinical outcome at week 12. Based on our data, we suggest measuring baseline LDLc levels in all patients with active GO and strongly considering cholesterol-lowering treatment before referring these patients to ivGC therapy.

AUTHOR CONTRIBUTIONS

RL conceptualized and designed the study. RL, AN, FG, MA, CR, FF, and DM collected the data. AN, RL, and FG performed the statistical analysis. RL and AN were in charge of the figures. RL, AB, FF, and AN wrote and revised the manuscript. All authors read and approved the final manuscript. All authors contributed to the article and approved the submitted version.

ACKNOWLEDGMENTS

The authors gratefully acknowledge the clinical support of the day-hospital staff coordinator (Dr. M. Arpi) who managed the patients' care and the chief of the department of ophthalmology (Dr. A. Marino) who handled the eye care.

REFERENCES

1. Bartalena L, Baldeschi L, Dickinson A, Eckstein A, Kendall-Taylor P, Marcocci C, et al. Consensus statement of the European Group on Graves' orbitopathy (EUGOGO) on management of GO. *Eur J Endocrinol* (2008) 158:273–85. doi: 10.1530/EJE-07-0666
2. Soeters MR, Van Zeijl CJJ, Boelen A, Kloos R, Saeed P, Vriesendorp TM, et al. Optimal management of Graves orbitopathy a multidisciplinary approach. *Neth J Med* (2011) 69:302–8.
3. Smith TJ, Hegedüs L, Douglas RS. Role of insulin-like growth factor-1 (IGF-1) pathway in the pathogenesis of Graves' orbitopathy. *Best Pract Res Clin Endocrinol Metab* (2012) 26:291–302. doi: 10.1016/j.beem.2011.10.002
4. Bartalena L, Baldeschi L, Boboridis K, Eckstein A, Kahaly GJ, Marcocci C, et al. The 2016 European Thyroid Association/European Group on Graves' Orbitopathy Guidelines for the Management of Graves' Orbitopathy. *Eur Thyroid J* (2016) 5:9–26. doi: 10.1159/000443828
5. Xing L, Ye L, Zhu W, Shen L, Huang F, Jiao Q, et al. Smoking was associated with poor response to intravenous steroids therapy in Graves' ophthalmopathy. *Br J Ophthalmol* (2015) 99:1686–91. doi: 10.1136/bjophthalmol-2014-306463
6. Shen L, Huang F, Ye L, Zhu W, Zhang X, Wang S, et al. Circulating microRNA predicts insensitivity to glucocorticoid therapy in Graves' ophthalmopathy. *Endocrine* (2015) 49:445–56. doi: 10.1007/s12020-014-0487-4
7. Stein JD, Childers D, Gupta S, Talwar N, Nan B, Lee BJ, et al. Risk factors for developing thyroid-associated ophthalmopathy among individuals with graves disease. *JAMA Ophthalmol* (2015) 133:290–6. doi: 10.1001/jamaophthalmol.2014.5103
8. Lanzolla G, Vannucchi G, Ionni I, Campi I, Sileo F, Lazzaroni E, et al. Cholesterol Serum Levels and Use of Statins in Graves' Orbitopathy: A New Starting Point for the Therapy. *Front Endocrinol (Lausanne)* (2020) 10:1–8. doi: 10.3389/fendo.2019.00933
9. Sabini E, Mazzi B, Profilo MA, Mautone T, Casini G, Rocchi R, et al. High Serum Cholesterol Is a Novel Risk Factor for Graves' Orbitopathy: Results of a Cross-Sectional Study. *Thyroid* (2018) 28:386–94. doi: 10.1089/thy.2017.0430
10. Busnelli M, Manzini S, Froio A, Vargiolu A, Cerrito MG, Smolenski RT, et al. Diet induced mild hypercholesterolemia in pigs: Local and systemic inflammation, effects on vascular injury - Rescue by high-dose statin treatment. *PloS One* (2013) 8:1–15. doi: 10.1371/journal.pone.0080588
11. Wang Y, Patel A, Douglas RS. Thyroid eye disease: How a novel therapy may change the treatment paradigm. *Ther Clin Risk Manage* (2019) 15:1305–18. doi: 10.2147/TCRM.S193018
12. Mourits MP, Prummel MF, Wiersinga WM, Koornneef L. Clinical activity score as a guide in the management of patients with Graves' ophthalmopathy. *Clin Endocrinol (Oxf)* (1997) 47:9–14. doi: 10.1046/j.1365-2265.1997.2331047.x
13. Martin SS, Giugliano RP, Murphy SA, Wasserman SM, Stein EA, Češka R, et al. Comparison of low-density lipoprotein cholesterol assessment by Martin/Hopkins estimation, friedewald estimation, and preparative ultracentrifugation insights from the FOURIER trial. *JAMA Cardiol* (2018) 3:749–53. doi: 10.1001/jamacardio.2018.1533
14. Van Isselt JW, De Klerk JMH, Van Rijk PP, Van Gils APG, Polman LJ, Kamphuis C, et al. Comparison of methods for thyroid volume estimation in patients with Graves' disease. *Eur J Nucl Med Mol Imaging* (2003) 30:525–31. doi: 10.1007/s00259-002-1101-1
15. Rosenthal R. *Meta-Analytic T Procedures Fob Social Research*. Sage Publications (1991) 6. doi: 10.4135/9781412984997
16. Box GEP, Tidwell PW. Transformation of the Independent Variables. *Technometrics* (1961) 4:531–50. doi: 10.1080/00401706.1962.10490038
17. Tabachnick BG, Fidell LS. *Using multivariate statistics. 6 t h* California State University Northridge (2013).
18. Menard S. *Applied logistic regression analysis*. Thousand Oaks: Sage University Paper. Sage Publications, Inc. (1995).
19. Myers RH. *Classical and modern regression with applications. 2nd ed.* Boston: PWS Publishing Company (1990).
20. Nagelkerke NJD. A note on a general definition of the coefficient of determination. *Biometrika* (1991) 78:691–2. doi: 10.1093/biomet/78.3.691
21. Hilbe JM. *Logistic regression models*. Boca Raton, Florida: Chapman and Hall/CRC (2009). doi: 10.1201/9781420075779
22. Youden WJ. Index for rating diagnostic tests. *Cancer* (1950) 3:32–5. doi: 10.1002/1097-0142(1950)3:1<32::AID-CNCR2820030106>3.0.CO;2-3
23. Hosmer DW, Lemershow S, Sturdiwant R. *Applied logistic regression*. New Jersey, US: John Willey & Sons Hoboken (2013). doi: 10.1002/9781118548387
24. Stan MN, Bahn RS. 2010 Risk factors for development or deterioration of Graves' ophthalmopathy. *Thyroid* (2010) 20:777–83. doi: 10.1089/thy.2010.1634
25. Wiersinga W, Žarković M, Bartalena L, Donati S, Perros P, Okosieme O, et al. Predictive score for the development or progression of Graves' orbitopathy in patients with newly diagnosed Graves' hyperthyroidism. *Eur J Endocrinol* (2018) 178:635–43. doi: 10.1530/EJE-18-0039
26. Le Moli R, Muscia V, Tumminia A, Frittitta L, Buscema M, Palermo F, et al. Type 2 diabetic patients with Graves' disease have more frequent and severe Graves' orbitopathy. *Nutr Metab Cardiovasc Dis* (2015) 25:452–7. doi: 10.1016/j.numecd.2015.01.003
27. Lanzolla G, Ricci D, Nicolì F, Sabini E, Sframeli A, Brancatella A, et al. Putative protective role of autoantibodies against the insulin-like growth factor-1 receptor in Graves' Disease: results of a pilot study. *J Endocrinol Invest* (2020) 43(12):1759–68. doi: 10.1007/s40618-020-01341-2
28. Marinò M, Rotondo GD, Ionni I, Lanzolla G, Sabini E, Ricci D, et al. Serum antibodies against the insulin-like growth factor- 1 receptor (IGF-1R) in Graves' disease and Graves' orbitopathy. *J Endocrinol Invest* (2019) 42:471–80. doi: 10.1007/s40618-018-0943-8
29. Douglas RS. Teprotumumab, an insulin-like growth factor-1 receptor antagonist antibody, in the treatment of active thyroid eye disease: a focus on proptosis *Eye (Lond)* (2019) 33:183–90. doi: 10.1038/s41433-018-0321-y
30. Boulanouar L, Grunenwald S, Imbert P, Khalifa J, Dekeister C, Boutault F, et al. Effect of orbital radiotherapy on the outcome of surgical orbital decompression for thyroid-associated orbitopathy (TAO): a retrospective study in 136 patients. *Endocrine* (2020) 67:605–12. doi: 10.1007/s12020-019-02113-6

31. Bartalena L, Veronesi G, Krassas GE, Wiersinga WM, Marcocci C, Marinò M, et al. Does early response to intravenous glucocorticoids predict the final outcome in patients with moderate-to-severe and active Graves' orbitopathy? *J Endocrinol Invest* (2017) 40:547–53. doi: 10.1007/s40618-017-0608-z
32. Perros P, Crombie AL, Matthews JNS, Kendall-Taylor P. Age and gender influence the severity of thyroid-associated ophthalmopathy: A study of 101 patients attending a combined thyroid-eye clinic. *Clin Endocrinol (Oxf)* (1993) 38:367–72. doi: 10.1111/j.1365-2265.1993.tb00516.x
33. Bereshchenko O, Bruscoli S, Riccardi C. Glucocorticoids, sex hormones, and immunity. *Front Immunol* (2018) 9:1–10. doi: 10.3389/fimmu.2018.01332
34. Baschant U, Tuckermann J. The role of the glucocorticoid receptor in inflammation and immunity. *J Steroid Biochem Mol Biol* (2010) 120:69–75. doi: 10.1016/j.jsbmb.2010.03.058
35. Rao X, Zhao S, Braunstein Z. Oxidized LDL upregulates macrophage DPP4 expression via TLR4/TRIF/CD36 pathways. *EBioMedicine* (2019) 41:50–61. doi: 10.1016/j.ebiom.2019.01.065
36. Enuka Y, Feldman ME, Chowdhury A, Srivastava S, Lindzen M, Sas-Chen A, et al. Epigenetic mechanisms underlie the crosstalk between growth factors and a steroid hormone. *Nucleic Acids Res* (2017) 45:12681–99. doi: 10.1093/nar/gkx865

13

Stimulatory Thyrotropin Receptor Antibodies are a Biomarker for Graves' Orbitopathy

*Augustine George, Tanja Diana, Jan Längericht and George J. Kahaly**

Molecular Thyroid Research Laboratory, Department of Medicine I, Johannes Gutenberg University (JGU) Medical Center, Mainz, Germany

Keywords: functional thyrotropin receptor antibodies, stimulatory TSH receptor antibodies, Graves' orbitopathy, thyroid eye disease, biomarker

***Correspondence:**
George J. Kahaly
George.kahaly@unimedizin-mainz.de

INTRODUCTION

Graves' Orbitopathy (GO) or thyroid eye disease (TED) is the most common and prominent extrathyroidal manifestation in patients diagnosed with Graves' disease (GD). Approximately 50% of patients diagnosed with GD develop GO, and with further orbital imaging, up to 80% of patients test positive for TED (1). Physical signs and symptoms (2), as well as the impact on the psychological well-being (3, 4) and quality of life (5, 6), underline the importance of effective disease management. Furthermore, the incidence of TED is linked to autoimmune gastritis and coeliac disease (7), implicating the importance of diagnosis of GO in patients, to identify risk factors for gastrointestinal autoimmunity.

Current evidence indicates that stimulating thyrotropin receptor IgG antibodies (stim. TSH-R-Ab or TSAb) are the main causative agent of GO, making its measurement a useful tool to predict and assess both clinical disease severity and activity.

TERMINOLOGY

Numerous terms have been established to describe TSH-R-Ab, the different nomenclature refers to various types of immunoassays (8). Total TSH-R-Ab also referred to as TRAb, are Ab that interact distinctively with the TSH-R. Routinely, these Ab are gauged by competitive immune binding assays and therefore are termed TSH-R-binding inhibitory immunoglobulins (TBII). Since binding assays only assess the binding of Ab to the TSH-R, it cannot display the function of the Ab it tests. Cell-based bioassays however differentiate between Ab that block or stimulate the TSH-R. Stimulating Ab are termed thyroid-stimulating Ab (TSAb) or thyroid-stimulating immunoglobulins (TSI), while blocking Ab are referred to as thyroid blocking Ab (TBAb) or thyroid blocking immunoglobulins (TBI). Further alternative terms for TBAb are TSH-R-stimulating-blocking Ab and TSH-R-blocking Ab or TRBAb.

DISTINCTION BETWEEN BLOCKING AND STIMULATING ANTIBODIES

TSH-R-Ab are found in patients with autoimmune thyroid disease (AITD) and play a major role in their pathogenesis and clinical presentation (9). TSH-R-Ab are divided into three groups since they have different ways to interact with the TSH-R. TSAb bind to the large extracellular amino-terminal and cause a stimulation of the TSH-R. This results in increased cyclic adenosine 3', 5'-monophosphate (cAMP), which increases the transcription of proteins necessary for the synthesis of thyroxine (T4), and triiodothyronine (T3). The outcome of this pathway is higher synthesis rates of thyroid-related hormones T3 and T4, and increased proliferation of the thyroid follicular endothelial cell. On the other hand, TBAb inhibit the function of the TSH-R, decreasing the synthesis rate of thyroid hormones, and inhibiting the proliferation and growth of the thyroid cell (10, 11). Other TSH-R-Ab neither block nor stimulate but rather have a neutral effect on the TSH-R. These Ab are referred to as neutral Ab or "cleavage" Ab and are not fully understood in their respective effect *in vivo*. Neutral Ab are able to induce various signaling cascades including some of which are initiated by TSAb, as well. However, neutral Ab can induce unique downstream signaling cascades including the activation of protein kinase C/mitogen activated protein kinase (MAPK), mammalian target of rapamycin (mTOR), nuclear factor 'kappa light chain enhancer' of activated B-cells (NF-κB), different cytokines, and reactive oxygen species (ROS). The initiation of these pathways is yet unclear, a recruitment of multiple G-proteins is possible. *In vitro* experiments show the expression of heat shock Proteins (p27, p107), endoplasmic reticulum stress protein (grp98), various oncogenes (p53, p73, retinoblastoma protein), and apoptosis of rat thyrocytes after a period of exposure to neutral Ab. It is unclear if ROS alone, or other signaling cascades play a role in the initiation of apoptosis (12, 13).

ROLE OF FUNCTIONAL TSH-R AUTOANTIBODIES IN GO

GO/TED is characterized by a protrusion of the eyes, upper lid retraction, diplopia, and irritation of the periorbital tissue and conjunctiva. In a study including 101 consecutive patients with TED, none tested positive for TBAb while 91 (90%) showed presence of TSAb of whom 90 were diagnosed with GD (14), concluding that not TBAb but rather TSAb are greatly prevalent in patients with TED. Current evidence suggests that TED is primarily caused by TSAb, which are present in patients with GD and Hashimoto's thyroiditis (HT). Animal models support the hypothesis of TSAb and TBAb, being synthesized as a result of immunization with the TSH-R, detected as an auto-antigen (15). The TSH-R is physiologically expressed in the soft tissue of the orbit, which was demonstrated in experiments where TSH-R mRNA was detected in affected tissue of the eye socket (16). Another study independently noted an overexpression of the TSH-R and human leukocyte antigen-DR (HLA-DR) in patients with GO (17). Produced by B- cells, TSAb enter the bloodstream and stimulate the TSH-R in various tissues e.g., the thyroid gland, orbital soft tissue, skin, and heart. In orbital fibroblasts, the Ab induce differentiation into pre-adipocytes and secretion of hydrophilic glycosaminoglycans (GAG), resulting in edema and later fibrosis (18, 19) (**Figure 1**).

Inflammatory cytokines play a major role in the pathogenesis of GO. By binding to the TSH-R, TSAb induces inflammation through inflammatory cytokines such as tumor necrosis factor-α (TNF-α), interferon-γ, and interleukin-1 which perpetuate the synthesis of collagen, GAG, and differentiation of orbital fibroblasts into adipocytes (20). Furthermore, by inducing the expression of heat shock proteins, prostaglandins, adhesion molecules, CD40, and major histocompatibility complex protein class two, cytokines amplify the inflammation cascade (21). The importance of inflammation explains the success of anti-inflammatory drugs like mycophenolate and glucocorticoids in the treatment of GO (22–24). The pathogenesis of GO is further supported by evidence, as high TSAb titers are associated with GO in patients with GD (25).

CLINICAL RELEVANCE OF TSAB AS A BIOMARKER FOR GO

Since the clinical presentation of GD and GO, especially the eye protrusion, is caused by stimulating TSH-R-Ab, measurement of TSAb is an excellent tool to manage patients with GD/GO. As there is a need to assess the function of the Ab, a cell-based bioassay rather than a binding assay is preferred (26, 27). In cell-based bioassays, IgG Ab are gauged through the signal transduction of cAMP, mediated through genetically engineered TSH-R on intact cells. Previously, the concentration of cAMP was measured through radiolabeled immunoassays (RIA). More recently, the amount of cAMP is assessed with cAMP-inducible reporter genes that express the luciferase enzyme. The enzyme concentration is then gauged with a luminometer after the luciferase substrate is added. TBAb are measured in an analogous bioassay while measuring their ability to competitively block the TSH-R against bovine TSH. In contrast, clinically employed immune binding assays assess the amount of TRAb, by measuring the displacement of a tracer, which is either radioiodine labeled bovine TSH or a monoclonal mouse antibody (MAb) with affinity to the TSH-R.

Previously, cell-based bioassays were toilsome and complicated procedures with varying specificity and sensitivity between laboratories, making it an unreliable way to measure Ab in comparison to binding assays. However, through major improvements in genetic engineering and molecular cloning, cell-based bioassays have become much more reliable and easier to perform. To improve reproducibility, the use of transfected cell lines of the Chinese ovarian hamster (CHO) was established, making the procedure more convenient with an improvement of assay sensitivity and specificity. Even though binding TSH-R-Ab or TBII can be used for differential diagnosis of GO (28), cell-based bioassays significantly outperform binding assays in terms of sensitivity and accuracy (27, 29–31), making it a better choice for management of GO.

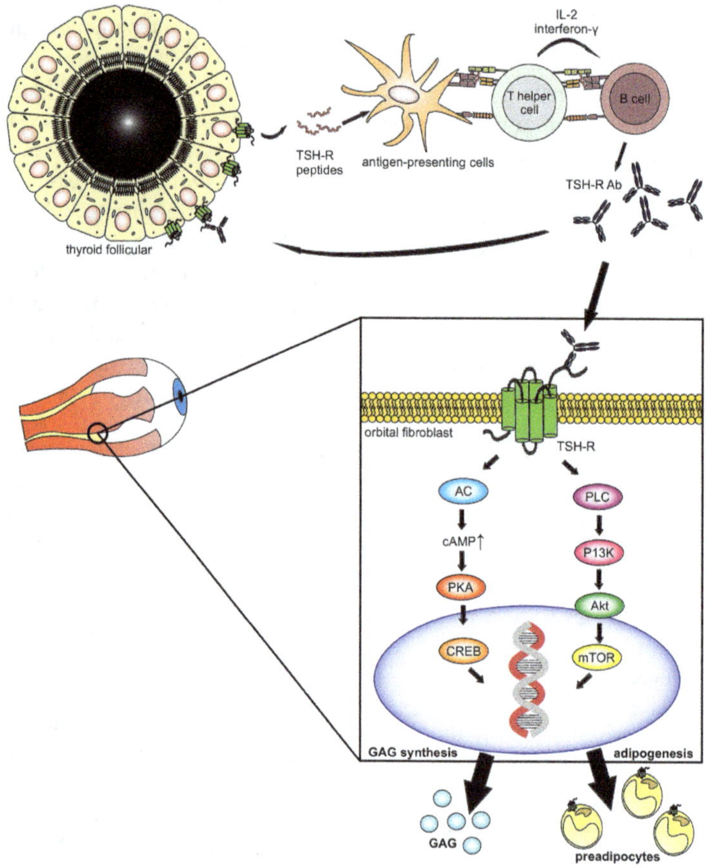

FIGURE 1 | The thyrotropin receptor (TSH-R) is the main autoantigen in Graves' hyperthyroidism and associated eye disease. TSH-R peptides are ingested by antigen-presenting cells (APC) through phagocytosis and expressed through MHC class II. T-helper cells recognize the antigen, by binding with the T-cell receptor, along with CD154 to its ligand CD40 on the surface of the APC. The activated T-helper cells bind to B-cells, transforming them into TSH-R antibody-secreting plasma cells through inflammatory cytokines interleukin II and gamma interferon. The synthesized TSAb bind to the TSH-R expressed by thyrocytes and orbital target cells (fibroblasts, pre-adipocytes), activating the Gαs adenylyl cyclase (AC) pathway. This stimulates protein kinase A which induces gene activation through the cAMP responsive element binding (CREB) protein. Additionally, the Gαq protein kinase C (PKC) pathway activates protein kinase B (Akt) inducing the mammalian target of rapamycin (mTOR) further inducing gene expression. The induction of gene expression lead to differentiation into pre-adipocytes and synthesis of hydrophilic mucopolysaccharides (glycosaminoglycans), hence leading to edema and later fibrosis in the orbital space, resulting in the clinical phenotype of thyroid eye disease.

Several studies were conducted to assess the reliability of TSAb as predictor for GO. A report investigating the relation of TSH-R-Ab and GO underlines the benefits of using functional Ab in the clinical routine (32). A total of 155 GD patients were tested for TSAb, using two different types of cell lines. All hyperthyroid patients with GD and TED tested positive for TSAb/TSI and TSAb were detected in 150 of 155 patients with TED. None of the 40 controls was Ab positive. TSAb levels in patients with GO were 3-fold and 8-fold higher than in GD patients and healthy controls, respectively.

To evaluate the relation between TSAb and the clinical presentation of TED, two standardized classifications were utilized. A clinical activity score (CAS), determined through an author unaware of the measured lab data, was used. To gauge the severity of TED, a clinical severity score (CSS) was utilized, based on the NOSPECS classification (33). TSAb titer correlated with both severity ($r = 0.87$, $p < 0.001$) and activity ($r = 0.87$, $p < 0.001$). In contrast, radiolabeled assays (RIA) showed weaker correlations at $r = 0.17$, $p < 0.015$ and $r = 0.54$, $p < 0.001$, respectively. Further, a cross-sectional trial assessing the clinical relevance of TSI in regards to TED, showed a similar correlation between severity ($r = 0.83$, $p < 0.001$) and activity ($r = 0.81$, $p < 0.001$) (34). A more significant association of TSAb with clinical features of GO was observed than TBII and thus TSAb may be regarded as functional biomarker for GO.

A multicenter cross-sectional study evaluated the relation of TSAb and TED in children with GD (35). 422 samples from 157 children with GD, 101 samples from non-thyroidal autoimmune diseases, and 50 healthy controls were tested. All patients with GD+GO tested positive for TSAb, compared to 96% in the binding assay (both $p < 0.001$). Further, in euthyroid children with GO, TBII were positive in 24 of 31 (77%) children only, while TSI were detected in all subjects (both $p = 0.016$). Additionally, in a different trial (36), children with GD+GO displayed the highest titers of TSAb (SRR% 417±135) in comparison to GD only (SRR% 320±157). Additionally, hyperthyroid children with GD+GO displayed higher TSI levels compared to children with GD only (median SRR%, 481 vs. 395%, both $p < 0.001$). TBII however, failed to differ between the two groups ($p < 0.125$). With the classification of disease severity, children were distinguished in moderate-to-severe and mild GO according to the classification of the European Group on Graves' Orbitopathy (EUGOGO). As in adults, children with moderate-to-severe GO exhibited higher TSAb titers compared to cases with mild GO (median SRR% 536 vs. 259, $p < 0.001$). Following the subjects during an average 3-year antithyroid drug (ATD) treatment, TSAb decreased by 69% and 20% in patients with GD and GD+GO, respectively. In contrast, TBII titers did not significantly differ between the two groups (90 vs. 89% in GD vs. GD+GO). Hence, TSAb is a strong indicator and predictor of GO in children (37), and supports the use of TSI/TSAb for management of pediatric GD/GO.

Furthermore, a 2-year prospective trial was conducted to evaluate the success of ATD treatment of one hundred consecutive hyperthyroid adults with GD, by measuring functional Ab and TBII (38). Forty-four of one hundred patients responded to ATD with Methimazole (MMI), of whom 43% suffered from GO. In the group with 56 non-responders, 66% of patients were diagnosed with GO. TSAb mirrored the activity of GD and was able to differentiate responders from non-responders. Additionally, and in contrast to TBII, TSAb titers were higher in adults with GO+GD, compared to GD alone. Finally, studies from Japan and Singapore also support the fact that TSAb correlate with the severity of GO. Indeed, increased TSAb titers are found in adults with higher GO scores (39), and in patients with GD+GO vs. GD only (40). As shown previously, GO activity did not correlate with serum TBII levels.

CLINICAL UTILITY OF FUNCTIONAL TSH-R-AB

Cell-based bioassays exclusively and solely differentiate between blocking and stimulating TSH-R-Ab and can measure TSH-R-Ab at very low concentrations (27). The presence of TSI/TSAb is predictive for GO (39). In contrast, TBII is not associated with GO. The utilization of TSAb facilitates rapid diagnosis of GD and allows differential diagnosis of thyrotoxicosis, being the only biomarker able to reliably differentiate GO+GD from patients with GD only. In the clinical routine, using early *in vitro* testing of TSAb showed a 46% faster time to diagnosis of GD and 47% cost savings since costly procedures and consultation of specialists was reduced (41). During specific treatment, TSAb detects patients with GO and can predict their responsiveness to therapy. Therefore, TSAb is the superior tool to manage GO in pediatric and adult patients (9, 20, 37, 42). Recently, an immunoassay has been developed to measure TSH-R-Ab using the bridge technology (43). It has been assumed that this assay detects TSAb only. The assay utilizes a pair of recombinant TSH-R and TSH-R-Ab are measured by binding one antibody arm to a capture receptor on the solid phase and bridging with the other arm to a detection receptor generating a signal. However, numerous comparative studies have proved that the bridge immunoassay is not able to differentiate between functional TSH-R-Ab (stimulating or blocking). Indeed, twenty hypothyroid Hashimoto's thyroiditis (HT) patients with high titers of TBAb measured in a blocking TSH-R-Ab cell-based bioassay, tested all positive in the bridge immunoassay (30). In another study, ten samples from TBAb-positive/TSAb-negative (both measured in bioassays) patients with GD or HT were positive in the bridge immunoassay (31). Further, various mixtures of monoclonal antibodies (MAb) of M22 and K1-70 were positive detected in the bridge assay. A recent study revealed that TBAb were present in one patient with HT and in two patients with GD and these patients were also positive in the bridge immunoassay but negative in the TSAb bioassay (29). Furthermore, all TBAb positive samples in a Graves' disease animal model were positive in the bridge assay without exception (15). Therefore, the bridge assay is a purely binding immunoassay. In conclusion, although not standardized yet and requiring more time and experienced lab personal, functional TSH-R-Ab in general and stimulatory Ab in particular are clinically useful and have been demonstrated to be a reliable and accurate biomarker for the diagnosis, differential diagnosis and monitoring of patients with GO.

AUTHOR CONTRIBUTIONS

Literature search, writing, text revision, layout: AG. Primary concept, writing, editing, critical evaluation, supervision: GK. Critical evaluation and editorial assistance: TD and JL. All authors contributed to the article and approved the submitted version.

ACKNOWLEDGMENTS

The authors thank the members of the Endocrine and Molecular Thyroid Laboratory, Department of Medicine I, JGU Medical Center for their technical support.

REFERENCES

1. Davies TF, Andersen S, Latif R, Nagayama Y, Barbesino G, Brito M, et al. Graves' disease. *Nat Rev Dis Primers* (2020) 6(1):52. doi: 10.1038/s41572-020-0184-y
2. Ponto KA, Merkesdal S, Hommel G, Pitz S, Pfeiffer N, Kahaly GJ. Public health relevance of Graves' orbitopathy. *J Clin Endocrinol Metab* (2013) 98 (1):145–52. doi: 10.1210/jc.2012-3119
3. Ponto KA, Binder H, Diana T, Matheis N, Otto AF, Pitz S, et al. Prevalence, Phenotype, and Psychosocial Well-Being in Euthyroid/Hypothyroid Thyroid-Associated Orbitopathy. *Thyroid* (2015) 25(8):942–8. doi: 10.1089/thy.2015.0031
4. Kahaly GJ, Petrak F, Hardt J, Pitz S, Egle UT. Psychosocial morbidity of Graves' orbitopathy. *Clin Endocrinol (Oxf)* (2005) 63(4):395–402. doi: 10.1111/j.1365-2265.2005.02352.x

5. Terwee CB, Dekker FW, Mourits MP, Gerding MN, Baldeschi L, Kalmann R, et al. Interpretation and validity of changes in scores on the Graves' ophthalmopathy quality of life questionnaire (GO-QOL) after different treatments. *Clin Endocrinol (Oxf)* (2001) 54(3):391–8. doi: 10.1046/j.1365-2265.2001.01241.x
6. Ponto KA, Kahaly GJ. Quality of life in patients suffering from thyroid orbitopathy. *Pediatr Endocrinol Rev* (2010) 7(Suppl 2):245–9.
7. Ponto KA, Schuppan D, Zwiener I, Binder H, Mirshahi A, Diana T, et al. Thyroid-associated orbitopathy is linked to gastrointestinal autoimmunity. *Clin Exp Immunol* (2014) 178(1):57–64. doi: 10.1111/cei.12395
8. Kahaly GJ, Diana T. TSH Receptor Antibody Functionality and Nomenclature. *Front Endocrinol (Lausanne)* (2017) 8:28. doi: 10.3389/fendo.2017.00028
9. Kahaly GJ. Management of Graves Thyroidal and Extrathyroidal Disease: An Update. *J Clin Endocrinol Metab* (2020) 105(12):3704–20. doi: 10.1210/clinem/dgaa646
10. Chiovato L, Vitti P, Santini F, Lopez G, Mammoli C, Bassi P, et al. Incidence of antibodies blocking thyrotropin effect in vitro in patients with euthyroid or hypothyroid autoimmune thyroiditis. *J Clin Endocrinol Metab* (1990) 71 (1):40–5. doi: 10.1210/jcem-71-1-40
11. Furmaniak J, Sanders J, Rees Smith B. Blocking type TSH receptor antibodies. *Auto- Immun Highlights* (2012) 4(1):11–26. doi: 10.1007/s13317-012-0028-1
12. Morshed SA, Ando T, Latif R, Davies TF. Neutral antibodies to the TSH receptor are present in Graves' disease and regulate selective signaling cascades. *Endocrinology* (2010) 151(11):5537–49. doi: 10.1210/en.2010-0424
13. Morshed SA, Ma R, Latif R, Davies TF. How one TSH receptor antibody induces thyrocyte proliferation while another induces apoptosis. *J Autoimmun* (2013) 47:17–24. doi: 10.1016/j.jaut.2013.07.009
14. Kampmann E, Diana T, Kanitz M, Hoppe D, Kahaly GJ. Thyroid Stimulating but Not Blocking Autoantibodies Are Highly Prevalent in Severe and Active Thyroid-Associated Orbitopathy: A Prospective Study. *Int J Endocrinol* (2015) 2015:678194. doi: 10.1155/2015/678194
15. Diana T, Holthoff H-P, Fassbender J, Wüster C, Kanitz M, Kahaly George J, et al. A Novel Long-Term Graves' Disease Animal Model Confirmed by Functional Thyrotropin Receptor Antibodies. *Eur Thyroid J* (2020) 9:1–8. doi: 10.1159/000508790
16. Kahaly GJ. The thyrocyte-fibrocyte link: closing the loop in the pathogenesis of Graves' disease? *J Clin Endocrinol Metab* (2010) 95(1):62–5. doi: 10.1210/jc.2009-2405
17. Hai YP, Lee ACH, Frommer L, Diana T, Kahaly GJ. Immunohistochemical analysis of human orbital tissue in Graves' orbitopathy. *J Endocrinol Invest* (2020) 43(2):123–37. doi: 10.1007/s40618-019-01116-4
18. Fatourechi V. Thyroid dermopathy and acropachy. *Best Pract Res Clin Endocrinol Metab* (2012) 26(4):553–65. doi: 10.1016/j.beem.2011.10.001
19. Kahaly G, Förster G, Hansen C. Glycosaminoglycans in thyroid eye disease. *Thyroid* (1998) 8(5):429–32. doi: 10.1089/thy.1998.8.429
20. Diana T, Kahaly GJ. Thyroid Stimulating Hormone Receptor Antibodies in Thyroid Eye Disease-Methodology and Clinical Applications. *Ophthalmic Plast Reconstr Surg* (2018) 34(4S Suppl 1):S13–S9. doi: 10.1097/IOP.0000000000001053
21. Cao HJ, Wang HS, Zhang Y, Lin HY, Phipps RP, Smith TJ. Activation of human orbital fibroblasts through CD40 engagement results in a dramatic induction of hyaluronan synthesis and prostaglandin endoperoxide H synthase-2 expression. Insights into potential pathogenic mechanisms of thyroid-associated ophthalmopathy. *J Biol Chem* (1998) 273(45):29615–25. doi: 10.1074/jbc.273.45.29615
22. Kahaly GJ, Riedl M, König J, Pitz S, Ponto K, Diana T, et al. Mycophenolate plus methylprednisolone versus methylprednisolone alone in active, moderate-to-severe Graves' orbitopathy (MINGO): a randomised, observer-masked, multicentre trial. *Lancet Diabetes Endocrinol* (2018) 6(4):287–98. doi: 10.1016/S2213-8587(18)30020-2
23. Zang S, Ponto KA, Kahaly GJ. Clinical review: Intravenous glucocorticoids for Graves' orbitopathy: efficacy and morbidity. *J Clin Endocrinol Metab* (2011) 96(2):320–32. doi: 10.1210/jc.2010-1962
24. Zang S, Ponto KA, Pitz S, Kahaly GJ. Dose of intravenous steroids and therapy outcome in Graves' orbitopathy. *J Endocrinol Invest* (2011) 34(11):876–80. doi: 10.1007/BF03346732
25. Kahaly GJ, Wuster C, Olivo PD, Diana T. High Titers of Thyrotropin Receptor Antibodies Are Associated With Orbitopathy in Patients With Graves Disease. *J Clin Endocrinol Metab* (2019) 104(7):2561–8. doi: 10.1210/jc.2018-02705
26. Diana T, Kanitz M, Lehmann M, Li Y, Olivo PD, Kahaly GJ. Standardization of a bioassay for thyrotropin receptor stimulating autoantibodies. *Thyroid* (2015) 25(2):169–75. doi: 10.1089/thy.2014.0346
27. Leschik JJ, Diana T, Olivo PD, Konig J, Krahn U, Li Y, et al. Analytical performance and clinical utility of a bioassay for thyroid-stimulating immunoglobulins. *Am J Clin Pathol* (2013) 139(2):192–200. doi: 10.1309/AJCPZUT7CNUEU7OP
28. Marinò M, Ionni I, Lanzolla G, Sframeli A, Latrofa F, Rocchi R, et al. Orbital diseases mimicking graves' orbitopathy: a long-standing challenge in differential diagnosis. *J Endocrinol Invest* (2020) 43(4):401–11. doi: 10.1007/s40618-019-01141-3
29. Allelein S, Diana T, Ehlers M, Kanitz M, Hermsen D, Schott M, et al. Comparison of a Bridge Immunoassay with Two Bioassays for Thyrotropin Receptor Antibody Detection and Differentiation. *Horm Metab Res* (2019) 51 (6):341–6. doi: 10.1055/a-0914-0535
30. Diana T, Wuster C, Kanitz M, Kahaly GJ. Highly variable sensitivity of five binding and two bio-assays for TSH-receptor antibodies. *J Endocrinol Invest* (2016) 39(10):1159–65. doi: 10.1007/s40618-016-0478-9
31. Diana T, Wuster C, Olivo PD, Unterrainer A, Konig J, Kanitz M, et al. Performance and Specificity of 6 Immunoassays for TSH Receptor Antibodies: A Multicenter Study. *Eur Thyroid J* (2017) 6(5):243–9. doi: 10.1159/000478522
32. Lytton SD, Ponto KA, Kanitz M, Matheis N, Kohn LD, Kahaly GJ. A novel thyroid stimulating immunoglobulin bioassay is a functional indicator of activity and severity of Graves' orbitopathy. *J Clin Endocrinol Metab* (2010) 95 (5):2123–31. doi: 10.1210/jc.2009-2470
33. Werner SC. Modification of the classification of the eye changes of Graves' disease: recommendations of the Ad Hoc Committee of the American Thyroid Association. *J Clin Endocrinol Metab* (1977) 44(1):203–4. doi: 10.1210/jcem-44-1-203
34. Ponto K, Kanitz M, Olivo P, Pitz S, Pfeiffer N, Kahaly G. Clinical Relevance of Thyroid-Stimulating Immunoglobulins in Graves' Ophthalmopathy. *Ophthalmology* (2011) 118:2279–85. doi: 10.1016/j.ophtha.2011.03.030
35. Diana T, Brown RS, Bossowski A, Segni M, Niedziela M, Konig J, et al. Clinical relevance of thyroid-stimulating autoantibodies in pediatric graves' disease-a multicenter study. *J Clin Endocrinol Metab* (2014) 99(5):1648–55. doi: 10.1210/jc.2013-4026
36. Stozek K, Bossowski A, Ziora K, Bossowska A, Mrugacz M, Noczynska A, et al. Functional TSH receptor antibodies in children with autoimmune thyroid diseases. *Autoimmunity* (2018) 51(2):62–8. doi: 10.1080/08916934.2018.1431776
37. Kahaly GJ, Diana T, Olivo PD. Tsh Receptor Antibodies: Relevance & Utility. *Endocr Pract* (2020) 26(1):97–106. doi: 10.4158/EP-2019-0363
38. Kahaly GJ, Diana T, Kanitz M, Frommer L, Olivo PD. Prospective Trial of Functional Thyrotropin Receptor Antibodies in Graves Disease. *J Clin Endocrinol Metab* (2020) 105(4):e1006–14. doi: 10.1210/clinem/dgz292
39. Noh JY, Hamada N, Inoue Y, Abe Y, Ito K, Ito K. Thyroid-Stimulating Antibody is Related to Graves' Ophthalmopathy, But Thyrotropin-Binding Inhibitor Immunoglobulin is Related to Hyperthyroidism in Patients with Graves' Disease. *Thyroid* (2000) 10(9):809–13. doi: 10.1089/thy.2000.10.809
40. Goh SY, Ho SC, Seah LL, Fong KS, Khoo DHC. Thyroid autoantibody profiles in ophthalmic dominant and thyroid dominant Graves' disease differ and suggest ophthalmopathy is a multiantigenic disease. *Clin Endocrinol* (2004) 60 (5):600–7. doi: 10.1111/j.1365-2265.2004.02033.x
41. McKee A, Peyerl F. TSI Assay Utilization: Impact on Costs of Graves' Hyperthyroidism Diagnosis. *Am J Managed Care* (2012) 18:e1–14.
42. Diana T, Ponto KA, Kahaly GJ. Thyrotropin receptor antibodies and Graves' orbitopathy. *J Endocrinol Invest* (2020). doi: 10.1007/s40618-020-01380-9
43. Frank CU, Braeth S, Dietrich JW, Wanjura D, Loos U. Bridge Technology with TSH Receptor Chimera for Sensitive Direct Detection of TSH Receptor Antibodies Causing Graves' Disease: Analytical and Clinical Evaluation. *Horm Metab Res* (2015) 47(12):880–8. doi: 10.1055/s-0035-1554662

14

Cytokines as Targets of Novel Therapies for Graves' Ophthalmopathy

Poupak Fallahi[1], Silvia Martina Ferrari[2], Giusy Elia[2], Francesca Ragusa[2], Sabrina Rosaria Paparo[2], Armando Patrizio[2], Stefania Camastra[2], Mario Miccoli[2], Gabriella Cavallini[1], Salvatore Benvenga[3,4,5] and Alessandro Antonelli[6]*

[1] Department of Translational Research of New Technologies in Medicine and Surgery, University of Pisa, Pisa, Italy, [2] Department of Clinical and Experimental Medicine, University of Pisa, Pisa, Italy, [3] Section of Endocrinology, Department of Clinical and Experimental Medicine, University of Messina, Messina, Italy, [4] Master Program on Childhood, Adolescent and Women's Endocrine Health, University of Messina, Messina, Italy, [5] Interdepartmental Program of Molecular & Clinical Endocrinology, and Women's Endocrine Health, University Hospital, A.O.U. Policlinico Gaetano Martino, Messina, Italy, [6] Department of Surgical, Medical and Molecular Pathology and Critical Care, University of Pisa, Pisa, Italy

***Correspondence:**
Alessandro Antonelli
alessandro.antonelli@med.unipi.it

Graves' disease (GD) is an organ-specific autoimmune disorder of the thyroid, which is characterized by circulating TSH-receptor (TSH-R) stimulating antibodies (TSAb), leading to hyperthyroidism. Graves' ophthalmopathy (GO) is one of GD extra-thyroidal manifestations associated with the presence of TSAb, and insulin-like growth factor-1 receptor (IGF-1R) autoantibodies, that interact with orbital fibroblasts. Cytokines are elevated in autoimmune (i.e., IL-18, IL-6) and non-autoimmune hyperthyroidism (i.e., TNF-α, IL-8, IL-6), and this could be associated with the chronic effects of thyroid hormone increase. A prevalent Th1-immune response (not related to the hyperthyroidism *per se*, but to the autoimmune process) is reported in the immune-pathogenesis of GD and GO; Th1-chemokines (CXCL9, CXCL10, CXCL11) and the (C-X-C)R3 receptor are crucial in this process. In patients with active GO, corticosteroids, or intravenous immunoglobulins, decrease inflammation and orbital congestion, and are considered first-line therapies. The more deepened understanding of GO pathophysiology has led to different immune-modulant treatments. Cytokines, TSH-R, and IGF-1R (on the surface of B and T lymphocytes, and fibroblasts), and chemokines implicated in the autoimmune process, are possible targets of novel therapies. Drugs that target cytokines (etanercept, tocilizumab, infliximab, adalimumab) have been tested in GO, with encouraging results. The chimeric monoclonal antibody directed against CD20, RTX, reduces B lymphocytes, cytokines and the released autoantibodies. A multicenter, randomized, placebo-controlled, double-masked trial has investigated the human monoclonal blocking antibody directed against IGF-1R, teprotumumab, reporting its effectiveness in GO. In conclusion, large, controlled and randomized studies are needed to evaluate new possible targeted therapies for GO.

Keywords: corticosteroids, cytokines, Graves' ophthalmopathy, rituximab, teprotumumab, tocilizumab

INTRODUCTION

Graves' disease (GD) is an organ-specific autoimmune disorder and it is the most frequent cause of hyperthyroidism in West Countries (1–3). It affects overall women, typically in their third to fifth decade, with an overall prevalence of 0.5% (4).

Clinical manifestations are linked to hyperthyroidism and to the autoimmune process. GD-associated signs and symptoms can vary markedly, influencing the overall well-being (5, 6).

GD is one of the principal autoimmune thyroid disorders (AITD), which are associated with the failure of immune tolerance against thyroid antigens [thyroid-stimulating hormone (TSH) receptor (TSH-R), thyroid peroxidase (TPO), and thyroglobulin (Tg)] (7, 8). At the basis of GD, an autoimmune multifactorial mechanism is present, which acts through environmental and endogenous factors in genetically predisposed individuals (9). GD is characterized by thyrotoxicosis, circulating anti-thyroid antibodies (ATA) and autoreactive lymphocytes into the thyroid (10).

The autoimmune reaction in GD induces the release of anti-TSH-R autoantibodies (TRAb) by B-cell clones, which infiltrate the thyroid, and are implicated in GD pathogenesis and its extrathyroidal manifestations, such as pretibial myxedema (PTM)/Graves' dermopathy and Graves' ophthalmopathy (GO). TRAb can be distinguished in: neutral antibodies; thyroid blocking antibodies (TBAb); thyroid stimulating antibodies (TSAb) (11). TSAb have similar downstream effects such as the binding of TSH to TSH-R, leading to thyrocytes proliferation, and secretion of thyroid hormones (TH; T4 and T3) (11, 12).

GD is associated to another autoimmune disease in ~20% of patients (13). A study evaluated prospectively the prevalence of other autoimmune diseases in GD patients (including some GO patients) vs. healthy controls, or patients with autoimmune thyroiditis (AT), or with multinodular goiter (MNG) (gender- and age-matched, and with a similar iodine intake). In 1.5% of GD, three associated autoimmune disorders were present. Patients with GO had a higher prevalence (18.9%) of another autoimmune disorder than GD patients without GO (15.6%) (13).

GRAVES' OPHTHALMOPATHY

According to the European Group on Graves' Orbitopathy (EUGOGO), GO has a prevalence of 10/10,000 persons and 16/10,000 persons in Europe and Japan, respectively (14, 15).

Approximately 30% to 50% of patients with GD develop GO. Tearing, proptosis, periorbital edema, and diplopia are the characteristic signs of Graves' orbitopathy (16).

Orbital fibroblasts (OF) are the target of a variety of autoimmune responses, that taking together induce proliferation, adipogenesis and overproduction of the extracellular matrix, that includes glycosaminoglycans [GAG; i.e., hyaluronan (HA) and chondroitin sulfate] (4).

GD is a phasic disorder characterized during the active phase by hyperthyroidism, which can go in remission both after therapy or sometimes spontaneously. The recurrence of hyperthyroidism can occur after weeks or decades of euthyroidism, overall owing to physical or psychological stressful events (2). Also, GO is characterized by the presence of moderate-severe inflammatory signs during the active phase that can remit after therapy or spontaneously. Mild GO disappears spontaneously in the majority of cases (17). The most frequent factors associated with the recurrence of GO are stressful life events (2), and smoking (18). Smoking cessation can improve the outcome for GO (3, 4). Components of cigarette smoke might induce adipogenesis and synthesis of GAG, through reactive oxygen species (ROS) production, and whether vaping could have some negative effects on GO is still to be clarified, as nicotine induces the release of pro-inflammatory cytokines (4, 19). As well as in GD, an autoimmune response is at the basis of GO. T cells, and autoantibodies recognizing a common autoantigen both for the thyroid and retro-ocular tissues (such as TSH-R, that is expressed also on fibroblasts and orbital preadipocytes), have a crucial role in this process (20). Moreover, another autoantigen, the insulin-like growth factor-1 (IGF-1) receptor (IGF-1R), has been suggested to be linked to GO (21). Autoantibodies against IGF-1R take part in the activation of GO OF, and its elevated expression has been shown in the thyroid and in orbital tissues in GD patients (20).

THERAPIES FOR GO

An anti-inflammatory treatment is suggested in the active phase of GO. A euthyroid state is mandatory for successful treatment and radioiodine therapy should be avoided in active progressive GO (15).

In patients with active GO, corticosteroids (CS), or high dose intravenous (iv) immunoglobulins, decrease inflammation and orbital congestion (22). A prospective, randomized trial compared the efficacy and safety of two protocols of iv 4.5 g methylprednisolone (MP) in 80 patients, randomized to receive iv MP weekly or daily. The weekly protocol of iv MP therapy was more efficient and safer than the daily protocol for patients with active moderate-to-severe GO (23).

According to randomized controlled trials, a meta-analysis reported in patients treated with iv glucocorticoids that a reduction of 1.14 mm of proptosis and of 33% of diplopia is present, while non-randomized studies reported a reduction of 1.58 mm of proptosis and of 25% of diplopia (24). After 6 weeks, in case of worsening of the disease the therapy should be supplemented or substituted with second-line treatments (15), such as orbital radiotherapy (25, 26). Orbital decompression should be done in severe GO (27).

Patients with severe GO can have a reduced quality of life (QoL) during standard therapies and, for this reason, novel treatments, targeting directly the pathogenic disease mechanisms in GO, are necessary to improve the clinical outcome in these patients.

At present, the more deepened understanding of GO pathophysiology has led to alternative immune-modulant therapies that target various antigens (28, 29).

The aim of new treatments for thyroidal and extrathyroidal GD is firstly to target the principal autoantigens of the disease and/or molecules that have a key role in the immunological response. Future treatments of GD, and GO, will involve monoclonal antibodies (mAb) or small molecules (15).

A mechanism for targeting the pathophysiology of GD, and GO, is to "mask" the TSH-R from the action of thyroid-stimulating immunoglobulin (TSI), through the TSH-R antagonist, K1-70 (15, 30, 31). An open-label clinical trial (clinical trial number NCT02904330) is currently in progress to assess its safety and tolerability in patients with hyperthyroidism in GD (32).

A small TSH-R antagonist (clinical trial number NCGC00229600) has been shown to reduce the synthesis of HA in retro-ocular fibroblasts/adipocytes in GO, with good results (33).

Furthermore, an encouraging treatment in GO patients is teprotumumab (RV 001, R1507), a recombinant, human mAb of the immunoglobulin G1 subclass. It binds to the cysteine-rich domain of human IGF-1R with high affinity, preventing the binding with endogenous ligands (IGF-1 and IGF-2), and leading to the internalization of the receptor, in this way stopping the IGF-1R signaling cascade (34–37).

As written above, active GO is linked to the autoimmune activation of OF. This causes the production of cytokines that promote T-cell infiltration into orbital tissues, triggering a local inflammatory process, and resulting in growth and differentiation of fibroblasts, and remodeling of orbital tissues. Teprotumumab blocks these pathophysiological responses (36).

Teprotumumab decreased *in vitro* TSH-R and IGF-1R, the TSH- and IGF-1–dependent phosphorylated Akt levels in fibrocytes, such as the TSH induction of IL-6 and IL-8 mRNA and protein (38).

A randomized, double-masked study was performed, to evaluate the effectiveness and safety of this drug in 88 patients with active, moderate-to-severe GO, administered with placebo, or the drug (eight infusions) (39). The primary end point was the response in the study eye. This response was defined as a reduction of two points or more in the Clinical Activity Score (CAS) and a reduction of 2 mm or more in proptosis at week 24. About 69% of patients taking teprotumumab, in comparison to 20% of those receiving placebo, had a response at week 24 ($P<0.001$). At week 6, 43% of patients administered with teprotumumab and 4% with placebo had a response ($P<0.001$). The reported findings in active GO demonstrated that teprotumumab, compared to placebo, is more effective in decreasing proptosis and CAS (39).

Another randomized, double-masked, phase III multicenter trial was done in patients with active GO in a 1:1 ratio to receive iv teprotumumab (10 mg/kg of body weight for the 1st infusion and 20 mg/kg for the following ones) or placebo once every 3 weeks for 21 weeks, for a total of 24 weeks (40). At week 24, the response in proptosis was higher in patients treated with teprotumumab than with placebo (83% vs. 10%, $P<0.001$). Secondary findings were significantly better with teprotumumab than with placebo ($P \leq 0.001$). The data demonstrated that teprotumumab led to better outcomes (than placebo) with regard to proptosis, CAS, diplopia, and QoL, with uncommon severe adverse events (40).

Teprotumumab attained the approval by the U.S. Food and Drug Administration (FDA) as first drug for thyroid eye disease in March 2020 (41, 42).

Another emerging therapy is rituximab (RTX), a chimeric mAb against CD20. It was approved by FDA in Wegener's granulomatosis, chronic lymphocytic leukemia, non-Hodgkin's lymphoma, and rheumatoid arthritis (RA), and it is an off-label drug in different autoimmune diseases (43). Since RTX reduces B lymphocytes, the cytokine burden and the produced autoantibodies, its use has been proposed also in GO.

Two randomized trials showed contrasting results regarding the use of RTX. In the 1st prospective, randomized, placebo-controlled trial, RTX was not effective in 25 GO patients, showing no improvement of CAS (44). In the other randomized, double-blinded study, 32 patients took iv MP or RTX, and CAS decreased in both cases, overall with RTX. After 24 weeks, all patients receiving RTX ameliorated with respect to 69% after ivMP, showing RTX was more effective than ivMP in GO patients (45).

More recently, a meta-analysis and systematic review was done in 293 GO patients, treated with RTX, or glucocorticoids, or saline, to evaluate the effectiveness of RTX. It was shown a significant decrease of CAS (vs. controls) in patients receiving RTX at 24 weeks, and a not significant one of proptosis (46).

In another study (47), 219 GO patients received pulse MP, and then oral steroids and/or orbital radiotherapy. At last, 15 (6.8%) were administered with 100 mg RTX (100–400 mg as cumulative dose) for the presence of active GO. A low dose of RTX had an anti-inflammatory effect in patients with active GO resistant to standard treatments (47). Another paper agreed with those results in 12 patients with active GO treated with a 100 mg RTX infusion; it reported that a low dose of RTX is effective in these patients, thus leading to a reduced administration of systemic steroid (48).

Furthermore, 14 patients with active and moderate-to-severe GO, of whom 11 CS-refractory, were administered with ivRTX (1000 mg twice with a 2-week interval), reporting that RTX was well-tolerated (49). A modest amelioration of CAS, and disease inactivation in half of the patients, were reported. At week 12, CAS ameliorated in 14.3% of patients and inactivation of GO in 28.6%. At week 24, total eye score and proptosis improved in 28.6% and 33% of patients, respectively.

CYTOKINES AND DRUGS TARGETING CYTOKINES, IN GD AND GO

Cytokines in GD and GO

Cytokines [including interleukins (IL), tumor necrosis factors (TNFs), interferons (IFNs), lymphokines, and chemokines] are small proteins, important in normal physiology, and in host responses to infection, trauma, reproduction, inflammation, sepsis, and tumors (10).

They are produced by different cell types, including immune cells (B and T lymphocytes, mast cells, macrophages), fibroblasts, endothelial cells, and different stromal cells, and act through receptors (**Table 1**).

Chemokines are "chemotactic cytokines", or signaling proteins, which can induce directed chemotaxis in the responsive cells. Chemokines exert their biological effects through the interaction with G-protein-linked transmembrane receptors, which are present on their target cells (10). The chemokine receptor (C-X-C)R3 binds Th1-chemokines [IFN-γ-inducible protein 10 (IP-10)/chemokine ligand 10 (C-X-C motif) (CXCL)10, IFN-inducible T-cell α chemoattractant (I-TAC)/ CXCL11 and monokine induced by IFN-γ (MIG)/CXCL9] (60). Th1 lymphocytes are attracted in inflamed tissues by Th1 chemokines, that are released there (61), and increase cytokines production, leading to Th1 chemokines secretion by different cells, establishing an amplification feedback loop (62). Raised serum and tissue Th1 chemokines levels have been demonstrated in specific autoimmune disorders [autoimmune thyroiditis (AT) (63–65), GD and GO (52), etc.], or systemic rheumatological diseases [systemic sclerosis, psoriasis or psoriatic arthritis (66, 67), etc.], hepatitis C virus infection related autoimmune disorders (68), and cancer (69, 70).

Certain serum cytokines are elevated in non-autoimmune (IL-8, TNF-α, and IL-6) (71) and autoimmune (IL-18 and IL-6) (72) hyperthyroidism, and this could be due to the chronic effects of TH excess, and not to the coexisting autoimmune condition at the basis of GD (73).

A Th1 immune response is more prevalent in the active phase of GD, and GO; CXCR3 and Th1 chemokines (CXCL9, CXCL10, CXCL11) are crucial in this process, while a switch in immune prevalence from a Th1 to a Th2 response is present in the inactive or later phases (1, 74).

Systemic hyperthyroidism and T cell infiltration into orbital tissue leads to ROS production, which can aggravate GO severity by increasing T cell proliferation, adipogenesis, and GAG production in OF (75). Recently, the role of the protein tyrosine phosphatase 1B (PTP1B), encoded by the PTPN1 gene, has been characterized in GO (76). PTP1B is known to be involved in immune cell signaling by regulating cytokines *via* dephosphorylation of janus kinase (JAK)2, signal transducer and activator of transcription (STAT)5, and tyrosine kinase (TYK)2. After 24 h of transfection with PTPN1 siRNA, the fibroblasts were exposed to IL-1β, cigarette smoke extract (CSE), H2O2, and transforming growth factor (TGF)-β stimulations. PTPN1 silencing ameliorated ROS generation in both CSE- and H_2O_2-stimulated cells. The changes in the phosphorylation level of multiple transcription factors after PTP1B inhibition in GO OF indicate a more complex network of signaling pathways. PTP1B inhibition suppressed IL-1β–induced Akt, and JNK phosphorylation, but p38 MAPK phosphorylation was reduced only in GO OF. As the p38 and JNK pathways, and the MAPK pathway, can mediate the transcription and translation of inflammatory cytokines, this study demonstrated that PTP1B mediates inflammatory reactions in GO OF (76).

Inflammation and cytokine production, adipogenesis, and HA synthesis are the prevailing processes implicated in the pathogenesis of GO (20). In the initial phases of GO, the prevalent Th1 immune response facilitates cell-mediated immunity, leading to the production of IFN-γ, TNF-α, IL-1β, and IL-2, that increase fibroblast proliferation and GAG synthesis. IFN-γ induces the secretion of Th1 chemokines by fibroblasts, and the migration of lymphocytes is promoted (54). IL-1β further stimulates the synthesis of GAG (77) and the production of CCL2, CCL5, IL-6, IL-16, IL-8, and neutrophils, by OF (78). Then, inflammation leads to Th2 lymphocytes activation, that release cytokines (i.e., IL-13, IL-10, IL-5, and IL-4), and to humoral reactions and the production of IgG (79). Tissue remodeling and fibrosis characterize the late phase of GO (20).

OF express also the costimulatory protein CD40, and its binding to the ligand CD154, on T cells, induces the production of different inflammatory mediators by OF [CCL2, IL-1α, prostaglandin E2 (PGE2), IL-6, and IL-8] (80–82).

GD OF include cell subsets with specific cellular markers, such as the CD34+ CXCR4 + Collagen 1+ phenotype (CD34+ OF), while CD34– OF do not display them. On the other hand, OF obtained from normal subjects are CD34– OF (55). The axon guidance glycoprotein Slit2 is produced by CD34– OF, and it inhibits fibrocyte differentiation and modulates their characteristic gene expression profile. Slit2 upregulates IL-12 expression and it attenuates that of IL-23, which are both involved in GD and GO (83). CD34+ fibrocytes obtained from peripheral blood mononuclear cells (PBMCs) produce low basal levels of HA, very few of which were affected by bovine thyrotropin (bTSH). On the other hand, GD OF synthesize higher levels of HA, both basally and after the treatment with bTSH. The treatment of confluent cultures with rhSlit2 increases HA production in fibrocytes, while the knock-down of Slit2 expression attenuates its synthesis in GD OF. Considering HA synthase isoenzymes (HAS1–3), low HAS1 levels are present in fibrocytes, while HAS2 is the most strongly expressed in GD OF. Slit2 alters the pattern of HAS and uridine diphosphate (UDP) glucose dehydrogenase (UDPGD) expression and cytokine production, both in GD OF and fibrocytes. The exogenous rhSlit2 causes a transition from HAS1 dominating expression to that of HAS2 in fibrocytes, decreasing also the expression of TNF-α and IL-6. These data suggest that HA synthesis in GD OF depends on the CD34– OF cell subset, while TNF-α and IL-6 expression is present in CD34+ OF. For these reasons GD OF, comprising both CD34+ OF and CD34– OF, can generate inflammatory factors (84, 85).

The activation of OF by TRAb suggests the link between GD and GO. The increased OF activity contributes to the fibrosis of the orbital tissues, causing inflammatory cell infiltration, and edema. Consequently, the optic nerve can be compressed leading to optic neuropathy. The inflammation and swelling of the eye muscles are involved in the final exophthalmos (20).

TABLE 1 | Main cytokines implicated in Graves' ophthalmopathy, the cells producing them and their biological effects.

Retrobulbar Cells	Main Cytokines	Biological effects	References
Fibroblasts/ preadipocytes	IFN-γ, TNF-α, IL-1α has been observed in tissue sections and in primary OF cultures of patients with active GO	IFN-γ, TNF-α, IL-1α in fibroblast stimulate: -the expression of a 72-kDa heat shock protein (HSP 72) -the expression of inter-cellular adhesion molecule-1 (ICAM-I). IFN-γ, TNF-α enhance the expression of HLA-DR	(50)
	IL-6, 8, 16, RANTES, MCP-1, IFN-γ, TNF-α, IL-1	IL-16 acts as a ligand for CD4+ cells, and it is important for T-cell trafficking. IL-16 production is believed to follow that of RANTES, and both are responsible for T-cell trafficking in orbital and thyroid fibroblasts	(51)
	In retrobulbar fibroblasts and preadipocytes obtained from GO patients: 1)IFN-γ induced CXCL10 secretion in a dose-dependent manner; 2)TNF-α alone was not able to induce chemokine secretion; 3)IFN-γ+TNF-α synergistically increased CXCL10 secretion	CXCL10 induces the migration of Th1 lymphocytes into the orbit, thereby perpetuating the autoimmune cascade	(52, 53)
	In retrobulbar fibroblasts and preadipocytes obtained from GO patients: 1) IFN-γ alone dose dependently induced the secretion of CXCL9 and CXCL11; 2) IFN-γ+TNF-α combination leads to a huge response of CXCL9	C-X-C chemokines participate in the self-perpetuation of inflammation	(54)
	-Cytokines detected *in situ* in GO include TNF-α, IL-1α, IL-6, IL-8, IL-10, IL-12, IL-13, and IFN-γ; -Several of these are more highly expressed in active vs stable disease and include IL-1β, IL-6, IL-8, and IL-10; -predominance of T helper (Th)1 cytokines in active GO	-Both IFN-γ and TNF-α induce B cell activating factor in GD OF -IL-1β induces both IL-16 and RANTES in GD OF, enhancing the release of T cell migration-promoting activity	(55)
	In cultured primary OF from GO patients: -IL-17A combined with CD40L could induce the production of RANTES in time- and dose-dependent modifications; -IL-17A alone was not enough sufficient to trigger RANTES release	Amplification of GO inflammatory process	(56)
	In primary cell cultures of GO fibroblasts and preadipocytes: 1)TNF-α increases the secretion of CXCL8 dose-dependently; 2) IFN-γ stimulates the secretion of CXCL10, but it inhibits that of CXCL8	This differential modulation of CXCL10 and CXCL8 chemokines could reflect a different role of the two chemokines during the course of the disease, as CXCL10 could be associated with the initial phase of the disease when a Th1 immune response (induced by IFN-γ) is preponderant, while CXCL8 could be associated with a later chronic phase of the disease, when there is a switch to a Th2 prevalent immune response (induced by TNF-α)	(57)
Adipocytes	High levels of MCP-1 mRNA in the orbital fat tissue of patients with GO have been reported	MCP-1 positively correlated with the degree of macrophage infiltration in patients with GO	(58)
Muscle cells	In primary extraocular muscle (EOM) cultures from patients with GO: 1)IFN-γ induced CXCL10 secretion in a dose-dependent manner; 2)IFN-γ+TNF-α synergistically increased CXCL10 secretion; 3)IFN-γ and TNF-α induce CCL2 secretion	Self-perpetuation of inflammation	(59)

GO, Graves' ophthalmopathy; IP-10, IFN-γ-inducible protein 10;C-X-C motif (CXCL)10, chemokine ligand 10; IFN-γ, interferon-γ; IL, interleukin; MCP-1/CCL2, monocyte chemoattractant protein-1; OF, orbital fibroblasts; TNF-α, tumor necrosis factor-α.

Furthermore, TSH-R–expressing T cells, which could be activated by TRAb, could stimulate adipogenesis of OF in GO through a peroxisome proliferator-activated receptor-γ (PPAR-γ) ligand produced *via* upregulated cyclooxygenase (4). CD34+ fibrocytes, such as OF, migrate from the circulation into sites of inflammation and injury and express two of the major GO thyroid autoantigens, TSH-R and thyroglobulin (4). Both CD4+ and CD8+ T cells, and B cells, are present in the majority of GO orbits, and the level of infiltration correlates with disease activity (86). Macrophages are found in the orbits in early disease, whereas monocytes and mast cells have been associated with secretion of platelet-derived growth factor, that stimulates OF proliferation and HA production, in particular the platelet-derived growth factor-BB isoform in OF from both patients with/without GO (4). Mast cells also produce prostaglandins, which are able to enhance adipogenesis (87). In light of the above, there are multiple overlapping factors in the development of GO, and cytokines are strongly involved in its pathogenesis.

DRUGS TARGETING CYTOKINES, IN GD AND GO

Drugs that target cytokines (etanercept, tocilizumab, infliximab, adalimumab) have been tested in GO, with encouraging results.

OF have an increased expression of TSH-R, and a strong up-regulation of TNF-α and IL-6, in the pathogenesis of GO (88).

The association between elevated circulating TNF-α levels and the severity of GO has led to the use of mAb against TNF-α, such as infliximab and etanercept (89, 90). The effectiveness of infliximab in severe steroid and surgical-resistant GO has recently been demonstrated in three cases, with complete resolution after three doses of 5 mg/kg body weight given 1 month apart (91, 92). Moreover, a positive effect of infliximab administration on active GO in a 58-year-old woman with GD has been described, in whom a single dose of this drug resulted in a reduction of inflammation and improvement of visual function, determined by magnetic resonance imaging and CAS and NO SPECS scales, with no noticeable short-term side effects (93).

Etanercept is usually used to treat RA (29). The use of etanercept has been evaluated as potential treatment in 10 patients with active GO, showing remission in 6/10 (89). Moreover, a paper reported the case of a woman, initially diagnosed with primary hypothyroidism (in substitutive treatment with levothyroxine) and subsequently with RA, who had insufficient therapeutic effectiveness with a conventional medication. After 3 years, she showed symptoms and signs of GO. Then, the patient received etanercept for RA, and after 4 months, the ocular symptoms ameliorated and exophthalmos decreased, showing that RA and GO can share similar pathogenic characteristics (88).

Furthermore adalimumab, that has been approved by FDA for psoriatic arthritis, ankylosing spondylitis, inflammatory bowel disease, RA, showed a significant amelioration in the inflammatory composite score in a retrospective review (94).

In patients with active GO, IL-6 and its soluble receptor are activated. Tocilizumab is a humanized mAb recognizing the IL-6R, which attained the approval in Castleman's disease, systemic juvenile idiopathic arthritis, and RA. A prospective non-randomized study has been conducted in 18 GO patients (refractory to CS) treated with tocilizumab (95). An amelioration of proptosis was reported in 13 patients, extraocular motility in 15, and 7/13 solved the problem of diplopia, with no relapse of GO at the end of the follow-up. These data suggested that tocilizumab might be effective in GO patients resistant to steroids (95). Furthermore, a reduction in extraocular muscle thickness and chemosis was reported after therapy with tocilizumab in patients with GO, by using an optical coherence tomography. Four women and one man with a median age of 52 years (range, 38–73 years) were enrolled. Median GO activity duration was 17 months (12–18). After tocilizumab, median muscle thicknesses and chemosis reduced. Median CAS decreased from 5 (4–8) to 1 (0–3) (96). More recently, a paper reported three GO patients refractory to CS or with advanced diplopia, receiving tocilizumab (8 mg/kg; monthly iv), and it showed a significant amelioration in eye symptoms (97).

CONCLUSION

GO is one of the extrathyroidal manifestations of GD. In patients with GO, OF can differentiate into myofibroblasts or adipocytes, able to interact with mononuclear cells, that produce chemoattractants and cytokines, in this way reiterating orbital inflammation.

Certain cytokines are elevated in autoimmune (i.e. IL-18 and IL-6) and non-autoimmune hyperthyroidism (i.e. TNF-α, IL-8, and IL-6), supporting the idea that this may be associated with the chronic effects of TH increase, and not with the GD inflammatory, autoimmune condition.

A prevalent Th1 immune response is reported in the immune-pathogenesis of GD and GO; Th1 chemokines (CXCL9, CXCL10, CXCL11), and the CXCR3, are crucial in this process

Patients with active, mild GO usually benefit from local therapies and selenium, whereas patients with moderate-to-severe disease generally need the addition of iv glucocorticoids. In case of an inadequate response to glucocorticoid therapy, different second-line therapies have been evaluated, such as orbital radiotherapy (with additional glucocorticoids), RTX, mycophenolate mofetil, cyclosporine, and methotrexate. Novel biologic agents, in particular teprotumumab and tocilizumab, have shown strong reductions in disease activity and severity. If these data are confirmed in the future, the treatment paradigm could be changed. Moreover, new immunotherapies are now evaluated for GD, that may have treatment implications also for GO (30).

At present, the more deepened understanding of GO pathophysiology has led to different immune-modulant treatments. Cytokines, TSH-R and IGF-1R (on the surface of B and T lymphocytes, and fibroblasts), and chemokines implicated in the autoimmune process, are possible targets of novel therapies.

The remodeled tissues in GO are dominated by adipogenesis, the increase of HA into the orbit, and the local synthesis of proinflammatory cytokines (including TNF-α and IL-6). There is a high complexity in the interactions among the cells of the heterogeneous population of GD OF in the GO orbit. Slit2 seems to play an important role in the determination of the pattern of HAS and UDPGD expression and IL-6, TNF-α, and HA production in these fibroblasts, and it could be considered as an interesting therapeutic target in GO (84, 85).

In the pathogenesis of GO, OF have an increased expression of TSH-R, and a strong up-regulation of TNF-α and IL-6. Drugs that target cytokines have been tested in GO, with encouraging results. The association between elevated circulating TNF-α levels and the severity of GO has led to the use of mAb against TNF-α, such as infliximab, adalimumab, and etanercept. Also tocilizumab (anti-IL6-R) have reached significant findings in GO.

In conclusion, large, controlled and randomized studies are needed to evaluate new possible targeted therapies for GO.

AUTHOR CONTRIBUTIONS

PF, SMF, SB, and AA conceived the paper. All authors contributed to the article and approved the submitted version.

REFERENCES

1. Antonelli A, Ferrari SM, Corrado A, Di Domenicantonio A, Fallahi P. Autoimmune thyroid disorders. *Autoimmun Rev* (2015) 14:174–80. doi: 10.1016/j.autrev.2014.10.016
2. Smith TJ, Hegedüs L. Graves' disease. *N Engl J Med* (2016) 375:1552–65. doi: 10.1056/NEJMra1510030
3. Antonelli A, Ferrari SM, Ragusa F, Elia G, Paparo SR, Ruffilli I, et al. Graves' disease: Epidemiology, genetic and environmental risk factors and viruses. *Best Pract Res Clin Endocrinol Metab* (2020) 34:101387. doi: 10.1016/j.beem.2020.101387
4. Taylor PN, Zhang L, Lee RWJ, Muller I, Ezra DG, Dayan CM, et al. New insights into the pathogenesis and nonsurgical management of Graves orbitopathy. *Nat Rev Endocrinol* (2020) 16:104–16. doi: 10.1038/s41574-019-0305-4
5. Vaidya B, Pearce SH. Diagnosis and management of thyrotoxicosis. *BMJ* (2014) 349:g5128. doi: 10.1136/bmj.g5128
6. Antonelli A, Fallahi P, Elia G, Ragusa F, Paparo SR, Ruffilli I, et al. Graves' disease: Clinical manifestations, immune pathogenesis (cytokines and chemokines) and therapy. *Best Pract Res Clin Endocrinol Metab* (2020) 34:101388. doi: 10.1016/j.beem.2020.101388
7. Romagnani S. The Th1/Th2 paradigm and allergic disorders. *Allergy* (1998) 53:12–5. doi: 10.1111/j.1398-9995.1998.tb04951.x
8. McLachlan SM, Rapoport B. Breaking tolerance to thyroid antigens: changing concepts in thyroid autoimmunity. *Endocr Rev* (2014) 35:59–105. doi: 10.1210/er.2013-1055
9. Wémeau JL, Klein M, Sadoul JL, Briet C, Vélayoudom-Céphise FL. Graves' disease: introduction, epidemiology, endogenous and environmental pathogenic factors. *Ann Endocrinol* (2018) 79:599–607. doi: 10.1016/j.ando.2018.09.002
10. Ferrari SM, Ruffilli I, Elia G, Ragusa F, Paparo SR, Patrizio A, et al. Chemokines in hyperthyroidism. *J Clin Transl Endocrinol* (2019) 16:100196. doi: 10.1016/j.jcte.2019.100196
11. Kotwal A, Stan M. Thyrotropin receptor antibodies-an overview. *Ophthalmic Plast Reconstr Surg* (2018) 34(4S Suppl 1):S20–7. doi: 10.1097/IOP.0000000000001052
12. Kahaly GJ, Diana T, Kanitz M, Frommer L, Olivo PD. Prospective Trial of Functional Thyrotropin Receptor Antibodies in Graves Disease. *J Clin Endocrinol Metab* (2020) 105:e1006–14. doi: 10.1210/clinem/dgz292
13. Ferrari SM, Fallahi P, Ruffilli I, Elia G, Ragusa F, Benvenga S, et al. The association of other autoimmune diseases in patients with Graves' disease (with or without ophthalmopathy): review of the literature and report of a large series. *Autoimmun Rev* (2019) 18:287–92. doi: 10.1016/j.autrev.2018.10.001
14. Perros P, Hegedüs L, Bartalena L, Marcocci C, Kahaly GJ, Baldeschi L, et al. Graves' orbitopathy as a rare disease in Europe: a European Group on Graves' Orbitopathy (EUGOGO) position statement. *Orphanet J Rare Dis* (2017) 12:72. doi: 10.1186/s13023-017-0625-1
15. Davies TF, Andersen S, Latif R, Nagayama Y, Barbesino G, Brito M, et al. Graves' disease. *Nat Rev Dis Primers* (2020) 6:52. doi: 10.1038/s41572-020-0184-y
16. Davies TF, Burch HB. *Clinical features and diagnosis of Graves' orbitopathy (ophthalmopathy)* (2019). Available at: https://www.uptodate.com/contents/pathogenesis-of-graves-disease/ (Accessed 14 Jan 2021).
17. Bartalena L, Baldeschi L, Boboridis K, Eckstein A, Kahaly GJ, Marcocci C, et al. The 2016 European Thyroid Association/European Group on Graves' Orbitopathy Guidelines for the Management of Graves' Orbitopathy. *Eur Thyroid J* (2016) 5(1):9–26. doi: 10.1159/000443828
18. Perricone C, Versini M, Ben-Ami D, Gertel S, Watad A, Segel MJ, et al. Smoke and autoimmunity: the fire behind the disease. *Autoimmun Rev* (2016) 15:354–74. doi: 10.1016/j.autrev.2016.01.001
19. Cawood TJ, Moriarty P, O'Farrelly C, O'Shea D. Smoking and thyroid-associated ophthalmopathy: a novel explanation of the biological link. *J Clin Endocrinol Metab* (2007) 92:59–64. doi: 10.1210/jc.2006-1824
20. Łacheta D, Miśkiewicz P, Głuszko A, Nowicka G, Struga M, Kantor I, et al. Immunological Aspects of Graves' Ophthalmopathy. *Biomed Res Int* (2019) 2019:7453260. doi: 10.1155/2019/7453260
21. Place RF, Krieger CC, Neumann S, Gershengorn MC. Inhibiting thyrotropin/insulin-like growth factor 1 receptor crosstalk to treat Graves' ophthalmopathy: studies in orbital fibro blasts in vitro. *Br J Pharmacol* (2017) 174:328–40. doi: 10.1111/bph.13693
22. Antonelli A, Saracino A, Alberti B, Canapicchi R, Cartei F, Lepri A, et al. High-dose intravenous immunoglobulin treatment in Graves' ophthalmopathy. *Acta Endocrinol (Copenh)* (1992) 126(1):13–23. doi: 10.1530/acta.0.1260013
23. Zhu W, Ye L, Shen L, Jiao Q, Huang F, Han R, et al. A prospective, randomized trial of intravenous glucocorticoids therapy with different protocols for patients with graves' ophthalmopathy. *J Clin Endocrinol Metab* (2014) 99(6):1999–2007. doi: 10.1210/jc.2013-3919
24. Zang S, Ponto KA, Kahaly GJ. J. Clinical review: intravenous glucocorticoids for Graves' orbitopathy: efficacy and morbidity. *J Clin Endocrinol Metab* (2011) 96:320–32. doi: 10.1210/jc.2010-1962
25. Bartalena L, Veronesi G, Krassas GE, Wiersinga WM, Marcocci C, Marinò M, et al. Does early response to intravenous glucocorticoids predict the final outcome in patients with moderate-to-severe and active Graves' orbitopathy? *J Endocrinol Invest* (2017) 40:547–53. doi: 10.1007/s40618-017-0608-z
26. Tanda ML, Bartalena L. Efficacy and safety of orbital radiotherapy for Graves' orbitopathy. *J Clin Endocrinol Metab* (2012) 97:3857–65. doi: 10.1210/jc.2012-2758
27. Currò N, Covelli D, Vannucchi G, Campi I, Pirola G, Simonetta S, et al. Therapeutic outcomes of high-dose intravenous steroids in the treatment of dysthyroid optic neuropathy. *Thyroid* (2014) 24:897–905. doi: 10.1089/thy.2013.0445
28. Fallahi P, Ferrari SM, Elia G, Nasini F, Colaci M, Giuggioli D, et al. Novel Therapies for Thyroid Autoimmune Diseases. *Expert Rev Clin Pharmacol* (2016) 9:853–61. doi: 10.1586/17512433.2016.1157468
29. Ferrari SM, Fallahi P, Elia G, Ragusa F, Camastra S, Paparo SR, et al. Novel therapies for thyroid autoimmune diseases: An update. *Best Pract Res Clin Endocrinol Metab* (2020) 34:101366. doi: 10.1016/j.beem.2019.101366
30. Genere N, Stan MN. Current and Emerging Treatment Strategies for Graves' Orbitopathy. *Drugs* (2019) 79:109–24. doi: 10.1007/s40265-018-1045-9
31. Sanders P, Young S, Sanders J, Kabelis K, Baker S, Sullivan A, et al. Crystal structure of the TSH receptor (TSHR) bound to a blocking-type TSHR autoantibody. *J Mol Endocrinol* (2011) 46:81–99. doi: 10.1530/JME-10-0127
32. Available at: https://clinicaltrials.gov/ct2/show/NCT02904330 (Accessed 14 Jan 2021).
33. Turcu AF, Kumar S, Neumann S, Coenen M, Iyer S, Chiriboga P, et al. A small molecule antagonist inhibits thyrotropin receptor antibody-induced orbital fibroblast functions involved in the pathogenesis of Graves ophthalmopathy. *J Clin Endocrinol Metabol* (2013) 98:2153–9. doi: 10.1210/jc.2013-1149
34. Smith TJ, Janssen JA. Building the case for insulin-like growth factor receptor-I involvement in thyroid-associated ophthalmopathy. *Front Endocrinol (Lausanne)* (2016) 7:167. doi: 10.3389/fendo.2016.00167
35. Smith TJ, Janssen J. Insulin-like growth factor-I receptor and thyroid-associated ophthalmopathy. *Endocr Rev* (2019) 40:236–67. doi: 10.1210/er.2018-00066
36. Kahaly GJ. Immunotherapies for thyroid eye disease. *Curr Opin Endocrinol Diabetes Obes* (2019) 26:250–5. doi: 10.1097/MED.0000000000000493
37. Mohyi M, Smith TJ. IGF1 receptor and thyroid-associated ophthalmopathy. *J Mol Endocrinol* (2018) 61:T29–43. doi: 10.1530/JME-17-0276

38. Chen H, Mester T, Raychaudhuri N, Kauh CY, Gupta S, Smith TJ, et al. Teprotumumab, an IGF-1R blocking monoclonal antibody inhibits TSH and IGF-1 action in fibrocytes. *J Clin Endocrinol Metab* (2014) 99:E1635–40. doi: 10.1210/jc.2014-1580
39. Smith TJ, Kahaly GJ, Ezra DG, Fleming JC, Dailey RA, Tang RA, et al. Teprotumumab for Thyroid-Associated Ophthalmopathy. *N Engl J Med* (2017) 376:1748–61. doi: 10.1056/NEJMoa1614949
40. Douglas RS, Kahaly GJ, Patel A, Sile S, Thompson EHZ, Perdok R, et al. Teprotumumab for the Treatment of Active Thyroid Eye Disease. *N Engl J Med* (2020) 382:341–52. doi: 10.1056/NEJMoa1910434
41. Smith TJ. Thyroid-associated ophthalmopathy: Emergence of teprotumumab as a promising medical therapy. *Best Pract Res Clin Endocrinol Metab* (2020) 34:101383. doi: 10.1016/j.beem.2020.101383
42. *Horizon therapeutics plc announces the FDA has granted priority review of the teprotumumab biologics license application (BLA) for the treatment of active thyroid eye disease (TED)* (2019). Available at: https://ir.horizontherapeutics.com/news-releases/news-release-details/horizon-therapeutics-plc-announces-fda-has-granted-priority (Accessed 14 Jan 2021).
43. Giuggioli D, Lumetti F, Colaci M, Fallahi P, Antonelli A, Ferri C. Rituximab in the treatment of patients with systemic sclerosis. Our experience and review of the literature. *Autoimmun Rev* (2015) 14:1072–8. doi: 10.1016/j.autrev.2015.07.008
44. Stan MN, Garrity JA, Carranza Leon BG, Prabin T, Bradley EA, Bahn RS. Randomized controlled trial of rituximab in patients with Graves' orbitopathy. *J Clin Endocrinol Metab* (2015) 100:432–41. doi: 10.1210/jc.2014-2572
45. Salvi M, Vannucchi G, Currò N, Campi I, Covelli D, Dazzi D, et al. Efficacy of B-cell targeted therapy with rituximab in patients with active moderate to severe Graves' orbitopathy: a randomized controlled study. *J Clin Endocrinol Metab* (2015) 100:422–31. doi: 10.1210/jc.2014-3014
46. Shen WC, Lee CH, Loh EW, Hsieh AT, Chen L, Tam KW. Efficacy and safety of rituximab for the treatment of graves' orbitopathy: a meta-analysis of randomized controlled trials. *Pharmacotherapy* (2018) 38:503–10. doi: 10.1002/phar.2111
47. Du Pasquier-Fediaevsky L, Andrei S, Berche M, Leenhardt L, Héron E, Rivière S. Low-dose rituximab for active moderate to severe graves' orbitopathy resistant to conventional treatment. *Ocul Immunol Inflamm* (2019) 27:844–50. doi: 10.1080/09273948.2018.1453078
48. Insull EA, Sipkova Z, David J, Turner HE, Norris JH. Early low-dose rituximab for active thyroid eye disease: an effective and well-tolerated treatment. *Clin Endocrinol* (2019) 91:179–86. doi: 10.1111/cen.13970
49. Eid L, Coste-Verdier V, Longueville E, Ribeiro E, Nicolescu-Catargi B, Korobelnik JF. The effects of Rituximab on Graves'orbitopathy: a retrospective study of 14 patients. *Eur J Ophthalmol* (2019) 30:1008–13. doi: 10.1177/1120672119845224
50. Heufelder AE, Bahn RS. Detection and localization of cytokine immunoreactivity in retro-ocular connective tissue in Graves' ophthalmopathy. *Eur J Clin Invest* (1993) 23:10–7. doi: 10.1111/j.1365-2362.1993.tb00712.x
51. Ludgate M, Baker G. Unlocking the immunological mechanisms of orbital inflammation in thyroid eye disease. *Clin Exp Immunol* (2002) 127:193–8. doi: 10.1046/j.1365-2249.2002.01792.x
52. Antonelli A, Ferrari SM, Fallahi P, Piaggi S, Paolicchi A, Franceschini SS, et al. Cytokines (interferon-γ- and tumor necrosis factor-α)-induced nuclear factor-κB activation and chemokine (C-X-C motif) ligand 10 release in Graves disease and ophthalmopathy are modulated by pioglitazone. *Metabolism* (2011) 60:277–83. doi: 10.1016/j.metabol.2010.02.002
53. Antonelli A, Rotondi M, Ferrari SM, Fallahi P, Romagnani P, Franceschini SS, et al. Interferon-gamma-inducible alpha-chemokine CXCL10 involvement in Graves' ophthalmopathy: modulation by peroxisome proliferator-activated receptor-gamma agonists. *J Clin Endocrinol Metab* (2006) 91:614–20. doi: 10.1210/jc.2005-1689
54. Antonelli A, Ferrari SM, Fallahi P, Frascerra S, Santini E, Franceschini SS, et al. Monokine induced by interferon gamma (IFNgamma) (CXCL9) and IFNgamma inducible T-cell alpha-chemoattractant (CXCL11) involvement in Graves' disease and ophthalmopathy: modulation by peroxisome proliferator-activated receptor-gamma agonists. *J Clin Endocrinol Metab* (2009) 94:1803–9. doi: 10.1210/jc.2008-2450
55. Smith TJ. Potential roles of CD34+ fibrocytes masquerading as orbital fibroblasts in thyroid-associated ophthalmopathy. *J Clin Endocrinol Metab* (2019) 104:581–94. doi: 10.1210/jc.2018-01493
56. Fang S, Huang Y, Zhong S, Zhang Y, Liu X, Wang Y, et al. IL-17A Promotes RANTES Expression, But Not IL-16, in Orbital Fibroblasts Via CD40-CD40L Combination in Thyroid-Associated Ophthalmopathy. *Invest Ophthalmol Vis Sci* (2016) 57:6123–33. doi: 10.1167/iovs.16-20199
57. Ferrari SM, Ragusa F, Paparo SR, Nasini F, Nardi M, Franceschini SS, et al. Differential modulation of CXCL8 versus CXCL10, by cytokines, PPAR-gamma, or PPAR-alpha agonists, in primary cells from Graves' disease and ophthalmopathy. *Autoimmun Rev* (2019) 18:673–8. doi: 10.1016/j.autrev.2019.05.004
58. Chen MH, Chen MH, Liao SL, Chang TC, Chuang LM. Role of macrophage infiltration in the orbital fat of patients with Graves' ophthalmopathy. *Clin Endocrinol (Oxf)* (2008) 69:332–7. doi: 10.1111/j.1365-2265.2008.03219.x
59. Antonelli A, Ferrari SM, Corrado A, Franceschini SS, Gelmini S, Ferrannini E, et al. Extra-ocular muscle cells from patients with Graves' ophthalmopathy secrete α (CXCL10) and β (CCL2) chemokines under the influence of cytokines that are modulated by PPARγ. *Autoimmun Rev* (2014) 13:1160–6. doi: 10.1016/j.autrev.2014.08.025
60. Lasagni L, Francalanci M, Annunziato F, Lazzeri E, Giannini S, Cosmi L, et al. An alternatively spliced variant of CXCR3 mediates the inhibition of endothelial cell growth induced by IP-10, Mig, and I-TAC, and acts as functional receptor for platelet factor 4. *J Exp Med* (2003) 197:1537–49. doi: 10.1084/jem.20021897
61. Tokunaga R, Zhang W, Naseem M, Puccini A, Berger MD, Soni S, et al. CXCL9, CXCL10, CXCL11/CXCR3 axis for immune activation – a target for novel cancer therapy. *Cancer Treat Rev* (2018) 63:40–7. doi: 10.1016/j.ctrv.2017.11.007
62. Antonelli A, Ferrari SM, Giuggioli D, Ferrannini E, Ferri C, Fallahi P. Chemokine (C-X-C motif) ligand (CXCL)10 in autoimmune diseases. *Autoimmun Rev* (2014) 13:272–80. doi: 10.1016/j.autrev.2013.10.010
63. Antonelli A, Ferrari SM, Frascerra S, Di Domenicantonio A, Nicolini A, Ferrari P, et al. Increase of circulating CXCL9 and CXCL11 associated with euthyroid or subclinically hypothyroid autoimmune thyroiditis. *J Clin Endocrinol Metab* (2011) 96:1859–63. doi: 10.1210/jc.2010-2905
64. Antonelli A, Ferrari SM, Fallahi P, Ghiri E, Crescioli C, Romagnani P, et al. Interferon-alpha, -beta and -gamma induce CXCL9 and CXCL10 secretion by human thyrocytes: modulation by peroxisome proliferator-activated receptor-gamma agonists. *Cytokine* (2010) 50:260–7. doi: 10.1016/j.cyto.2010.01.009
65. Fallahi P, Ferrari SM, Ruffilli I, Elia G, Biricotti M, Vita R, et al. The association of other autoimmune diseases in patients with autoimmune thyroiditis: review of the literature and report of a large series of patients. *Autoimmun Rev* (2016) 15:1125–8. doi: 10.1016/j.autrev.2016.09.009
66. Antonelli A, Ferri C, Fallahi P, Colaci M, Giuggioli D, Ferrari SM, et al. Th1 and Th2 chemokine serum levels in systemic sclerosis in the presence or absence of autoimmune thyroiditis. *J Rheumatol* (2008) 35:1809–11.
67. Antonelli A, Fallahi P, Delle Sedie A, Ferrari SM, Maccheroni M, Bombardieri S, et al. High values of alpha (CXCL10) and beta (CCL2) circulating chemokines in patients with psoriatic arthritis, in presence or absence of autoimmune thyroiditis. *Autoimmunity* (2008) 41:537–42. doi: 10.1080/08916930802170401
68. Ferrari SM, Fallahi P, Mancusi C, Colaci M, Manfredi A, Ferri C, et al. HCV-related autoimmune disorders in HCV chronic infection. *Clin Ter* (2013) 164:e305–12. doi: 10.7417/CT.2013.1594
69. Antonelli A, Ferrari SM, Fallahi P, Piaggi S, Di Domenicantonio A, Galleri D, et al. Variable modulation by cytokines and thiazolidinediones of the prototype Th1 chemokine CXCL10 in anaplastic thyroid cancer. *Cytokine* (2012) 59:218–22. doi: 10.1016/j.cyto.2012.04.042
70. Ferrari SM, Fallahi P, Galdiero MR, Ruffilli I, Elia G, Ragusa F, et al. Immune and Inflammatory Cells in Thyroid Cancer Microenvironment. *Int J Mol Sci* (2019) 20:4413. doi: 10.3390/ijms20184413
71. Siddiqi A, Monson JP, Wood DF, Besser GM, Burrin JM. Serum cytokines in thyrotoxicosis. *J Clin Endocrinol Metab* (1999) 84:435–9. doi: 10.1210/jcem.84.2.5436
72. Salvi M, Pedrazzoni M, Girasole G, Giuliani N, Minelli R, Wall JR, et al. Serum concentrations of proinflammatory cytokines in Graves' disease: effect of

treatment, thyroid function, ophthalmopathy and cigarette smoking. *Eur J Endocrinol* (2000) 143:197–202. doi: 10.1530/eje.0.1430197

73. Antonelli A, Fallahi P, Rotondi M, Ferrari SM, Romagnani P, Grosso M, et al. Increased serum CXCL10 in Graves' disease or autoimmune thyroiditis is not associated with hyper- or hypothyroidism per se, but is specifically sustained by the autoimmune, inflammatory process. *Eur J Endocrinol* (2006) 154:651–8. doi: 10.1530/eje.1.02137
74. Fallahi P, Ferrari SM, Ragusa F, Ruffilli I, Elia G, Paparo SR, et al. Th1 Chemokines in Autoimmune Endocrine Disorders. *J Clin Endocrinol Metab* (2020) 105:dgz289. doi: 10.1210/clinem/dgz289
75. Venditti P, Di Meo S. Thyroid hormone-induced oxidative stress. *Cell Mol Life Sci* (2006) 63:414–34. doi: 10.1007/s00018-005-5457-9
76. Byeon HJ, Kim JY, Ko J, Lee EJ, Don K, Yoon JS. Protein tyrosine phosphatase 1B as a therapeutic target for Graves' orbitopathy in an in vitro model. *PloS One* (2020) 15:e0237015. doi: 10.1371/journal.pone.0237015
77. Han R, Smith TJ. T helper type 1 and type 2 cytokines exert divergent influence on the induction of prostaglandin E2 and hyaluronan synthesis by interleukin-1β in orbital fibroblasts: implications for the pathogenesis of thyroidassociated ophthalmopathy. *Endocrinology* (2006) 147:13–9. doi: 10.1210/en.2005-1018
78. Chen B, Tsui S, Smith TJ. IL-1 beta induces IL-6 expression in human orbital fibroblasts: identification of an anatomic-site specific phenotypic attribute relevant to thyroid- associated ophthalmopathy. *J Immunol* (2005) 175:1310–9. doi: 10.4049/jimmunol.175.2.1310
79. Mikoś H, Mikoś M, Obara-Moszyńska M, Niedziela M. The role of the immune system and cytokines involved in the pathogenesis of autoimmune thyroid disease (AITD). *Endokrynol Pol* (2014) 65:150–5. doi: 10.5603/EP.2014.0021
80. Hwang CJ, Afifiyan N, Sand D, Naik V, Said J, Pollock SJ, et al. Orbital fibroblasts from patients with thyroid-associated ophthalmopathy overexpress CD40: CD154 hyper induces IL-6, IL-8, and MCP-1. *Invest Ophthalmol Vis Sci* (2009) 50:2262–8. doi: 10.1167/iovs.08-2328
81. Kuehn HS, Jung MY, Beaven MA, Metcalfe DD, Gilfillan AM. Prostaglandin E2 activates and utilizes mTORC2 as a central signaling locus for the regulation of mast cell chemotaxis and mediator release. *J Biol Chem* (2011) 286:391–402. doi: 10.1074/jbc.M110.164772
82. Zhao LQ, Wei RL, Cheng JW, Cai JP, Li Y. The expression of intercellular adhesion molecule-1 induced by CD40-CD40L ligand signaling in orbital fibroblasts in patients with Graves' ophthalmopathy, Invest. *Opthalmol Vis Sci* (2010) 51:4652–60. doi: 10.1167/iovs.09-3789
83. Fernando R, Atkins SJ, Smith TJ. Slit2 may underlie divergent induction by thyrotropin of IL-23 and IL-12 in human fibrocytes. *J Immunol* (2020) 204:1724–35. doi: 10.4049/jimmunol.1900434
84. Fernando R, Smith TJ. Slit2 regulates hyaluronan & cytokine synthesis in fibrocytes: Potential relevance to thyroid associated ophthalmopathy. *J Clin Endocrinol Metab* (2020) 106:e20–33. doi: 10.1210/clinem/dgaa684
85. Antonelli A, Ferrari SM, Fallahi P. Slit2 regulation of hyaluronan & cytokine synthesis in fibrocytes in thyroid associated ophthalmopathy. *J Clin Endocrinol Metab* (2020) 136:dgaa959. doi: 10.1210/clinem/dgaa959
86. Rotondo Dottore G, Torregrossa L, Caturegli P, Ionni I, Sframeli A, Sabini E, et al. Association of T and B cells infiltrating orbital tissues with clinical features of graves orbitopathy. *JAMA Ophthalmol* (2018) 136:613–9. doi: 10.1001/jamaophthalmol.2018.0806
87. Draman MS, Ludgate M. Thyroid eye disease — an update. *Expert Rev Ophthalmol* (2016) 11:273–84. doi: 10.1080/17469899.2016.1202113
88. Boskovic O, Medenica S, Radojevic N, Zarkovic M. Etanercept in the treatment of Graves' ophthalmopathy with primary hypothyroidism and rheumatoid arthritis. *Cent Eur J Immunol* (2019) 44:463–5. doi: 10.5114/ceji.2019.92803
89. Paridaens D, van den Bosch WA, van der Loos TL, Krenning EP, van Hagen PM. The effect of etanercept on Graves' ophthalmopathy: a pilot study. *Eye (Lond)* (2005) 19:1286–9. doi: 10.1038/sj.eye.6701768
90. Kumari R, Chandra Saha B. Advances in the management of thyroid eye diseases: An overview. *Int Ophthalmol* (2018) 38:2247–55. doi: 10.1007/s10792-017-0694-0
91. Strianese D. Update on Graves disease: advances in treatment of mild, moderate and severe thyroid eye disease. *Curr Opin Ophthalmol* (2017) 28:505–13. doi: 10.1097/ICU.0000000000000402
92. Strianese D. Efficacy and Safety of Immunosuppressive Agents for Thyroid Eye Disease. *Ophthalmic Plast Reconstr Surg* (2018) 34(4S Suppl 1):S56–9. doi: 10.1097/IOP.0000000000001131
93. Komorowski J, Jankiewicz-Wika J, Siejka A, Lawnicka H, Kłysik A, Goś R, et al. Monoclonal anti-TNF-alpha antibody (infliximab) in the treatment of patient with thyroid associated ophthalmopathy. *Klin Oczna* (2007) 109:457–60.
94. Ayabe R, Rootman DB, Hwang CJ, Ben-Artzi A, Goldberg R. Adalimumab as steroid-sparing treatment of inflammatory-stage thyroid eye disease. *Ophthalmic Plast Reconstr Surg* (2014) 30:415–9. doi: 10.1097/IOP.0000000000000211
95. Pérez-Moreiras JV, Alvarez-López A, Gómez EC. Treatment of active corticosteroid-resistant graves' orbitopathy. *Ophthalmic Plast Reconstr Surg* (2014) 30:162–7. doi: 10.1097/IOP.0000000000000037
96. de-Pablo-Gómez-de-Liaño L, Fernández-Vigo JI, Troyano-Rivas J, Niño-Rueda C, Romo-López Á, Gómez-de-Liaño R. Response to tocilizumab treatment in Graves' ophthalmopathy by measuring rectus muscle thickness and chemosis using optical coherence tomography. *Arch Soc Esp Oftalmol* (2018) 93:386–91. doi: 10.1016/j.oftal.2018.04.011
97. Maldiney T, Deschasse C, Bielefeld P. Tocilizumab for the Management of Corticosteroid-Resistant Mild to Severe Graves' Ophthalmopathy, a Report of Three Cases. *Ocul Immunol Inflamm* (2020) 28:281–4. doi: 10.1080/09273948.2018.1545914

15

Antioxidant Therapy in Graves' Orbitopathy

*Giulia Lanzolla, Claudio Marcocci and Michele Marinò**

Department of Clinical and Experimental Medicine, Endocrinology Unit II, University of Pisa and University Hospital of Pisa, Pisa, Italy

Correspondence:
Michele Marinò
michele.marino@med.unipi.it

The balance of the cell redox state is a key point for the maintenance of cellular homeostasis. Increased reactive oxygen species (ROS) generation leads to oxidative damage of tissues, which is involved in the development of several diseases, including autoimmune diseases. Graves' Orbitopathy (GO) is a disfiguring autoimmune-related condition associated with Graves' Disease (GD). Patients with active, moderate-to-severe GO, are generally treated with high doses intravenous glucocorticoids (ivGCs) and/or orbital radiotherapy. On the contrary, up to recently, local ointments were the treatment most frequently offered to patients with mild GO, because the risks related to ivGCs does not justify the relatively poor benefits expected in mild GO. However, a medical treatment for these patients is heavily wanted, considering that GO can progress into more severe forms and also patients with mild GO complain with an impairment in their quality of life. Thus, based on the role of oxidative stress in the pathogenesis of GO, a therapy with antioxidant agents has been proposed and a number of studies have been performed, both *in vitro* and *in vivo*, which is reviewed here.

Keywords: Graves' orbitopathy (GO), oxidative stress, Quercetin, Enalapril, Vitamin C, N-acetyl-l-cysteine, melatonin, β-carotene

INTRODUCTION

Graves' Orbitopathy (GO) is an autoimmune, disfiguring disease observed in ~25%–30% of patients with Graves' Disease (GD). More rarely, GO can be found in patients with hypothyroid autoimmune thyroiditis or in subjects with subclinical evidence of thyroid autoimmunity, but with no thyroid dysfunction, and the pathogenesis of these conditions is still a matter of debate (1, 2). Patients affected with moderate-to-severe and active GO are generally treated with high dose intravenous glucocorticoids (ivGCs), orbital radiotherapy, surgical procedures (3) as well as new medications, including Rituximab, an anti-CD20 monoclonal antibody (4), Teprotumumab, an anti-insulin-like growth factor-1 receptor (IGF1R) monoclonal antibody (5, 6), Tocilizumab, an interleukin 6 (IL-6) receptor antagonist (7) and mycophenolate (8). Fortunately, the majority of GO patients have a mild disease and are typically treated with local measures (3), because the risks carried by the above-mentioned therapies is not justified in view of the relatively poor benefits in mild GO, unless there is an important impairment of the quality of life of patients (9–11). Nevertheless, patients affected with mild GO still complain with a significant impairment in their quality of life, and although GO can improve spontaneously in up to 50% of them, it can worsen in ~15% of patients, thereby leading to the search for treatments that are suitable for these patients (2, 12). Oxidative stress plays an important role in the pathogenesis of GO, being involved in the production of pro-inflammatory cytokines and hyaluronic acid (HA), as well as in promoting proliferation of fibroblasts and their differentiation into adipocytes (13). Keeping in mind that an ideal treatment for mild GO should be effective, well tolerated and widely available, several antioxidant agents have been investigated as new possible approaches for the management of these patients. The role and efficacy of selenium have been well demonstrated, as extensively discussed in another review in the same issue of this journal. In addition to selenium, various antioxidant agents, namely pentoxifylline, nicotinamide, allopurinol, quercetin, enalapril, vitamin C, N-acetyl-L-cysteine and melatonin, have been proposed to play a potential therapeutic role in GO (14–18).

OXIDATIVE STRESS IN GRAVES' ORBITOPATHY

Oxidative stress is defined as the disruption of the balance between the production and the elimination of reactive oxygen species (ROS), which causes a remarkable damage of several cell components, namely proteins, lipids, membranes, and nucleic acids (19, 20). The process ultimately results in mitochondrial dysfunction and loss of enzymatic activity. The ultimate pathogenetic mechanisms of GO are still unclear, but the most popular hypothesis implies an interplay between cellular and humoral immunity against the thyrotropic hormone (TSH) receptor (TSH-R) and possibly other autoantigens expressed by thyrocytes and orbital fibroblasts (OFs) (2). Following recognition of these antigens by autoreactive T lymphocytes, they infiltrate fibroadipose orbital tissue, thereby triggering the production of pro-inflammatory cytokines, growth factors and chemokines. The inflammatory response and the consequent local cell damage cause a dysregulated production of ROS, with saturation of the antioxidant systems. The interplay between cellular and humoral immunity, as well as the uncontrolled release of inflammatory molecules and ROS, leads to the increased proliferation of OFs, the differentiation of connective orbital cells into pre-adipocytes and then adipocytes, and the synthesis of great amounts of glycosaminoglycans (GAGs), especially hyaluronic acid (HA). The resulting orbital remodeling is characterized by extraocular muscle enlargement and orbital fat expansion, which are ultimately responsible for the clinical manifestations of the disease (12, 21, 22). Among the various players involved in the pathogenesis of GO, oxidative stress is believed to have a major role. Tissue hypoxia, as well as ROS, are involved in the typical changes of fibroadipose orbital tissue and of the perimysium of extraocular muscles (23) (**Figure 1**). ROS, and the consequent antioxidant defense mobilization, are present at sites of inflammation in general and, in the case of GO, together with edema and tissue hypoxia, contribute the damage of orbital tissue. A role of oxidative stress in GO is supported by a number of basic studies suggesting that ROS promote the proliferation of OFs and the release of GAGs, the synthesis and secretion of cytokines, and the expression of other factors involved in the pathogenesis of GO, namely heat shock protein 72 (HSP-72), HLA-DR and ICAM-1 (14).

In this context, a number of studies, performed both *in vitro* and *in vivo*, investigated the effects of antioxidant agents in GO, including selenium, pentoxifylline, quercetin, enalapril, vitamin C, N-acetyl-L-cysteine and melatonin (14–18, 24, 25). Some of these studies have provided convincing or at least promising results, and in the case of selenium, have led to the clinical use of these antioxidant agents. In addition to the above mentioned compounds, statins (3-hydroxy-3-methylglutaryl-coenzyme reductase inhibitors), because of their anti-oxidative actions, have also been considered for GO treatment (26).

Oxidative Stress and Proliferation of Orbital Fibroblasts

Burch et al. performed a study on primary culture of OFs obtained from GO patients and control subjects, demonstrating that superoxide radicals induced an increased proliferation of OFs from GO patients compared with control fibroblasts (27). Moreover, preincubation of OFs with anti-thyroid drugs (ATD) and antioxidant agents as allopurinol and nicotinamide inhibited the proliferation induced by ROS (27).

The hypothesis that oxidative stress contributes GO pathogenesis was also suggested by studies performed by Tsai et al. and Hondur et al. (28, 29). They both showed that H_2O_2, a potent ROS-inducer, and superoxide dismutase (SOD), a natural antioxidant agent, were higher in GO then control OFs, whereas the ROS antagonist glutathione peroxidase (GPX) was reduced, with a reduced ratio between glutathione and oxidized glutathione, suggesting the presence of a remarkable state of oxidative stress (28–31).

Glycosaminoglycan Production and Heat Shock Protein 72 Expression in Orbital fibroblasts

As mentioned above, the release of GAGs plays an important role in the pathogenesis of GO. The phenomenon is triggered by a number of cytokines, among which interleukin-1 (IL-1) is mostly involved (1, 2). Lu et al. reported that IL-1β promotes an increase in ROS release in OFs from patients with GO (32). SOD and catalase, another ROS antagonist, to some extent reduced the secretion of GAGs induced by IL-1β, suggesting that ROS may be involved in the IL-1β-dependent release of GAGs. In addition, pentoxifylline, which has antioxidant properties, was found to be able to inhibit GAG accumulation in GO OFs (33). HSP-72 is involved in antigen recognition and T-lymphocyte activation in orbital tissue, and its expression in GO fibroblasts is promoted by H_2O_2 (34),. The effects of H_2O_2 were reduced by anti-oxidative agents or ATD (35), suggesting that ROS play a role in the aberrant expression of HSP-72 in OFs of GO.

Clinical Evidence of a Role of Oxidative Stress in Graves' Orbitopathy

In addition to basic studies, the importance of oxidative stress in GO is supported by clinical investigations. Cigarette smoking is

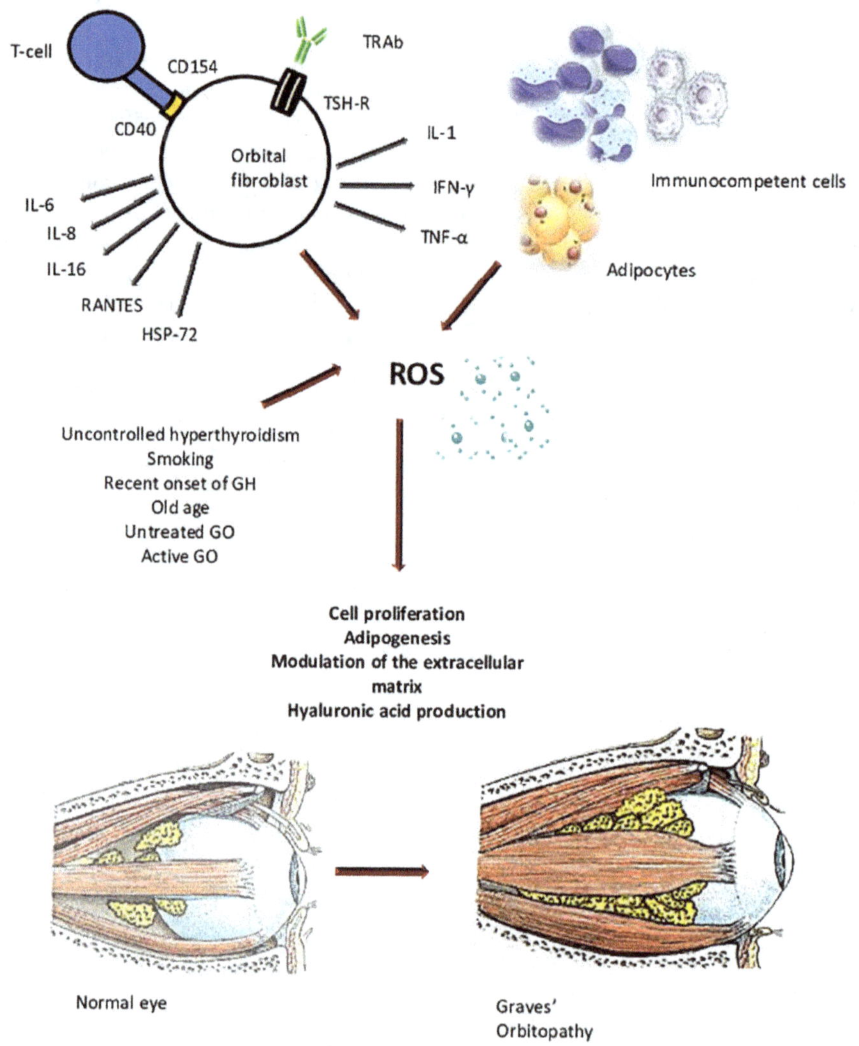

FIGURE 1 | Orbital fibroblasts (OFs) are activated by both cellular and humoral immune responses against autoantigens, among which the thyrotropic hormone (TSH) receptor (TSH-R) is the main involved. The inflammatory process triggers the production of pro-inflammatory cytokines, growth factors, chemokines, and ROS, which contribute the increased proliferation of OFs, the differentiation of connective orbital cells into pre-adipocytes and then adipocytes, and the synthesis of great amounts of glycosaminoglycans (GAGs), especially hyaluronic acid. The resulting orbital remodeling is characterized by extraocular muscle enlargement and orbital fat expansion, which are ultimately responsible for the clinical manifestations of the disease. IL-6, interleukin-6; IL-8, interleukin-8; IL-16, interleukin-16; RANTES, regulated upon activation, normal T-cell expressed and presumably secreted; HSP-72, heat shock protein-72; IL-1, interleukin-1; IFN-γ, interferon γ; TNF-α, tumor necrosis factor α; GH, Graves' hyperthyroidism; GO, Graves' orbitopathy.

the most important environmental risk factors for GO. Thus, cigarette smoke enhances the *in vitro* generation of ROS and reduces the antioxidant machinery (36). Patients with a recent onset Graves' hyperthyroidism (GH) have higher plasma levels of SOD and catalase than control subjects, regardless of the presence of GO (37). No differences in serum GPX and thioredoxin reductase (TRs), another ROS antagonist, were observed. However, the normalization of oxidative markers following restoration of euthyroidism was observed only in patients without GO, suggesting that orbital inflammation contributes the increased serum markers of oxidative stress (38–40). Moreover, higher urinary levels of 8-hydroxy-2'-deoxyguanosine (8-OHdG), a marker of oxidative DNA damage, were found in patients with active GO (29, 31). Interestingly, urinary 8-OHdG was higher in smokers and in patients with GO relapse, and oral glucocorticoid (GC) administration led to a significant decrease of 8-OHdG levels, which was also associated with a reduction of GO activity and severity. These data were confirmed by a subsequent study performed in a larger cohort of GO patients, where there was a significant positive correlation between the GO Clinical Activity Score (CAS) and urinary levels of 8-OHdG. The relationship between oxidative stress and GC has also been studied (30) Akarsu et al. reported a significant reduction in the serum levels of malondealdyde (MAD), a marker of oxidative stress, following GC administration in GO patients (41). Similar findings were obtained by Abalovich et al. (38) and Bednarek et al. (39), in line with an involvement of oxidative stress in the pathogenesis of GO.

ANTIOXIDANT AGENTS IN GRAVES' ORBITOPATHY

According to the guidelines of the European Thyroid Association and of the European Group on Graves' Orbitopathy (EUGOGO), a number of therapies can be offered to patients with moderate-to-severe and active GO. Even though mild GO often improve spontaneously (in ~50% of cases), it worsens in up to 15% of patients (3, 12) and, because of the disfiguring features of the disease and the impairment in the quality of life, also patients with mild GO ask for some sort of treatment, which has been searched for over the last decades. Keeping in mind that an ideal treatment for mild GO should be effective, well tolerated and widely available, antioxidant agents have been proposed as a reasonable approach. Selenium has been largely investigated and currently used in the clinical practice but will not be mentioned in this review article as it is treated largely elsewhere in this special issue. In addition to selenium, a protective role in GO has been suggested by studies on other antioxidant agents, as reported below and summarized in **Table 1**.

Nicotinamide and Allopurinol

Allopurinol is a drug widely used in the management of hyperuricemia and gout, with powerful antioxidant activities, being an inhibitor of the enzyme xanthine oxidase (45). Vitamin nicotinamide is a largely studied nicotinamide adenine dinucleotide (NAD^+) precursor, which is a coenzyme involved in a number of metabolic pathways and in the balance of cell redox state (46). The effects of nicotinamide are currently being investigated by some clinical trials (46). The potential role of allopurinol and nicotinamide in pathophysiologic conditions involving oxidative stress led to the investigation of their effects in GO. As mentioned above, Burch et al. reported that allopurinol and nicotinamide inhibit the proliferation of OFs induced by superoxide (27). This evidence was confirmed by a subsequent *in vitro* study performed in cultured OFs from patients with GO, incubated with interferon γ (IFN-γ) and tumor necrosis factor α (TNF-α) in the presence of nicotinamide (47). The authors reported an inhibitory effect of nicotinamide on cytokine production and OF proliferation. Moreover, nicotinamide was also able to reduce HSP-72 and HLA-DR as well as the expression of ICAM-1 expression, which is involved in the recruitment of T-lymphocytes to the orbit and enhances immune reactions and cytotoxicity (47–50). Bouzas et al. performed the first clinical, pilot study on antioxidants, which included 22 consecutive patients with mild or moderately severe GO treated with placebo or allopurinol (200 mg daily) plus nicotinamide (300 mg daily) for 3 months (42). All patients recruited had an active GO of recent onset (<6 months) and were euthyroid for at least 2 months. The response to treatment was evaluated by a complete ophthalmologic examination 1 and 3 months after the beginning of treatment. A significant improvement of GO was observed in 9 (82%) and 3 (27%) patients who respectively received antioxidant agents or placebo. The inflammation of soft tissue was the feature that responded more to the treatment, whereas proptosis was little affected. Clearly, further studies in larger series of patients are needed to confirm these promising results.

Pentoxifylline

Pentoxifylline is an analog of the methylaxantine theobromine with anti-inflammatory and antioxidant properties (51). It is commonly used in the management of patients with vascular diseases (52). It has been demonstrated that pentoxifylline inhibits the synthesis of GAG and the proliferation of human skin fibroblasts (53). Similar results were reported in primary cultures of fibroblasts derived from patients with fibrotic diseases, including hypertrophic scar, scleroderma and keloid (54). In 1993 Chang et al. reported that treatment with pentoxifylline inhibits GAG release and fibroblast proliferation in primary cultures of OFs derived from patients with GO and control subjects, with no significant difference between them (33). Based on this evidence, some clinical studies investigated the potential beneficial effect of pentoxifylline in patients with GO. Balazs et al. performed a pilot study, neither randomized nor controlled, in 10 patients with GO selected for having contraindications to GCs (43). They were euthyroid for at least 4 weeks and they had a mild or moderate-to-severe GO. The patients were treated with a daily infusion of pentoxifylline (200 mg/die) for 10 days, following which treatment was continued orally (1800 to 1200 mg/day) and stopped after 3 months. At the end of treatment, a significant improvement of GO was observed in 8 of 10 patients. The beneficial effect was more evident on soft tissue inflammation whereas diplopia and proptosis were less affected by treatment. The randomized clinical trial performed by Marcocci et al. which opened for the clinical use of selenium in patients with GO, also investigated the effects of pentoxifylline. The authors showed that pentoxifylline was not associated with a significant improvement of the eye disease in terms of overall clinical outcome as well as the quality of life of patients (44).

Quercetin

Quercetin is a member of the flavonoid family contained in vegetables and fruits, which assures an adequate intake with diet (16). Quercetin has anti-inflammatory, antioxidant, anti-viral activity, and is also able to promote apoptosis in tumor cells (55, 56). It has been reported that quercetin blocks the transforming factor-β (TGF β)/Smad signaling pathway, leading to the inhibition of the proliferation of scar-derived fibroblasts (57, 58). In addition, an antifibrotic activity in fibroblasts and adipocytes from GO patient has been reported, and quercetin seems also to be able to reduce the adipogenesis induced by cigarette smoke-extract in GO fibroblasts. Based on these evidences, a number of *in vitro* studies evaluated the possibility that quercetin may reduce the proliferation of OFs in GO. A study performed in primary cultures of OFs from GO patients and control subjects demonstrated that quercetin exerts an inhibitory effect on fibroblasts proliferation and HA release, with no difference between GO and control fibroblasts (16).

TABLE 1 | Antioxidant agents in Graves' orbitopathy (GO).

Compound	Main finding	Methods	Results	Reference
Nicotinamide and Allopurinol	Clinically significant improvement of GO	A pilot study including 22 consecutive patients with mild or moderately severe, active GO of recent onset (<6 months). They were treated with placebo or allopurinol (200 mg daily) plus nicotinamide (300 mg daily) for 3 months.	After 3 months, a significant improvement of GO was observed in 9 (82%) and 3 (27%) patients who respectively received antioxidant agents or placebo. The inflammation of soft tissue was the feature that responded more, whereas proptosis was little affected.	(42) Bouzas EA. et al.
Pentoxifylline	Inhibition of GAG release and fibroblast proliferation	Primary cultures of OFs from GO patients and control subjects were obtained. Cell proliferation and GAG production were measured after the addition of pentoxifylline (0.1–1,000 mg/L).	The exposure of OFs cultures to pentoxifylline resulted in a dose-dependent inhibition of fibroblast proliferation and GAG synthesis.	(33) Chang C.C et al.
	Clinically significant improvement of GO	A pilot study, neither randomized nor controlled, which involved 10 patients with active, mild or moderate-to-severe GO. Patients were treated with a daily infusion of pentoxifylline (200 mg/die) for 10 days, following which treatment was continued orally (1,800 to 1,200 mg/day) and stopped after 3 months.	At the end of treatment, a significant improvement of GO was observed in 8 of 10 patients. The beneficial effect was more evident on soft tissue inflammation, whereas diplopia and proptosis were less affected.	(43) Balazs C. et al.
	No improvement of GO	A prospective, multicenter, placebo-controlled clinical trial in which 159 patients with mild GO were randomized to receive sodium selenite (100 μg twice daily orally), pentoxifylline (600 mg twice daily orally) or placebo for 6 months.	Unlike selenium, no beneficial effects of pentoxifylline were observed	(44) Marcocci NEJM
Quercetin	Reduction of cell proliferation and HA release in GO fibroblasts	Primary cultures of OFs from GO patients and control subjects were obtained. Cell proliferation, cell necrosis, apoptosis and HA release were measured after incubation with medium without compounds, or containing: i) quercetin, ii) quercitrin, or iii) rutin. (at concentrations ranging between 1 and 150 μMCell).	Beginning at a 30 μM concentration, quercetin reduced cell proliferation and HA release, acting by the induction of necrosis and cell cycle blockade. No difference between GO and control fibroblasts was observed.	(16) Lisi S. et al.
N-acetyl-cysteine, vitamin C and melatonine .	Reduction of proliferation and release of cytokines in GO fibroblasts	Primary cultures of OFs from GO patients and control subjects. Oxidative stress was induced by H_2O_2. Cells were pretreated with N-acetylcysteine (100 and 200 μM) or vitamin C (250 and 500 μM). Cell proliferation, cell necrosis, apoptosis and HA release were measured	Treatment with H_2O_2 at low concentrations of H_2O_2 (3.125–25 μM) increased the survival of GO fibroblasts. 6.25 μM H_2O_2 led to a significant elevation of TGF β, IL-1 β and superoxide anion in GO fibroblasts, in GO, but not in control OFs. Pretreatment with N-acetylcysteine or vitamin C reversed the enhanced proliferation and the production of TGF-β, IL-1β and superoxide anion of GO fibroblasts in response to 6.25 μM H_2O_2.	(24) Tsai CC. et al.
	Reduction of cell proliferation and HA release in GO fibroblasts	GSSG, as a measure of oxidative stress, cell proliferation, HA, TNFα, IFNγ, and IL-1β were measured in primary cultures of GO and control OFs treated with H_2O_2 and incubated with N-acetyl-cysteine, vitamin C and melatonine	Oxidative stress was reduced by all of the three antioxidant agents. Vitamin C reduced proliferation in GO, but not in control fibroblasts. N-acetyl-l-cysteine reduced proliferation and IFNγ in GO, and HA and IL-1β in both GO and control fibroblasts. Melatonin reduced IL-1β and HA in GO and control fibroblasts, and IFNγ only in GO fibroblasts.	(17) Rotondo Dottore G. et al
Enalapril .	Reduction of cell proliferation and HA release in GO fibroblasts	Primary cultures of GO and control fibroblasts were treated with enalapril (2 or 5 mM, for 3 or 5 days) or with a control compound (lisinopril). Cell proliferation assays, lactate dehydrogenase release assays (as a measure of cell necrosis), apoptosis assays, and measurement of HA in the cell media were performed	Enalapril reduced OFs proliferation and HA release in the cell media in both GO and control fibroblasts. Because enalapril did not affect cell necrosis and apoptosis, the effects on proliferation probably reflected an inhibition of cell growth and/or a delay in cell cycle.	(15) Botta R. et al.
Retinol, β-carotene, vitamin E	Reduction of cell proliferation in GO fibroblasts	Primary cultures of GO and control fibroblasts. Oxidative stress was induced by treatment with H_2O_2. Cells were pre-incubated for 2 days at 37°C with complete medium without compounds, or with medium containing either one of the compounds investigated at various concentrations. GSSG, cell proliferation, HA, TNFα, IFNγ, and IL1β were measured	Retinol, β-carotene and vitamin E significantly reduced the release of GSSG and IL-1β induced by H_2O_2 in GO, but not in control fibroblasts. β-carotene reduced OFs proliferation in GO, but not in control fibroblasts, whereas retinol and vitamin E had no effect. Retinol reduced IFNγ in GO and control fibroblasts.	(16) Rotondo Dottore G. et al

OFs, orbital fibroblasts; GAG, glycosaminoglycans; HA, hyaluronic acid; H_2O_2, hydrogen peroxide; TGF β, transforming growth factor β; IL-1β, interleukin-1β, IFNγ, interferon γ, GSSG, Glutathione disulfide; TNFα, tumor necrosis factor α.

The reduction of cell proliferation was likely due to a pro-necrotic, rather than to a pro-apoptotic, effect of quercetin. These findings suggest that quercetin may have a therapeutic role in GO, but *in vivo* studies are needed to confirm this hypothesis, also considering that quercetin seems to act through necrosis, which may worsen autoimmunity against orbital antigens due to antigen exposure to the immune system.

Enalapril

Enalapril is a rather common anti-hypertensive medication, and it has been reported to inhibit fibroblasts proliferation and HA production in cheloid scars (59, 60). In view of these effects, a study was carried out using primary cultures of OFs from patients with GO and control subjects, which were treated with enalapril or with a control compound (lisinopril) (15). Cell proliferation, apoptosis, cell necrosis and HA release were measured. A significant reduction of OFs proliferation and HA release upon enalapril, but not lisinopril treatment, was observed in both GO and control OFs. Because enalapril did not cause an increase in necrosis or apoptosis, its inhibitory effects on proliferation were interpreted as the consequence of a direct action on cell growth and/or of a delay in cell cycle. No clinical studies are available on the use of this promising medication in GO.

Vitamin C, N-Acetyl-l-Cysteine, and Melatonin

Additional antioxidant agents, namely Vitamin C, N-acetyl-l-cysteine and melatonin, were tested in another *in vitro* study performed in primary cultures of OFs from six GO patients and six control subjects (17). After treatment with H_2O_2 to induce oxidative stress, primary cultures were incubated with the various compounds. Glutathione disulfide (GSSG), as gage of oxidative stress, cell proliferation, HA, TNF-α, IFN-γ, and interleukin 1- β (IL1-β) were measured (17). H_2O_2 induced oxidative stress, as demonstrated by an increase in GSSG, and promoted cell proliferation and cytokine release, but did not affect HA. Vitamin C reduced proliferation in GO, but not in control fibroblasts. N-acetyl-l-cysteine reduced fibroblasts proliferation and release of IFN-γ, a cytokine involved in the pathogenesis of GO, in OFs from GO patients, and it was also able to inhibit HA and IL1-β secretion in both GO and control OFs. Melatonin reduced IL1-β and HA release in GO and control OFs, whereas its inhibitory effect on IFN-γ release was significant only in GO OFs (17). Overall, the results of this study support a beneficial role of Vitamin C and N-acetyl-L-cysteine, suggesting a possible clinical use of these compounds. Furthermore, this study showed, for the first time, a beneficial effect of melatonin in terms of cytokines and HA synthesis. However, based on the lack of an inhibitory effect on fibroblasts proliferation, melatonin does not seem to be a strong candidate for a clinical use.

β-carotene, Retinol, and Vitamin E

Among other bio-available substances with antioxidant effects, β-carotene seems to be rather promising for a use in GO patients. In a study performed in our laboratory (18), again using primary cultures of OFs from GO patients and control subjects, cells were pre-incubated with medium containing β-carotene, retinol or Vitamin E, or with medium without compounds, following induction of oxidative stress with H_2O_2. As in previous studies (17), oxidative stress promoted fibroblast proliferation, but it did not affect HA release. All of the three substances were able to reduce oxidative stress in GO, but not in control OFs (18). Cell proliferation, HA synthesis, as well as of pro-inflammatory cytokines were measured. Cell proliferation was reduced only by β-carotene. No effects in terms of HA synthesis were observed, whereas all of the cytokines measured, namely IL-1β, IFN-γ and TNF-α, which were increased by H_2O_2, were reduced by β-carotene as well as by retinol and Vitamin E (18). We can speculate that Vitamin E and retinol might not have an effect on GO *in vivo*, because they do not affect cell proliferation. On the contrary, β-carotene displayed antiproliferative effects in addition to an antioxidant and anti-inflammatory action, making it the most suitable candidate, among the three compounds studied, for a clinical use. Clearly, clinical studies are needed.

CONCLUSIONS

The balance of the cell redox state is a key point in cellular homeostasis. The disruption of the balance between oxidative and reductive activities in the cells leads to oxidative stress, by an increase in ROS production and a reduction of their scavenging. ROS interfere with intracellular reactions, thereby damaging various cellular components. Oxidative stress is involved in a number of diseases and seems to play an important role in GO. The management of patients with mild GO represents a challenge for endocrinologists and ophthalmologists. In addition to selenium, studies *in vitro* on the effect of other antioxidant agents provided, at least in part, interesting results which, unfortunately, have not been yet completely confirmed by clinical studies. Nicotinamide and allopurinol seem to be effective in reducing the inflammation of soft tissue but the data sustaining this conclusion were obtained in a rather small sample of GO patients affected with both moderate-to-severe and mild GO (42). The *in vitro* results on the use of pentoxifylline are promising, but clinical studies provided conflicting results (43, 44). Among the other compounds, because of the *in vitro* findings reported above, one can speculate that quercetin and β-carotene might be the most promising, but clinical trials are needed to confirm this hypothesis.

AUTHOR CONTRIBUTIONS

GL wrote the manuscript. CM and MM contributed to the conception of the manuscript and revised the paper critically. All authors contributed to the article and approved the submitted version.

REFERENCES

1. Leporati P, Groppelli G, Zerbini F, Rotondi M, Chiovato L. Etiopathogenesis of Basedow's disease. Trends and current aspects. *Nuklearmedizin* (2015) 54 (5):204–10. doi: 10.3413/Nukmed-0739-15-04
2. Smith TJ, Hegedüs L. Graves' Disease. *N Engl J Med* (2016) 375(16):1552–65. doi: 10.1056/NEJMra1510030
3. Bartalena L, Baldeschi L, Boboridis K, Eckstein A, Kahaly GJ, Marcocci C, et al. The 2016 European Thyroid Association/European Group on Graves' Orbitopathy Guidelines for the Management of Graves' Orbitopathy. *Eur Thyroid J* (2016) 5(1):9–26. doi: 10.1159/000443828
4. Stan MN, Salvi M. MANAGEMENT OF ENDOCRINE DISEASE: Rituximab therapy for Graves' orbitopathy - lessons from randomized control trials. *Eur J Endocrinol* (2017) 176(2):R101–9. doi: 10.1530/EJE-16-0552
5. Douglas RS, Kahaly GJ, Patel A, Sile S, Thompson EHZ, Perdok R, et al. Teprotumumab for the Treatment of Active Thyroid Eye Disease. *N Engl J Med* (2020) 382(4):341–52. doi: 10.1056/NEJMoa1910434
6. Smith TJ, Kahaly GJ, Ezra DG, Fleming JC, Dailey RA, Tang RA, et al. Teprotumumab for Thyroid-Associated Ophthalmopathy. *N Engl J Med* (2017) 376(18):1748–61. doi: 10.1056/NEJMoa1614949
7. Pérez-Moreiras JV, Alvarez-López A, Gómez EC. Treatment of active corticosteroid-resistant graves' orbitopathy. *Ophthal Plast Reconstr Surg* (2014) 30(2):162–7. doi: 10.1097/IOP.0000000000000037
8. Kahaly GJ, Riedl M, König J, Pitz S, Ponto K, Diana T, et al. Mycophenolate plus methylprednisolone versus methylprednisolone alone in active, moderate-to-severe Graves' orbitopathy (MINGO): a randomised, observer-masked, multicentre trial. *Lancet Diabetes Endocrinol* (2018) 6(4):287–98. doi: 10.1016/S2213-8587(18)30020-2
9. Sisti E, Coco B, Menconi F, Leo M, Rocchi R, Latrofa F, et al. Intravenous glucocorticoid therapy for Graves' ophthalmopathy and acute liver damage: an epidemiological study. *Eur J Endocrinol* (2015) 172(3):269–76. doi: 10.1530/EJE-14-0712
10. Marcocci C, Watt T, Altea MA, Rasmussen AK, Feldt-Rasmussen U, Orgiazzi J, et al. Fatal and non-fatal adverse events of glucocorticoid therapy for Graves' orbitopathy: a questionnaire survey among members of the European Thyroid Association. *Eur J Endocrinol* (2012) 166(2):247–53. doi: 10.1530/EJE-11-0779
11. Sisti E, Coco B, Menconi F, Leo M, Rocchi R, Latrofa F, et al. Age and Dose Are Major Risk Factors for Liver Damage Associated with Intravenous Glucocorticoid Pulse Therapy for Graves' Orbitopathy. *Thyroid* (2015) 25 (7):846–50. doi: 10.1089/thy.2015.0061
12. Piantanida E, Tanda ML, Lai A, Sassi L, Bartalena L. Prevalence and natural history of Graves' orbitopathy in the XXI century. *J Endocrinol Invest* (2013) 36(6):444–9. doi: 10.3275/8937
13. Marcocci C, Leo M, Altea MA. Oxidative stress in graves' disease. *Eur Thyroid J* (2012) 1(2):80–7. doi: 10.1159/000337976
14. Bartalena L, Tanda ML, Piantanida E, Lai A. Oxidative stress and Graves' ophthalmopathy: in vitro studies and therapeutic implications. *Biofactors* (2003) 19(3–4):155–63. doi: 10.1002/biof.5520190308
15. Botta R, Lisi S, Marcocci C, Sellari-Franceschini S, Rocchi R, Latrofa F, et al. Enalapril reduces proliferation and hyaluronic acid release in orbital fibroblasts. *Thyroid* (2013) 23(1):92–6. doi: 10.1089/thy.2012.0373
16. Lisi S, Botta R, Lemmi M, Sellari-Franceschini S, Altea MA, Sisti E, et al. Quercetin decreases proliferation of orbital fibroblasts and their release of hyaluronic acid. *J Endocrinol Invest* (2011) 34(7):521–7. doi: 10.3275/7321
17. Rotondo Dottore G, Ionni I, Menconi F, Casini G, Sellari-Franceschini S, Nardi M, et al. Action of three bioavailable antioxidants in orbital fibroblasts from patients with Graves' orbitopathy (GO): a new frontier for GO treatment? *J Endocrinol Invest* (2018) 41(2):193–201. doi: 10.1007/s40618-017-0718-7
18. Rotondo Dottore G, Ionni I, Menconi F, Casini G, Sellari-Franceschini S, Nardi M, et al. Antioxidant effects of β-carotene, but not of retinol and vitamin E, in orbital fibroblasts from patients with Graves' orbitopathy (GO). *J Endocrinol Invest* (2018) 41(7):815–20. doi: 10.1007/s40618-017-0809-5
19. Halliwell B, Gutteridge JM. Lipid peroxidation, oxygen radicals, cell damage, and antioxidant therapy. *Lancet (Lond Engl)* (1984) 1(8391):1396–7. doi: 10.1016/S0140-6736(84)91886-5
20. Valko M, Leibfritz D, Moncol J, Cronin MTD, Mazur M, Telser J. Free radicals and antioxidants in normal physiological functions and human disease. *Int J Biochem Cell Biol* (2007) 39(1):44–84. doi: 10.1016/j.biocel.2006.07.001
21. Marinò M, Rotondo Dottore G, Ionni I, Lanzolla G, Sabini E, Ricci D, et al. Serum antibodies against the insulin-like growth factor-1 receptor (IGF-1R) in Graves' disease and Graves' orbitopathy. *J Endocrinol Invest* (2019) 42 (4):471–80. doi: 10.1007/s40618-018-0943-8
22. Bartalena L, Fatourechi V. Extrathyroidal manifestations of Graves' disease: a 2014 update. *J Endocrinol Invest* (2014) 37(8):691–700. doi: 10.1007/s40618-014-0097-2
23. Görtz G-E, Horstmann M, Aniol B, Reyes BD, Fandrey J, Eckstein A, et al. Hypoxia-Dependent HIF-1 Activation Impacts on Tissue Remodeling in Graves' Ophthalmopathy-Implications for Smoking. *J Clin Endocrinol Metab* (2016) 101(12):4834–42. doi: 10.1210/jc.2016-1279
24. Tsai C-C, Wu S-B, Kao S-C, Kau H-C, Lee F-L, Wei Y-H. The protective effect of antioxidants on orbital fibroblasts from patients with Graves' ophthalmopathy in response to oxidative stress. *Mol Vis* (2013) 19:927–34.
25. Marinò M, Marcocci C, Vitti P, Chiovato L, Bartalena L. Selenium in the Treatment of Thyroid Diseases. *Eur Thyroid J* (2017) 6(2):113–4. doi: 10.1159/000456660
26. Lanzolla G, Vannucchi G, Ionni I, Campi I, Sileo F, Lazzaroni E, et al. Cholesterol Serum Levels and Use of Statins in Graves' Orbitopathy: A New Starting Point for the Therapy. *Front Endocrinol (Lausanne)* (2019) 10:933. doi: 10.3389/fendo.2019.00933
27. Burch HB, Lahiri S, Bahn RS, Barnes S. Superoxide radical production stimulates retroocular fibroblast proliferation in Graves' ophthalmopathy. *Exp Eye Res* (1997) 65(2):311–6. doi: 10.1006/exer.1997.0353
28. Hondur A, Konuk O, Dincel AS, Bilgihan A, Unal M, Hasanreisoglu B. Oxidative stress and antioxidant activity in orbital fibroadipose tissue in Graves' ophthalmopathy. *Curr Eye Res* (2008) 33(5):421–7. doi: 10.1080/02713680802123532
29. Tsai C-C, Wu S-B, Cheng C-Y, Kao S-C, Kau H-C, Chiou S-H, et al. Increased oxidative DNA damage, lipid peroxidation, and reactive oxygen species in cultured orbital fibroblasts from patients with Graves' ophthalmopathy: evidence that oxidative stress has a role in this disorder. *Eye (Lond)* (2010) 24(9):1520–5. doi: 10.1038/eye.2010.31
30. Tsai C-C, Kao S-C, Cheng C-Y, Kau H-C, Hsu W-M, Lee C-F, et al. Oxidative stress change by systemic corticosteroid treatment among patients having active graves ophthalmopathy. *Arch Ophthalmol (Chicago Ill 1960)* (2007) 125 (12):1652–6. doi: 10.1001/archopht.125.12.1652
31. Tsai C-C, Wu S-B, Cheng C-Y, Kao S-C, Kau H-C, Lee S-M, et al. Increased response to oxidative stress challenge in Graves' ophthalmopathy orbital fibroblasts. *Mol Vis* (2011) 17:2782–8.
32. Lu R, Wang P, Wartofsky L, Sutton BD, Zweier JL, Bahn RS, et al. Oxygen free radicals in interleukin-1beta-induced glycosaminoglycan production by retro-ocular fibroblasts from normal subjects and Graves' ophthalmopathy patients. *Thyroid* (1999) 9(3):297–303. doi: 10.1089/thy.1999.9.297
33. Chang CC, Chang TC, Kao SC, Kuo YF, Chien LF. Pentoxifylline inhibits the proliferation and glycosaminoglycan synthesis of cultured fibroblasts derived from patients with Graves' ophthalmopathy and pretibial myxoedema. *Acta Endocrinol (Copenh)* (1993) 129(4):322–7. doi: 10.1530/acta.0.1290322
34. Burch HB, Wartofsky L. Graves' ophthalmopathy: current concepts regarding pathogenesis and management. *Endocr Rev* (1993) 14(6):747–93. doi: 10.1210/edrv-14-6-747
35. Heufelder AE, Wenzel BE, Bahn RS. Methimazole and propylthiouracil inhibit the oxygen free radical-induced expression of a 72 kilodalton heat shock protein in Graves' retroocular fibroblasts. *J Clin Endocrinol Metab* (1992) 74(4):737–42. doi: 10.1210/jcem.74.4.1532179
36. Wiersinga WM. Smoking and thyroid. *Clin Endocrinol (Oxf)* (2013) 79 (2):145–51. doi: 10.1111/cen.12222
37. Cetinkaya A, Kurutas EB, Buyukbese MA, Kantarceken B, Bulbuloglu E. Levels of malondialdehyde and superoxide dismutase in subclinical hyperthyroidism. *Mediators Inflamm* (2005) 2005(1):57–9. doi: 10.1155/MI.2005.57
38. Abalovich M, Llesuy S, Gutierrez S, Repetto M. Peripheral parameters of oxidative stress in Graves' disease: the effects of methimazole and 131 iodine treatments. *Clin Endocrinol (Oxf)* (2003) 59(3):321–7. doi: 10.1046/j.1365-2265.2003.01850.x
39. Bednarek J, Wysocki H, Sowiński J. Oxidative stress peripheral parameters in Graves' disease: the effect of methimazole treatment in patients with and without infiltrative ophthalmopathy. *Clin Biochem* (2005) 38(1):13–8. doi: 10.1016/j.clinbiochem.2004.09.015

40. Rybus-Kalinowska B, Zwirska-Korczala K, Kalinowski M, Kukla M, Birkner E, Jochem J. Activity of antioxidative enzymes and concentration of malondialdehyde as oxidative status markers in women with newly diagnosed Graves-Basedow disease and after thiamazole therapy leading to euthyroidism. *Pol Arch Med Wewn* (2008) 118(7–8):420–5. doi: 10.20452/pamw.438
41. Akarsu E, Buyukhatipoglu H, Aktaran S, Kurtul N. Effects of pulse methylprednisolone and oral methylprednisolone treatments on serum levels of oxidative stress markers in Graves' ophthalmopathy. *Clin Endocrinol (Oxf)* (2011) 74(1):118–24. doi: 10.1111/j.1365-2265.2010.03904.x
42. Bouzas EA, Karadimas P, Mastorakos G, Koutras DA. Antioxidant agents in the treatment of Graves' ophthalmopathy. *Am J Ophthalmol* (2000) 129 (5):618–22. doi: 10.1016/S0002-9394(00)00359-7
43. Balazs C, Kiss E, Vamos A, Molnar I, Farid NR. Beneficial effect of pentoxifylline on thyroid associated ophthalmopathy (TAO)*: a pilot study. *J Clin Endocrinol Metab* (1997) 82(6):1999–2002. doi: 10.1210/jcem.82.6.9995
44. Marcocci C, Kahaly GJ, Krassas GE, Bartalena L, Prummel M, Stahl M, et al. Selenium and the course of mild Graves' orbitopathy. *N Engl J Med* (2011) 364 (20):1920–31. doi: 10.1056/NEJMoa1012985
45. Glantzounis GK, Tsimoyiannis EC, Kappas AM, Galaris DA. Uric acid and oxidative stress. *Curr Pharm Des* (2005) 11(32):4145–51. doi: 10.2174/138161205774913255
46. Mehmel M, Jovanović N, Spitz U. Nicotinamide Riboside-The Current State of Research and Therapeutic Uses. *Nutrients* (2020) 12(6):1616. doi: 10.3390/nu12061616
47. Hiromatsu Y, Yang D, Miyake I, Koga M, Kameo J, Sato M, et al. Nicotinamide decreases cytokine-induced activation of orbital fibroblasts from patients with thyroid-associated ophthalmopathy. *J Clin Endocrinol Metab* (1998) 83(1):121–4. doi: 10.1210/jcem.83.1.4478
48. Hiromatsu Y, Sato M, Yamada K, Nonaka K. Inhibitory effects of nicotinamide on recombinant human interferon-gamma-induced intercellular adhesion molecule-1 (ICAM-1) and HLA-DR antigen expression on cultured human endothelial cells. *Immunol Lett* (1992) 31 (1):35–9. doi: 10.1016/0165-2478(92)90007-B
49. Hiromatsu Y, Sato M, Yamada K, Nonaka K. Nicotinamide and 3-aminobenzamide inhibit recombinant human interferon-gamma-induced HLA-DR antigen expression, but not HLA-A, B, C antigen expression, on cultured human thyroid cells. *Clin Endocrinol (Oxf)* (1992) 36(1):91–5. doi: 10.1111/j.1365-2265.1992.tb02907.x
50. Heufelder AE, Smith TJ, Gorman CA, Bahn RS. Increased induction of HLA-DR by interferon-gamma in cultured fibroblasts derived from patients with Graves' ophthalmopathy and pretibial dermopathy. *J Clin Endocrinol Metab* (1991) 73(2):307–13. doi: 10.1210/jcem-73-2-307
51. Bhat VB, Madyastha KM. Antioxidant and radical scavenging properties of 8-oxo derivatives of xanthine drugs pentoxifylline and lisofylline. *Biochem Biophys Res Commun* (2001) 288(5):1212–7. doi: 10.1006/bbrc.2001.5922
52. Kamphuis J, Smits P, Thien T. Vascular effects of pentoxifylline in humans. *J Cardiovasc Pharmacol* (1994) 24(4):648–54. doi: 10.1097/00005344-199410000-00016
53. Isaac C, Mathor MB, Bariani G, Paggiaro AO, Herson MR, Goldenstein-Schainberg C, et al. Pentoxifylline modifies three-dimensional collagen lattice model contraction and expression of collagen types I and III by human fibroblasts derived from post-burn hypertrophic scars and from normal skin. *Burns* (2009) 35(5):701–6. doi: 10.1016/j.burns.2008.11.017
54. Berman B, Duncan MR. Pentoxifylline inhibits the proliferation of human fibroblasts derived from keloid, scleroderma and morphoea skin and their production of collagen, glycosaminoglycans and fibronectin. *Br J Dermatol* (1990) 123(3):339–46. doi: 10.1111/j.1365-2133.1990.tb06294.x
55. Cushnie TPT, Lamb AJ. Antimicrobial activity of flavonoids. *Int J Antimicrob Agents* (2005) 26(5):343–56. doi: 10.1016/j.ijantimicag.2005.09.002
56. Woodman OL, Chan EC. Vascular and anti-oxidant actions of flavonols and flavones. *Clin Exp Pharmacol Physiol* (2004) 31(11):786–90. doi: 10.1111/j.1440-1681.2004.04072.x
57. Phan TT, See P, Tran E, Nguyen TTT, Chan SY, Lee ST, et al. Suppression of insulin-like growth factor signalling pathway and collagen expression in keloid-derived fibroblasts by quercetin: its therapeutic potential use in the treatment and/or prevention of keloids. *Br J Dermatol* (2003) 148(3):544–52. doi: 10.1046/j.1365-2133.2003.05174.x
58. Phan T-T, Lim IJ, Chan S-Y, Tan E-K, Lee S-T, Longaker MT. Suppression of transforming growth factor beta/smad signaling in keloid-derived fibroblasts by quercetin: implications for the treatment of excessive scars. *J Trauma* (2004) 57(5):1032–7. doi: 10.1097/01.TA.0000114087.46566.EB
59. Iannello S, Milazzo P, Bordonaro F, Belfiore F. Low-dose enalapril in the treatment of surgical cutaneous hypertrophic scar and keloid–two case reports and literature review. *MedGenMed* (2006) 8(4):60.
60. Kim S, Ohta K, Hamaguchi A, Omura T, Yukimura T, Miura K, et al. Angiotensin II type I receptor antagonist inhibits the gene expression of transforming growth factor-beta 1 and extracellular matrix in cardiac and vascular tissues of hypertensive rats. *J Pharmacol Exp Ther* (1995) 273 (1):509–15.

16

Immunological Features of Paranasal Sinus Mucosa in Patients with Graves' Orbitopathy

Yi Lu[1,2†], *Yu Wu*[1,2†], *Yazhuo Huang*[1,2], *Sijie Fang*[1,2], *Yinwei Li*[1,2], *Jing Sun*[1,2] *and Huifang Zhou*[1,2*]

[1] Department of Ophthalmology, Shanghai Ninth People's Hospital, Shanghai JiaoTong University School of Medicine, Shanghai, China, [2] Shanghai Key Laboratory of Orbital Diseases and Ocular Oncology, Shanghai Ninth People's Hospital, Shanghai, China

***Correspondence:**
Huifang Zhou
fangzzfang@163.com

†These authors have contributed equally to this work

Background: Previous studies showed that patients with Graves' orbitopathy (GO) had concomitant mucosal abnormality within the paranasal sinuses. It remains unknown whether the immunological reactions in sinus mucosa affect the orbit inflammation in GO.

Methods: Patients with GO underwent sinus computed tomography (CT) scans for sinus mucosal disease by two independent reviewers using the Lund-MacKay systems. Ethmoid mucosal samples were collected during orbital decompression surgeries for patients with GO and correction surgeries for patients with old orbital fractures as controls. Histological analysis and immunofluorescence were performed in all sinus mucosa tissues. Flow cytometry analysis was used to examine the immunological features of sinus mucosa in both GO and control groups.

Results: Immunohistochemistry showed that the paranasal sinus mucosa of patients with GO grew swelling, with goblet cell and small vessel proliferation, endothelial cell swelling, and inflammatory cell infiltration. The number of T helper (Th)1, Th17, and gamma-delta T cells in nasal sinus mucosa of patients with GO increased significantly compared with those from controls. Further, the proportion of Th1 cells was significantly correlated with clinical activity score. In addition, there was a decreased number of regulatory T cells in patients with GO. The number of Th2 cells showed no significant difference between the two groups. Finally, the proportion of interleukin-22-producing cell subsets in gamma-delta T cells of patients with GO was significantly increased compared with those from controls.

Conclusions: Our observations illustrated a potential pathogenic role of mucosal-infiltrating T cells, which may have the possibility to aggravate inflammatory responses in GO.

Keywords: immune, T cells, paranasal sinus, mucosa, Graves' orbitopathy

INTRODUCTION

Graves' orbitopathy (GO) is an autoimmune disorder ranking first in orbital diseases. GO is also the most common extrathyroidal manifestation of Graves' disease (GD) (1). Orbital tissue remodeling is a major pathological feature of GO, which includes extraocular muscle swelling, adipogenesis, fibrosis, and extracellular matrix deposition such as glycosaminoglycan (2). It is generally accepted that the bony orbit confines the orbital soft tissues on all sides except anteriorly. Intriguingly, the two most frequently enlarged extraocular muscles are the inferior and medial rectus muscles, which are next to ethmoid and maxillary sinus, respectively. Both muscles overlie the thinnest bones of the orbit (3). Gouveris et al. reported that patients with GD had concomitant mucosal thickening within the paranasal sinuses. Patients with GO who underwent orbital decompression surgeries exhibited a higher prevalence (29.4%) of sinus mucosal thickening on CT scan. Histological exams showed chronic rhinosinusitis in 45.5% of GO patients (4). These findings may be explained by circulating autoantibodies targeting autoantigens, namely thyrotropin receptor and insulin-like growth factor-1 receptor, associated with GD and found to be expressed in sinus mucosa (5).

Until today, the pathogenesis of GO is not fully understand. Many studies have indicated that T cells are critical in GO autoimmune responses. They have confirmed that at least three T helper (Th) cell groups are involved in the development of GO, which are Th1 cells, Th2 cells, and Th17 cells. Early studies mainly focused on Th1/Th2 subsets and their related cytokines in the inflammation of GO. It is recognized that Th1 cells play a significant role in inducing cytokine release in early active GO, and the chronic fibrotic phase of GO is dominated by Th2-type immune responses (6–9). Furthermore, Th17 cells have been proved to be an important proinflammatory and profibrotic cell subsets. In GO patients, the level of interleukin (IL)-17A and the number of IL-17A-producing T cells in the peripheral blood were higher than those of healthy controls. IL-17A was shown to promote inflammation and fibrosis of orbital fibroblasts (OF) derived from GO patients (10–12). Moreover, Th17 cells could stimulate the expression of proinflammatory cytokines such as IL-6, IL-8, monocyte chemoattractant protein-1, tumor necrosis factor-α, etc., and costimulatory molecules to regulate the balance of fibrosis and adipogenesis in different OF subsets (13). In this current study, we raise a hypothesis that there is a relationship between nasal sinuses inflammation and GO pathology. We sought to investigate why there is a higher prevalence of sinus mucosa disorder in GO patients and to unravel the potential immunological features of paranasal sinus mucosa in GO.

MATERIALS AND METHODS

Subjects and Samples

A collection of 58 ethmoid sinus mucosa tissues (38 samples of patients with GO undergoing orbital decompression surgery and 20 samples of patients with old orbital fracture undergoing orbital repair surgery) were included in the study. Informed consent was provided by all participants. Use of these samples was approved by the Ethical Committee of Shanghai Ninth People's Hospital, Shanghai JiaoTong University School of Medicine. All 38 GO patients were in inactive stage. Steroid or immunosuppressive treatment was discontinued for at least 3 months before surgery, and all patients were clinically euthyroid at the time of surgery. Exclusion criteria included age less than 18 years old, and patients with history of sinus surgery. Patients with rheumatic or hemolymph diseases were also excluded. Based on the findings of pre-operative computer tomography (CT) scans, scores based on the Lund-Mackay staging systems (**Table 1**) were calculated for each patient and control subject.

Histology and Immunofluorescence

For histological analysis, nasal sinus mucosa tissues were fixed in 4% formalin and paraffin-embedded. The specimens were cut in 4-μm-thick sections before staining with hematoxylin and eosin (HE). The sections were then examined with a light microscope. The expression of CD4 and CD8 was determined by immunofluorescence analysis. Cryostat sections (4 μm thick) were fixed with 4% paraformaldehyde fixative at room temperature for 20 min and washed in PBS for three times. The sections were then incubated with a blocking solution (normal goat serum) at room temperature for another 20 min. Next, they were incubated with rabbit anti-CD4 and mouse anti-CD8 (Abcam, USA) primary antibodies overnight at 4°C. After being washed in PBS for three times, the sections were incubated with secondary antibodies for 1 h at room temperature. Finally, coverslip-mounted slides were observed and photographed under a fluorescence microscope.

Flow Cytometry Analysis

The ethmoid sinus mucosa tissues were digested with 5% Type IV collagenase into single cell suspensions, and were stimulated with phorbol 12-myristate 13-acetate (50ng/ml; Sigma-Aldrich, USA) and ionomycin (1 μg/ml; Sigma-Aldrich, USA) in the presence of

TABLE 1 | Lund-Mackay Scoring System.

Anatomic Location	Scoring Criteria*
Maxillary sinuses	0: No abnormality 1: Partial opacification 2: Total opacification
Anterior ethmoid sinuses	0: No abnormality 1: Partial opacification 2: Total opacification
Posterior ethmoid sinuses	0: No abnormality 1: Partial opacification 2: Total opacification
Sphenoid sinuses	0: No abnormality 1: Partial opacification 2: Total opacification
Frontal sinuses	0: No abnormality 1: Partial opacification 2: Total opacification
Ostiomeatal complex (OMC)	0: Not occluded 2: Occluded

Total score can range from 0 to 24.

Golgi Plug (1 μl/ml; BD Biosciences, USA) at 37°C for 6 h before flow cytometry. To analyze T cell subsets in sinus mucosa, cells were incubated with APC-Cy7-Fixable Viability Dye (eBioscience, USA) before staining for surface markers (FITC-anti-CD3, AF700-anti-CD8, BV650-anti-γδTCR) (All from BD Biosciences, USA). Then, cells were treated with Fixation/Permeabilization reagents (eBioscience, USA) and stained with intracellular markers (BV711-anti-IFN-γ, BV421-anti-IL-13; BD Biosciences, USA; PE-anti-IL-17A, APC-anti-FOXP3, PE-Cy7-anti-IL-22; eBioscience, USA). A BD LSRFortessa X-20 was applied for sample sorting. The data were analyzed after adjusting the fluorescence compensation with FlowJoV10.

Statistical Analysis

All values are expressed as the mean ± standard deviation (SD). Statistical analyses were performed by one-way ANOVA, analysis of Spearman's correlation and t-test followed by the appropriate tests with the statistical analysis program GraphPad Prism 6.0 (GraphPad Prism Software, USA) and SPSS 25 (IBM SPSS Software, USA). A P value less than 0.05 was considered to indicate a statistically significant difference.

RESULTS

Clinical Characteristic and Radiographic Findings of GO Patients

Clinical characteristics of patients and controls were described in **Table 2**. As expected, the GO group had more proptosis reflected in higher exophthalmometry readings than controls (23.37 ± 2.44 vs. 15.24 ± 2.73, $P < 0.0001$) mm. CT scans demonstrated a higher score in patients with GO compared with controls for Lund-MacKay system (4.00 ± 1.94 vs. 1.67 ± 0.58, $P < 0.0001$). Among GO patients, the most common location for mucosal thickening was in the ethmoid sinuses (69.2%), followed by the maxillary (53.8%), OMC (46.2%), and sphenoid sinuses (30.8%). The representative CT scanning was showed in **Figure 1A**. When comparing the extent of sinus mucosal thickening to the degree of orbital proptosis as measured by exophthalmometry, higher Lund-MacKay scores did not correlate with greater orbital proptosis (r=-0.1386, P =0.582).

TABLE 2 | Clinical Characteristic and Radiographic Finding of GO and normal control.

	GO	Control	*P* value
Number, n	38	20	
Male/Female, n/n	16/22	11/9	0.41
Age(years), mean ± SD	44.80 ± 11.64	40.91 ± 12.21	0.38
Smoker, n (%)	13 (34.2%)	11 (55.5%)	0.16
Proptosis(mm), mean ± SD	23.65 ± 2.31	15.24 ± 2.73	<0.0001
Course of disease (months), mean ± SD	23.84 ± 20.62	/	
Sinus mucosal thickening, n (%)	15 (39.5%)	3 (15%)	0.08
Lund-Mackay Score, mean ± SD	3.84 ± 1.83	1.67 ± 0.58	<0.0001
Involved nasal sinuses, n (%)			
Ethmoid	11 (73.3%)	1 (33.3%)	0.25
Maxillary	9 (60.0%)	3 (100%)	0.51
OMC	6(40.0%)	0	0.51
Frontal	0	0	1
Sphenoid	4 (26.7%)	1 (33.3%)	1

Mucosal thickening defined as Lund-MacKay score≥1.
GO, Graves' orbitopathy; CT, computed tomography; SD, standard deviation; OMC, osteomeatal complex.

Histological Changes of Paranasal Sinus Mucosa in GO Patients

Histological changes of the sinus mucosa were found in 21 out of the 38 GO patients (60%). The mucosa showed thickening in GO patients. Compared with normal nasal sinus, typical histological changes include mucosal swelling and epithelial cell proliferation. Some cases show goblet cell proliferation and mucus over-secretion; chronic inflammatory cell infiltration and small vessel proliferation (**Figure 1B**). $CD4^+$ and $CD8^+$ T cells infiltration can be found in GO patients' mucosa, which was detected by immunofluorescence staining (**Figure 1C**). There was a significant increase of $CD4^+$ (29.78 ± 15.16 vs. 10.60 ± 3.78, P=0.024)/HPF and $CD8^+$ T cells (29.00 ± 10.33 vs. 15.33 ± 4.76, P=0.013)/HPF in GO mucosa compared with controls (**Figure 1D**).

Immunological Characteristics of Paranasal Sinuses Mucosa in GO

T cell populations present in the nasal mucosa from GO patients and normal controls were identified as CD4/CD8/γδ T cells by using flow cytometric analysis. The proportion (%) of $CD3^+$ to total living cells (**Figure 2A**) was higher in GO patients compared with normal controls. (33.69 ± 15.84% vs.17.15 ± 9.04%, P<0.001). Th1 cells were defined as $CD3^+CD8^-IFN\text{-}\gamma^+$ subsets and Th2 cells as $CD3^+CD8^-IL\text{-}13^+$ subsets. Our data indicated that Th1 cells increased significantly in GO patients' mucosa (7.19 ± 4.69% vs. 1.74 ± 1.67%, P<0.01), while Th2 cells showed no difference between GO patients and normal controls (9.37 ± 6.70% vs. 6.90 ± 5.10%, P=0.16) (**Figure 2B**). In patients with GO, the mucosa was also characterized by significantly increased Th17 cells ($CD3^+CD8^-IL\text{-}17A^+$) (1.91 ± 0.99% vs. 0.84 ± 0.63%, P<0.001) (**Figure 2C**) and decreased Treg cells ($CD3^+CD8^-FOXP3^+$) (1.38 ± 1.39% vs. 3.04 ± 1.62%, P<0.001) (**Figure 3A**), which suggested a similar Th-driven inflammation to orbital connective tissue. In addition to the changes of Th cells in the mucosa, we further investigated into the difference of γδ T cells between the two groups, which play an important role in mucosal immunity. Our results showed that γδT cells was significantly elevated in GO patients' mucosa (1.47 ± 1.05% vs. 0.60 ± 0.38, P<0.01) (**Figure 3B**). Additionally, we examined IL-17A expression in those sinus mucosal γδT cells and found that there was no difference between the two groups. Intriguingly, we observed a significantly augmented amount of IL-22-secreting γδT cells in the mucosa of GO patients compare with controls (24.32 ± 14.76% vs. 8.42 ± 6.30%, P=0.04) (**Figure 3C**).

The Relationship Between Th1, Th2, Th17 Cells in Nasal Sinus Mucosa and Clinical Characteristics of GO

The proportion of different subtypes of T cells was further analyzed with GO clinical activity score (CAS). Our data

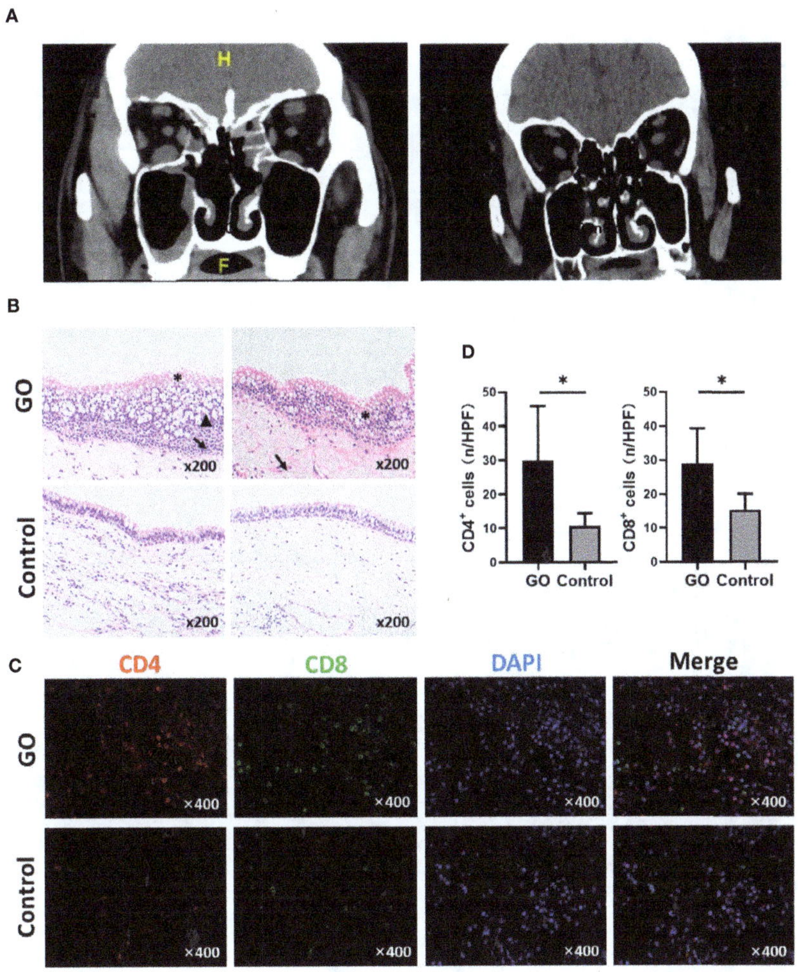

FIGURE 1 | Orbital computed tomography (CT) images and nasal sinus mucosa histological presentation of Graves' orbitopathy (GO) patients and controls. **(A)** Left: A GO patient shows mucosal thickening of maxillary sinus and ethmoid sinus on both sides; Right: Normal control with right orbital fracture. **(B)** Typical changes include mucosal swelling and epithelial cells proliferation. *Disorder of ciliary columnar epithelial; ↑epithelial cell proliferation; ▲ Mucus over-secretion. (HE staining, ×200). **(C)** Immunofluorescence staining results of CD4 and CD8 positive cells in GO and control mucosa. **(D)** Statistical analyses of CD4 and CD8 positive cells, the mucosa of GO has a significant increase compared with control. Significance (*P*) values after t-test was represented by *$P < 0.05$.

indicated that the proportion of Th1 cells was significantly correlated with disease activity (R^2 = 0.11, *P*=0.0474), while there was no correlation between the number of Th2 cells (R^2 = 0.07, *P*=0,136) or Th17cells (R^2 = 0.02, *P*=0.446) and CAS (**Figure 4A**). The study cohort was then divided into two groups according to the time course of GO. One group was longer than 2 years, and the other was less than 2 years. The subtypes of T cells were re-analyzed on the basis of disease course. Our data indicated that the average proportion of Th1 cells (8.23 ± 5.03% vs. 5.62 ± 3.40%) and Th17 cells (2.04 ± 1.16% vs. 1.74 ± 0.62%) declined with the extension of disease course, while Th2 cells (8.27 ± 5.77% vs. 11.11 ± 8.02%) slightly increased with GO duration. However, there was no significant difference in any of the T cell subtypes between these two groups (*P*=0.11, 0.40, 0.24) (**Figure 4B**), which may attribute to the limited number of cases.

DISCUSSION

Previous studies suggested that disorders of the paranasal sinus mucosa were associated with a number of systemic autoimmune diseases. Patients with GD were reported to have significantly greater paranasal sinus mucosal thickening on CT scan than normal controls. The presence of autoantigens TSHR and IGF-1R were also identified in paranasal sinus mucosa (5). These studies hold the opinion that autoantibodies circulating in the blood of patients with GD would be expected to bind to either TSHR or IGF-1R in the sinus mucosa, as occurs in the thyroids and orbital connective tissues, resulting in the localized mucosal edema and inflammatory cell infiltration.

T cell immunity plays an important role in the pathogenesis of GO (14). The frequency of Th1 cells and the Th1/Th2 ratio

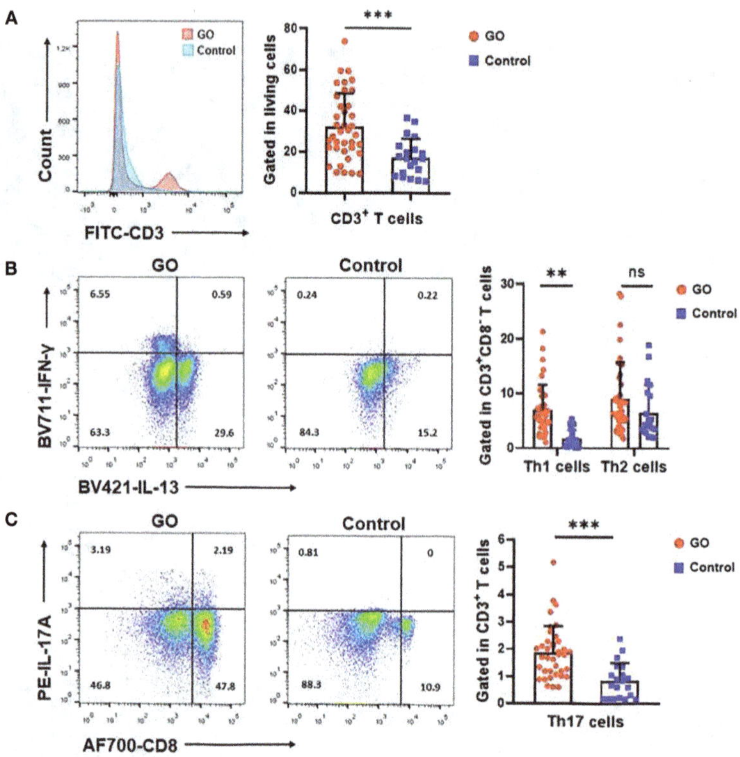

FIGURE 2 | Th1, Th17 but not Th2 cells varied in Graves' orbitopathy (GO) patients compared with controls. **(A)** The percentage (%) of CD3+ cells to total living cells was higher in GO patients compared with controls. **(B)** Flow cytometry showed that Th1 cells increased significantly in GO patients' mucosa, while Th2 cells showed no significant difference between GO patients and controls. Significance (*P*) values after t-test was represented by $^{**}P < 0.01$, $^{***}P < 0.001$. **(C)** Flow cytometry showed that Th17 cells increased significantly in GO patients' mucosa. Significance (*P*) values after t-test was represented by $^{***}P < 0.001$.

were positively correlated with the inflammatory activity score of GO (8). Wakelkamp et al. (15) found that active GO patients were characterized by Th1 type cytokines and there was no direct correlation between Th2 type cytokines and disease progression. Han *et al.* further demonstrated that IFN-γ secreted by Th1 cells and IL-4 secreted by Th2 cells can promote the production of hyaluronic acid by orbital fibroblasts. However, our research did find that there was no difference between GO and control groups in Th2 population. Some studies have revealed that Th1 cells may predominate in the orbit in early GO and Th2 cells might play a greater role in later stages of the disease (16, 17). Yet, others studies have indicated that the active phase is characterized by the presence of proinflammatory and Th1-derived cytokines, whereas other cytokines, including Th2-derived cytokines, do not seem to be linked to a specific stage of GO (18, 19). However, we found most of the studies outdated. Notably, these studies defined Th2 cells by means of establishing T cell clones or examining bulk RNA expression of cytokines within orbital connective tissues due to technical limitation at that time, which made their results not convincing enough. In order to explain the phenomenon, the characteristics of chronic sinusitis should be considered. Chronic rhinosinusitis (CRS) is a persistent inflammatory disease affecting paranasal sinuses. CRS is categorized into two distinct subgroups defined as CRS with nasal polyps (CRSwNP) and CRS without nasal polyps (CRSsNP) (20). Th1 cytokines are mostly found in CRSsNP and Th2 cytokines in CRSwNP. The sinus mucosal abnormality in GO patients isn't usually accompanied by polyps, which might explain the Th1 but not Th2 dominance observed in our study cohort.

We and other groups reported that in GO patients the level of IL-17A and the number of IL-17A-producing T cells were higher than those of healthy controls in the periphery blood as well as in orbital connective tissues (10–12, 21, 22). These results indicate that the $CD4^+$ T cells may contribute to the immunopathological process in GO. In this current study, we also found that there was a higher proportion of both Th1 cells and Th17 cells in the sinus mucosa of GO patients. Combined with previous studies, we suspect that these lymphocytes in nasal sinus may infiltrate into the orbit through the very thin bone walls and blood vessels.

Furthermore, we studied Treg cells in the sinus. Treg cells are a suppressive subset of $CD4^+$ T subsets important for the regulation of immune responses in various autoimmune diseases. Treg cell dysfunction also contributes to the development of autoimmune thyroid disease (23–25). A study showed that patients with improved GO were more likely to have higher proportion of Treg

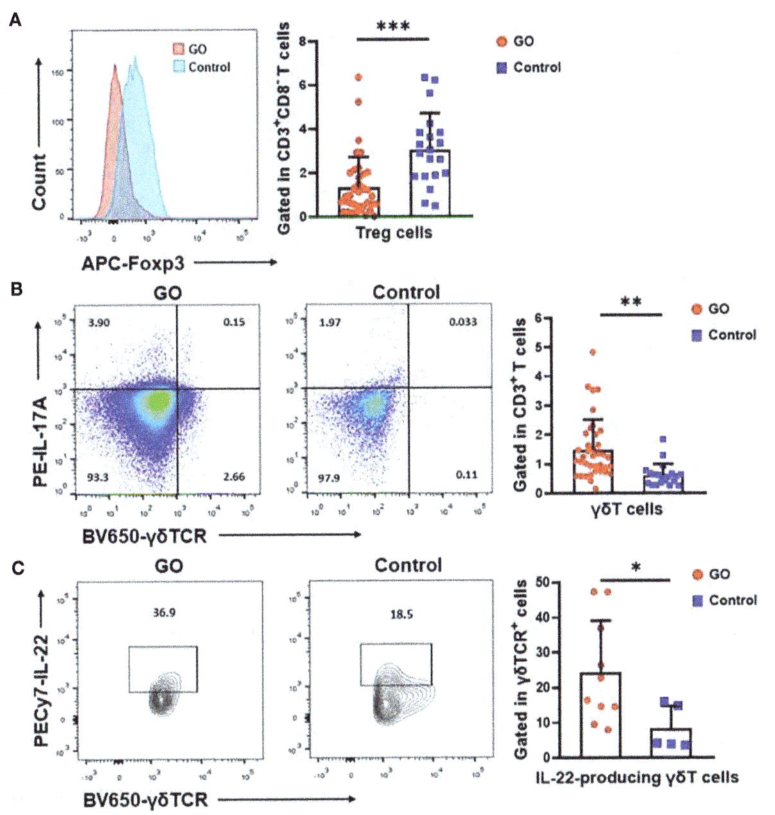

FIGURE 3 | The significant change of Treg cells and γδT cells in the nasal sinus mucosa of Graves' orbitopathy (GO) patients. **(A)** There was also a significant decrease in the percentage (%) of Treg cells in GO patients. Significance (*P*) values after t-test was represented by $^{***}P < 0.001$. **(B)** Flow cytometry showed that γδT cells increased significantly in GO patients' mucosa. Significance (*P*) values after t-test was represented by $^{**}P < 0.01$. **(C)** There was also a significant increase in the percentage (%) of IL-22 secreting γδT cells in GO patients. Significance (*P*) values after t-test was represented by $^{*}P < 0.05$.

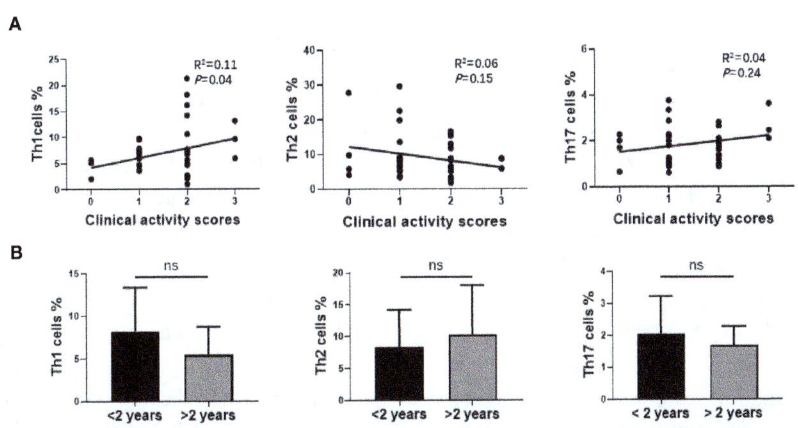

FIGURE 4 | The relationship between Th1, Th2, Th17 cells in nasal sinus mucosa and clinical characteristics of Graves' orbitopathy (GO). **(A)** The analysis of Spearman's correlation between Th1, Th2, Th17 cells and CAS of GO patients. Th1 cells amount was correlated with CAS of GO patients significantly. **(B)** There was no significant difference between two groups of different disease course in Th1, Th2 or Th17 cells.

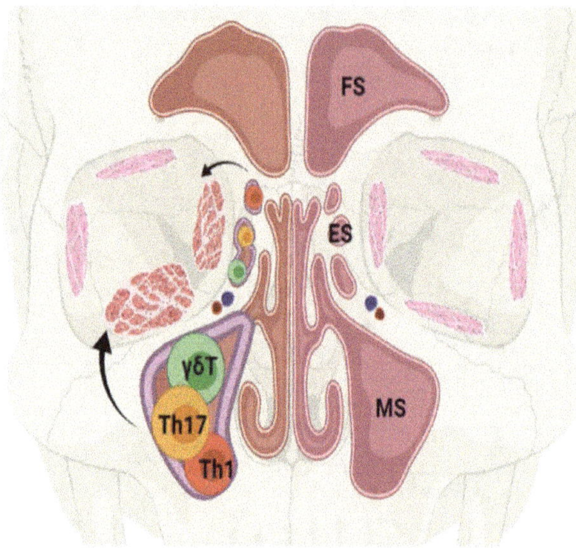

FIGURE 5 | Theoretic model for the relationship between immunological abnormality in nasal sinus of Graves' orbitopathy (GO) patients and orbital inflammation. FS, frontal sinus; ES, ethmoid sinus; MS, maxillary sinus (Declaration: this figure was designed by the first author Yi Lu with the help of drawing website "https://biorender.com").

cells than those with stable or deteriorated GO. Thus, the number of Treg cells in the peripheral blood of GO patients can be used as a predictor of clinical course (26). Kahaly et al. (27) demonstrated that the proportion of Treg cells in the peripheral blood leukocytes derived from GO patients increased after incubation with rabbit polyclonal anti-T lymphocyte globulin. Taken together, our findings reinforced the point of view that the decline of Treg cells might be responsible for the activation of inflammatory cells in GO.

Despite $CD4^+$ and $CD8^+$ T cells, γδT cells are a distinctive subset of T cells that were first recognized by Brenner in 1986. These cells primarily colonize in the mucosa and skin where they play an important role in immune regulation (28). In autoimmune disorders, γδT cells have immunoregulatory properties and secrete both IL-17A and IL-22 (29). A previous study showed that orbital-infiltrating T cells were primarily γδT cells, while the classic αβT helper cells were rare (30). Intriguingly, we previously confirmed an elevated subset of IL-17A-producing γδT cells in the circulation of GO patients compared with healthy controls (12). However, in this current study, we did not find the up-regulation of IL-17A-producing γδT cells, while IL-22-producing γδT cells were observed to be increased in GO sinus mucosa. IL-22 can affect the fibroblasts in the skins, intestines, and joints. Proliferation of synovial fibroblasts in rheumatoid arthritis patients as well as monocyte chemoattractant protein-1-dependent recruitment of monocytes to the sites of inflammation are driven by IL-22 (31). Furthermore, IL-22 can increase the production of anti-inflammatory factors such as IL-11 as well as inflammatory mediators such as IL-6 and CXCLs chemokines in human colonic myofibroblast cells (32, 33). These results indicate that the infiltration of γδT cells in sinus mucosa might be associated with the complicated and refined regulation of orbital inflammation in patients with GO.

This research helps us build a preliminary understanding of the relationship between sinus disorder and GO. It could represent the local effects of sinus for the adjacent orbital inflammation. Inflammatory cells and cytokines may spread from the sinus to the orbit *via* natural dehiscence in adjacent bony walls or by hematogenous spread through common blood vessels (**Figure 5**). All in all, the immune abnormality of the nasal sinus mucosa in GO patients may not only be a clinical manifestation of Graves' disease, but also be involved in the pathogenesis of GO.

AUTHOR CONTRIBUTIONS

Research conception and design: YLu, YW, SF, HZ. Experiment implementation: YLu, YW, JS, YLi. Analysis and interpretation of data: YLu, YH, SF. Drafting of manuscript: YLu, YW. Critical revision: SF, HZ. All authors contributed to the article and approved the submitted version.

FUNDING

This work was supported by the National Natural Science Foundation of China (81930024, 82071003, 82000879, 81761168037, 81770974, 81800695, 81570883, 81600766, 31701046, 31600971, and 31500714), the Shanghai Sailing Program (18YF1412300), the Research Grant of the Shanghai Science and Technology Committee (20DZ2270800, 14JC1493103, 12419A9300, and 16411950600), the Shanghai Municipal Hospital Emerging Frontier Technology Joint Research Project (SHDC12012107), the Shanghai JiaoTong University School of Medicine Summit Plan, and the Shanghai JiaoTong University Medical and Engineering Cross Fund (YG2014MS03), the National Key R&D Program of China (2018YFC1106100, 2018YFC1106101), the Shanghai Municipal Hospital Emerging Frontier Technology Joint Research Project (16CR1004A), the Shanghai Municipal Education Commission—Gaofeng Clinical Medicine Grant Support (20152228), the Shanghai JiaoTong University Translational Medicine Crossed ResearchGrant (ZH2018ZDA12), and the Sample Database Project of Shanghai Ninth People's Hospital (YBKB201901), the Joint Innovation Team for Young Physicians of Shanghai Ninth People's Hospital (QC202002).

REFERENCES

1. Perros P, Krassas GE. Graves orbitopathy: a perspective. *Nat Rev Endocrinol* (2009) 5(6):312–8. doi: 10.1038/nrendo.2009.61
2. Bahn RS. Current Insights into the Pathogenesis of Graves' Ophthalmopathy. *Horm. Metab Res* (2015) 47(10):773–8. doi: 10.1055/s-0035-1555762
3. Dutton JJ. Anatomic Considerations in Thyroid Eye Disease. *Ophthalmic Plast Reconstr Surg* (2018) 34(4S Suppl 1):S7–S12. doi: 10.1097/IOP.0000000000001122
4. Gouveris HT, Al-Homsi J, Gosepath J, Mann WJ. Histological and radiological signs indicative for chronic sinus mucosal inflammation in Graves' ophthalmopathy. *Rhinology* (2009) 47(2):144–7.
5. Soler ZM, Platt MP, Leung MK, Mong S, Metson R. Sinonasal abnormalities in patients with Graves' orbitopathy. *Laryngoscope* (2011) 121(3):656–60. doi: 10.1002/lary.21392
6. Pappa A, Lawson JM, Calder V, Fells P, Lightman S. T cells and fibroblasts in affected extraocular muscles in early and late thyroid associated ophthalmopathy. *Br J Ophthalmol* (2000) 84(5):517–22. doi: 10.1136/bjo.84.5.517
7. Han R, Smith TJ. T helper type 1 and type 2 cytokines exert divergent influence on the induction of prostaglandin E2 and hyaluronan synthesis by interleukin-1beta in orbital fibroblasts: implications for the pathogenesis of thyroid-associated ophthalmopathy. *Endocrinology* (2006) 147(1):13–9. doi: 10.1210/en.2005-1018
8. Xia N, Zhou S, Liang Y, Xiao C, Shen H, Pan H, et al. CD4+ T cells and the Th1/Th2 imbalance are implicated in the pathogenesis of Graves' ophthalmopathy. *Int J Mol Med* (2006) 17(5):911–6. doi: 10.3892/ijmm.17.5.911
9. Lehmann GM, Feldon SE, Smith TJ, Phipps RP. Immune mechanisms in thyroid eye disease. *Thyroid* (2008) 18(9):959–65. doi: 10.1089/thy.2007.0407
10. Kim SE, Yoon JS, Kim KH, Lee SY. Increased serum interleukin-17 in Graves' ophthalmopathy. *Graefes Arch Clin Exp Ophthalmol* (2012) 250(10):1521–6. doi: 10.1007/s00417-012-2092-7
11. Shen J, Li Z, Li W, Ge Y, Xie M, Lv M, et al. Th1, Th2, and Th17 Cytokine Involvement in Thyroid Associated Ophthalmopathy. *Dis Markers* (2015) 2015:609593. doi: 10.1155/2015/609593
12. Fang S, Huang Y, Wang S, Zhang Y, Luo X, Liu L, et al. IL-17A Exacerbates Fibrosis by Promoting the Proinflammatory and Profibrotic Function of Orbital Fibroblasts in TAO. *J Clin Endocrinol Metab* (2016) 101(8):2955–65. doi: 10.1210/jc.2016-1882
13. Fang S, Huang Y, Zhong S, Li Y, Zhang Y, Li Y, et al. Regulation of Orbital Fibrosis and Adipogenesis by Pathogenic Th17 Cells in Graves Orbitopathy. *J Clin Endocrinol Metab* (2017) 102(11):4273–83. doi: 10.1210/jc.2017-01349
14. Huang Y, Fang S, Li D, Zhou H, Li B, Fan X. The involvement of T cell pathogenesis in thyroid-associated ophthalmopathy. *Eye (Lond)* (2019) 33 (2):176–82. doi: 10.1038/s41433-018-0279-9
15. Wakelkamp IM, Bakker O, Baldeschi L, Wiersinga WM, Prummel MF. TSH-R expression and cytokine profile in orbital tissue of active vs. inactive Graves' ophthalmopathy patients. *Clin Endocrinol (Oxf)* (2003) 58(3):280–7. doi: 10.1046/j.1365-2265.2003.01708.x
16. Aniszewski JP, Valyasevi RW, Bahn RS. Relationship between disease duration and predominant orbital T cell subset in Graves' ophthalmopathy. *J Clin Endocrinol Metab* (2000) 85(2):776–80. doi: 10.1210/jcem.85.2.6333
17. Hiromatsu Y, Yang D, Bednarczuk T, Miyake I, Nonaka K, Inoue Y. Cytokine profiles in eye muscle tissue and orbital fat tissue from patients with thyroid-associated ophthalmopathy. *J Clin Endocrinol Metab* (2000) 85(3):1194–9. doi: 10.1210/jcem.85.3.6433
18. Wakelkamp IM, Bakker O, Baldeschi L, Wiersinga WM, Prummel MF. TSH-R expression and cytokine profile in orbital tissue of active vs. inactive Graves' ophthalmopathy patients. *Clin Endocrinol (Oxf)* (2003) 58(3):280–7. doi: 10.1046/j.1365-2265.2003.01708.x
19. Yang D, Hiromatsu Y, Hoshino T, Inoue Y, Itoh K, Nonaka K. Dominant infiltration of T(H)1-type CD4+ T cells at the retrobulbar space of patients with thyroid-associated ophthalmopathy. *Thyroid* (1999) 9(3):305–10. doi: 10.1089/thy.1999.9.305
20. Scheckenbach K, Wagenmann M. Cytokine Patterns and Endotypes in Acute and Chronic Rhinosinusitis. *Curr Allergy Asthma Rep* (2016) 16(1):3 doi: 10.1007/s11882-015-0583-4
21. Wei H, Guan M, Qin Y, Xie C, Fu X, Gao F, et al. Circulating levels of miR-146a and IL-17 are significantly correlated with the clinical activity of Graves' ophthalmopathy. *Endocr J* (2013) 61(11):1087–92. doi: 10.1507/endocrj.ej14-0246
22. Fang S, Huang Y, Wang N, Zhang S, Zhong S, Li Y, et al. Insights onto local orbital immunity: evidence for the involvement of the Th17 cell pathway in thyroid-associated ophthalmopathy. *J Clin Endocrinol Metab* (2019) 104 (5):1697–711. doi: 10.1210/jc.2018-01626
23. González-Amaro R, Marazuela M. T regulatory (Treg) and T helper 17 (Th17) lymphocytes in thyroid autoimmunity. *Endocrine* (2016) 52(1):30–8. doi: 10.1007/s12020-015-0759-7
24. Marazuela M, García-López MA, Figueroa-Vega N, de la Fuente H, Alvarado-Sánchez B, Monsiváis-Urenda A, et al. Regulatory T cells in human autoimmune thyroid disease. *J Clin Endocrinol Metab* (2006) 91(9):3639–46. doi: 10.1210/jc.2005-2337
25. Roncarolo MG, Gregori S, Bacchetta R, Battaglia M. Tr1 cells and the counter-regulation of immunity: natural mechanisms and therapeutic applications. *Curr Top Microbiol Immunol* (2014) 380:39–68. doi: 10.1007/978-3-662-43492-5_3
26. Matsuzawa K, Izawa S, Okura T, Fujii S, Matsumoto K, Shoji K, et al. Implications of FoxP3-positive and -negative CD4(+) CD25(+) T cells in Graves' ophthalmopathy. *Endocr J* (2016) 63(8):755–64. doi: 10.1507/endocrj.EJ16-0108
27. Kahaly GJ, Shimony O, Gellman YN, Lytton SD, Eshkar-Sebban L, Rosenblum N, et al. Regulatory T-cells in Graves' orbitopathy: baseline findings and immunomodulation by anti-T lymphocyte globulin. *J Clin Endocrinol Metab* (2011) 96(2):422–9. doi: 10.1210/jc.2010-1424
28. Brenner MB, McLean J, Dialynas DP, Strominger JL, Smith JA, Owen FL, et al. Identification of a putative second T-cell receptor. *Nature* (1986) 322 (6075):145–9. doi: 10.1038/322145a0
29. Sutton CE, Lalor SJ, Sweeney CM, Brereton CF, Lavelle EC, Mills KH. Interleukin-1 and IL-23 induce innate IL-17 production from gammadelta T cells, amplifying Th17 responses and autoimmunity. *Immunity* (2009) 31 (2):331–41. doi: 10.1016/j.immuni.2009.08.001
30. Eckstein AK, Quadbeck B, Tews S, Mann K, Krüger C, Mohr CH, et al. Thyroid associated ophthalmopathy: evidence for CD4(+) gammadelta T cells; de novo differentiation of RFD7(+) macrophages, but not of RFD1(+) dendritic cells; and loss of gammadelta and alphabeta T cell receptor expression. *Br J Ophthalmol* (2004) 88(6):803–8. doi: 10.1136/bjo.2003.035915
31. Ikeuchi H, Kuroiwa T, Hiramatsu N, Kaneko Y, Hiromura K, Ueki K, et al. Expression of interleukin-22 in rheumatoid arthritis: potential role as a proinflammatory cytokine. *Arthritis Rheumatol* (2005) 52(4):1037–46. doi: 10.1002/art.20965
32. Andoh A, Zhang Z, Inatomi O, Fujino S, Deguchi Y, Araki Y, et al. Interleukin-22, a member of the IL-10 subfamily, induces inflammatory responses in colonic subepithelial myofibroblasts. *Gastroenterology* (2005) 129(3):969–84. doi: 10.1053/j.gastro.2005.06.071
33. Lo Re S, Dumoutier L, Couillin I, Van Vyve C, Yakoub Y, Uwambayinema F, et al. IL-17A-producing gammadelta T and Th17 lymphocytes mediate lung inflammation but not fibrosis in experimental silicosis. *J Immunol* (2010) 184 (11):6367–77. doi: 10.4049/jimmunol.0900459

17

Orbital Signaling in Graves' Orbitopathy

Mohd Shazli Draman [1,2], Lei Zhang [1], Colin Dayan [1] and Marian Ludgate [1†]*

[1] *Thyroid Research Group, Cardiff University School of Medicine, Cardiff, United Kingdom,* [2] *KPJ Healthcare University College, Nilai, Malaysia*

***Correspondence:**
Lei Zhang
zhangL14@cf.ac.uk*

†Senior Author: Marian Ludgate

Graves' orbitopathy (GO) is a complex and poorly understood disease in which extensive remodeling of orbital tissue is dominated by adipogenesis and hyaluronan production. The resulting proptosis is disfiguring and underpins the majority of GO signs and symptoms. While there is strong evidence for the thyrotropin receptor (TSHR) being a thyroid/orbit shared autoantigen, the insulin-like growth factor 1 receptor (IGF1R) is also likely to play a key role in the disease. The pathogenesis of GO has been investigated extensively in the last decade with further understanding of some aspects of the disease. This is mainly derived by using *in vitro* and *ex vivo* analysis of the orbital tissues. Here, we have summarized the features of GO pathogenesis involving target autoantigens and their signaling pathways.

Keywords: thyroid eye disease, adipogenesis, hyaluronan, TSAB, TSHR, IGF1R

INTRODUCTION

Graves' orbitopathy (GO) or thyroid eye disease is the most common overt thyroidal manifestation of Graves' disease (GD) with substantial morbidity and socioeconomic impact (1–4). Extensive orbital tissue remodelling in GO is mainly shown as adipose tissue expansion and tissue edema *via* increased adipogenesis and hyaluronan production, respectively. These pathogenetic processes produce disfiguring proptosis and underpin all GO signs and symptoms. There is a close clinical and temporal association between GD and GO suggesting an autoimmune response to common antigen/s in the orbit and thyroid gland. The thyrotropin receptor (TSHR) is expressed in orbital adipose tissue (OAT) (5–8) and virtually all patients with hyperthyroid GO have thyroid stimulating antibodies (TSAB). Therefore, the TSHR is the most logical candidate (9), which is further supported by the existence of TSHR-induced GO in an animal model (10). The incidence of GO is estimated to be 16/100,000 in females and 2.9/100,000 in males (11). On the other hand, the prevalence estimate is about 10/10,000 (12). A recent meta-analysis reported that current GD patients have a milder phenotype than in the past; as a consequence, a smaller proportion display

---

Abbreviations: GO, Graves' orbitopathy; TSAB, thyroid stimulating antibodies; TSHR, thyrotropin receptor; IGF1, insulin like growth factor 1; IBMX, 3-isobutyl-1-methylxanthine; PPARγ, peroxisome proliferator-activated receptors gamma; PI3 kinase Phosphoinositide-3- kinase; MAP, mitogen-activated protein kinase; FOXO, Forkhead Box O1; C/EBP-δ, CCAAT-enhancer-binding proteins Delta; cAMP, Cyclic adenosine monophosphate; PKA, protein kinase A; GCRP, G protein coupled receptors; FRET, fluorescence resonance energy transfer; CREB, cAMP responsive element binding protein; TG, thyroglobulin; TPO, thyroid peroxidase; NIS, sodium iodide symporter (NIS), TTF, thyroid transcription factors; PKC, Protein kinase C; PLC phospholipase C; DAG, di-acyl-glycerol; NFAT, Nuclear factor of activated T-cells; HA, hyaluronic acid; GAG, glycosaminoglycan; SNP, single nucleotide polymorphism.

GO symptoms (13). As with other autoimmune conditions there is female preponderance towards the condition with 6:1 female to male ratio, although in GO the ratio is less skewed than in GD. In addition, most patients with GO have reduced quality of life (QOL) (14) and suffer long-term psychological distress due to the disfiguring appearance of the proptosis, also known as exophthalmos (15). Available treatments for GO are unsatisfactory and more research is needed to address the pathophysiology of the disease which may lead to early pre-clinical diagnosis promoting preventative/early interventions. This in turn will improve long-term morbidity and socioeconomic impact.

ADIPOGENESIS

Adipogenesis is a process in which preadipocytes differentiate into mature adipocytes to form adipose tissues. Our current understanding of adipogenesis has been largely derived by using the murine 3T3L1 cell line. This cell line can spontaneously differentiate into adipocytes when maintained in a high concentration of fetal calf serum for several weeks but the process can be accelerated by employing adipogenic cocktails including insulin, steroid and 3- isobutyl-1-methylxanthine (IBMX) (16). Further components of the differentiation cocktails may also include proliferation-activated receptor gamma (PPARγ) agonists such as pioglitazone and indomethacin (17). Insulin, in common with insulin-like growth factor-1 (IGF-1) activates PI3 kinase (18) and MAP (mitogen-activated protein kinase) (19) pathways. Phosphorylation of protein kinase B (PKB/Akt) in turn phosphorylates forkhead box protein O1 (FOXO1) causing it to exit from the nucleus leading to increased transcription of adipogenic genes (20). Steroids induce the expression of the early adipogenic gene, CCAAT enhancer binding protein delta (C/EBP-δ). This transcription factor contributes to an increase in PPAR-γ expression and production of prostacyclin leading to elevated intracellular cAMP. IBMX is a nonselective phosphodiesterase inhibitor whose presence further elevates levels of intracellular cAMP and protein kinase A (PKA). IBMX is thus required for transcriptional activation of the master regulator of adipogenesis, PPARγ.

Adipogenesis contributes to OAT expansion because a fibroblast has an approximate diameter of 30 microns, whereas the diameter of a mature adipocyte is approximately 150 microns, i.e. 5 times larger. The increased adipogenesis has been demonstrated by using *in vitro* cultures of human fibroblasts and analysis of *ex vivo* samples from patients with GO (21). By using both *in vitro* lineage specific differentiation protocols and flow cytometry, studies have indicated that orbital fibroblasts (OF) possess mesenchymal stem cell (MSC) properties including positivity for Thy-1 (CD90) which is a marker of MSC (22–25). In the orbit, Thy-1 negative OF can be induced to differentiate when cultured in appropriate adipogenic medium whereas Thy-1 positive cells are more likely to undergo differentiation to myofibroblasts and cause fibrosis (23, 24). The orbital fibroblast is also able to undergo neurogenesis, myogenesis, osteogenesis and chondrogenesis *in vitro*, indicating their pluripotency (22, 25).

EXTRA-CELLULAR MATRIX

Several extracellular matrix (ECM) components are overproduced in GO including collagens and glycosaminoglycans (GAGs). The excess ECM accumulation in OAT and extraocular muscle (EOM) lead to oedema with consequent proptosis and diplopia respectively (26). The main GAG produced in GO is hyaluronic acid, which is generated by three synthase enzymes (HAS1, HAS2 and HAS3) and broken down by hyaluronidases. Activation of cAMP-protein kinase A signaling *via* the TSHR, increases cAMP response element binding protein (CREB) at CREB binding sites in the promoters of HAS1 and HAS2 genes, thereby enhancing hyaluronan production (27).

TSHR INTRACELLULAR PATHWAYS

Several studies, including from our group, have shown that activation of the TSHR in OF leads to an increase in hyaluronan production and adipogenesis (20, 28). TSHR expression has been shown to increase during adipogenesis (5). We demonstrated that 'neutral' TSHR antibodies were capable of binding but had no effect on traditional TSHR signaling pathways (described below) (29). Indeed, TSHR signaling may be far more complex than initially thought (30). Little is known about the effects of TSHR activation at various stages during differentiation. The downstream cascade triggered by TSHR will depend on the types and abundance of guanine-nucleotide binding proteins (G proteins) available in the cell (31). G protein coupled receptors (GPCR) can exist as monomers or oligomers. Oligomerization is the term used to describe dimeric, tetrameric, or higher-order complexes between GPCR monomers. The activation of different GPCR complexes will have major influence on subsequent G protein signaling pathways. The evidence that TSHR may exist in an oligomeric state was initially provided by studies using antibodies (32) and more recently by fluorescence resonance energy transfer (FRET) technology (33). Interestingly, the presence of dimerization influences TSHR behavior. Unstimulated TSHRs have been shown to form oligomers that return to the monomer state with TSH (34). TSHR autoantibodies with stimulating properties are (TSAB) proposed to favor formation of TSHR dimers, whilst TSHR blocking antibodies, are unable to bring about this conformational change. After TSH binding, a constitutively oligomeric TSHR dissociates into active monomers (or dimers when TSAB bind). Subsequently the monomers or dimers are recruited to the lipid rafts and interact with G proteins, thereby initiating the signaling cascade. In the case of TSH, the signal is rapid and brief because of faster movement of monomers into the lipid rafts, in contrast to the slow motion of the dimers. Multivalent blocking TSHR antibodies may cross-link the oligomers, thus preventing them from dissociating and impeding their entry into lipid rafts (35). In cells with low levels of TSHR expression, homo-heterodimer formation is less likely. This may change during adipogenesis, as TSHR expression increases, and may lead to activation of different signaling cascades from that predominating in orbital fibroblasts.

TSHR is known to activate mainly the guanine-nucleotide protein alpha stimulation (Gs)-cAMP pathway. In addition, TSHR may activate several other G protein subtypes, as detailed below (36, 37), non G protein pathways such as β-arrestin-1 (38) and other signalling pathways (39, 40). When TSH binds to its receptor, GTP replaces GDP in the heterotrimeric G protein, which dissociates into Gsα and Gβγ subunits with the former activating all isoforms of adenylate cyclase (41). This enzyme increases levels of cAMP in the cell and activates PKA, also known as cAMP-dependent protein kinase. The activated PKA phosphorylates multiple downstream target proteins one of which is cAMP responsive element binding protein (CREB). CREB then binds to its receptors on the promoter region of the DNA exerting various gene transcription processes including expression of thyroglobulin (TG), thyroid peroxidase (TPO), sodium iodide symporter (NIS), the thyroid transcription factors TTF1/NKx2.1, TTF2/FoxE1, and PAX (42, 43). Every intermediary in the pathway described above may additionally interact with different molecules belonging to other pathways.

In human thyrocytes and rat FRTL-5, guanidine binding protein alpha a/alpha 11 (Gαq/α11) coupling has been shown to stimulate Protein kinase C (PKC) pathways by generating phospholipase C (PLCβ). The PKC pathways has been associated with hyaluronan generation in GO (44). Activation of PKC pathways requires supraphysiological TSH concentrations although not all research agrees with this finding (45). PLC catalyses hydrolysis of phosphatidylinositol in cell membranes yielding di-acyl-glycerol (DAG) and inositol tri phosphate (IP3) as second messengers. DAG directly stimulates PKC. IP3 increases cytosolic Ca+2 levels which act through a number of effectors including PKC itself (46) and Nuclear Factor of Activated T-cells (NFAT) transcription factor protein. NFAT plays an important role in cytokine gene transcription regulation (47). Calcium *via* calmodulin –a calcium sensor protein - activates the serine/threonine phosphatase calcineurin (inhibited by cyclosporin and FK506). This in turn rapidly dephosphorylates NFAT proteins, resulting in a conformational change that exposes a nuclear localization signal leading to NFAT nuclear import (48). TSHR may also couple to guanine nucleotide binding protein alpha inhibition (Gαi1), which inhibits adenylyl cyclase and decreases cAMP levels. The accompanying Gβγ dimers may induce multitudes of other pathways, including adenylyl cyclase, PI3K/Akt (PKB)-FOXO and PLC cascades (49–51). Others have reported that TSHR activation of OF signals *via* p70s6 kinase (52). The finding may explain our lack of success when using gain-of-function mutants of the TSHR, which signal predominantly *via* Gsα, to stimulate adipogenesis (28) and concurs with the study from van Ziejl et al. who investigated TSH/TSAB induced hyaluronan production (53). It contrasts with the studies of Neumann and colleagues, who report increased M22-mediated cAMP, even at baseline. However, these authors maintain their OF in a semi-adipogenic medium which likely increases TSHR expression (54).

Our previous work has demonstrated that adipogenesis and HA production, are linked in the orbit. HA accumulation increases in the orbit during adipogenesis but not in other fat depots (55). In this study, adipogenesis in orbital preadipocytes was accompanied by HA accumulation and significantly increased *HAS2* transcripts (but not *HAS 1* and *3*). In contrast, adipogenic differentiation in subcutaneous preadipocyte-fibroblasts significantly decreased secreted HA and *HAS2* transcript levels. IGF-I alone did not increase *HAS2* levels, but inhibition of PKB/Akt increased orbital *HAS2* transcripts but not subcutaneous preadipocytes. Furthermore, our study suggested that mTORC1 negative feedback in IGF1–PI3K–Akt signalling is absent in OF but present in subcutaneous adipose tissue (55). The difference might be explained by the fact that human OF originate from neural crest, while subcutaneous adipose tissue is of mesodermal origin. In addition, our most recent studies demonstrated a depot specific fatty acid-uptake driven adipogenesis with unique gene signatures in OAT. These result in hyperplastic-type expansion of adipocytes in GO (56, 57). Taken together, these findings suggest a very distinctive mechanism underlying the orbital adipogenesis process.

INSULIN LIKE GROWTH FACTOR -1 RECEPTOR SIGNALLING

While there is strong evidence supporting the role of TSHR in GO, IGF1R is also likely to play a key role in the disease progress. The IGF1R was first proposed by Weightman and colleagues who demonstrated high affinity IGF1 binding sites in OF (58). More recently extensive work from Terry Smith and his colleagues has confirmed this finding and further showed that TSHR and IGF1R co-localize to orbital cell membranes (59). The same group has further reported a wide range of IGF1R mediated effects in OF including increases in proliferation, GAG production and cytokine production (60, 61). Our own study demonstrated that activation of TSHR and IGR1R has additive effect on HAS2 transcripts/HA production (62). Krieger et al. found that M22 stimulation of HA secretion by OF involves cross talk between IGF-1R and TSHR. The relationship relies on TSHR activation per se rather than direct activation of IGF-1R which leads to synergistic stimulation of HA secretion (63). TSH induced ERK phosphorylation can be blocked by an IGF-1R-blocking monoclonal antibody suggesting that IGF-1R might mediate some TSH-provoked signalling. Further studies have highlighted the importance of down stream factors of IGF1–PI3K signalling and revealed that FOXOs, may mediate both TSHR and IGF1R signalling pathways in GO (64). The notion is further supported by recent successful trial of teprotumumab-monoclonal antibody which blocks IGF1R - in reducing proptosis in patients with GO (65, 66). Whilst effective medical treatment for GO is welcome, some concerns have been raised about these trials including the lack of orbital imaging and the fact that despite QOL scores being improved in the teprotumumab group, all patients scores remained low (67). Furthermore, the activation of Fibroblast Growth factor (FGF) and its receptor has been shown to increase the expression of Insulin like growth factor-2 (IGF-2) in mesenchymal stem cells *via* IGF-2 and IGF1-R (68). The FGF signalling pathway has also been shown to play a role in OAT expansion in GO (69). Our most recent study used RNA-seq analysis to demonstrate that FGFs, FGFR2, IGF-2 and IGF1-R were highly expressed in OAT compared with white adipose tissue, supporting the aforementioned successful trial of IGF1R inhibition in GO (56).

TSHR VARIANTS

To add to the complexity of the molecular events associated with GO, several TSHR variants have been described which lack the transmembrane domain. If the variants are expressed as protein, they would yield soluble receptor products which could serve as TSH/TRAB binding proteins or even as autoantigens. Early northern blot analysis of thyroid tissue identified the expected full-length transcript plus 2 additional transcripts at 1.3 and 1.6 kb (70); the transcripts were also detected in OF (71). Of interest, the exon 1-8 variant is similar in structure to the TSHR A subunit which is generated following cleavage of the full-length receptor (72, 73). Furthermore, induced murine models of GD and GO are more effective when immunizing with the A subunit than with the complete TSHR (74, 75). We have reported that the 1.3 variant is expressed as a protein and can affect TSHR activation (76). Thus, these variants could have impact on the pathogenesis of GO by inducing further production of TSAB or protect against GO by 'neutralizing' TSAB, respectively.

DISCUSSION

TSHR and IGF1 signaling are important in orbital tissues (summarized in **Figure 1**) but more complex than generally thought. Although these signals are mainly activated through G protein signalling pathways, other cascades may also be involved.

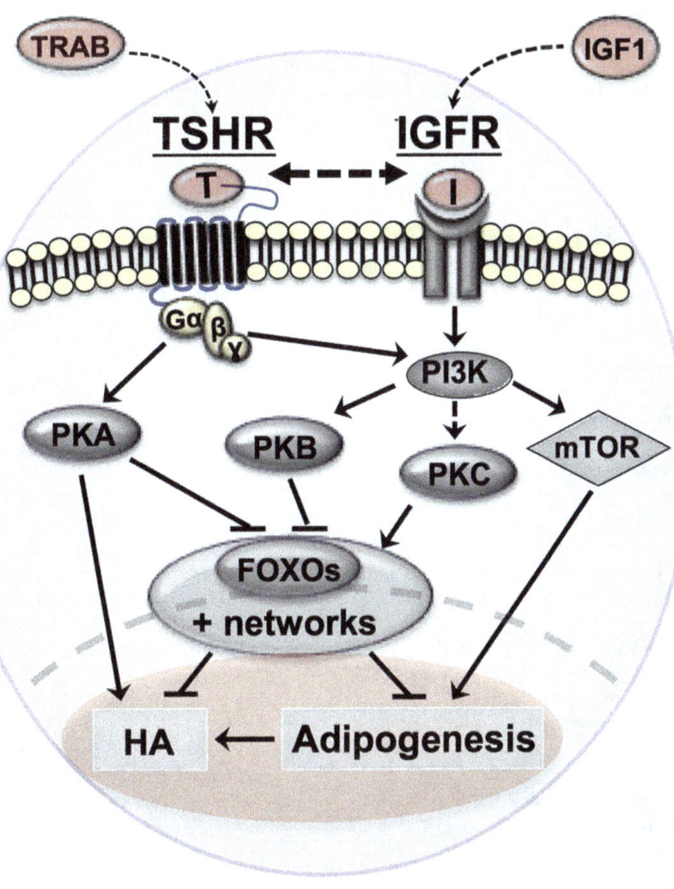

FIGURE 1 | Cartoon summarizing orbital fibroblast signaling cascades in Graves' orbitopathy (GO) and how they affect pathogenetic mechanisms (adipogenesis and hyaluronan production). TSHR/TRAB and IGFR/IGF are shown in red with arrows indicating the possible crosstalk between the pathways in GO. thyrotropin receptor (TSHR, serpentine structure); TSHR auto-antibodies (TRAB); Insulin-like growth factor 1 receptor (IGF-1R) and IGF1; protein kinase A (PKA); protein kinase B (PKB/Akt); protein kinase C (PKC); phosphoinositide 3-kinase (PI3K); forkhead box protein O (FOXO); hyaluronan production (HA).

As our understanding expands, additional extracellular or intracellular factors, which regulate signaling, may be identified. The abundance of the receptors may also dictate which pathways are activated. The recent success of TSHR extracellular domain crystallization is likely to catapult these areas of research and may lead to further alternative treatment strategies for GO (77).

As discussed above, a human monoclonal anti-IGF-1R-blocking antibody, Teprotumumab has been approved by FDA for treatment of patients with GO specifically in reducing proptosis and has recently been reported to be highly effective in active GO (65). The potential for treatments based on TSHR antagonism, which have been demonstrated to be effective *in vitro*, is keenly anticipated either with blocking antibodies or small molecule antagonists which in theory could inhibit both TSHR and IGF-1R related and/or unrelated pathways (78). The beneficial effects on GD and GO following administration of a monoclonal TSHR blocking antibody (TBAB) in a patient with thyroid cancer has recently been described (79). Furthermore, manipulating the two pathways concomitantly may provide even more effective treatment for GO and merits investigation.

AUTHOR CONTRIBUTIONS

MD and LZ wrote the manuscript with input from ML. CD and ML reviewed the manuscript. All authors contributed to the article and approved the submitted version.

REFERENCES

1. Reddy SV, Jain A, Yadav SB, Sharma K, Bhatia E. Prevalence of Graves' Ophthalmopathy in Patients With Graves' Disease Presenting to a Referral Centre in North India. *Indian J Med Res* (2014) 139(1):99–104.
2. Tellez M, Cooper J, Edmonds C. Graves' Ophthalmopathy in Relation to Cigarette Smoking and Ethnic Origin. *Clin Endocrinol* (1992) 36(3):291–4. doi: 10.1111/j.1365-2265.1992.tb01445.x
3. Wiersinga WM, Bartalena L. Epidemiology and Prevention of Graves' Ophthalmopathy. *Thyroid* (2002) 12(10):855–60. doi: 10.1089/105072502761016476
4. Tanda ML, Piantanida E, Liparulo L, Veronesi G, Lai A, Sassi L, et al. Prevalence and Natural History of Graves' Orbitopathy in a Large Series of Patients With Newly Diagnosed Graves' Hyperthyroidism Seen at a Single Center. *J Clin Endocrinol Metab* (2013) 98(4):1443–9. doi: 10.1210/jc.2012-3873
5. Crisp M, Starkey KJ, Lane C, Ham J, Ludgate M. Adipogenesis in Thyroid Eye Disease. *Invest Ophthalmol Visual Sci* (2000) 41(11):3249–55.
6. Kumar S, Coenen MJ, Scherer PE, Bahn RS. Evidence for Enhanced Adipogenesis in the Orbits of Patients With Graves' Ophthalmopathy. *J Clin Endocrinol Metab* (2004) 89(2):930–5. doi: 10.1210/jc.2003-031427
7. Bahn RS, Dutton CM, Natt N, Joba W, Spitzweg C, Heufelder AE. Thyrotropin Receptor Expression in Graves' Orbital Adipose/Connective Tissues: Potential Autoantigen in Graves' Ophthalmopathy. *J Clin Endocrinol Metab* (1998) 83(3):998–1002. doi: 10.1210/jc.83.3.998
8. Roselli-Rehfuss L, Robbins LS, Cone RD. Thyrotropin Receptor Messenger Ribonucleic Acid Is Expressed in Most Brown and White Adipose Tissues in the Guinea Pig. *Endocrinology* (1992) 130(4):1857–61. doi: 10.1210/endo.130.4.1547715
9. Khoo DH, Ho SC, Seah LL, Fong KS, Tai ES, Chee SP, et al. The Combination of Absent Thyroid Peroxidase Antibodies and High Thyroid-Stimulating Immunoglobulin Levels in Graves' Disease Identifies a Group at Markedly Increased Risk of Ophthalmopathy. *Thyroid* (1999) 9(12):1175–80. doi: 10.1089/thy.1999.9.1175
10. Banga JP, Moshkelgosha S, Berchner-Pfannschmidt U, Eckstein A. Modeling Graves' Orbitopathy in Experimental Graves' Disease. *Horm Metab Res* (2015) 47(10):797–803. doi: 10.1055/s-0035-1555956
11. Lazarus JH. Epidemiology of Graves' Orbitopathy (GO) and Relationship With Thyroid Disease. *Best Pract Res Clin Endocrinol Metab* (2012) 26 (3):273–9. doi: 10.1016/j.beem.2011.10.005
12. Perros P, Hegedus L, Bartalena L, Marcocci C, Kahaly GJ, Baldeschi L, et al. Graves' Orbitopathy as a Rare Disease in Europe: A European Group on Graves' Orbitopathy (EUGOGO) Position Statement. *Orphanet J Rare Dis* (2017) 12(1):72. doi: 10.1186/s13023-017-0625-1
13. Ippolito S, Cusini C, Lasalvia P, Gianfagna F, Veronesi G, Gallo D, et al. Change in Newly Diagnosed Graves' Disease Phenotype Between the Twentieth and the Twenty-First Centuries: Meta-Analysis and Meta-Regression. *J Endocrinol Invest* (2021) 44(8):1707–18. doi: 10.1007/s40618-020-01479-z
14. Wiersinga WM. Quality of Life in Graves' Ophthalmopathy. *Best Pract Res Clin Endocrinol Metab* (2012) 26(3):359–70. doi: 10.1016/j.beem.2011.11.001
15. Coulter I, Frewin S, Krassas GE, Perros P. Psychological Implications of Graves' Orbitopathy. *Eur J Endocrinol Eur Fed Endocrine Societies* (2007) 157 (2):127–31. doi: 10.1530/EJE-07-0205
16. Rosen ED, Spiegelman BM. Molecular Regulation of Adipogenesis. *Annu Rev Cell Dev Biol* (2000) 16:145–71. doi: 10.1146/annurev.cellbio.16.1.145
17. Tontonoz P, Hu E, Spiegelman BM. Stimulation of Adipogenesis in Fibroblasts by PPAR Gamma 2, a Lipid-Activated Transcription Factor. *Cell* (1994) 79(7):1147–56. doi: 10.1016/0092-8674(94)90006-x
18. Xu J, Liao K. Protein Kinase B/AKT 1 Plays a Pivotal Role in Insulin-Like Growth Factor-1 Receptor Signaling Induced 3T3-L1 Adipocyte Differentiation. *J Biol Chem* (2004) 279(34):35914–22. doi: 10.1074/jbc.M402297200
19. Qiu Z, Wei Y, Chen N, Jiang M, Wu J, Liao K. DNA Synthesis and Mitotic Clonal Expansion Is Not a Required Step for 3T3-L1 Preadipocyte Differentiation Into Adipocytes. *J Biol Chem* (2001) 276(15):11988–95. doi: 10.1074/jbc.M011729200
20. Zhang L, Paddon C, Lewis MD, Grennan-Jones F, Ludgate M. Gsalpha Signalling Suppresses PPARgamma2 Generation and Inhibits 3T3L1 Adipogenesis. *J Endocrinol* (2009) 202(2):207–15. doi: 10.1677/JOE-09-0099
21. Starkey KJ, Janezic A, Jones G, Jordan N, Baker G, Ludgate M. Adipose Thyrotrophin Receptor Expression Is Elevated in Graves' and Thyroid Eye Diseases *Ex Vivo* and Indicates Adipogenesis in Progress *In Vivo*. *J Mol Endocrinol* (2003) 30(3):369–80. doi: 10.1677/jme.0.0300369
22. Brandau S, Bruderek K, Hestermann K, Gortz GE, Horstmann M, Mattheis S, et al. Orbital Fibroblasts From Graves' Orbitopathy Patients Share Functional and Immunophenotypic Properties With Mesenchymal Stem/Stromal Cells. *Invest Ophthalmol Visual Sci* (2015) 56(11):6549–57. doi: 10.1167/iovs.15-16610
23. Smith TJ, Koumas L, Gagnon A, Bell A, Sempowski GD, Phipps RP, et al. Orbital Fibroblast Heterogeneity May Determine the Clinical Presentation of Thyroid-Associated Ophthalmopathy. *J Clin Endocrinol Metab* (2002) 87 (1):385–92. doi: 10.1210/jcem.87.1.8164
24. Sorisky A, Pardasani D, Gagnon A, Smith TJ. Evidence of Adipocyte Differentiation in Human Orbital Fibroblasts in Primary Culture. *J Clin Endocrinol Metab* (1996) 81(9):3428–31. doi: 10.1210/jcem.81.9.8784110
25. Kozdon K, Fitchett C, Rose GE, Ezra DG, Bailly M. Mesenchymal Stem Cell-Like Properties of Orbital Fibroblasts in Graves' Orbitopathy. *Invest Ophthalmol Visual Sci* (2015) 56(10):5743–50. doi: 10.1167/iovs.15-16580
26. Laurberg P, Berman DC, Pedersen IB, Andersen S, Carle A. Double Vision Is a Major Manifestation in Moderate to Severe Graves' Orbitopathy, But It Correlates Negatively With Inflammatory Signs and Proptosis. *J Clin Endocrinol Metab* (2015) 100(5):2098–105. doi: 10.1210/jc.2014-4557
27. Zhang L, Bowen T, Grennan-Jones F, Paddon C, Giles P, Webber J, et al. Thyrotropin Receptor Activation Increases Hyaluronan Production in Preadipocyte Fibroblasts: Contributory Role in Hyaluronan Accumulation in Thyroid Dysfunction. *J Biol Chem* (2009) 284(39):26447–55. doi: 10.1074/jbc.M109.003616

28. Zhang L, Baker G, Janus D, Paddon CA, Fuhrer D, Ludgate M. Biological Effects of Thyrotropin Receptor Activation on Human Orbital Preadipocytes. *Invest Ophthalmol Visual Sci* (2006) 47(12):5197–203. doi: 10.1167/iovs.06-0596
29. Metcalfe R, Jordan N, Watson P, Gullu S, Wiltshire M, Crisp M, et al. Demonstration of Immunoglobulin G, A, and E Autoantibodies to the Human Thyrotropin Receptor Using Flow Cytometry. *J Clin Endocrinol Metab* (2002) 87(4):1754–61. doi: 10.1210/jcem.87.4.8411
30. Latif R, Morshed SA, Zaidi M, Davies TF. The Thyroid-Stimulating Hormone Receptor: Impact of Thyroid-Stimulating Hormone and Thyroid-Stimulating Hormone Receptor Antibodies on Multimerization, Cleavage, and Signaling. *Endocrinol Metab Clinics North Am* (2009) 38(2):319–41. doi: 10.1016/j.ecl.2009.01.006
31. Wess J. Molecular Basis of Receptor/G-Protein-Coupling Selectivity. *Pharmacol Ther* (1998) 80(3):231–64. doi: 10.1016/S0163-7258(98)00030-8
32. Graves PN, Vlase H, Bobovnikova Y, Davies TF. Multimeric Complex Formation by the Thyrotropin Receptor in Solubilized Thyroid Membranes. *Endocrinology* (1996) 137(9):3915–20. doi: 10.1210/endo.137.9.8756566
33. Latif R, Graves P, Davies TF. Oligomerization of the Human Thyrotropin Receptor: Fluorescent Protein-Tagged hTSHR Reveals Post-Translational Complexes. *J Biol Chem* (2001) 276(48):45217–24. doi: 10.1074/jbc.M103727200
34. Latif R, Graves P, Davies TF. Ligand-Dependent Inhibition of Oligomerization at the Human Thyrotropin Receptor. *J Biol Chem* (2002) 277(47):45059–67. doi: 10.1074/jbc.M206693200
35. Moffett S, Brown DA, Linder ME. Lipid-Dependent Targeting of G Proteins Into Rafts. *J Biol Chem* (2000) 275(3):2191–8. doi: 10.1074/jbc.275.3.2191
36. Allgeier A, Offermanns S, Van Sande J, Spicher K, Schultz G, Dumont JE. The Human Thyrotropin Receptor Activates G-Proteins Gs and Gq/11. *J Biol Chem* (1994) 269(19):13733–5.
37. Laugwitz KL, Allgeier A, Offermanns S, Spicher K, Van Sande J, Dumont JE, et al. The Human Thyrotropin Receptor: A Heptahelical Receptor Capable of Stimulating Members of All Four G Protein Families. *Proc Natl Acad Sci USA* (1996) 93(1):116–20. doi: 10.1073/pnas.93.1.116
38. Boutin A, Eliseeva E, Gershengorn MC, Neumann S. Beta-Arrestin-1 Mediates Thyrotropin-Enhanced Osteoblast Differentiation. *FASEB J* (2014) 28(8):3446–55. doi: 10.1096/fj.14-251124
39. Büch TRH, Biebermann H, Kalwa H, Pinkenburg O, Hager D, Barth H, et al. G13-Dependent Activation of MAPK by Thyrotropin. *J Biol Chem* (2008) 283 (29):20330–41. doi: 10.1074/jbc.M800211200
40. Laurent E, Mockel J, Van Sande J, Graff I, Dumont JE. Dual Activation by Thyrotropin of the Phospholipase C and Cyclic AMP Cascades in Human Thyroid. *Mol Cell Endocrinol* (1987) 52(3):273–8. doi: 10.1016/0303-7207(87) 90055-4
41. Raspe E, Dumont JE. Robert Feulgen Lecture 1991. Control and Role of Major Signalling Cascades of the Thyrocyte. *Prog Histochem Cytochem* (1992) 26(1-4):1–29. doi: 10.1016/s0079-6336(11)80074-4
42. Postiglione MP, Parlato R, Rodriguez-Mallon A, Rosica A, Mithbaokar P, Maresca M, et al. Role of the Thyroid-Stimulating Hormone Receptor Signaling in Development and Differentiation of the Thyroid Gland. *Proc Natl Acad Sci USA* (2002) 99(24):15462–7. doi: 10.1073/pnas.242328999
43. Vassart G, Dumont JE. The Thyrotropin Receptor and the Regulation of Thyrocyte Function and Growth. *Endocrine Rev* (1992) 13(3):596–611. doi: 10.1210/edrv-13-3-596
44. Wang HS, Tung WH, Tang KT, Wong YK, Huang GJ, Wu JC, et al. TGF-Beta Induced Hyaluronan Synthesis in Orbital Fibroblasts Involves Protein Kinase C betaII Activation *In Vitro*. *J Cell Biochem* (2005) 95(2):256–67. doi: 10.1002/jcb.20405
45. D'Arcangelo D, Silletta MG, Di Francesco AL, Bonfitto N, Di Cerbo A, Falasca M, et al. Physiological Concentrations of Thyrotropin Increase Cytosolic Calcium Levels in Primary Cultures of Human Thyroid Cells. *J Clin Endocrinol Metab* (1995) 80(4):1136–43. doi: 10.1210/jcem.80.4.7714082
46. Jhon DY, Lee HH, Park D, Lee CW, Lee KH, Yoo OJ, et al. Cloning, Sequencing, Purification, and Gq-Dependent Activation of Phospholipase C-Beta 3. *J Biol Chem* (1993) 268(9):6654–61. doi: 10.1016/S0021-9258(18) 53300-7
47. Macian F. NFAT Proteins: Key Regulators of T-Cell Development and Function. *Nat Rev Immunol* (2005) 5(6):472–84. doi: 10.1038/nri1632
48. Luo C, Shaw KT, Raghavan A, Aramburu J, Garcia-Cozar F, Perrino BA, et al. Interaction of Calcineurin With a Domain of the Transcription Factor NFAT1 That Controls Nuclear Import. *Proc Natl Acad Sci USA* (1996) 93(17):8907–12. doi: 10.1073/pnas.93.17.8907
49. Sunahara RK, Dessauer CW, Gilman AG. Complexity and Diversity of Mammalian Adenylyl Cyclases. *Annu Rev Pharmacol Toxicol* (1996) 36:461–80. doi: 10.1146/annurev.pa.36.040196.002333
50. Vanhaesebroeck B, Leevers SJ, Panayotou G, Waterfield MD. Phosphoinositide 3-Kinases: A Conserved Family of Signal Transducers. *Trends Biochem Sci* (1997) 22(7):267–72. doi: 10.1016/S0968-0004(97) 01061-X
51. Rhee SG, Bae YS. Regulation of Phosphoinositide-Specific Phospholipase C Isozymes. *J Biol Chem* (1997) 272(24):15045–8. doi: 10.1074/jbc.272.24.15045
52. Bell A, Gagnon A, Grunder L, Parikh SJ, Smith TJ, Sorisky A. Functional TSH Receptor in Human Abdominal Preadipocytes and Orbital Fibroblasts. *Am J Physiol Cell Physiol* (2000) 279(2):C335–40. doi: 10.1152/ajpcell.2000.279.2.C335
53. van Zeijl CJ, Fliers E, van Koppen CJ, Surovtseva OV, de Gooyer ME, Mourits MP, et al. Thyrotropin Receptor-Stimulating Graves' Disease Immunoglobulins Induce Hyaluronan Synthesis by Differentiated Orbital Fibroblasts From Patients With Graves' Ophthalmopathy Not Only *via* Cyclic Adenosine Monophosphate Signaling Pathways. *Thyroid* (2011) 21 (2):169–76. doi: 10.1089/thy.2010.0123
54. Neumann S, Pope A, Geras-Raaka E, Raaka BM, Bahn RS, Gershengorn MC. A Drug-Like Antagonist Inhibits Thyrotropin Receptor–Mediated Stimulation of cAMP Production in Graves' Orbital Fibroblasts. *Thyroid* (2012) 22:839–43. doi: 10.1089/thy.2011.0520
55. Zhang L, Grennan-Jones F, Lane C, Rees DA, Dayan CM, Ludgate M. Adipose Tissue Depot-Specific Differences in the Regulation of Hyaluronan Production of Relevance to Graves' Orbitopathy. *J Clin Endocrinol Metab* (2012) 97(2):653–62. doi: 10.1210/jc.2011-1299
56. Zhang L, Evans A, von Ruhland C, Draman MS, Edkins S, Vincent AE, et al. Distinctive Features of Orbital Adipose Tissue (OAT) in Graves' Orbitopathy. *Int J Mol Sci* (2020) 21(23):9145–62. doi: 10.3390/ijms21239145
57. Zhang L, Rai P, Miwa S, Draman MS, Rees DA, Haridas AS, et al. The Role of Mitochondria Linked Fatty-Acid Uptake-Driven Adipogenesis in Graves' Orbitopathy. *Endocrinology* (2021) 162(12):bqab188. doi: 10.1210/endocr/bqab188
58. Weightman DR, Perros P, Sherif IH, Kendall-Taylor P. Autoantibodies to IGF-1 Binding Sites in Thyroid Associated Ophthalmopathy. *Autoimmunity* (1993) 16(4):251–7. doi: 10.3109/08916939309014643
59. Tsui S, Naik V, Hoa N, Hwang CJ, Afifiyan NF, Sinha Hikim A, et al. Evidence for an Association Between Thyroid-Stimulating Hormone and Insulin-Like Growth Factor 1 Receptors: A Tale of Two Antigens Implicated in Graves' Disease. *J Immunol (Baltimore Md 1950)* (2008) 181(6):4397–405. doi: 10.4049/jimmunol.181.6.4397
60. Smith TJ, Janssen JA. Building the Case for Insulin-Like Growth Factor Receptor-I Involvement in Thyroid-Associated Ophthalmopathy. *Front Endocrinol (Lausanne)* (2016) 7:167. doi: 10.3389/fendo.2016.00167
61. Smith TJ, Janssen J. Insulin-Like Growth Factor-I Receptor and Thyroid-Associated Ophthalmopathy. *Endocrine Rev* (2019) 40(1):236–67. doi: 10.1210/er.2018-00066
62. Zhang L, Grennan-Jones F, Draman MS, Lane C, Morris D, Dayan CM, et al. Possible Targets for Nonimmunosuppressive Therapy of Graves' Orbitopathy. *J Clin Endocrinol Metab* (2014) 99(7):E1183–90. doi: 10.1210/jc.2013-4182
63. Krieger CC, Neumann S, Place RF, Marcus-Samuels B, Gershengorn MC. Bidirectional TSH and IGF-1 Receptor Cross Talk Mediates Stimulation of Hyaluronan Secretion by Graves' Disease Immunoglobins. *J Clin Endocrinol Metab* (2015) 100(3):1071–7. doi: 10.1210/jc.2014-3566
64. Zhang L, Ji QH, Ruge F, Lane C, Morris D, Tee AR, et al. Reversal of Pathological Features of Graves' Orbitopathy by Activation of Forkhead Transcription Factors, FOXOs. *J Clin Endocrinol Metab* (2016) 101(1):114–22. doi: 10.1210/jc.2015-2932
65. Kahaly GJ, Douglas RS, Holt RJ, Sile S, Smith TJ. Teprotumumab for Patients With Active Thyroid Eye Disease: A Pooled Data Analysis, Subgroup Analyses, and Off-Treatment Follow-Up Results From Two Randomised, Double-Masked, Placebo-Controlled, Multicentre Trials. *Lancet Diabetes Endocrinol* (2021) 9(6):360–72. doi: 10.1016/S2213-8587(21)00056-5

66. Smith TJ, Kahaly GJ, Ezra DG, Fleming JC, Dailey RA, Tang RA, et al. Teprotumumab for Thyroid-Associated Ophthalmopathy. *N Engl J Med* (2017) 376(18):1748–61. doi: 10.1056/NEJMoa1614949
67. Piantanida E, Bartalena L. Teprotumumab: A New Avenue for the Management of Moderate-to-Severe and Active Graves' Orbitopathy? *J Endocrinol Invest* (2017) 40(8):885–7. doi: 10.1007/s40618-017-0717-8
68. Bendall SC, Stewart MH, Menendez P, George D, Vijayaragavan K, Werbowetski-Ogilvie T, et al. IGF and FGF Cooperatively Establish the Regulatory Stem Cell Niche of Pluripotent Human Cells. *Vitro Nat* (2007) 448(7157):1015–21. doi: 10.1038/nature06027
69. Schrijver B, Kooiman MA, Kasteleijn E, van Holten-Neelen C, Virakul S, Paridaens D, et al. Basic Fibroblast Growth Factor Induces Adipogenesis in Orbital Fibroblasts: Implications for the Pathogenesis of Graves' Orbitopathy. *Thyroid* (2019) 29(3):395–404. doi: 10.1089/thy.2018.0544
70. Graves PN, Tomer Y, Davies TF. Cloning and Sequencing of a 1.3 KB Variant of Human Thyrotropin Receptor mRNA Lacking the Transmembrane Domain. *Biochem Biophys Res Commun* (1992) 187(2):1135–43. doi: 10.1016/0006-291x(92)91315-h
71. Paschke R, Metcalfe A, Alcalde L, Vassart G, Weetman A, Ludgate M. Presence of Nonfunctional Thyrotropin Receptor Variant Transcripts in Retroocular and Other Tissues. *J Clin Endocrinol Metab* (1994) 79(5):1234–8. doi: 10.1210/jcem.79.5.7962314
72. Quellari M, Desroches A, Beau I, Beaudeux E, Misrahi M. Role of Cleavage and Shedding in Human Thyrotropin Receptor Function and Trafficking. *Eur J Biochem* (2003) 270(17):3486–97. doi: 10.1046/j.1432-1033.2003.03718.x
73. Rapoport B, McLachlan SM. The Thyrotropin Receptor in Graves' Disease. *Thyroid* (2007) 17(10):911–22. doi: 10.1089/thy.2007.0170
74. Zhao SX, Tsui S, Cheung A, Douglas RS, Smith TJ, Banga JP. Orbital Fibrosis in a Mouse Model of Graves' Disease Induced by Genetic Immunization of Thyrotropin Receptor cDNA. *J Endocrinol* (2011) 210(3):369–77. doi: 10.1530/joe-11-0162
75. Moshkelgosha S, So PW, Deasy N, Diaz-Cano S, Banga JP. Cutting Edge: Retrobulbar Inflammation, Adipogenesis, and Acute Orbital Congestion in a Preclinical Female Mouse Model of Graves' Orbitopathy Induced by Thyrotropin Receptor Plasmid-*In Vivo* Electroporation. *Endocrinology* (2013) 154(9):3008–15. doi: 10.1210/en.2013-1576
76. Draman MS, Grennan-Jones F, Taylor P, Muller I, Evans S, Haridas A, et al. Expression of Endogenous Putative TSH Binding Protein in Orbit. *Curr Issues Mol Biol* (2021) 43:1794–804. doi: 10.3390/cimb43030126
77. Miller-Gallacher J, Sanders P, Young S, Sullivan A, Baker S, Reddington SC, et al. Crystal Structure of a Ligand-Free Stable TSH Receptor Leucine-Rich Repeat Domain. *J Mol Endocrinol* (2019) 62(3):117–28. doi: 10.1530/JME-18-0213
78. Neumann S, Krieger CC, Gershengorn MC. Targeting TSH and IGF-1 Receptors to Treat Thyroid Eye Disease. *Eur Thyroid J* (2020) 9(Suppl 1):59–65. doi: 10.1159/000511538
79. Ryder M, Wentworth M, Algeciras-Schimnich A, Morris JC, Garrity J, Sanders J, et al. Blocking the TSH Receptor With K1-70™ in a Patient With Follicular Thyroid Cancer, Graves' Disease and Graves' Ophthalmopathy. *Thyroid* (2021) 31(10):1597–602. doi: 10.1089/thy.2021.0053

18

Role of Proprotein Convertase Subtilisin/Kexin Type 9 in the Pathogenesis of Graves' Orbitopathy in Orbital Fibroblasts

Ga Eun Lee[1], Jinjoo Kim[2], Jihei Sara Lee[2], JaeSang Ko[2], Eun Jig Lee[3] and Jin Sook Yoon[2]*

[1] Yonsei University College of Medicine, Seoul, South Korea, [2] Department of Ophthalmology, Severance Hospital, Institute of Vision Research, Yonsei University College of Medicine, Seoul, South Korea, [3] Department of Endocrinology, Severance Hospital, Yonsei University College of Medicine, Seoul, South Korea

***Correspondence:**
Jin Sook Yoon
yoonjs@yuhs.ac

Background: The proprotein convertase subtilisin/kexin type 9 (PCSK9) has been implicated in the pathogenesis of inflammatory diseases. We sought to investigate the role of PCSK9 in the pathogenesis of Graves' orbitopathy (GO) and whether it may be a legitimate target for treatment.

Methods: The *PCSK9* was compared between GO (n=11) and normal subjects (n=7) in orbital tissue explants using quantitative real-time PCR, and in cultured interleukin-1β (IL-1β)-treated fibroblasts using western blot. Western blot was used to identify the effects of PCSK9 inhibition on IL-1β-induced pro-inflammatory cytokines production and signaling molecules expression as well as levels of adipogenic markers and oxidative stress-related proteins. Adipogenic differentiation was identified using Oil Red O staining. The plasma PCSK9 concentrations were compared between patients with GO (n=44) and healthy subjects (n=26) by ELISA.

Results: The *PCSK9* transcript level was higher in GO tissues. The depletion of PCSK9 blunted IL-1β-induced expression of intercellular adhesion molecule 1 (ICAM-1), IL-6, IL-8, and cyclooxygenase-2 (COX-2) in GO and non-GO fibroblasts. The levels of activated nuclear factor kappa-light-chain-enhancer of activated B cells (NF-κB) and phosphorylated forms of Akt and p38 were diminished when PCSK9 was suppressed in GO fibroblasts. Decreases in lipid droplets and attenuated levels of peroxisome proliferator-activated receptor gamma (PPARγ), CCAAT/enhancer-binding protein β (C/EBPβ), and leptin as well as hypoxia-inducible factor 1α (HIF-1α), manganese superoxide dismutase (MnSOD), thioredoxin (Trx), and heme oxygenase-1 (HO-1) were noted when PCSK9 was suppressed during adipocyte differentiation. The plasma PCSK9 level was significantly higher in GO patients and correlated with level of thyrotropin binding inhibitory immunoglobulin (TBII) and the clinical activity score (CAS).

Conclusions: PCSK9 plays a significant role in GO. The PCSK9 inhibition attenuated the pro-inflammatory cytokines production, oxidative stress, and fibroblast differentiation into adipocytes. PCSK9 may serve as a therapeutic target and biomarker for GO.

Keywords: adipogenesis, Graves' orbitopathy, inflammation, oxidative stress, proprotein convertase subtilisin/kexin type 9, PCSK9, thyroid eye disease

INTRODUCTION

Graves' orbitopathy (GO) is an inflammatory autoimmune disorder, and it is the most frequent extrathyroidal manifestation of Graves' disease (1). Clinical features of GO include upper eyelid retraction, edema and erythema of the periorbital tissue and conjunctiva, proptosis, corneal ulceration, and optic neuropathy. Three cell types which predominantly contribute to the development and progression of GO are B cells, T cells, and orbital fibroblasts (2). Stimulated by interactions with T cells and autoantibodies produced by B cells, orbital fibroblasts play a key role in the establishment of inflammation by producing cytokines, chemokines, and lipid mediators. Furthermore, they proliferate, synthesize extracellular matrix, and differentiate into adipocytes, leading to tissue remodeling characteristic of GO. The mainstay treatment for moderate-to-severe GO is systemic glucocorticoids therapy (3). Due to inadequate responses and adverse effects to glucocorticoids, however, there have been several investigations for other possible biological therapies (3).

The proprotein convertase subtilisin/kexin type 9 (PCSK9), which was first reported in 2003, is the ninth member of the protein convertase family (4). PCSK9 targets low density lipoprotein receptors (LDLR) on the hepatic cell surface, toward lysosomes for degradation, resulting in elevated serum LDL cholesterol levels (5). Now, PCSK9 inhibitors have emerged as novel therapeutics to treat cardiovascular diseases (6). However, current data suggest that PCSK9 inhibitors may have pleiotropic effects, affecting targets beyond LDLR (7–9). According to other studies, PCSK9 may be a key molecule in the pathophysiology of diseases such as atherosclerosis, myocardial ischemia, Alzheimer's disease, psoriasis, and fatty liver disease (10–14). Studies on the PCSK9 in atherosclerosis, a chronic inflammatory disorder of vessel walls, showed that PCSK9 inhibition suppressed inflammatory cytokines production and decreased the activity of nuclear factor kappa-light-chain-enhancer of activated B cells (NF-κB) and intracellular cell adhesion molecule 1 (ICAM-1). Additionally, silencing PCSK9 decreased oxidative stress, apoptosis, proliferative capacity, and accumulation of macrophages (10, 14, 15). Numerous studies reporting the benefit of PCSK9 suppression *in vivo* and *in vitro* suggest that PCSK9 may be an attractive target in chronic inflammatory disorders (16). However, no previous studies have reported the effect of PCSK9 inhibition in GO.

In light of what is said above, this study was designed to investigate the role of PCSK9 in the pathogenesis of GO. We used small interfering RNA (siRNA) to promote cleavage of intracellular PCSK9 mRNA in orbital fibroblasts obtained from GO and normal subjects. We tested whether PCSK9 siRNA counteracts inflammation, proliferation, and adipocyte differentiation in orbital fibroblasts, the main pathogenic mechanisms in GO. In addition, we examined whether the plasma PCSK9 levels reflect the presence and the activity of GO using the clinical activity score (CAS).

MATERIALS AND METHODS

Reagents

The antibodies were purchased from Santa Cruz Biotechnology (Santa Cruz, CA, USA), Cell Signaling Technology (Beverly, MA, USA), Novus Biologicals (Centennial, CO, USA), and Abcam (Cambridge, UK). The antibodies used in the study are listed in detail in **Supplementary Table 1**. PCSK9 siRNA and control siRNA were obtained from Santa Cruz Biotechnology, Inc. (Dallas, TX, USA). TransIT-siQUEST siRNA Transfection reagent was purchased from Mirus Bio, Inc. (Madison, WI, USA). The 3-(4,5-dimethyl-thiazol-2-yl)-2,5-diphenyl-tetrazolium bromide (MTT) assay and Oil Red O were products from Sigma-Aldrich, Inc. (Merck KGaA, Darmstadt, Germany). Dulbecco's modified Eagle's medium (DMEM), fetal bovine serum (FBS), penicillin, and gentamicin were purchased from Hyclone Laboratories, Inc. (Logan, UT, USA). Recombinant human interleukin-1β (IL-1β) and the enzyme-linked immunosorbent assay (ELISA) kit for PCSK9 were obtained from R&D Systems (Minneapolis, MN, USA).

Subjects and Preparation of Tissues and Cells

Orbital tissue specimens were collected from GO subjects during orbital decompression surgery (nine females and two males; age 38–54 years). Non-GO orbital tissue was obtained during the course of upper (n=3) and lower lid (n=4) blepharoplasty from patients without history or clinical evidence of any thyroid disease (5 females and 2 males; age 36–57 years). Out of 11 GO and seven non-GO tissues, three GO and three non-GO tissues were randomly chosen for primary orbital fibroblast cultures. For gene expression analysis, nine out of 11 GO tissues were randomly selected, while all seven non-GO tissues were used. The study protocol was approved by the Institutional Review Board of Severance Hospital, and all participants provided written informed consent. This research adhered to the tenets of the Declaration of Helsinki. At the time of surgery, all GO patients were in euthyroid state and had not been administered steroid or radiation therapy for at least three months.

For plasma PCSK9 evaluation, 70 subjects were recruited: 22 with active GO (15 females and 7 males; age 42.41 ± 17.91 years), 22 with inactive GO (16 females and 6 males; age 40.64 ± 16.91 years), and 26 healthy volunteers (23 females and three males; age 36.69 ± 14.20 years). GO was considered "active" based on CAS, a grading system based on the seven classic features of inflammation in GO (17). Out of seven, GO was considered "active" if the CAS was ≥3. **Table 1** shows the demographic, clinical, and serologic data of the subjects.

Orbital fibroblasts were isolated from the harvested tissue and cultured as described previously (18). After being minced, the tissue was placed directly in DMEM/F12 (in 1:1 ratio) medium containing 20% FBS, penicillin (100 U/ml), and gentamycin (20 µg/ml). Following incubation, tissues were maintained in solution containing DMEM, antibiotics, and 10% FBS. Once the growth of the fibroblasts was confirmed, the cells were treated with trypsin/ethylenediaminetetraacetic acid and passaged in

TABLE 1 | Clinical and serological characteristics of patient population for ELISA.

	Active GO (n=22)	Inactive GO (n=22)	Non-GO (n=26)	p-value
Sex (male/female)	7/15	6/16	3/23	0.213
Age (years), *M* ± *SD*	42.41 ± 17.91	40.64 ± 16.91	36.69 ± 14.20	0.575
Smokers, n (%)	6 (27.27)	4 (18.18)	2 (7.69)	0.202
PCSK9 (ng/ml)	256.46 ± 53.49	223.48 ± 36.42	190.83 ± 28.77	<0.001
CAS	4.45 ± 1.47	1.36 ± 0.66	–	<0.001
Duration GD (months), median (IQR)	8.55 (2–16)	7.18 (2–22)	–	0.396
T3 (0.58–1.59 ng/dl), *M* ± *SD*	1.17 ± 0.25	1.17 ± 0.26	–	0.796
Free T4 (0.70–1.48 ng/dl), *M* ± *SD*	1.19 ± 0.22	1.23 ± 0.21	–	0.751
TSH (0.35–4.94 μIU/ml), *M* ± *SD*	1.40 ± 0.84	1.36 ± 1.00	–	0.605
TBII (0–1.75 IU/L), *M* ± *SD*	18.09 ± 12.26	12.99 ± 7.42	–	0.231

ELISA, enzyme-linked immunosorbent assay; GO, Graves' orbitopathy; SD, standard deviation; PCSK9, proprotein convertase subtilisin/kexin type 9; CAS, clinical activity score; GD, Graves' disease; IQR, interquartile ranges; T3, triiodothyronine; T4, thyroxine; TSH, thyrotropin; TBII, thyrotropin-binding inhibitory immunoglobulin.

monolayers. Strains were stored in liquid nitrogen and only those between the third and fifth passages were used for experiments.

Cell Viability Assay

Cell viability was assessed with an MTT assay, following the manufacturer's protocol (Sigma-Aldrich, Inc.). Orbital fibroblasts obtained from GO patients were seeded into 24-well culture plates (1×10^5 cells/well) and treated with PCSK9 and control siRNAs (50 nM) for 10, 24, and 48 h. Thereafter, cells were washed and incubated in MTT solution (5 mg/ml) for 3 h at 37°C. Dimethyl sulfoxide (DMSO) was applied for solubilization and the absorbance of the converted dye was measured with a microplate reader (EL 340 Bio Kinetics Reader; Bio-Tek Instruments, Winooski, VT, USA) at 540 nm, with background subtraction at 630 nm.

Quantitative Real-Time PCR

The RNA was extracted from cells using TriZol (Invitrogen, Carlsbad, CA, USA). Out of the extract, 1 μg was reverse-transcribed into cDNA (Qiagen, Valencia, CA, USA) and amplified with SYBR green real-time PCR master mix in a StepOne Plus real-time PCR thermocycler (Applied Biosystems, Foster City, CA, USA). The sequence of primers is listed in **Supplementary Table 2**. The PCR results for each type of mRNA were normalized to the level of GAPDH, and expressed as fold-change in the Ct value relative to the control group using the $2^{-\Delta\Delta Ct}$ method (19).

Western Blot Assay

Equal amounts of protein (50 μg) were separated by 10% SDS polyacrylamide gel electrophoresis. The resolved proteins were transferred to nitrocellulose membranes and incubated overnight with primary antibodies at 4°C. Then, the membranes were probed with horseradish peroxidase-conjugated secondary antibodies. The bands were detected on X-ray films (GE Healthcare, Piscataway, NJ), and their intensities were quantified and normalized to that of the β-actin in the same sample.

Adipogenesis

Using a previously published protocol, adipocyte differentiation of GO fibroblasts was induced (20). Cells were cultured in serum-free DMEM supplemented with T3, insulin (Boehringer-Mannheim, Mannheim, Germany), carbaprostaglandin (cPGI2; Calbiochem, La Jolla, CA, USA), and dexamethasone, along with proliferator-activated receptor gamma (PPARγ) agonist, rosiglitazone (10 μM; Cayman, Ann Arbor, MI, USA) for 7 days. To evaluate the effect of PCSK9 siRNA on adipogenesis, cells were transfected with PCSK9 siRNA for the entire 7-day differentiation period according to the manufacturer's instructions.

Oil Red O Staining

Cells were stained with Oil Red O as described by Green and Kehinde (21). A working solution was prepared by diluting 6 ml of a stock solution (0.5% Oil red O in isopropanol) with 4 ml of distilled water. The cells were fixed with 3.7% formalin at 4°C for 1 h before being washed with PBS and mixed with Oil Red O solution for 1 h at room temperature. The cell-solution mixture was visualized under on a light microscope (Olympus BX60; Olympus Corp., Melville, NY, USA).

Blood Sampling and Measurement of Plasma PCSK9 and TBII Concentrations

Blood samples were drawn into test tubes containing sodium citrate. Platelet-free plasma was obtained after centrifugation at 1,500 g for 15 min at 4°C and stored at −80°C until analysis. Plasma PCSK9 levels were determined with a commercially available ELISA kit. All samples were tested in triplicate, and all sera were run in the same assay. The average value of three repeated assays was used for statistical analyses. Thyrotropin (TSH) binding inhibitory immunoglobulin (TBII) was measured with a third-generation TBII assay using the automated Cobas electrochemiluminescence immunoassay (Elecsys; Roche Diagnostics GmbH, Penzberg, Germany).

Statistical Analysis

All experiments were performed in duplicate or triplicate on samples from each patient, and the results were expressed as mean ± standard deviation (SD). Comparisons of data between groups were performed with the independent *t*-test or ANOVA. The Bonferroni test was performed as a *post hoc* test. The Mann–Whitney *U*-test and Kruskal–Wallis test were used for nonparametric or not normally distributed data. Spearman's rank correlation coefficient was used to analyze the correlation of plasma PCSK9 concentrations with CAS and plasma TBII levels. The SPSS for Windows, version 20.0 (SPSS, Inc.,

Chicago, IL, USA) was used. A p-value < 0.05 denoted statistical significance.

RESULTS

GO Tissues Show Increased Expression of PCSK9, LDLR, and HIF-1α

To investigate its potential role in GO, we measured the expression of PCSK9 in orbital tissues taken from GO and non-GO subjects. The RT-PCR results showed that PCSK9 transcript levels were greater in GO tissues (n=9) than in non-GO tissues (n=7) (**Figure 1A**). Additionally, the mRNA levels of LDLR and hypoxia-inducible factor 1α (HIF-1α) were higher in GO tissues (n=9) than in non-GO tissues (n=7) (**Figures 1B, C**).

IL-1β Induces PCSK9 and LDLR in Orbital Fibroblasts

We challenged GO and non-GO orbital fibroblasts with IL-1β, a key mediator in GO (18, 22), for 1, 3, 6, 16, and 24 h. The western blot results showed that IL-1β led the GO and non-GO fibroblasts to increase PCSK9 and LDLR expression in a time-

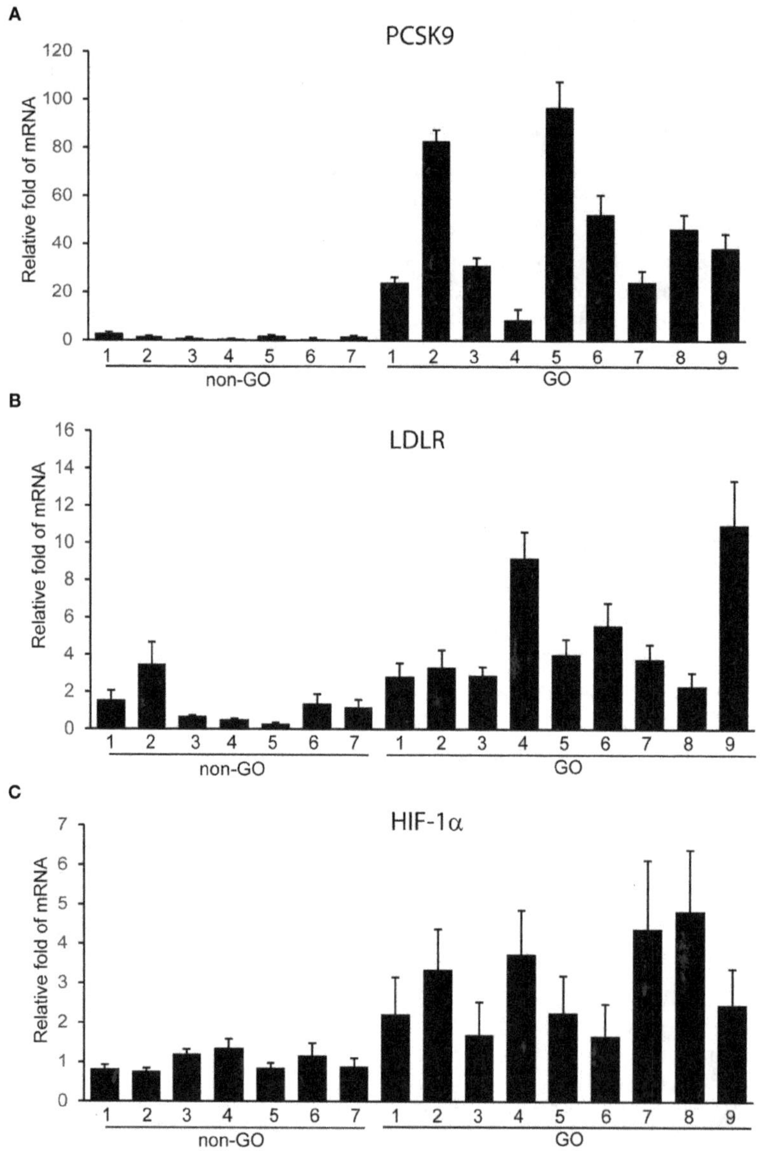

FIGURE 1 | Expression of proprotein convertase subtilisin/kexin type 9 (PCSK9), low density lipoprotein receptor (LDLR), and hypoxia-inducible factor 1a (HIF-1a) mRNAs in Graves' orbitopathy (GO) and non-GO orbital tissues. The RNA extracted from GO (n=9) and non-GO (n=7) orbital tissues was reverse-transcribed by real-time PCR and quantified. Experiments were performed in triplicate for each donor. The results showed elevated transcript levels of PCSK9 **(A)**, LDLR **(B)**, and HIF-1a **(C)** in GO tissues than in non-GO tissues. Data in the column indicate the mean ± SD fold elevation relative to the control.

dependent manner (**Figure 2**). The increase in PCSK9 and LDLR was more prominent in GO than in non-GO fibroblasts.

Silencing PCSK9 Suppresses IL-1β-Induced Expression of Pro-Inflammatory Mediators

The western blot results showed that when orbital fibroblasts were transfected with PCSK9 siRNA, the production of pro-inflammatory mediators, ICAM-1, IL-6, IL-8, and cyclooxygenase-2 (COX-2), in response to the challenge with IL-1β was significantly suppressed in GO and non-GO fibroblasts (**Figure 3**).

Silencing PCSK9 Reduces Activation of Signaling Molecules

As shown in **Figure 4**, the IL-1β-treatment (10 ng/ml for 60 min) increased levels of nuclear NF-κB p65 and phosphorylated (p-) forms of Akt and p38 in GO and non-GO fibroblasts in western blot analyses. In GO fibroblasts, PCSK9 interference with siRNA reduced IL-1β-stimulated expression of nuclear NF-κB p65, p-Akt, and p-p38. In non-GO fibroblasts, the PCSK9 inhibition suppressed IL-1β-stimulated expression of p-Akt, but not NF-κB p65 and p-p38.

Silencing PCSK9 Inhibits Proliferation of GO Fibroblasts

The enhanced proliferative capacity of GO fibroblasts at baseline and in response to certain cytokines may play a role in the pathogenesis of GO (23). According to the MTT assay results, the proliferation of GO fibroblasts slowed down 48 h after being transfected with PCSK9 siRNA compared to control siRNA-treated group (**Supplementary Figure 1**).

PCSK9 Inhibition Suppresses Adipocyte Differentiation and Oxidative Stress-Related Protein Production in GO Fibroblasts

The transfection of differentiating fibroblasts with PCSK9 siRNA attenuated adipogenesis on day 7 according to the Oil Red O staining (**Figure 5A**). When quantified by measuring optical density of Oil Red O-stained cell lysates at 490 nm, the same pattern was identified (**Figure 5B**). Throughout adipogenic differentiation, the PCSK9 levels gradually increased (**Figure 5C**), but PCSK9 siRNA substantially diminished levels of adipogenic transcription factors, PPARγ and CCAAT/enhancer-binding protein β (C/EBPβ), and mature adipocyte marker, leptin. In addition, silencing PCSK9 markedly decreased the levels of oxidative stress-related protein, HIF-1α, and antioxidant proteins, manganese superoxide dismutase (MnSOD), thioredoxin (Trx), and heme oxygenase-1 (HO-1) (**Figure 5C**).

Plasma PCSK9 Protein Levels Are Elevated in GO and Plasma PCSK9 Concentrations Show Positive Correlations With Plasma TBII Levels and CAS

The plasma PCSK9 levels were measured in GO and healthy subjects by ELISA (**Figure 6A**). The mean plasma PCSK9 level was significantly higher in GO patients (n=44, 239.97 ± 48.20 ng/ml) than in healthy subjects (n=26, 190.83 ± 28.77 ng/ml; $p < 0.01$). Additionally, the mean plasma PCSK9 level was significantly higher in patients with active GO (n=22, 256.46 ± 53.49 ng/ml) than in patients with inactive GO (n=22, 223.48 ± 36.42 ng/ml; p=0.01). The plasma PCSK9 level was correlated

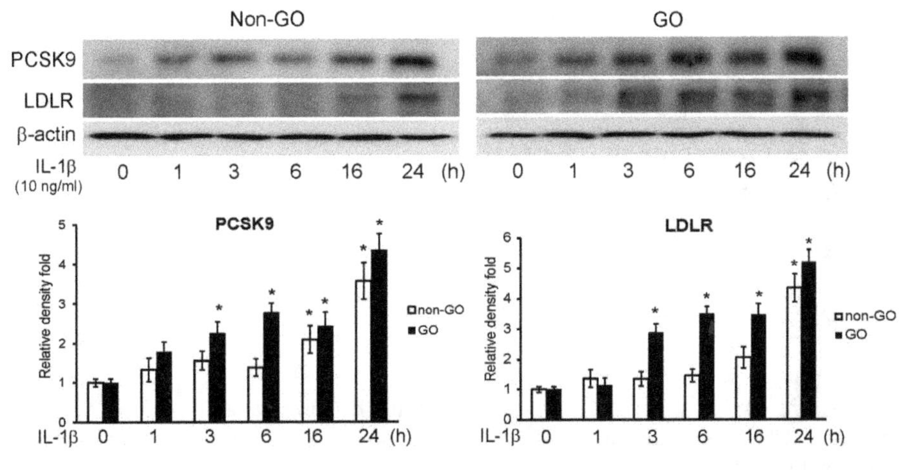

FIGURE 2 | Western blot of proprotein convertase subtilisin/kexin type 9 (PCSK9) and low density lipoprotein receptor (LDLR) after interleukin-1β (IL-1β) treatment. Confluent orbital fibroblasts obtained from Graves' orbitopathy (GO) (n=3) and non-GO subjects (n=3) were treated with 10 ng/ml of IL-1β for increasing lengths of time (0–24 h). Western blot analyses were performed to investigate the levels of PCSK9 and LDLR. The treatment with IL-1β increased the levels of PCSK9 and LDLR in both GO and non-GO tissues in a time-dependent manner. Representative gel images are shown. Data in the columns indicate the mean density ratio ± SD, normalized to the level of β-actin in the same sample (*$p < 0.05$ vs. 0 h in each group).

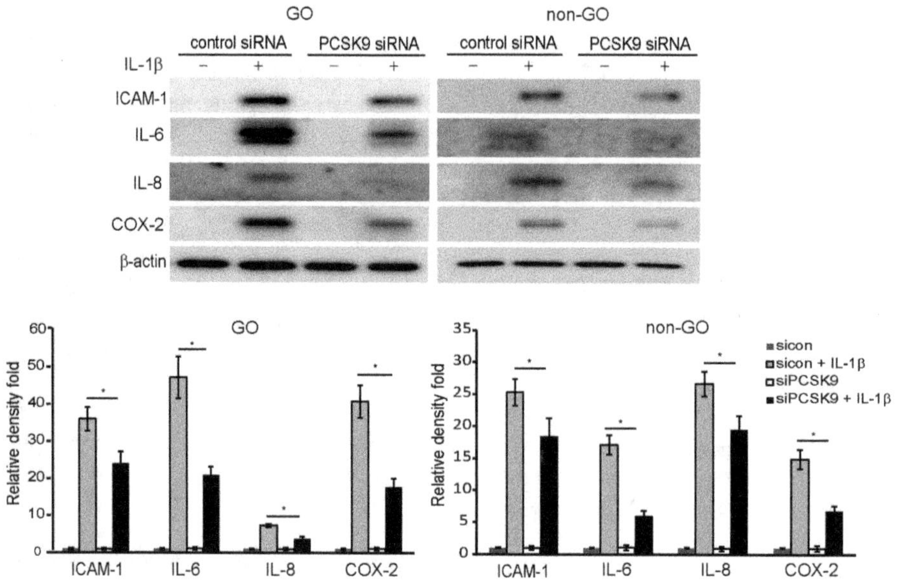

FIGURE 3 | Effect of silencing proprotein convertase subtilisin/kexin type 9 (PCSK9) on the expression of pro-inflammatory cytokines protein. Confluent fibroblasts obtained from Graves' orbitopathy (GO) patients (n=3) were treated with either control siRNA or PCSK9 siRNA (50 nM, 24 h). Then, they were challenged with 10 ng/ml of interleukin-1β (IL-1β) and compared to non-IL-1β-treated counterparts. Western blot analyses were conducted to compare the levels of pro-inflammatory cytokines, intercellular adhesion molecule 1 (ICAM-1), IL-6, IL-8, and cyclooxygenase-2 (COX-2). The same experiment was repeated with fibroblasts obtained from non-GO subjects (n=3). Representative gel images are shown. The mean density ratio ± SD from fibroblasts were normalized to the level of *β*-actin in the same sample (**p* < 0.05 between sicon + IL-1β and siPCSK9 + IL-1β; sicon, control siRNA; siPCSK9, PCSK9 siRNA).

with TBII ($r = 0.576$, $p < 0.001$, n = 44; **Figure 6B**) and CAS ($r = 0.631$, $p < 0.001$, n = 44; **Figure 6C**).

DISCUSSION

In this study, we examined the role of PCSK9 in GO pathogenesis. GO tissues showed increased expression of *PCSK9*, *LDLR*, and *HIF-1α*. The IL-1β challenge and adipogenic stimulation led to the increase of PCSK9 and LDLR. PCSK9 silencing with siRNA significantly decreased pro-inflammatory cytokines production, oxidative stress-related proteins, adipogenic transcription factors, and adipocyte differentiation. Importantly, the plasma level of PCSK9 was elevated in GO patients when compared to the non-GO subjects. It also showed a positive correlation with CAS, a measure of GO activity as well as TBII, a predictor of GO severity (17, 24).

Numerous studies have attempted to clarify the pro-inflammatory roles of PCSK9 in a variety of disorders including atherosclerosis, sepsis, psoriasis, steatosis, and myocardial ischemia (12–14, 25–30). For example, Tang et al. suggested an atherogenic role of PCSK9 as the suppression of PCSK9 expression in *apoE* null mice by means of small hairpin RNA decreased expression of TNF-α, IL-1β, monocyte chemotactic protein 1, Toll-like receptor 4, and NF-κB and reduced macrophage infiltration in the atherosclerotic plaques (26). In other *in vivo* and *in vitro* studies, the PCSK9 inhibition diminished pro-inflammatory cytokines production and macrophage accumulation by inhibiting NF-κB activation (12, 27, 30). In the context of GO, however, there have been no studies on the role of PCSK9. To the best of our knowledge, this study is the first of its kind to identify the pro-inflammatory properties of PCSK9 in GO. Based on our results, silencing PCSK9 ameliorated inflammation by modulating NF-κB pathway. Furthermore, the PCSK9 level was higher in GO tissues compared to the control at baseline, and IL-1β, a key mediator in GO inflammation (18, 22), increased PCSK9 levels more prominently in GO fibroblasts than in the control. Our study suggests that PCSK9 may serve as a therapeutic target for GO inflammation.

Mounting evidence has shown the anti-adipogenic effects of PCSK9 depletion (13, 31–33). Currently, PPARγ and C/EBPβ are believed to be responsible for terminal differentiation of fibroblasts into adipocytes (34). The PPARγ activation leads to the expression of adipogenic markers including leptin and fatty acid synthase (FAS) (35). Upstream of PPARγ, molecules such as E2F1 is thought to be involved (36). Recently, a study on rat models with alcohol-induced steatosis showed that the treatment with alirocumab, a human PCSK9 monoclonal antibody, attenuated expression of FAS and alleviated alcohol-induced lipid accumulation. Moreover, PCSK9 inhibition reduced mRNA expression of E2F1 as well as sterol regulatory element-binding protein (SREBP)-1 and SREBP-2 (13). SREBP-1 and SREBP-2 have been found to regulate cholesterol- and fatty acid metabolism-related genes (37). Ruscica et al. also showed that, in

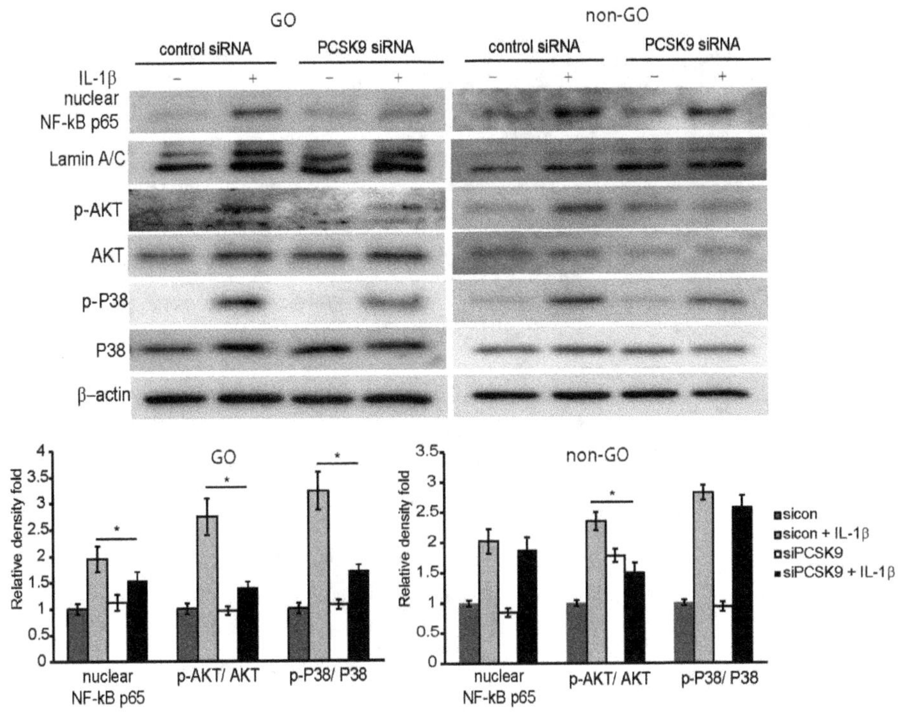

FIGURE 4 | Effect of silencing proprotein convertase subtilisin/kexin type 9 (PCSK9) on the activation of signal molecules by interleukin-1β (IL-1β) treatment. Confluent orbital fibroblasts obtained from Graves' orbitopathy (GO) patients (n=3) were treated with or without 10 ng/ml of IL-1β after transfection with control siRNA or PCSK9 siRNA (50 nM, 24 h). Treatment with IL-1β (10 ng/ml, 60 min) resulted in an increase in the levels of nuclear NF-κB p65 and phosphorylated forms of Akt and p38. The treatment with PCSK9 siRNA in GO cells significantly blunted the increases in the transcription factors. However, in fibroblasts from non-GO subjects (n=3), the PCSK9 inhibition only suppressed the phosphorylated Akt. Representative gel images are shown. Data in the columns indicate the mean density ratio ± SD of the bands obtained from the GO patients, normalized to the level of *β*-actin in the same sample (**p* < 0.05 between sicon + IL-1β and siPCSK9 + IL-1β).

201 patients with suspected nonalcoholic steatosis, hepatic PCSK9 mRNA levels were correlated with hepatic SREBP-1 and FAS expression (31). These results are consistent with the those of our own study; the PCSK9 inhibition attenuated adipogenesis as identified by Oil Red O and blunted the expression of PPARγ, C/EBPβ, and leptin. Furthermore, the PCSK9 expression gradually increased throughout the adipogenic differentiation. In this study, we present the evidence for the adipogenic role of PCSK9 in GO. However, whether PCSK9 directly modulates PPARγ or C/EBPβ activity needs to be further investigated. Furthermore, as PPARγ agonists have recently been suggested to modulate helper T cell-related chemokine production in GO (38), further studies are needed to examine if PCSK9 intervention modulates PPARγ-mediated inflammation.

Adipogenesis is thought to be closely associated with oxidative stress (39), and both are found by our study to be significantly suppressed by the PCSK9 inhibition. Multiple studies have proven the anti-oxidative effects of PCSK9 suppression in several disorders including atherosclerosis and myocardial infarction (14, 40). Locally produced reactive oxygen species (ROS) leads to the oxidation of LDL and contributes to atherogenesis (41). Transfection of endothelial cells and vascular smooth muscle cells with PCSK9 siRNA substantially decreased the production of ROS (40). In several *in vitro* studies, PCSK9 inhibition reduced ROS generation, while PCSK9 overexpression produced the opposite results (14, 42–44). In an *in vivo* study, PCSK9 knockout mice expressed significantly less NADPH oxidase and subsequently less ROS in aorta (40). These results are in line with those of our study. As antioxidants, Trx, MnSOD, and HO-1 are induced by oxidative stress and protect tissues from oxidative injuries (45–47). Under hypoxia, HIF-1α is activated to increase the expression of genes involved in adipogenesis and tissue remodeling in GO (39). Our results demonstrated that PCSK9 inhibition blunted the level of oxidative stress-related proteins which was induced by adipocyte differentiation. Previously, we have found that quercetin inhibits cigarette smoke extract-induced adipogenesis in GO fibroblasts by reducing ROS (48). Additionally, we have reported several molecules with anti-oxidative properties such as resveratrol, caffeine, and curcumin suppress adipogenesis in GO fibroblasts (49–51). Given that oxidative stress contributes to the proliferation of orbital fibroblasts (52), the impeded proliferation of GO fibroblasts by PCSK9 inhibition demonstrated in this study may be attributed to the anti-oxidative property of the PCSK9 inhibitor.

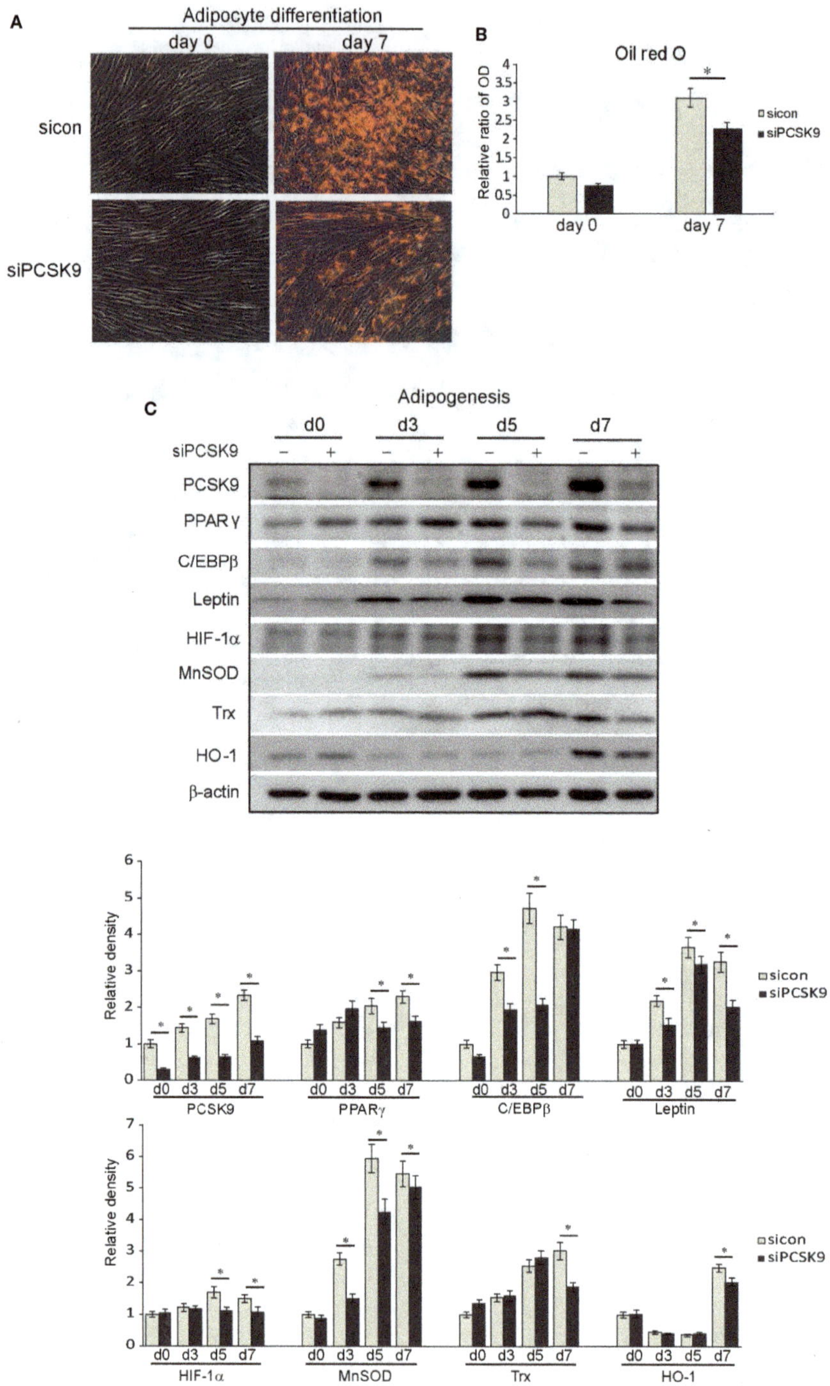

FIGURE 5 | Proprotein convertase subtilisin/kexin type 9 (PCSK9) siRNA suppresses adipogenesis and oxidative stress in Graves' orbitopathy (GO) fibroblasts. Orbital fibroblasts from GO (n=3) patients were cultured in adipogenic medium to induce differentiation into adipocytes for 7 days. **(A)** Oil red O staining showed treatment with PCSK9 siRNA (50 nM, 24 h) attenuated adipogenesis. **(B)** Quantification by measurements of optical density of cell lysates at 490nm echoed the histochemical results. The results are presented as the mean optical ratio ± SD ($^*p < 0.05$ between sicon and siPCSK9). **(C)** Western blot analyses showed that throughout the 7-day period of adipogenesis, the cell lysates of fibroblasts collected at different time points showed a gradual increase in production of PCSK9, which was markedly decreased when PCSK9 siRNA (50 nM, 24 h) was treated. The levels of adipogenic transcription factors, peroxisome proliferator-activated receptor gamma (PPARγ) and CCAAT/enhancer-binding protein β (C/EBPβ), were substantially curtailed in fibroblasts transfected with PCSK9 siRNA. The levels of mature adipocyte marker, leptin, were also significantly reduced in the PCSK9 siRNA-treated group. The levels of antioxidants, manganese superoxide dismutase (MnSOD), thioredoxin (Trx), and heme oxygenase-1 (HO-1), and oxidative stress-related protein, hypoxia-inducible factor 1α (HIF-1α) were significantly decreased in the PCSK9 siRNA-transfected group. Data in the columns indicate the mean density ratio ± SD, normalized to the level of β-actin in the same sample, and representative gel images are shown ($^*p < 0.05$ between sicon and siPCSK9 on days 0, 3, 5, and 7 of adipogenesis).

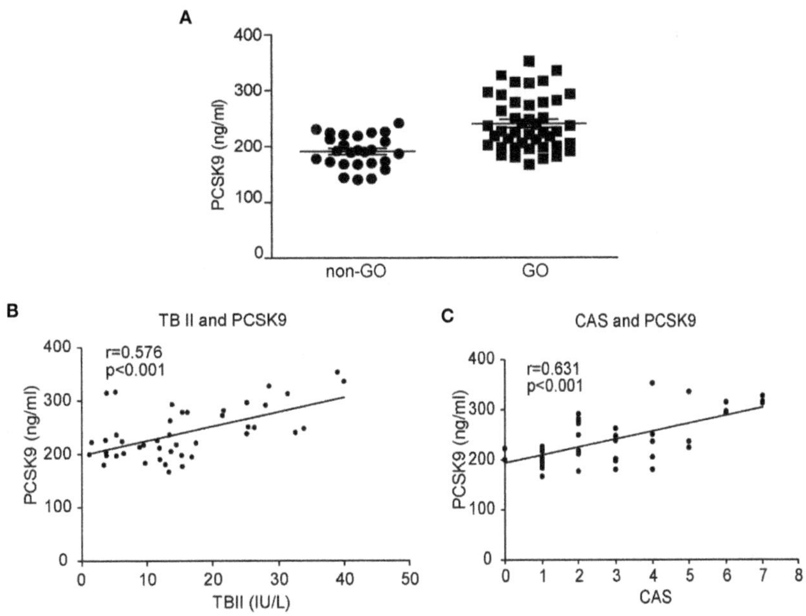

FIGURE 6 | Comparison of plasma levels of proprotein convertase subtilisin/kexin type 9 (PCSK9) between Graves' orbitopathy (GO) patients and non-GO subjects, and correlation analyses between plasma levels of PCSK9, thyrotropin-binding inhibitor immunoglobulin and clinical activity score (CAS). The plasma levels of PCSK9 were measured in GO patients and non-GO subjects using ELISA. The samples were assayed in triplicate. **(A)** The mean PCSK9 plasma level was significantly higher in the GO patients (n=44, 239.97 ± 48.20 ng/ml) than the healthy subjects (n=26, 190.83 ± 28.77 ng/ml; $p < 0.01$). A single dot represents the value obtained from a single donor. The results of Spearman's rank correlation test between plasma levels of PCSK9 (GO patients, n=44) and **(B)** plasma levels of thyrotropin binding inhibitory immunoglobulin (TBII) (GO patients, n=44) or **(C)** clinical activity score (CAS) (GO patients, n=44) are shown. The plasma PCSK9 concentrations showed significant associations with the plasma TBII levels ($r = 0.576$, $p < 0.001$) and CAS ($r = 0.631$, $p < 0.001$).

The changes in the level of phosphorylated forms of transcription factors upon the transfection of PCSK9 siRNA in GO fibroblasts indicate that a complex network of signaling pathways may exist. In this study, the PCSK9 inhibition decreased the activation of Akt and attenuated adipogenesis in GO fibroblasts. Our study with siRNA transfection is limited by the lack of mRNA data, which would have provided additional insights to its effect at transcriptional or translational level. However, like other studies that have employed similar methods (53, 54), we believe that we have shown a concrete evidence with western blot and ELISA that PCSK9, regardless of the mechanism with which its level is modified, affects inflammation and adipogenesis in GO. In line with our study, Kumar et al. have previously reported that an autoantibody against TSH receptor stimulated the phosphoinositide 3-kinase (PI3K)/Akt pathway and induced adipogenesis of orbital preadipocytes in GO (55). They asserted that this pathway triggered the terminal stages of adipogenesis. Another recent study by our group has presented that an Akt inhibitor suppressed adipogenesis in GO orbital fibroblasts (56). Another downstream effector of PI3K/Akt pathway, Forkhead box O (FOXOs), has also been demonstrated to repress excessive adipogenesis and hyaluronan overproduction in GO fibroblasts (57). As multiple studies, including our own, continue to highlight the importance of the PI3K/Akt pathway in the GO pathogenesis, further studies are necessary to identify the interaction between the signaling molecules as well as PCSK9.

Finally, we show that plasma PCSK9 levels were significantly higher in active GO patients than inactive GO patients as well as healthy subjects. These results, along with the higher PCSK9 mRNA levels in GO tissues, strongly suggest the involvement of PCSK9 in GO pathogenesis. Moreover, the plasma PCSK9 level revealed a strong correlation with plasma TBII level as well as CAS. Its role in many other inflammatory and autoimmune diseases such as systemic lupus erythematosus, rheumatoid arthritis, and type 1 diabetes demonstrates its complex biological activity (58–60). Identifying new biomarkers and therapeutic targets such as PCSK9 can further our knowledge of these disorders and lead to the development of effective treatments.

In conclusion, we demonstrated that PCSK9 inhibition countered pro-inflammatory cytokines production, oxidative stress-related proteins, adipogenic transcription factors, and adipocyte formation in GO fibroblasts. The PCSK9 level was increased during the IL-1β challenge and adipogenic stimulation. The plasma PCSK9 level was elevated in GO patients and positively correlated with clinical inflammation and thyrotropin receptor antibody titer, indicating that PCSK9 is a potential biomarker for diagnosis and prognosis of GO. Further studies are needed to establish the response to PCSK9 inhibitors *in vivo* and explore the use of the inhibitor as an effective therapeutic strategy for GO.

AUTHOR CONTRIBUTIONS

GL drafted the manuscript; JiK acquired and interpreted the data. JL, JaK, and EL revised the work. JY designed the study and revised the work. All authors contributed to the article and approved the submitted version.

SUPPLEMENTARY MATERIAL

SUPPLEMENTARY FIGURE 1 | siRNA-mediated knockdown of PCSK9 in GO and non-GO fibroblasts. GO (n=3) and non-GO (n=3) orbital fibroblasts were transfected with PCSK9 siRNA (50, 100 nM) for 24 h. As shown in western blot results, the level of PCSK9 was significantly decreased following RNA interference. β-actin was included as a loading control. NC, normal control.

SUPPLEMENTARY FIGURE 2 | Effect of PCSK9 siRNA on viability of GO fibroblasts. Orbital fibroblasts of GO patients (n=3) were seeded in 24-well culture plates, 1×10^5 cells per well. PCSK9 siRNA (50 nM) were applied to wells for 10, 24, and 48 h and MTT assay was conducted to test cell viability. Results are presented as mean ± SD. Assays were carried out in triplicate and repeated at least three times. The proliferation of GO fibroblasts was impeded in PCSK9 siRNA-treated fibroblasts compared to the control.

REFERENCES

1. Bahn RS. Graves' ophthalmopathy. *New Engl J Med* (2010) 362(8):726–38. doi: 10.1056/NEJMra0905750
2. Lehmann GM, Feldon SE, Smith TJ, Phipps RP. Immune mechanisms in thyroid eye disease. *Thyroid* (2008) 18(9):959–65. doi: 10.1089/thy.2007.0407
3. Genere N, Stan MN. Current and Emerging Treatment Strategies for Graves' Orbitopathy. *Drugs* (2019) 79(2):109–24. doi: 10.1007/s40265-018-1045-9
4. Seidah NG, Benjannet S, Wickham L, Marcinkiewicz J, Jasmin SB, Stifani S, et al. The secretory proprotein convertase neural apoptosis-regulated convertase 1 (NARC-1): liver regeneration and neuronal differentiation. *Proc Natl Acad Sci* (2003) 100(3):928–33. doi: 10.1073/pnas.0335507100
5. Horton JD, Cohen JC, Hobbs HH. PCSK9: a convertase that coordinates LDL catabolism. *J Lipid Res* (2009) 50 Suppl:S172–7. doi: 10.1194/jlr.R800091-JLR200
6. Filippatos TD, Christopoulou EC, Elisaf MS. Pleiotropic effects of proprotein convertase subtilisin/kexin type 9 inhibitors? *Curr Opin Lipidol* (2018) 29 (4):333–9. doi: 10.1097/MOL.0000000000000523
7. Seidah NG. New developments in proprotein convertase subtilisin–kexin 9's biology and clinical implications. *Curr Opin Lipidol* (2016) 27(3):274–81. doi: 10.1097/MOL.0000000000000295
8. Poirier S, Mayer G, Benjannet S, Bergeron E, Marcinkiewicz J, Nassoury N, et al. The proprotein convertase PCSK9 induces the degradation of low density lipoprotein receptor (LDLR) and its closest family members VLDLR and ApoER2. *J B ol C e m*(2008) 283(4):2363–72. doi: 10.1074/jbc.M708098200
9. Shan L, Pang L, Zhang R, Murgolo NJ, Lan H, Hedrick JA. PCSK9 binds to multiple receptors and can be functionally inhibited by an EGF-A peptide. *Biochem Biophys Res Commun* (2008) 375(1):69–73. doi: 10.1016/ j.bbrc.2008.07.106
10. Karagiannis AD, Liu M, Toth PP, Zhao S, Agrawal DK, Libby P, et al. Pleiotropic Anti-atherosclerotic Effects of PCSK9 InhibitorsFrom Molecular Biology to Clinical Translation. *Curr Atheroscler Rep* (2018) 20(4):20. doi: 10.1007/s11883-018-0718-x
11. Brown M, Ahmed S. Emerging role of proprotein convertase subtilisin/kexin type-9 (PCSK-9) in inflammation and diseases. *Toxicol Appl Pharmacol* (2019) 370:170–7. doi: 10.1016/j.taap.2019.03.018
12. Luan C, Chen X, Zhu Y, Osland JM, Gerber SD, Dodds M, et al. Potentiation of Psoriasis-Like Inflammation by PCSK9. *J Invest Dermatol* (2019) 139 (4):859–67. doi: 10.1016/j.jid.2018.07.046
13. Lee JS, Mukhopadhyay P, Matyas C, Trojnar E, Paloczi J, Yang YR, et al. PCSK9 inhibition as a novel therapeutic target for alcoholic liver disease. *Sci Rep* (2019) 9(1):17167. doi:10.1038/s41598-019-53603-6
14. Ding Z, Wang X, Liu S, Shahanawaz J, Theus S, Fan Y, et al. PCSK9 expression in the ischaemic heart and its relationship to infarct size, cardiac function, and development of autophagy. *Cardiovasc Res* (2018) 114(13):1738–51. doi: 10.1093/cvr/cvy128
15. Tang ZH, Li TH, Peng J, Zheng J, Li TT, Liu LS, et al. PCSK9: A novel inflammation modulator in atherosclerosis? *J Cell Physiol* (2019) 234(3):2345-55. doi:10.1002/jcp.27254
16. Koch CA, Krabbe S, Hehmke B. Statins, metformin, proprotein-convertase-subtilisin-kexin type-9 (PCSK9) inhibitors and sex hormones: Immunomodulatory properties? *Rev Endocr Metab Disord* (2018) 19 (4):363–95. doi: 10.1007/s11154-018-9478-8
17. Mourits MP, Prummel MF, Wiersinga WM, Koornneef L. Clinical activity score as a guide in the management of patients with Graves' ophthalmopathy. *Clin Endocrinol* (1997) 47(1):9–14. doi: 10.1046/j.1365-2265.1997.2331047.x
18. Yoon JS, Lee HJ, Choi SH, Chang E-J, Lee SY, Lee EJ. Quercetin inhibits IL-1β-induced inflammation, hyaluronan production and adipogenesis in orbital fibroblasts from Graves' orbitopathy. *PloS One* (2011) 6(10):e26261. doi: 10.1371/journal.pone.0026261
19. Livak KJ, Schmittgen TD. Analysis of relative gene expression data using real-time quantitative PCR and the 2– ΔΔCT method. *methods* (2001) 25(4):402–8. doi: 10.1006/meth.2001.1262
20. Kim SE, Lee JH, Chae MK, Lee EJ, Yoon JS. The role of sphingosine-1-phosphate in adipogenesis of Graves' orbitopathy. *Invest Ophthalmol Vis Sci* (2016) 57:(2):301–11. doi: 10.1167/iovs.15-17863
21. Green H, Kehinde O. An established preadipose cell line and its differentiation in culture II. Factors affecting the adipose conversion. *Cell* (1975) 5(1):19–27. doi: 10.1016/0092-8674(75)90087-2
22. Li H, Yuan Y, Zhang Y, He Q, Xu R, Ge F, et al. Celastrol inhibits IL-1β-induced inflammation in orbital fibroblasts through the suppression of NF-κB activity. *Mol Med Rep* (2016) 14(3):2799–806. doi: 10.3892/mmr.2016.5570
23. Heufelder AE, Bahn RS. Modulation of Graves' orbital fibroblast proliferation by cytokines and glucocorticoid receptor agonists. *Invest Ophthalmol Visual Sci* (1994) 35(1):120–7.
24. Eckstein AK, Plicht M, Lax H, Neuhäuser M, Mann K, Lederbogen S, et al. Thyrotropin receptor autoantibodies are independent risk factors for Graves' ophthalmopathy and help to predict severity and outcome of the disease. *J Clin Endocrinol Metab* (2006) 91(9):3464–70. doi: 10.1210/jc.2005-2813
25. Giunzioni I, Tavori H, Covarrubias R, Major AS, Ding L, Zhang Y, et al. Local effects of human PCSK9 on the atherosclerotic lesion. *J Pathol* (2016) 238 (1):52–62. doi: 10.1002/path.4630
26. Tang Z, Jiang L, Peng J, Ren Z, Wei D, Wu C, et al. PCSK9 siRNA suppresses the inflammatory response induced by oxLDL through inhibition of NF-kappaB activation in THP-1-derived macrophages. *Int J Mol Med* (2012) 30 (4):931–8. doi: 10.3892/ijmm.2012.1072
27. Ricci C, Ruscica M, Camera M, Rossetti L, Macchi C, Colciago A, et al. PCSK9 induces a pro-inflammatory response in macrophages. *Sci Rep* (2018) 8 (1):2267. doi: 10.1038/s41598-018-20425-x
28. Walley KR, Thain KR, Russell JA, Reilly MP, Meyer NJ, Ferguson JF, et al. PCSK9 is a critical regulator of the innate immune response and septic shock outcome. *Sci Trans Med* (2014) 6(258):258ra143–258ra143. doi: 10.1126/ scitranslmed.3008782
29. Dwivedi DJ, Grin PM, Khan M, Prat A, Zhou J, Fox-Robichaud AE, et al. Differential Expression of PCSK9 Modulates Infection, Inflammation, and Coagulation in a Murine Model of Sepsis. *Shock* (2016) 46(6):672–80. doi: 10.1097/SHK.0000000000000682

30. Tang Z-H, Peng J, Ren Z, Yang J, Li T-T, Li T-H, et al. New role of PCSK9 in atherosclerotic inflammation promotion involving the TLR4/NF-κB pathway. *Atherosclerosis* (2017) 262:113–22. doi: 10.1016/j.atherosclerosis.2017.04.023
31. Ruscica M, Ferri N, Macchi C, Meroni M, Lanti C, Ricci C, et al. Liver fat accumulation is associated with circulating PCSK9. *Ann Med* (2016) 48 (5):384–91. doi: 10.1080/07853890.2016.1188328
32. Lee S, Zhang C, Liu Z, Klevstig M, Mukhopadhyay B, Bergentall M, et al. Network analyses identify liver-specific targets for treating liver diseases. *Mol Syst Biol* (2017) 13(8):938. doi: 10.15252/msb.20177703
33. Tavori H, Giunzioni I, Predazzi IM, Plubell D, Shivinsky A, Miles J, et al. Human PCSK9 promotes hepatic lipogenesis and atherosclerosis development via apoE- and LDLR-mediated mechanisms. *Cardiovasc Res* (2016) 110(2):268–78. doi: 10.1093/cvr/cvw053
34. Kim HJ, Yoon BK, Park H, Seok JW, Choi H, Yu JH, et al. Caffeine inhibits adipogenesis through modulation of mitotic clonal expansion and the AKT/GSK3 pathway in 3T3-L1 adipocytes. *BMB Rep* (2016) 49(2):111. doi: 10.5483/BMBRep.2016.49.2.128
35. Lee J-H, Kim T, Lee J-J, Lee KJ, Kim H-K, Yun B, et al. The herbal medicine KBH-1 inhibits fat accumulation in 3T3-L1 adipocytes and reduces high fat diet-induced obesity through regulation of the AMPK pathway. *PloS One* (2015) 10(12):e0142041. doi: 10.1371/journal.pone.0142041
36. Fajas L, Landsberg RL, Huss-Garcia Y, Sardet C, Lees JA, Auwerx J. E2Fs regulate adipocyte differentiation. *Dev Cell* (2002) 3(1):39–49. doi: 10.1016/S1534-5807(02)00190-9
37. Inoue J, Kumagai H, Terada T, Maeda M, Shimizu M, Sato R. Proteolytic activation of SREBPs during adipocyte differentiation. *Biochem Biophys Res Commun* (2001) 283(5):1157–61. doi: 10.1006/bbrc.2001.4915
38. Ferrari SM, Fallahi P, Vita R, Antonelli A, Benvenga S. Peroxisome proliferator-activated receptor-γ in thyroid autoimmunity. *Ppar Res* (2015) 2015:232818. doi: 10.1155/2015/232818
39. Görtz G-E, Horstmann M, Aniol B, Reyes BD, Fandrey J, Eckstein A, et al. Hypoxia-dependent HIF-1 activation impacts on tissue remodeling in Graves' ophthalmopathy—implications for smoking. *J Clin Endocrinol Metab* (2016) 101(12):4834–42. doi: 10.1210/jc.2016-1279
40. Ding Z, Liu S, Wang X, Deng X, Fan Y, Sun C, et al. Hemodynamic shear stress via ROS modulates PCSK9 expression in human vascular endothelial and smooth muscle cells and along the mouse aorta. *Antioxid Redox Signal* (2015) 22(9):760–71. doi: 10.1089/ars.2014.6054
41. Yang X, Li Y, Li Y, Ren X, Zhang X, Hu D, et al. Oxidative stress-mediated atherosclerosis: mechanisms and therapies. *Front Physiol* (2017) 8:600. doi: 10.3389/fphys.2017.00600
42. Ding Z, Liu S, Wang X, Theus S, Deng X, Fan Y, et al. PCSK9 regulates expression of scavenger receptors and ox-LDL uptake in macrophages. *Cardiovasc Res* (2018) 114(8):1145–53. doi: 10.1093/cvr/cvy079
43. Ding Z, Liu S, Wang X, Mathur P, Dai Y, Theus S, et al. Cross-Talk Between PCSK9 and Damaged mtDNA in Vascular Smooth Muscle Cells: Role in Apoptosis. *Antioxid Redox Signal* (2016) 25(18):997–1008. doi: 10.1089/ars.2016.6631
44. Ding Z, Liu S, Wang X, Deng X, Fan Y, Shahanawaz J, et al. Cross-talk between LOX-1 and PCSK9 in vascular tissues. *Cardiovasc Res* (2015) 107 (4):556–67. doi: 10.1093/cvr/cvv178
45. Yun Y-S, Lee Y-N. Production of superoxide dismutase by Deinococcus radiophilus. *BMB Rep* (2003) 36(3):282–7. doi: 10.5483/BMBRep. 2003.36.3.282
46. Guo H-c, Zhang Z, Zhang L-n, Xiong C, Feng C, Liu Q, et al. Chronic intermittent hypobaric hypoxia protects the heart against ischemia/reperfusion injury through upregulation of antioxidant enzymes in adult guinea pigs. *Acta Pharmacol Sin* (2009) 30(7):947–55. doi: 10.1038/aps.2009.57
47. Takahashi T, Morita K, Akagi R, Sassa S. Heme oxygenase-1: a novel therapeutic target in oxidative tissue injuries. *Curr Med Chem* (2004) 11 (12):1545–61. doi: 10.2174/0929867043365080
48. Yoon JS, Lee HJ, Chae MK, Lee SY, Lee EJ. Cigarette smoke extract-induced adipogenesis in Graves' orbital fibroblasts is inhibited by quercetin via reduction in oxidative stress. *J Endocrinol* (2013) 216(2):145–56. doi: 10.1530/JOE-12-0257
49. Lee JS, Kim J, Lee EJ, Yoon JS. Therapeutic Effect of Curcumin, a Plant Polyphenol Extracted From Curcuma longae, in Fibroblasts From Patients With Graves' Orbitopathy. *Invest Ophthalmol Vis Sci* (2019) 60(13):4129–40. doi: 10.1167/iovs.19-27376
50. Kim CY, Lee HJ, Chae MK, Byun JW, Lee EJ, Yoon JS. Therapeutic effect of resveratrol on oxidative stress in Graves' orbitopathy orbital fibroblasts. *Invest Ophthalmol Visual Sci* (2015) 56(11):6352–61. doi: 10.1167/iovs.15-16870
51. Ko J, Kim J-Y, J-w K, Yoon JS. Anti-oxidative and anti-adipogenic effects of caffeine in an in vitro model of Graves' orbitopathy. *Endocrine J* (2020) 67 (4):439–47. doi: 10.1507/endocrj.EJ19-0521
52. Zarkovic M. The role of oxidative stress on the pathogenesis of graves' disease. *J Thyroid Res* (2012) 2012:302537. doi: 10.1155/2012/302537
53. Ko J, Kim JY, Lee EJ, Yoon JS. Role of binding immunoglobulin protein (BiP) in Graves' orbitopathy pathogenesis. *J Mol Endocrinol* (2020). doi: 10.1530/JME-20-0155
54. Byeon HJ, Kim J-Y, Ko J, Lee EJ, Don K, Yoon JS. Protein tyrosine phosphatase 1B as a therapeutic target for Graves' orbitopathy in an in vitro model. *PloS One* (2020) 15(8):e0237015. doi: 10.1371/journal.pone.0237015
55. Kumar S, Nadeem S, Stan MN, Coenen M, Bahn RS. A stimulatory TSH receptor antibody enhances adipogenesis via phosphoinositide 3-kinase activation in orbital preadipocytes from patients with Graves' ophthalmopathy. *J Mol Endocrinol* (2011) 46(3):155. doi: 10.1530/JME-11-0006
56. Ko J, Kim J-Y, Lee EJ, Yoon JS. Inhibitory effect of idelalisib, a selective phosphatidylinositol 3-kinase δ inhibitor, on adipogenesis in an in vitro model of Graves' orbitopathy. *Invest Ophthalmol Visual Sci* (2018) 59(11):4477–85. doi: 10.1167/iovs.18-24509
57. Zhang L, Ji QH, Ruge F, Lane C, Morris D, Tee AR, et al. Reversal of Pathological Features of Graves' Orbitopathy by Activation of Forkhead Transcription Factors, FOXOs. *J Clin Endocrinol Metab* (2016) 101(1):114–22. doi: 10.1210/jc.2015-2932
58. Fang C, Luo T, Lin L. Elevation of serum proprotein convertase subtilisin/kexin type 9 (PCSK9) concentrations and its possible atherogenic role in patients with systemic lupus erythematosus. *Ann Transl Med* (2018) 6 (23):452. doi: 10.21037/atm.2018.11.04
59. Du Q, Yu X, Li H, Guan S, Zhang Z, Mei Y. The expression and clinical significance of proprotein convertase subtilisin kexin 9 in rheumatoid arthritis. *Zhonghua Nei Ke Za Zhi* (2017) 56(9):655–9. doi: 10.3760/cma.j.issn.0578-1426.2017.09.007
60. Levenson AE, Wadwa RP, Shah AS, Khoury PR, Kimball TR, Urbina EM, et al. PCSK9 Is Increased in Youth With Type 1 Diabetes. *Diabetes Care* (2017) 40 (7):e85–e7. doi: 10.2337/dc16-2563

19

Use of Rituximab after Orbital Decompression Surgery in Two Grave's Ophthalmopathy Patients Progressing to Optic Neuropathy

Benping Zhang[1], Yaling Li[2], Weijie Xu[1], Bei Peng[3] and Gang Yuan[1*]

[1] Department of Endocrinology, Tongji Hospital, Tongji Medical College, Huazhong University of Science and Technology, Wuhan, China, [2] Department of Critical Care Medicine, Wuhan No.1 Hospital, Wuhan, China, [3] Department of Endocrinology, Taikang Tongji (Wuhan) Hospital, Wuhan, China

***Correspondence:**
Gang Yuan
yuangang88@hotmail.com

Background: While orbital decompression can alleviate optic nerve compression and prevent further vision loss in dysthyroid optic neuropathy (DON), it cannot relieve inflammatory symptoms. Very high doses of intravenous glucocorticoids (GCs) are the first-line therapy for DON; however, the effective rate is only 40% and might be much lower in patients who fail high-dose GC pulse therapy and progressed to DON. The results of two case series studies indicated that rituximab treatment had a much better curative effect compared to very high doses of intravenous GCs, but some patients required urgent orbital decompression after rituximab injection because rituximab might lead to the release of cytokines, aggravated intraorbital edema, and further vision loss.

Methods: We retrospectively studied the therapeutic process of two Grave's ophthalmopathy (GO) patients complicated with DON who failed high-dose GC pulse therapy and underwent orbital decompression. Both patients received single-dose (500 mg) rituximab treatment.

Results: During more than 2 years of follow-up, rituximab treatment exhibited significant improvement in inflammatory symptoms, as manifested by a substantial decrease in Clinical Activity Score (CAS); meanwhile, the vision of both patients improved significantly and their diplopia was relieved.

Conclusions: The results of this study were consistent with those of two previous case series studies indicating the significant and lasting effect of rituximab treatment on DON, especially for patients with GC resistance or recurrence after GC therapy. Orbital decompression before rituximab treatment might reduce the incidence of rapid vision loss and urgent orbital decompression surgery caused by aggravated orbital edema after rituximab injection; however, the necessity for preventive decompression surgery requires further study.

Keywords: Grave's disease, Grave's ophthalmopathy, Dysthyroid optic neuropathy, orbital decompression, rituximab

INTRODUCTION

Grave's disease (GD) is an autoimmune disease involving the thyroid, skin, and orbit, with an incidence in the adult population of 1–2% (1). Grave's ophthalmopathy (GO) is the most frequent extrathyroidal manifestation of GD, occurring in up to 50% of GD patients throughout the course of the disease (2). GO is generally self-limiting, with the signs and symptoms improving naturally or following thyrotoxicosis control, smoking cessation, and local treatment (3). However, for some patients, the signs and symptoms persist or aggravate gradually, which require specific treatment besides smoking cessation and anti-thyroid drug administration (4).

The pathogenesis of GO is incompletely understood, although immunological cross-reactivity between the thyroid and orbital antigens may play a key role, and disorders of inflammatory cytokines, thyrotropin receptor autoantibodies, and immunoglobulins targeting the insulin-like growth factor 1 receptor may be correlated with GO (2, 5). Hence, the current internal medicine treatments for GO mostly target immunological disorders, especially for moderate-to-severe and sight-threatening GO.

High-dose intravenous glucocorticoid (GC) pulse treatment is the first-line treatment for moderate-to-severe and active GO, with a 4.5 g cumulative dose of methylprednisolone divided into 12 weekly intravenous injections recommended. A higher dose is acceptable for severe forms; however, the cumulative doses should not exceed 8.0 g (4, 6). The response rate of high-dose intravenous GCs pulse treatment is 70–80% (4, 6, 7); however, in clinical practice, many patients responding well to intravenous GCs may re-develop active disease after therapy completion. For patients with a recurrence or poor response to intravenous GCs, shared decision-making with patients to select an appropriate second-line treatment is recommended (6). A second course of intravenous GCs, orbital radiotherapy, combination use of cyclosporine and oral GCs, and rituximab are the most common second-line treatments (6).

As an alternative second-line treatment for GO, rituximab has been proven to be effective and safe in patients with GO who fail high-dose intravenous GC pulse treatment and shows potential to become a first-line treatment (6). For GO patients progressing to DON, non-control studies have also shown that rituximab was effective in relieving DON; however, a small number of patients in the studies required urgent orbital decompression surgery after receiving rituximab injection as rituximab may have aggravated intraorbital edema (8–10). This finding is consistent with the recommendation in the 2016 European Group of Graves' Orbitopathy Guidelines for the Management of GO that rituximab should not be used in patients with impending DON (6). Thus, the use of rituximab in patients with GO complicated with DON requires further clinical studies.

This study retrospectively analyzed the therapeutic processes of two GO patients who failed high-dose intravenous GC pulse treatment and progressed to DON. Although a very high dose of intravenous GCs is the first-line treatment for DON, patient 1 was not sensitive to GCs and the cumulative doses of GCs exceeded 8 g. Two patients underwent orbital decompression surgery first to avoid further vision loss. However, there was no significant improvement, especially the clinical activity score (CAS) and diplopia. Moreover, the recovery of vision was not ideal. Thus, rituximab treatment was initiated. During 2 years of follow-up after rituximab treatment, both patients achieved stable and significant remission.

Abbreviations: CAS, Clinical Activity Score; DON, dysthyroid optic neuropathy; GC, glucocorticoid; GD, Grave's disease; GO, Grave's ophthalmopathy.

CASE DESCRIPTIONS

Both patients were initially diagnosed with moderate-to-severe and active GO and received high-dose intravenous GC pulse treatment. The patients also received basic treatments including selenium supplementation and artificial tears. Orbital decompression surgery and sequential rituximab were initiated when the patients suffered from DON and resisted to GCs or the total methylprednisolone dose exceeded 8g. All patients received a single dose of 500 mg rituximab as a slow intravenous infusion, with 5 mg of dexamethasone to prevent allergic reactions.

Case 1: A 54-year-old man (non-smoker) was diagnosed with GD and GO in December 2017 at a local hospital, where he received methimazole treatment only. Three months later, he was transferred to Tongji Hospital, Wuhan, China, for further treatment due to rapidly declining vision (OD 0.3, OS 0.08), eyeball movement disorder, and inability to close his eyelid. The patient was then diagnosed with DON, with a CAS of 7/7. Two days after transfer to this hospital, we initiated high-dose intravenous GC pulse treatment (0.5 g methylprednisolone seven times) and performed bilateral orbital decompression and eyelid margin suture surgery as ophthalmologic examination showed persisting DON with no significant improvement in vision. The orbital decompression surgery was balanced decompression of the inner and outer orbital walls combined with lipectomy, part of the bone in both medial and lateral orbital walls and about 3ml of adipose tissue were removed in the surgery. After the above treatment, the patient's CAS decreased to 5/7, and ophthalmologic examination showed normal intraocular tension; however, the eyeball movement disorder remained and his vision did not improve (OD 0.1, OS 0.1). The patient then left the hospital and received oral GC treatment at home (methylprednisolone 40 mg/d for 1 week and 36 mg/d for another week). Two weeks later, the patient returned to the hospital. Ophthalmologic examination showed a CAS of 6/7; therefore, we administered an eighth intravenous GC treatment (0.5 g methylprednisolone). His vision improved 7 days after the intravenous GC treatment (OD 0.5, OS 0.6), but the CAS was still 6/7, and the eyeball movement disorder and inability to close the eyelids did not improve. Finally, we decided to administer rituximab treatment (a single dose of 500 mg) and oral GC treatment simultaneously.

Case 2: A 58-year-old man (smoker, quit smoking 10 years ago) was diagnosed with hyperthyroidism and moderate-to-severe GO in March 2017 at the local hospital, where he received methimazole and intravenous GC treatment (11

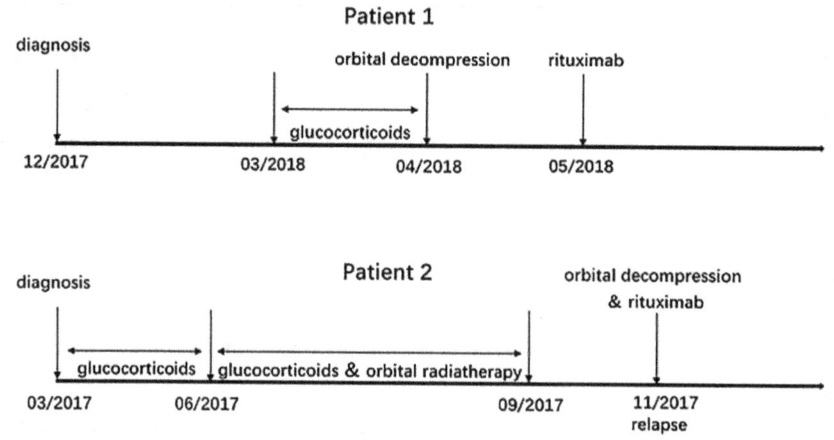

FIGURE 1 | Treatment process: corticosteroids, orbital decompression, and rituximab for patient 1 and patient 2.

weekly intravenous injections of 0.5 g methylprednisolone), without significant improvement. The patient was then transferred to Tongji Hospital, Wuhan, China. Ophthalmologic examination showed eyeball movement disorder; both eyes had 1.0 vision, and his CAS was 5/7. We administered intravenous GC treatment (12 weekly intravenous injections of 0.25 g methylprednisolone) combined with right orbital radiotherapy (2 Gy daily for 10 days). After the above treatment, his vision was normal (OD 1.2, OS 1.2), the intraocular tension was also normal, and the CAS decreased to 2/7. However, the disease relapsed approximately 2 months after completion of intravenous GC therapy, which manifested as severe exophthalmos, diplopia, vision decrease (OD 0.1, OS 1.0), and inability to close his eyelid. The CAS increased to 7/7. The patient was then diagnosed with DON and right orbital decompression surgery was performed. The surgical type and methods were similar to those described for patient 1. After orbital decompression surgery, his vision improved slightly (OD 0.4, OS 1.0); however, the CAS and diplopia did not improve. Therefore, we decided to administer rituximab treatment (a single dose of 500 mg) and oral GC treatment.

The treatment process of patient 1 and patient 2 was summarized in **Figure 1**. **Table 1** showed the baseline data of patients before rituximab treatment, **Table 2** showed in detail the patients undergoing orbital decompression surgery and rituximab treatment, and **Table 3** showed the changes in patients' vision before rituximab treatment.

RESULTS

As shown in **Table 4** and **Figure 2**, rituximab treatment was administered after orbital decompression and showed significant improvement in inflammatory symptoms, as manifested by a substantial decrease in CAS. Meanwhile, the vision of both patients improved significantly, and their diplopia was relieved after rituximab treatment.

In patient 1, the CAS decreased from 5/7 to 2/7 (OD) and from 6/7 to 3/7 (OS) 5 months after rituximab treatment, with a final CAS of both eyes of 2/7 at the last follow-up to 24 months after rituximab treatment. His vision had improved from 0.5 to 1.0 OD and from 0.6 to 0.8 (OS) at the last follow-up. The

TABLE 1 | Description of the two patients treated with Rituximab.

Patient number	Patient 1	Patient 2
Age (year)	54	58
Gender	Male	Male
Smoking	No	Yes
Quit smoking	N/A	10 years ago
Endocrinological treatment of GD	Methimazole	Methimazole
Chronology of GO in relation to GD	With GD	With GD
Corticosteroids therapy (time relative to GO diagnosis)	3 months	0 month
Corticosteroids therapy (duration time)	8 weeks	23 weeks
Total dose of intravenous corticosteroids dose (methylprednisolone, MPS)	4.0g	8.5g
Other immunosuppressive treatments before RTX	Oral MPS for 2 weeks, total dose 532mg	None
Orbital radiotherapy	None	2Gy/time × 10 times
Additional treatments	Selenium supplements	Selenium supplements

GD, Grave's disease; GO, Grave's ophthalmopathy; RTX, rituximab; MPS, methylprednisolone; N/A, not available.

TABLE 2 | Orbital decompression and Rituximab treatment details of the two patients.

Patient number	Patient 1	Patient 2
Reason for orbital decompression	DON, no improvement after intravenous MPS	Relapse and DON developed after intravenous MPS and orbital radiotherapy
Total dose of MPS before orbital decompression	3.5g	8.5g
Duration of MPS use before orbital decompression	7 weeks	23 weeks
Orbital decompression (time relative to DON diagnosis)	At 7 weeks	At 1 week
Immunosuppressive treatments after orbital decompression	Intravenous MPS 0.5g and oral MPS	None (prior to RTX)
RTX therapy (time related to orbital decompression)	At 52 days	At 4 days
RTX therapy (time related to diagnosisi)	5 months	8 months
Reason for RTX therapy	Failure of glucocorticoids treatment	MPS dose exceeded 8g
RTX dose	500mg only once	500mg only once
Immunosuppressive treatments after RTX	Oral MPS	Oral MPS

DON, dysthyroid optic neuropathy; MPS, methylprednisolone; RTX, rituximab.

TABLE 3 | Summary of changes in vision before RTX treatment.

	Vision	
	Right	Left
Patient 1		
Before high-dose GCs pulse treatment	0.3	0.08
After 7 times high-dose GCs pulse treatment	0.1	0.1
After bilateral orbital decompression and the eighth high-dose GCs pulse treatment (before RTX)	0.5	0.6
Patient 2		
Before high-dose GCs pulse treatment combined with right orbital radiotherapy	1.0	1.0
After high-dose GCs pulse treatment combined with right orbital radiotherapy	1.2	1.2
Disease relapse	0.1	1.0
After right orbital decompression (before RTX)	0.4	1.0

RTX, rituximab; GCs, glucocorticoids.

TABLE 4 | Results of the therapy with rituximab.

	CAS score (/7)		Vision		IPO (mmHg)		Proptosis (mm)		Diplopia
	Right	Left	Right	Left	Right	Left	Right	Left	
Patient 1									
Before RTX	5	6	0.5	0.6	19	15	21	20	Yes
5 months after RTX	2	3	1.0	0.8	18	14	20	21	Alleviated
Last examination 24 months after RTX	2	2	1.0	0.8	18	15	19	20	Alleviated
Patient 2									
Before RTX	7	3	0.4	1.0	21	19	19	19	Yes
6 months after RTX	2	0	0.8	1.0	19	17	18	18	Alleviated
Last examination 26 months after RTX	0	0	1.0	1.2	19	17	18	19	No

CAS, Clinical Activity Score; IPO, intraocular pressure; RTX, rituximab.

severity of diplopia decreased but persisted until the last follow-up. Slight improvements in intraocular pressure and proptosis were also observed.

In patient 2, similar to patient 1, inflammatory signs and vision improved significantly after rituximab treatment, while intraocular pressure and proptosis improved slightly. Specifically, the CAS decreased from 7/7 to 2/7 (OD) 6 months after rituximab treatment, with a final CAS of 0/7 (OD) at the last follow-up. The patient's vision had improved from 0.4 to 1.0 OD and from 1.0 to 1.2 (OS) at 26 months after rituximab treatment. In addition, diplopia was alleviated at 6 months and completely relieved at 26 months after rituximab treatment.

DISCUSSION

Rituximab is a mouse anti-human monoclonal antibody that directly targets CD20, a B-lymphocyte-specific antigen (11). It was initially developed and used in patients with CD20-expressing lymphoid malignancies, including chronic lymphocytic leukemia and B-cell non-Hodgkin lymphoma. Rituximab induces cell apoptosis by binding to the CD20 membrane antigen in both normal and malignant B cells (12). In addition, it significantly depletes lymphocytes not only in the blood but also in the target tissue, and the effect remained significant 2 months after rituximab infusion (13). Based on the pharmacological mechanism of

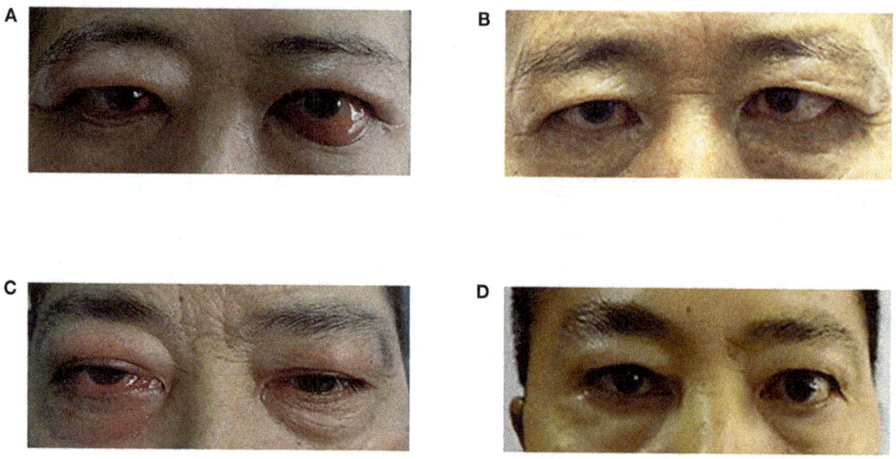

FIGURE 2 | Changes in the appearance of the two patients' eyes. **(A)** Before rituximab treatment (patient 1); **(B)** 24 months after rituximab treatment; **(C)** Before rituximab treatment (patient 2); **(D)** 26 months after rituximab treatment (patient 2).

rituximab, clinical trials on autoimmune diseases have indicated the potential use of rituximab as a candidate treatment for autoimmune diseases (14).

In 2006, two case reports indicated that corticosteroid-resistant GO might be significantly relieved after treatment with rituximab (15, 16). Following the two successful treatment cases, several non-controlled studies on the effects of rituximab in GO have been published, with most showing that rituximab can be used in active moderate-to-severe GO, especially when intravenous methylprednisolone therapy fails (5). In one study, Salvi et al. reported good therapeutic effects after rituximab treatment and improved activity and severity of GO in 98 and 91% of 43 GO patients who failed to respond to corticosteroids, respectively (17). In recent years, the results of two randomized clinical trials of rituximab as a first-line treatment in moderate-to-severe and active GO were published. In one study, Salvi et al. reported that GO was more significantly inactivated after 500 or 2,000 mg (administered twice over 2 weeks) rituximab injection (100 *vs.* 69% after 7.5 g intravenous methylprednisolone) at 24 weeks (18). However, another study by Stan et al. did not observe differences in either short- or long-term (24- or 52-week) outcomes between rituximab and placebo; meanwhile, two patients developed DON after rituximab. One possible explanation for the occurrence of DON is that the release of cytokines induced by rituximab treatment resulted in aggravated intraorbital edema, which transformed subclinical DON to DON (5, 19). The contradictory results of the two clinical trials suggest the need for more evidence before rituximab can be implemented as a first-line treatment for GO. However, the 2016 European Group of Graves' Orbitopathy Guidelines for the Management of Graves' orbitopathy recommended that, although it is still difficult to say which second-line option is more effective because of the limited evidence regarding differences in efficiency difference, treatment has relatively more evidence suggesting that rituximab is a good option for active moderate-to-severe GO when high-dose intravenous GC pulse treatment fails (6).

In GO patients progressing to DON, very high doses of intravenous GCs (*e.g.* 500–1,000 mg of methylprednisolone for 3 consecutive days) is the first-line therapy; however, the effective rate is only 40%, and many patients require urgent decompression surgery when the response is poor (6). In the formulation of the patients' treatment plans in the present report, we considered that very high doses of intravenous GCs might be ineffective in patient 1 as he showed resistance GCs, which manifested as non-remission of the disease after seven intravenous GC treatments. Meanwhile, very high doses of intravenous GCs might have led to serious side effects in patient 2 as the cumulative doses of GCs exceeded 8 g. To relieve compression of the optic nerve and avoid further loss of vision, we performed orbital decompression surgery first instead of administering very high doses of intravenous GCs. However, as it was predictable before the surgery that the patients' condition, especially the inflammatory symptoms and eye movement disorder, did not significantly improve as orbital decompression could only relieve orbital pressure and optic nerve compression; thus, further drug treatment was urgently required.

No evidence-based medical recommendations exist regarding the further treatment of GO patients complicated with DON who fail high-dose GC pulse therapy and require orbital decompression. We finally decided to administer rituximab based on the results of several non-control studies that indicated a better curative effect for rituximab treatment than for first-line therapy in GO patients with DON (8–10). Among these studies, Chong et al. successfully treated four patients who failed to respond to GCs and developed DON. In these patients, the CAS decreased significantly 2 months after rituximab treatment and remained so in all patients. The vision also improved bilaterally in all four patients. One of the four patients received decompression surgery and fractionated orbital irradiation 2 months before rituximab infusion, and another patient received urgent decompression surgery 12 days after the first rituximab infusion due to continued DON (8). Two other studies by Salvi et al. and Mitchell et al. also reported the successful treatment of five patients with DON, with significantly improved disease activity and vision in all five patients, similar to Chong's study. One of the five patients received urgent decompression surgery after the first rituximab infusion (9, 10). The longest interval between rituximab infusion and orbital decompression surgery was 2 months. Gess et al. administered rituximab to a patient with GO with DON who had failed very high-dose intravenous GCs. The patient improved initially but subsequently worsened 2 months later and underwent orbital decompression surgery (13).

The common characteristics of both patients in this study were significant enlarged extraocular muscle and orbital fat, which led to optic nerve compression and progression of DON. Previous studies revealed that the enlargement of extraocular muscle and orbital fat was associated with hyaluronic acid (HA) accumulation in the muscles and connective tissues and adipogenesis (20, 21). B cells play an important role in HA accumulation and adipogenesis. Briefly, B cells can present self-antigen and activate T cells through the complement receptor 2 (CR2, CD35), then activate helper T cells, recognize TSHR, ligate TSHR and TRAb together, and enhance hyaluronic acid (HA) production and adipogenesis (21, 22). Therefore, rituximab inhibits the activation of T cells by B-cell depletion and blockade of antigen presentation, which may be the main reason why rituximab is more effective compared with GC.

In conclusion, the treatment processes of these two patients indicated that rituximab might be safe and persistently effective for GO patients complicated with DON who fail high-dose GC pulse therapy and require orbital decompression. This finding is consistent with those of two previous non-control studies suggesting that rituximab treatment may have a better curative effect than very high doses of intravenous GCs. However, rituximab treatment may lead totherereleaseofcytokines, aggravated intraorbital edema, and rapid vision loss. Orbital decompression before rituximab injection might mitigate this side effect of rituximab; thus, the patients in this study might have obtained additional benefits from orbital decompression, although the surgeries were not performed preventively. The necessity for prophylactic orbital decompression surgery before rituximab injection requires additional evidence.

AUTHOR CONTRIBUTIONS

BZ: Data curation, Project administration, Formal analysis, Writing—original draft, Writing—review and editing. YL: Data curation, Writing—review and editing. WX: Data curation, Writing—review and editing. BP: Data curation, Writing—review and editing. GY: Conceptualization, Data curation, Project administration, Formal analysis, Investigation, Methodology, Project administration, Validation, Writing—review and editing.

REFERENCES

1. Weetman AP. Graves' disease. *N Engl J Med* (2000) 343(17):1236–48. doi: 10.1056/NEJM200010263431707
2. Minakaran N, Ezra DG. Rituximab for thyroid-associated ophthalmopathy. *Cochrane Database Syst Rev* (2013) (5):CD009226. doi: 10.1002/14651858.CD009226.pub2
3. Dolman PJ. Evaluating Graves' orbitopathy. *Best Pract Res Clin Endocrinol Metab* (2012) 26(3):229–48. doi: 10.1016/j.beem.2011.11.007
4. Zang S, Ponto KA, Kahaly GJ. Clinical review: Intravenous glucocorticoids for Graves' orbitopathy: efficacy and morbidity. *J Clin Endocrinol Metab* (2011) 96(2):320–32. doi: 10.1210/jc.2010-1962
5. Campi I, Vannucchi G, Salvi M. THERAPY OF ENDOCRINE DISEASE: Endocrine dilemma: management of Graves' orbitopathy. *Eur J Endocrinol* (2016) 175(3):R117–33. doi: 10.1530/EJE-15-1164
6. Bartalena L, Baldeschi L, Boboridis K, Eckstein A, Kahaly GJ, Marcocci C, et al. The 2016 European Thyroid Association/European Group on Graves' Orbitopathy Guidelines for the Management of Graves' Orbitopathy. *Eur Thyroid J* (2016) 5(1):9–26. doi: 10.1159/000443828
7. Stiebel-Kalish H, Robenshtok E, Hasanreisoglu M, Ezrachi D, Shimon I, Leibovici L. Treatment modalities for Graves' ophthalmopathy: systematic review and metaanalysis. *J Clin Endocrinol Metab* (2009) 94(8):2708–16. doi: 10.1210/jc.2009-0376
8. Khanna D, Chong KK, Afifiyan NF, Hwang CJ, Lee DK, Garneau HC, et al. Rituximab treatment of patients with severe, corticosteroid-resistant thyroid-associated ophthalmopathy. *Ophthalmology* (2010) 117(1):133–9.e2. doi: 10.1016/j.ophtha.2009.05.029
9. Salvi M, Vannucchi G, Campi I, Curro N, Simonetta S, Covelli D, et al. Rituximab treatment in a patient with severe thyroid-associated ophthalmopathy: effects on orbital lymphocytic infiltrates. *Clin Immunol* (2009) 131(2):360–5. doi: 10.1016/j.clim.2008.12.005
10. Mitchell AL, Gan EH, Morris M, Johnson K, Neoh C, Dickinson AJ, et al. The effect of B cell depletion therapy on anti-TSH receptor antibodies and clinical outcome in glucocorticoid-refractory Graves' orbitopathy. *Clin Endocrinol (Oxf)* (2013) 79(3):437–42. doi: 10.1111/cen.12141
11. Engel P, Gomez-Puerta JA, Ramos-Casals M, Lozano F, Bosch X. Therapeutic targeting of B cells for rheumatic autoimmune diseases. *Pharmacol Rev* (2011) 63(1):127–56. doi: 10.1124/pr.109.002006
12. Salles G, Barrett M, Foa R, Maurer J, O'Brien S, Valente N, et al. Rituximab in B-Cell Hematologic Malignancies: A Review of 20 Years of Clinical Experience. *Adv Ther* (2017) 34(10):2232–73. doi: 10.1007/s12325-017-0612-x
13. Gess AJ, Silkiss RZ. Orbital B-Lymphocyte Depletion in a Treatment Failure of Rituximab for Thyroid Eye Disease. *Ophthal Plast Reconstr Surg* (2014) 30 (1):e11–3. doi: 10.1097/IOP.0b013e31828956a8
14. Anolik JH, Barnard J, Owen T, Zheng B, Kemshetti S, Looney RJ, et al. Delayed memory B cell recovery in peripheral blood and lymphoid tissue in

systemic lupus erythematosus after B cell depletion therapy. *Arthritis Rheum* (2007) 56(9):3044–56. doi: 10.1002/art.22810

15. El FD, Nielsen CH, Hasselbalch HC, Hegedus L. Treatment-resistant severe, active Graves' ophthalmopathy successfully treated with B lymphocyte depletion. *Thyroid* (2006) 16(7):709–10. doi: 10.1089/thy.2006.16.709

16. Salvi M, Vannucchi G, Campi I, Rossi S, Bonara P, Sbrozzi F, et al. Efficacy of rituximab treatment for thyroid-associated ophthalmopathy as a result of intraorbital B-cell depletion in one patient unresponsive to steroid immunosuppression. *Eur J Endocrinol* (2006) 154(4):511–7. doi: 10.1530/eje.1.02119

17. Salvi M, Vannucchi G, Beck-Peccoz P. Potential utility of rituximab for Graves' orbitopathy. *J Clin Endocrinol Metab* (2013) 98(11):4291–9. doi: 10.1210/jc.2013-1804

18. Salvi M, Vannucchi G, Curro N, Campi I, Covelli D, Dazzi D, et al. Efficacy of B-cell targeted therapy with rituximab in patients with active moderate to severe Graves' orbitopathy: a randomized controlled study. *J Clin Endocrinol Metab* (2015) 100(2):422–31. doi: 10.1210/jc.2014-3014

19. Stan MN, Garrity JA, Carranza LB, Prabin T, Bradley EA, Bahn RS. Randomized controlled trial of rituximab in patients with Graves' orbitopathy. *J Clin Endocrinol Metab* (2015) 100(2):432–41. doi: 10.1210/jc.2014-2572

20. Blandford AD, Zhang D, Chundury RV, Perry JD. Dysthyroid optic neuropathy: update on pathogenesis, diagnosis, and management. *Expert Rev Ophthal* (2017) 12(2):111–21. doi: 10.1080/17469899.2017.1276444

21. Bahn RS. Current Insights into the Pathogenesis of Graves' Ophthalmopathy. *Horm Metab Res* (2015) 47:773–8. doi: 10.1055/s-0035-1555762

22. Hegedus L, Smith TJ, Douglas RS, Nielsen CH. Targeted biological therapies for Graves' disease and thyroidassociated ophthalmopathy. Focus on B-cell depletion with Rituximab. *Clin Endocrinol* (2011) 74:1–8. doi: 10.1111/j.1365-2265.2010.03806.x

20

Selenium in the Treatment of Graves' Hyperthyroidism and Eye Disease

*Giulia Lanzolla, Michele Marinò and Claudio Marcocci**

Department of Clinical and Experimental Medicine, Endocrinology Unit II, University of Pisa and University Hospital of Pisa, Pisa, Italy

Correspondence:
Claudio Marcocci
claudio.marcocci@med.unipi.it

Based on the role of oxidative stress in the pathogenesis of Graves' hyperthyroidism (GH) and Graves' Orbitopathy (GO), a therapy with the antioxidant agent selenium has been proposed and a number of studies have been performed, both *in vitro* and *in vivo*. In GH, reactive oxygen species (ROS) contribute to the thyroid and peripheral tissues damage. In GO, tissue hypoxia, as well as ROS, are involved in the typical changes that occur in fibroadipose orbital tissue and the perimysium of extraocular muscles. Antioxidants have been proposed to improve the effects of antithyroid drugs in GH patients, as well as the remodeling of orbital tissues in patients with GO. Here, we reviewed the literature on the possible beneficial effects and clinical use of selenium in the management of patients with GH and GO. A randomized clinical trial on the use of selenium in patients with mild GO provided evidence for a beneficial effect; no data are available on more severe forms of GO. Although the real effectiveness of selenium in patients with GH remains questionable, its use in the management of mild GO is generally believed to be beneficial, and selenium administration has been included in the clinical practice for the patients with mild eye disease.

Keywords: Graves' hyperthyroidism, Graves' orbitopathy, oxidative stress, reactive oxygen species, selenium, selenocysteine, selenoproteins

INTRODUCTION

Selenium has been proposed for the management of thyroid diseases, including Graves' disease (GD), Graves' Orbitopathy (GO), and chronic autoimmune thyroiditis (1–7). The efficacy of selenium in GD and GO is based on its anti-oxidant properties, being oxidative stress involved in the pathogenesis of both conditions (8–12).

GD is an autoimmune disease with a prevalence of ~1% (13), which affects mainly the thyroid. Extrathyroidal manifestations, including GO, pretibial myxedema, and acropachy, can be observed to various extents (13–17). The major pathogenetic mechanism of GD is the stimulation of the thyroid stimulating hormone receptor (TSH-R) by autoantibodies that bind to it and promote thyrocyte proliferation and activity, resulting in thyroid hyperfunction (13). The symptoms of thyrotoxicosis are often nonspecific, so patients with GD may present in various ways. Heat intolerance, tachycardia, inappropriate feelings of anxiety and apprehension, hyperactivity and weight loss are common. A diffuse goiter can be visible or palpable, with a systolic phase bruit found over it. Systolic blood pressure may be elevated, and hepatomegaly or splenomegaly may be observed (16). The complex pathogenetic interplay of GD includes, among others, oxidative stress (16–18), because of which selenium and other antioxidant agents have been proposed for the management of Graves' hyperthyroidism (GH). In this paper we review the role of oxidative stress in GH, as well as the most significant studies on the use of selenium in the management of patients with GH and GO. The molecular mechanisms by which the disruption of the cell redox state plays a role in the pathogenesis of GO, as well as the potential beneficial effect of other antioxidant agents in patients with GO, are largely discussed in another review article in this issue of the journal.

CELL REDOX STATE AND EVALUATION OF OXIDATIVE STRESS

The balancing of the cell redox state is a key point in cellular homeostasis. Reactive oxygen species (ROS), including hydroxyl radicals (OH^-), hydrogen peroxide (H_2O_2), superoxide anions (O^2), and lipid peroxides, are molecules highly reactive because of the presence of unpaired electrons (19, 20). The increase in ROS production, as well as the decrease in their elimination, can disrupt the balance of the cell redox state, resulting in oxidative stress and breaking of cellular homeostasis (19, 20). As oxidizing agents, ROS interfere with intracellular functions, being capable of damaging various cellular elements, including cell membranes, proteins, lipids and nucleic acids, and ultimately resulting in mitochondrial dysfunction and loss of enzymatic activity (19, 20). Under physiological conditions, antioxidant agents, namely glutathione (GSH), superoxide dismutase (SOD), glutathione peroxidase (GPX) and catalase, act as ROS antagonists, therefore contributing to the maintenance of the cell redox state (21).

The oxidant/antioxidant cell balance can by evaluated by several plasma and/or erythrocyte markers (20, 21). In healthy subjects, markers of oxidative stress, as well as of the antioxidant system, are lowly represented. The induction of an oxidative stress state promotes two different reactions in the cells, depending on how long it lasts. Initially, an increase in oxidative markers is accompanied by an increase in antioxidant markers, the latter being a homeostatic response aimed at avoiding cell damage. A long-lasting state of oxidative stress is however characterized by low levels of antioxidant markers, because of exhaustion of the antioxidant cell systems (20, 21).

OXIDATIVE STRESS IN GH

Thyrotoxicosis is a hypermetabolic state characterized by high consumption of intracellular ATP and oxygen, and by dysfunction of the mitochondrial respiratory chain, which leads to saturation of the physiological antioxidant systems, resulting in an uncontrolled production of ROS in peripheral tissues as well as in the thyroid (22–25). Studies in thyrotoxic rats suggest that the oxidative stress may be involved in the pathogenesis of thyrotoxic myopathy and cardiomyopathy (26) and *in vitro* studies have shown that exposure of thyroid cell to H_2O_2, particularly when made selenium-deficient, induces DNA double strand breaks, apoptosis, necrosis and mutagenesis (24). On this basis, we might speculate that the oxidative stress might exert a dual action in patients with GH. The ROS-induced damage of thyroid epithelial cells could lead to an increased release of autoantigens and production of TSH-R autoantibodies (TRAb), and the peripheral tissue damage might contribute the clinical manifestations of hyperthyroidism.

Animal Studies

Studies in animal models suggest that thyrotoxicosis, induced by the administration of triiodothyronine (T3) or thyroxine (T4), promotes oxidative stress as well as the response of the physiological antioxidant machinery (22–25). It has been demonstrated that MDA, is significantly higher in thyrotoxic than in control and euthyroid rats (25, 26). Moreover, the oxidative stress induced by thyrotoxicosis promotes an increase in erythrocyte antioxidant parameters, namely SOD and GPX. Interestingly, the administration of Vitamin E, which has antioxidant properties, reduces MDA, SOD and GPX in hyperthyroid rats (26), and it seems also to be protective against a thyroxine-induced increase of lipid peroxidation in cardiac and skeletal muscles (27).

Human Studies

The most relevant clinical studies on the role of oxidative stress in thyroid diseases have been performed in GH patients, either with uncontrolled hyperthyroidism, or after restoration of euthyroidism with antithyroid drugs (ATD) or radioiodine (28–33). It has been reported that the levels of oxidative stress markers, including hydrogen, lipid peroxides, MDA and thiobarbituric acid-reacting substances (TBARS) in the serum, plasma and erythrocytes of hyperthyroid patients were higher than in euthyroid subjects (28–33). Moreover, a correlation between serum thyroid hormones and lipid peroxidation products was observed in hyperthyroid patients (28–33). These findings do not seem to be specific for GH, but rather for hyperthyroidism in general, having been observed also in patients with subclinical hyperthyroidism due to multinodular goiter (31). The evaluation of the antioxidant defense system in thyrotoxic patients resulted in conflicting findings (10, 28, 29, 33). Komosinska-Vassev et al. reported higher levels of SOD, CAT and GPX in the erythrocytes of GH patients than in age-matched controls. However, no differences in serum glutathione reductase (an antioxidant enzyme involved in GSH synthesis) and in the total antioxidant status were found, likely suggesting rapid exhaustion of the antioxidant system (10). Bednarek et al. reported an increase in plasma SOD and catalase in patients with GH of short duration (1–2 months) compared with healthy subjects, but not of GPX and glutathione reductase, which were, conversely, decreased (29). On the contrary, Aslan et al. reported a significant reduction of the total antioxidant activity in 36 hyperthyroid patients with an average duration of hyperthyroidism of 2.3 ± 1.5 months compared with controls

(33). Finally, a study involving 69 GD patients with hyperthyroidism lasting more than 6 months showed decreased levels of erythrocyte SOD and catalase activities compared with controls, with no difference in erythrocyte GPX and total antioxidant activities (28). The duration of the hyperthyroid status at the time of the evaluation can explain, at least in part, the conflicting data on antioxidant activity in patients with GD. Probably, patients with hyperthyroidism of longer duration have exhausted the antioxidant defense system, which leads to the reduction of the antioxidant capacity (34, 35). It has been also reported that the monoclonal thyroid stimulating antibody M22 as well as polyclonal serum thyroid stimulating antibodies (TSAbs) from patients with GH, promote ROS generation and lipid peroxidation in HEK cells that stably overexpressed the human TSHR (HEK-293 TSHR) (36). ATD reduce the levels of oxidative stress markers, thereby improving the activity of the intra- and extracellular antioxidant defense systems, due to restoration of euthyroidism and possibly to their antioxidant properties (28–30, 32). As discussed in another review on the same issue of this journal, oxidative stress also plays a role in GO, and the beneficial effect of antioxidant agents are supported by *in vitro* and human studies (1–6, 11, 37–46).

SELENIUM

Selenium is a trace mineral which acts following incorporation as selenocysteine into selenoproteins, among which thioredoxin reductases (TRs), GPX, and iodothyronine deiodinases (D1, D2 or D3) are the best known (3–5, 47). In this regard, D1-3 are homologous proteins consisting of 250-300 amino acids, with a single transmembrane domain located at the N-terminus. They are involved in the reductive deiodination of thyroid hormones. The most remarkable feature of all three deiodinases is the presence of a selenocysteine residue in the center of the amino acid sequence. D1, encoded by DIO1 gene, is predominantly expressed in the liver, kidney and thyroid. It catalyzes the outer and inner ring deiodination of iodothyronine derivatives, with a preference for reverse T3 (rT3) and iodothyronine sulfates. D2, encoded by DIO2 gene, is primarily expressed in the thyroid, brain, anterior pituitary and brown adipose tissue, where contributes local conversion of T4 in T3. Moreover, the pituitary enzyme is involved in the negative feedback regulation of TSH and TRH secretion. The DIO3 gene codes for D3, which is detected in brain, skin, liver, intestine, placenta and pregnant uterus, where it catalyzes the inactivation of T4 and T3. Since D1-3 are selenoproteins, selenium deficiency would be expected to result in their reduced activities in different tissues, although this effect is observed only for D1 in the liver and kidney and not for D2 and D3 in other tissues (48).

Selenoproteins have antioxidant and enzymatic capacity (47) and, in the thyroid, where they are highly expressed, influence the balance of the cell reduction-oxidation activities (49). Furthermore, selenoproteins are essential for activated T-cell function, being involved in the proliferation of T-cells in response to T-cell receptor stimulation. It has been also reported that selenium supplementation promotes differentiation of CD4+ T cells into T-helper-1 (Th1) rather than T-helper-2 (Th2) effector. Among the immunomodulating functions, selenoproteins increased cytotoxic lymphocyte-mediated tumour cytotoxicity and natural killer activity (50). It has been also reported that selenium may regulate the inflammatory response by reducing the release of tumor necrosis factor α (TNFα) and cyclooxygenase (COX2), as well as the activation of nuclear factor κB (NF-κB) which is one of the transcriptional factors involved in the immune and pro-inflammatory response. Elevated selenium levels increase GPX, which inhibits IκB-α phosphorylation and consequently the translocation of NF-κB (51).

Dietary sources of selenium include meat, seafood, shellfish, offal, eggs and cereals (47, 49). The bioavailability of selenium varies depending on the type of food and content in the soil for growing crops and fodder. Furthermore, additional factors, such as selenium speciation, soil pH or the presence of ions complexed with selenium, play a role in the bioavailability of the mineral (47). Selenium dietary intake is followed by absorption in the gastrointestinal tract and transport to the liver, where it is incorporated into selenoglycoproteins containing up to 10 selenium residues per molecule. Selenoglycoproteins finally reach peripheral tissues, where their concentration is proportional to the degree of oxidative stress (47–50).

The measurement of total serum selenium concentration or circulating selenoproteins, including GPX-3 and selenoprotein P, can be used to evaluate the selenium status, which is variable depending on the geographical area, being high in North America and relatively low in most European countries, in particular in the Eastern Europe (50–52). The Office of Dietary Supplements has established that the recommended daily allowance (RDA) is 55 µg in men and women. Selenium intake in several European countries is lower than in the USA, because of its lower content in the soil. Values range from around 30 µg in UK, Germany, Sweden and Slovakia to around 70 in Netherlands and Switzerland (47, 50). To properly interpret these data, we need to have appropriate standards against which to compare them. There is no consensus on this issue. The UK reference nutrient intake of 75 µg per day in men and 60 in women has been determined as the amount needed to maximize the activity of the GPX in plasma (which occurs at a selenium concentration of about 95 µg/L). Current UK intake are about half the value. On the other hand, selenium excess has been suggested to increase the risk of type 2 diabetes and of malignancies (50, 52). However, the issue is still matter of debate and no adverse events for selenium doses not exceeding 200 µg/day were reported by a number of studies, including one in which relatively high levels of selenium were reached with supplementation (~190 µg/L after 90 days of treatment) (3, 50). It is therefore possible that selenium might lead to subclinical alterations, for example on glucose metabolism, in selected patients, with no real clinical impact (1, 4, 53, 54).

In this regard, several trials have shown a benefit of selenium supplementation on the risk of cancer incidence and death, as well as the risk of developing hyperglycemia. However, two large trials performed in USA have shown that these benefits are no longer seen in patients whose baseline serum selenium concentration was above 122 μg/L, in whom, conversely, these risks were increased. On this basis, Rayman proposed that 122 μg/L represents the concentration of baseline serum selenium that "delineates a change in risk, from lower to higher, of developing cancer and type 2 diabetes in patients treated with selenium supplementation of 200 μg per day" (50). This observation may be relevant for individuals living in countries, like the USA, where a large proportion of people has a serum selenium concentration above this cut-off. Therefore, it has been proposed to measure serum selenium concentrations before administering the supplement, in order to avoid overdosage in subjects with baseline serum concentrations higher than 122 μg/L (53). In our opinion, the measurement of serum selenium before supplementation might be useful in individual living in countries with high selenium intake, like the USA, to avoid the risk of potential disadvantages, but not individuals living in countries, like most European countries, where dietary selenium intake is low and high concentrations of serum selenium are very unlikely to be achieved with supplementation.

Selenium supplements contain sodium selenite or selenomethionine, and the main difference between them is that, after saturation of selenoproteins, selenite is excreted whereas selenomethionine can further increase serum selenium through its incorporation into proteins (1, 4). Consequently, the effect of selenite is strictly linked to the individual state of selenium, whereas using selenomethionine as a supplement, the concentration of plasma selenium increases also in subjects with a sufficient selenium concentration to begin with.

USE OF SELENIUM IN GH

Based on the above described role of oxidative stress in GH and the antioxidant activity of selenium, clinical studies were performed to investigate its effect in GH patients. The hypothesis is that selenium deficiency could enhance oxidative stress in thyrotoxicosis, by worsening the antioxidant machinery in response to ROS. To address this issue, a number of studies have tested selenium, either alone or within a mixture containing other antioxidant agents, in GH patients treated with ATD (2, 3, 55–57) (**Table 1**). These investigations did not provide clear-cut results. Vrca et al. performed a study in Croatia, an area characterized by moderate selenium deficiency, randomizing GH patients to therapy with methimazole (MMI) plus an antioxidant mixture containing β-carotene, Vitamin C and Vitamin E and a relatively low dose of selenium (60 μg), or MMI alone (55). The main difference between the two groups was that euthyroidism was more rapidly reached in the former group, likely reducing the period of exposure to oxidative stress. Moreover, a better response to treatment in terms of improvement of LDL-cholesterol levels was found in patients treated with the antioxidant mixture compared with those given MMI alone (55). Similar date on thyroid function were reported by Guerra et al. in patients given a mixture containing low doses of selenium (15 μg/day), compared to MMI alone (57).

Three studies were performed using "pure" selenium rather than a mixture of antioxidants (2, 3, 56) (**Table 1**). In one of these studies (56), hyperthyroid, selenium-deficient patients were randomized to receive a block-and-replace regimen (MMI plus levothyroxine), plus 200 μg/day of selenium or placebo. A slightly better control of hyperthyroidism was observed in the selenium group (56). Two additional randomized clinical trials performed in GH patients treated with MMI alone did not show beneficial effects on thyroid function and peripheral manifestations of hyperthyroidism in patients given selenium compared with placebo (2, 3). The conflicting results between the first study and the subsequent two can be explained, at least in part, by the different levels of baseline selenium, which was insufficient only in the first one. These findings support the main hypothesis of a role of ROS in GH, which might be relevant especially in patients with selenium deficiency. Thus, a supplementation with selenium can be considered in these cases, whereas, in our opinion, there is no sufficient evidence to recommend the routine addition of selenium to ATD in the management of all patients with GH.

USE OF SELENIUM IN GO

Over the last few years, in addition to the most common treatment for the management of moderate-to-severe and active GO, namely high dose oral and intravenous glucocorticoids (GC), orbital irradiation and surgical procedures (58), other medications have been proven effective to various extents, including rituximab (59), the recently FDA-approved teprotumumab (60, 61), mycophenolate (62), and tocilizumab (63). Until recently, the treatment of mild GO was typically limited to local measures (19 but ~15% of patients GO progress to an extent that requires specific treatments (13, 58). In general, major treatments are not recommended for mild GO, unless there is a sufficient impairment in the quality of life, which justifies the risk of GC-related adverse events (58, 64–66). In view of the role of oxidative stress in GO, antioxidant supplements have been proposed as a possible therapeutic approach, and basic and clinical studies have investigated the effect of selenium, due to its antioxidant and immunomodulating actions.

In Vitro Studies

A couple of *in vitro* studies have provided evidence for a beneficial effect of selenium in primary cultures of orbital fibroblasts (OFs) (38, 65, 66) (**Table 2**). In a first study (38), after induction of oxidative stress by treating OFs with H_2O_2, GPX activity, glutathione disulfide (GSSG), cell proliferation, HA and pro-inflammatory cytokines were measured, in the presence or absence of selenium-(Methyl)-selenocysteine (SeMCys). H_2O_2 induced oxidative stress in OFs, reflected by a dose-dependent increase in GSSG, a known measure of cell response to ROS (**Figure 1**). SeMCys reduced the effects of H_2O_2, providing evidence for an antioxidant action of selenium in OFs. The effect of selenium was observed in OFs from both GO patients and control subjects, which should not be seen as a limitation for its clinical use. Thus, in the same study the authors reported that proliferation of OFs, as well as the production of HA, were significantly greater in GO than in control fibroblasts. Moreover, SeMCys significantly reduced cell proliferation and hyaluronic acid (HA) release in GO OFs, whereas no effects were observed in control OFs (38). These findings might suggest that fibroblasts from GO patients are somehow different, leading to a different response to oxidative stress and selenium activity.

In a subsequent study, the same authors reported a dual effect of H_2O_2 on cell proliferation, depending on dose used (67). At low concentrations, H_2O_2 promoted cell proliferation, whereas at high concentration progressively decreased cell vitality and cell proliferation. The effects of both high and low dose H_2O_2 were inhibited by SeMCys which, interestingly,

TABLE 1 | Selenium in Graves' Hyperthyroidism (GH).

Reference	Journal and years	Type of study	Methods	Dosage of compounds used	Results
Vrca VB. et al. (53)	Acta Pharm. 2012	Prospective, placebo-controlled, clinical trial	Fifty-five patients with newly diagnosed GH were randomized to receive methimazole alone or methimazole plus a fixed combination of antioxidant agents	The mixture of antioxidants contained: **β-carotene** (6 mg), **selenium** (60 µg), **vitamins C** (200 mg) **and E** (36 mg)	**Beneficial effect on GH** Better and faster normalization of thyroid function was observed in patients with GH treated with methimazole plus the mixture of antioxidant agents compared with control group. In addition, a better response to treatment, in terms of improvement of LDL-cholesterol levels, was found in patients treated with the antioxidant mixture compared with those given methimazole alone
Calissendorff J. et al. (2)	Eur Thyroid J 2015	Prospective, placebo-controlled, clinical trial	Thirty-eight consecutive patients with newly diagnosed and untreated GH were randomized to receive "block and replace" treatment with methimazole and levothyroxine, plus Selenium or alone for 9 months	**Selenium** (200 µg daily orally)	**Beneficial effect on GH** Patients treated with selenium had a better control of hyperthyroidism: at 18 weeks, the serum levels of FT4 were lower in the selenium group compared to the placebo (14 vs. 17 pmol/l group, p = 0.01). Similar results were observed also at 36 weeks (15 vs. 18 pmol/l, p = 0.01). In accordance, the TSH levels increased more in the selenium group at 18 weeks (0.05 vs. 0.02 mIU/l, p = 0.04)
Leo M. et al. (3)	J Endocrinol Invest 2017	Prospective, placebo-controlled, clinical trial	Thirty consecutive patients with untreated GH were randomized to receive Methimazole plus Selenium vs methimazole alone for 3 months	**L-seleno-methionine** (166 µg daily orally)	**No beneficial effect on GH**. Administration of Methimazole leads to the normalization of FT3 and FT4, with no difference between groups. Serum levels of malondialdehyde, a marker of oxidative stress, was similarly high in the two groups and decreased significantly after therapy, with no difference between groups. The results suggested that selenium had not significant effect on short-term control of hyperthyroidism
Kahaly GJ. et al. (54)	J Clin Endocrinol Metab. 2017	Prospective, placebo-controlled, clinical trial	Sixty-one consecutive patients with untreated GH were randomized to receive Methimazole plus Selenium or methimazole alone for 6 months	**Sodium selenite** (300 µg daily orally)	**No beneficial effect on GH.** The response to treatment, in terms of thyroid function normalization of thyroid hormones, was very similar in the two groups at week 24. During a 12-week follow-up, GH relapsed in 48% of patients included in the selenium group and in 44% of patients of the placebo group. Serum concentrations of Selenium and selenoprotein P were unrelated to response or recurrence rates. At week 36, 12 of 29 patients (41%) and 15 of 33 patients (45%) were responders and still in remission in the selenium and placebo groups, respectively.

TABLE 2 | Selenium in Graves' Orbitopathy (GO).

Reference	Journal and years	Type of study	Methods	Dosage of compounds used	Results
Rotondo Dottore G. et al. (65)	Thyroid 2016	*In vitro* study	Primary cultures of orbital fibroblasts from 6 GO patients and 6 control subjects were obtained. To induce oxidative stress, cells were incubated for 24 h with medium containing H_2O_2 at various concentrations. The primary objective was to assess the effects of selenium in GO fibroblasts.	Cells were pre-incubated for 2 days with medium without compounds or containing **Se-methyl-selenocysteine hydrochloride (SeMCys)** or, as control, **methyl-cysteine** at various concentrations. Cell proliferation, hyaluronic acid (HA) and pro-inflammatory cytokines production were measured	**Selenium reduced proliferation and release of HA and cytokines in GO fibroblasts.** H_2O_2 promoted an increased release of glutathione disulfide (GSSG), a marker of oxidative stress, and of fibroblast proliferation, which were reduced by selenium. H_2O_2 promoted the production of cytokines involved in GO pathogenesis, namely TNF-α, IL1-β and IFN-γ. The increase in TNF-α and IFN-γ was rescued by selenium. Whereas the effects of selenium were similar in GO and control fibroblasts concerning oxidative stress and cytokines, they were exclusive to GO fibroblasts concerning proliferation and HA production.
Rotondo Dottore G. et al. (66)	Endocrine. 2017		Primary cultures of orbital fibroblasts from 6 patients with long lasting inactive GO and 6 control subjects were obtained. To induce oxidative stress, cells were incubated for 90 min at 37°C with medium containing H_2O_2 50 μM. The aim of the study was to evaluate the effects of selenium in GO fibroblasts.	Cells were preincubated for 2 days at 37°C with medium without compounds containing **SeMCys** or, as control, **methyl-cysteine** (MCys) at a 10 μM concentration. Cell vitality, lactate dehydrogenase production (as a measure of cell necrosis) and apoptosis were measured	**Selenium reduced cell damage in GO fibroblasts** SeMCys rescued from H_2O_2-dependent cytotoxicity, by reducing necrosis and apoptosis, with no difference between GO and control fibroblasts. MCys had no effect. To determine whether the findings reflected the antioxidant actions of selenium, the assessment of GSSG was performed. H_2O_2 promoted the increased production of GSSG, which was counteracted by SeMCys, but not by MCys, with no differences between GO and control fibroblasts.
Marcocci C. et al. (4)	N Engl J Med 2011	Prospective, multicenter, placebo-controlled clinical trial	One hundred fifty-nine patients with mild GO were randomized to receive sodium selenite or compared with placebo for 6 months	**Sodium selenite** (100 μg twice daily orally), or **pentoxifylline** (600 mg twice daily orally)	**Beneficial effect of selenium in mild GO.** Compared with placebo, Selenium, but not pentoxifylline, leads to the improvement of quality of life ($P < 0.001$), eye overall outcome ($P = 0.01$) and slowed the progression of GO ($P = 0.01$), at the 6 months evaluation.

inhibited HA synthesis in GO, but not in control fibroblasts, even though H_2O_2 did not affect HA release (67). This observation suggests that selenium may influence HA release, at least in part, regardless of the oxidative stress induced by H_2O_2, through mechanisms that are still to be clarified. Furthermore, a reduction in the release of pro-inflammatory cytokines induced by low dose H_2O_2, namely interferon-γ (IFNγ) and TNFα, was found in both GO and control OFs treated with SeMCys (67, 68), contributing the beneficial effects of selenium in GO OFs.

Clinical Studies

The first clinical, pilot study on antioxidants, showed an improvement of GO soft tissue involvement in patients treated with an antioxidant mixture containing allopurinol plus nicotinamide, compared with those given placebo (54). After these promising results, the European Group on Graves' Orbitopathy (EUGOGO) performed a randomized, placebo-controlled, multicenter, clinical trial in European countries known to have marginal selenium-deficiency, to investigate the effect of selenium and pentoxifylline in mild GO (4). One hundred and fifty-nine patients with mild GO were randomized to receive sodium selenite (100 mcg twice/day, equivalent to 91.3 μg of selenium), pentoxifylline (600 mg twice/day), or placebo (twice/day) for 6 months, followed by a follow-up period of 6 months. The overall eye outcome—assessed at the end of treatment by a change in a composite score including exophthalmometry, clinical activity score (CAS), measurement of eyelid aperture, diplopia and visual acuity—as well as the quality of life were significantly better in the selenium group. GO improved in 61% of patients treated with selenium and in 36% of patients receiving placebo, whereas the eye disease worsened in 7 and 26% of patients in the selenium and placebo group, respectively (**Figure 2**). The effect of pentoxifylline was not relevant compared to placebo. Similarly, at 6 months, the scores of the quality of life of GO

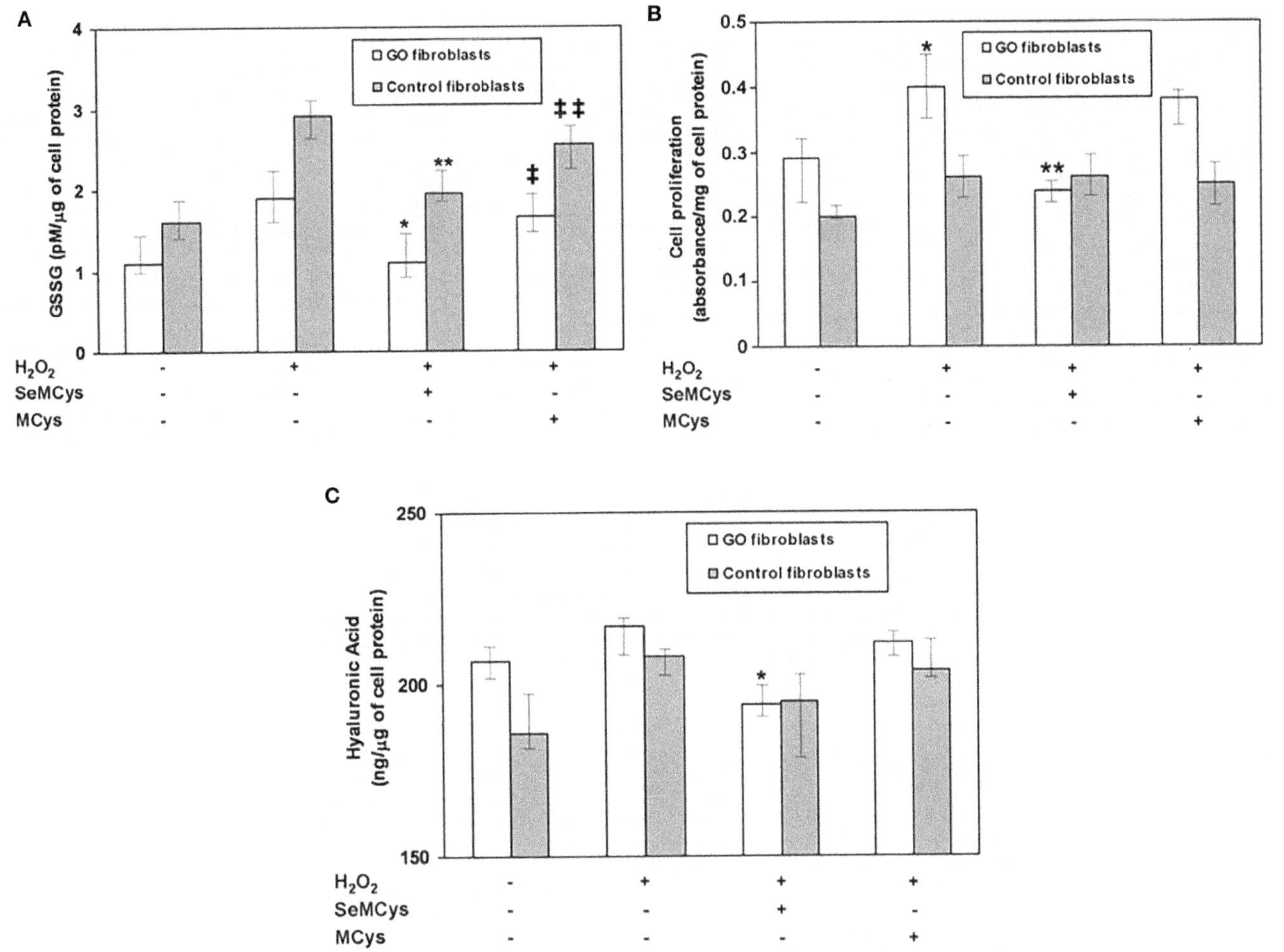

FIGURE 1 | (A) Effect of selenium (10 µMol) or of the negative control methylcysteine (MCys) (10 µMol) on Glutathione disulfide (GSSG), released after treatment with H_2O_2 (5 µMol), in fibroblasts from patients with Graves' orbitopathy (GO fibroblasts) or from control patients. P* and **P = 0.02 vs H_2O_2; ‡ and ‡‡ P = NS vs H_2O_2; P = NS between GO and control fibroblasts; **(B)** Effect of selenium (10 µMol) or methylcysteine (MCys) (10 µMol) on cell proliferation, induced by H_2O_2 treatment (5 µMol), in GO and control fibroblasts. *P = 0.02 vs untreated cells; **P = 0.02 vs H_2O_2; P = 0.003 between GO and control fibroblasts; **(C)** Effect of selenium (10 µMol) or methylcysteine (MCys) (10 µMol) on hyaluronic acid (HA) release in GO and control fibroblasts. *P = 0.02 vs H_2O_2; P = 0.02 between Graves' Orbitopathy and control fibroblasts.

(GO-QOL) increased from baseline by 6 or more points for visual functioning in 33 patients (62%) and for appearance in 40 patients (75%). Interestingly, the majority of selenium-treated patients who had a positive change in eyelid aperture, soft tissue involvement, or both, also had an improvement of 6 points or more on the appearance subscale of GO-QOL [84%; 95% confidence interval (CI), 67 to 95] and on visual functioning subscale (72%; 95% CI, 53 to 86), as well as in the overall score (81%; 95% CI 63 to 93). The GO improvement following treatment with selenium was maintained also at 12 months, suggesting that the beneficial effect of selenium is persistent after treatment withdrawal. A limit of this study is that neither baseline not end of treatment selenium concentrations were not measured. Therefore, it remains unclear whether correction of selenium deficiency accounted for the beneficial effects of selenium administration.

CONCLUSIONS

The redox state is a key point in cellular homeostasis and its unbalance leads to the disruption of intracellular reactions, thereby damaging cell structures. Oxidative stress plays an important role in both GH and GO but the question of whether the use of selenium in the management of patients with GH and GO can be truly effective is still to be clarified. Studies performed so far regarding the use of antioxidant agents, especially as

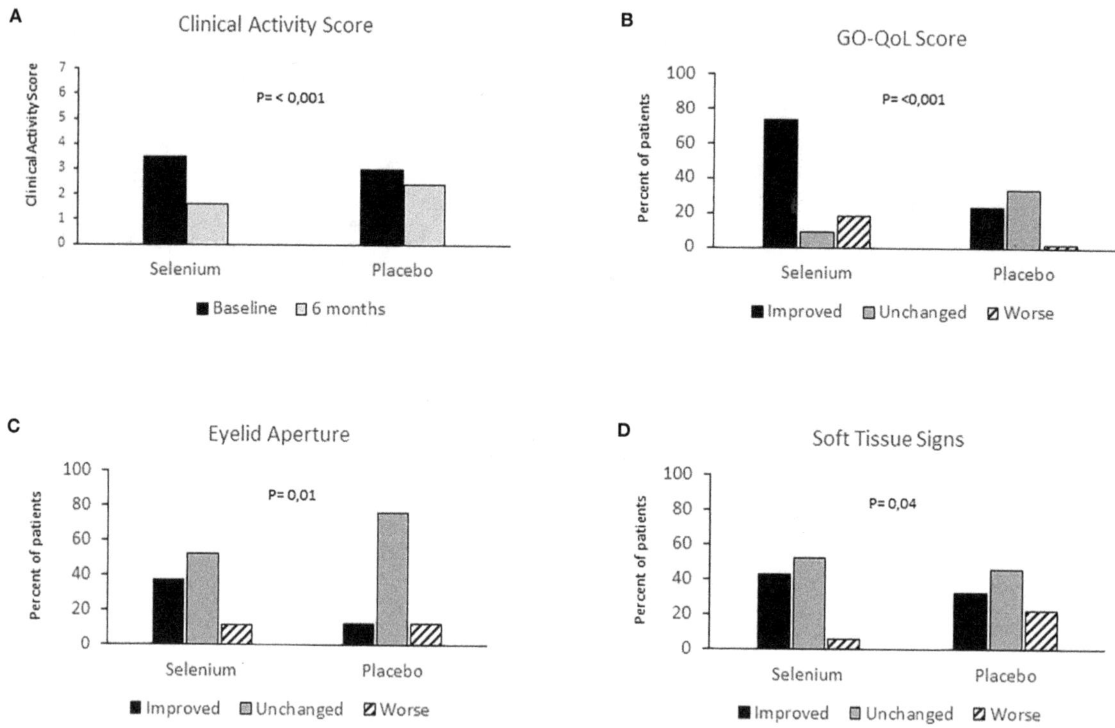

FIGURE 2 | **(A)** Clinical Activity Score (CAS) evaluation at baseline and 6 months in patients with mild Graves' Orbitopathy treated with selenium or placebo; **(B)** Graves' orbitopathy-specific quality-of-life questionnaire (GO-QOL) at baseline and 6 months in patients with mild Graves' Orbitopathy treated with selenium, placebo or Pentoxifylline; **(C)** Eyelid aperture at baseline and 6 months in patients with mild Graves' Orbitopathy treated with selenium, placebo or Pentoxifylline; **(D)** Soft tissue signs at baseline and 6 months in patients with mild Graves' Orbitopathy treated with selenium, placebo or Pentoxifylline. Redrawn from the Engl J Med 2011; 364: 1920-1931.

selenium, provided conflicting results on the possibility of a new therapeutic approach. The real effectiveness of selenium in patients with GH is very dubious and at this moment there is not enough evidence to use it. Current evidence on selenium supplementation in patients with mild GO provided promising results, suggesting that selenium may improve the quality of life and the course of GO and opening to the possibility of its clinical use. It is also possible that selenium may have beneficial effects in moderate-to-severe GO, especially when patients are selenium-deficient. The action of selenium for the long-term outcome remains to be well cleared. Further clinical studies are needed to define these issues.

AUTHOR CONTRIBUTIONS

GL wrote the manuscript. CM and MM contributed to the conception of the manuscript and revised the paper critically. All authors contributed to the article and approved the submitted version.

REFERENCES

1. Hegedüs L, Bonnema SJ, Winther KH. Selenium in the Treatment of Thyroid Diseases: An Element in Search of the Relevant Indications? *Eur Thyroid J* (2016) 5:149–51. doi: 10.1159/000448002
2. Calissendorff J, Mikulski E, Larsen EH, Möller M. A Prospective Investigation of Graves' Disease and Selenium: Thyroid Hormones, Auto-Antibodies and Self-Rated Symptoms. *Eur Thyroid J* (2015) 2:93–8. doi: 10.1159/000381768
3. Leo M, Bartalena L, Rotondo Dottore G, Piantanida E, Premoli P, Ionni I, et al. Effects of selenium on short-term control of hyperthyroidism due to Graves' disease treated with methimazole: Results of a randomized clinical trial. *J Endocrinol Invest* (2017) 40:281–7. doi: 10.1007/s40618-016-0559-9
4. Marcocci C, Kahaly GJ, Krassas GE, Bartalena L, Prummel M, Stahl M, et al. European Group on Graves' Orbitopathy. Selenium and the Course of Mild Graves' Orbitopathy. *N Engl J Med* (2011) 364:1920–31. doi: 10.1056/NEJMoa1012985
5. Köhrle J. Selenium and the thyroid. *Curr Opin Endocrinol Diabetes Obes* (2015) 22:392–401. doi: 10.1097/MED.0000000000000190
6. Esposito D, Rotondi M, Accardo G, Vallone G, Conzo G, Docimo G, et al. Influence of short-term selenium supplementation on the natural course of Hashimoto's thyroiditis: Clinical results of a blinded placebo-controlled randomized prospective trial. *J Endocrinol Invest* (2017) 40:83–9. doi: 10.1007/s40618-016-0535-4
7. De Farias CR, Cardoso BR, de Oliveira GM, de Mello Guazzelli IC, Catarino RM, Chammas MC, et al. A randomized-controlled, double-blind study of the impact of selenium supplementation on thyroid autoimmunity and inflammation with focus on the GPx1 genotypes. *J Endocrinol Invest* (2015) 38:1065–74. doi: 10.1007/s40618-015-0285-8
8. Leporati P, Groppelli G, Zerbini F, Rotondi M, Chiovato L. Etiopathogenesis of Basedow's disease. Trends and current aspects. *Nuklearmedizin* (2015) 54:204–10. doi: 10.3413/Nukmed-0739-15-04

9. Marinò M, Latrofa F, Menconi F, Chiovato L, Vitti P. Role of genetic and non-genetic factors in the etiology of Graves' disease. *J Endocrinol Invest* (2015) 38:283–94. doi: 10.1007/s40618-014-0214-2
10. Komosinska-Vassev K, Olczyk K, Kucharz EJ, Marcisz C, Winsz-Szczotka K, Kotulska A. Free radical activity and antioxidant defense mechanisms in patients with hyperthyroidism due to Graves' disease during therapy. *Clin Chim Acta* (2000) 300:7–117. doi: 10.1016/S0009-8981(00)00306-5
11. Duntas LH, Boutsiadis A, Tsakris A. Impaired Metabolism of Selenomethionine in Graves' Disease: A Biokinetics Study of Soft Gel Capsule Formulation. *Horm Metab Res* (2017) 49:589–94. doi: 10.1055/s-0043-113573
12. Wilson R, Chopra M, Bradley H, McKillop JH, Smith WE, Thomson JA. Free radicals and Graves' disease: the effects of therapy. *Clin Endocrinol (Oxf)* (1989) 30:429–33. doi: 10.1111/j.1365-2265.1989.tb00442.x
13. Smith TJ, Hegedus L. Graves' Disease. *N Engl J Med* (2016) 375:1552–65. doi: 10.1056/NEJMra1510030
14. Menconi F, Marcocci C, Marinò M. Diagnosis and classification of Graves' disease. *Autoimmun Rev* (2014) 13:398–402. doi: 10.1016/j.autrev.2014.01.013
15. Bartalena L, Fatourechi V. Extrathyroidal manifestations of Graves' disease: a 2014 update. *J Endocrinol Invest* (2014) 37:691–700. doi: 10.1007/s40618-014-0097-2
16. Papi G, Corsello MS, Pontecorvi A. Clinical concepts on thyroid emergencies. *Front Endocrinol* (2014) 5. article 102. doi: 10.3389/fendo.2014.00102
17. Marinò M, Latrofa F, Menconi F, Chiovato L, Vitti P. An update on the medical treatment of Graves' hyperthyroidism. *J Endocrinol Invest* (2014) 37:1041–8. doi: 10.1007/s40618-014-0136-z
18. Lanzolla G, Vannucchi G, Ionni I, Campi I, Sikahaly F, Lazzaroni E, et al. Cholesterol serum levels and use of statins in Graves' Orbitopathy: A new starting point for the therapy. *Front Endocrinol* (2020) 10:933. doi: 10.3389/fendo.2019.00933
19. Halliwell B, Gutteridge JM. Lipid peroxidation, oxigen radicals, cell damage, and antioxidante therapy. *Lancet* (1984) 1:1396–7. doi: 10.1016/S0140-6736(84)91886-5
20. Valko M, Leibfritz D, Moncol J. Cronin MT, Mazur M, Telser J. Free radicals and antioxidants in normal physiological function and human disease. *Int J Biochem Cell Biol* (2007) 39:44–84. doi: 10.1016/j.biocel.2006.07.001
21. Halliwell B, Gutteridge JMC. Cellular responses to oxidative stress: adaption, damage, repair, senescence and death. *Free Radicals Biol Med* (2007) 376 (18):1748–61. doi: 10.1056/NEJMoa1614949
22. Venditti P, Balestrini M, Di Meo S, De Leo T. Effect of thyroid state on lipid peroxidation, antioxidant defenses, and susceptibility to oxidative stress in rat tissues. *J Endocrinol* (1997) 155:151–7. doi: 10.1677/joe.0.1550151
23. Yamada T, Mishima T, Sakamoto M, Sugiyama M, Matsunaga S, Wada M. Oxidation of myosin heavy chain and reduction in force production in hyperthyroid rat soleus. *J Appl Physiol* (2006) 100:1520–6. doi: 10.1152/japplphysiol.01456.2005
24. Miot F, Van Sande J, Many MC, Dumont JE. Roles of hydrogen peroxide in thyroid physiology and disease. *J Clin Endocrinol Metab* (2007) 92:3764–73. doi: 10.1210/jc.2007-0660
25. Asayama K, Dobashi H, Hayashibe H, Megata Y, Kato K. Lipid peroxidation and free radical scavengers in thyroid dysfunction in the rat: a possible mechanism of injury to hearth and skeletal muscle in hyperthyroidism. *Endocrinology* (1987) 121:2112–8. doi: 10.1210/endo-121-6-2112
26. Chehade J, Kim J, Pinas JL, Mooradian AD. Age-related changes in the thyroid hormone effects on malondialdehyde modified proteins in the rat heart. *Proc Soc Exp Biol Med* (1999) 222:59–64. doi: 10.1111/j.1525-1373.1999.09995.x
27. Asayama K, Dobashi K, Hayashibe H, Kato K. Vitamin E protects against thyroxine-induced acceleration of lipid peroxidation in cardiac and skeletal muscles in rats. *J Nutr Sci Vitaminol (Tokyo)* (1989) 35:407–18. doi: 10.3177/jnsv.35.407
28. Abalovich M, Llesuy S, Gutierrez S, Repetto M. Peripheral parameters of oxidative stress in Graves disease: the effect of methimazole and 131 I iodine treatment. *Clin Endocrinol (Oxf)* (2003) 59:321–7. doi: 10.1046/j.1365-2265.2003.01850.x
29. Bednarek J, Wysocki H, Sowiński J. Oxidative stress peripheral parameters in Graves' disease: the effect of methimazole treatment in patients with and without infiltrative ophthalmopathy. *Clin Biochem* (2005) 38:13–8. doi: 10.1016/j.clinbiochem.2004.09.015
30. Rybus-Kalinowska B, Zwirska-Korczala K, Kalinowski M, Kukla M, Birkner E, Jochem J. Activity of antioxidative enzymes and concentration of malondialdehyde as oxidative status markers in women with newly diagnosed Graves-Basedow disease and after thiamazole therapy leading to euthyroidism. *Pol Arch Med Wewn* (2008) 118:420–5. doi: 10.20452/pamw.438
31. Cetinkaya A, Kurutas EB, Buyukbese MA, Kantarceken B, Bulbuloglu E. Levels of malondialdehyde and superoxide dismutase in subclinical hyperthyroidism. *Mediators Inflammation* (2005) 59(3):321–7. doi: 10.1155/MI.2005.57
32. Weetman AP. Effect of the anti-thyroid drug methimazole on interleukin-1 and interleukin- 2 levels in vitro. *Clin Endocrinol (Oxf)* (1986) 25:133–42. doi: 10.1111/j.1365-2265.1986.tb01674.x
33. Aslan M, Cosar N, Celik H, Aksoy N, Dulger AC, Begenik H, et al. Evaluation of oxidative status in patients with hyperthyroidism. *Endocrine* (2011) 40:285–29. doi: 10.1007/s12020-011-9472-3
34. Bartalena L, Tanda ML, Piantanida E, Lai A. Oxidative stress and Graves' ophthalmopathy: in vitro studies and therapeutic implications. *Biofactors* (2003) 19:155–63. doi: 10.1002/biof.5520190308
35. Marcocci C, Leo M, Altea MA. Oxidative stress in Graves' disease. *Eur Thyroid J* (2012) 2:80–7. doi: 10.1159/000337976
36. Diana T, Daiber A, Oelze M, Neumann S, Olivo PD, Kanitz M, et al. Stimulatory TSH-Receptor antibodies and oxidative stress in Graves' Disease. *JCEM* (2018) 103:3668–77. doi: 10.1210/jc.2018-00509
37. Heufelder AE, Wenzel BE, Bahn RS. Methimazole and propylthiouracil inhibit the oxygen free radical-induced expression of a 72 kilodalton heat shock protein in Graves' retroocular fibroblasts. *J Clin Endocrinol Metab* (1992) 74:737–42. doi: 10.1002/biof.5520190308
38. Rotondo Dottore G, Leo M, Casini G, Latrofa F, Cestari L, Sellari-Franceschini S, et al. Anti-oxidant actions of selenium in orbital fibroblasts: a basis for the effects of selenium in Graves' orbitopathy. *Thyroid* (2016) 27:271–8. doi: 10.1089/thy.2016.0397
39. Burch HB, Lahiri S, Bahn RS, Barnes S. Superoxide radical production stimulates retroocular fibroblast proliferation in Graves' ophthalmopathy. *Exp Eye Res* (1997) 65:311–6. doi: 10.1006/exer.1997.0353
40. Lu R, Wang P, Wartofsky L, Sutton BD, Zweier JL, Bahn RS, et al. Oxygen free radicals in interleukin-1beta-induced glycosaminoglycan production by retro-ocular fibroblasts from normal subjects and Graves' ophthalmopathy patients. *Thyroid* (1999) 9:297–303. doi: 10.1089/thy.1999.9.297
41. Hondur A, Konuk O, Dincel AS, Bilgihan A, Unal M, Hasanreisoglu B. Oxidative stress and antioxidant activity in orbital fibroadipose tissue in Graves' ophthalmopathy. *Curr Eye Res* (2008) 33:421–7. doi: 10.1080/02713680802123532
42. Tsai CC, Wu SB, Cheng CY, Kao SC, Kau HC, Chiou SH, et al. Increased oxidative DNA damage, lipid peroxidation, and reactive oxygen species in cultured orbital fibroblasts from patients with Graves' ophthalmopathy: evidence that oxidative stress has a role in this disorder. *Eye (Lond)* (2010) 24:1520–5. doi: 10.1038/eye.2010.31
43. Tsai CC, Wu SB, Cheng CY, Kao SC, Kau HC, Lee SM, et al. Increased response to oxidative stress challenge in Graves' ophthalmopathy orbital fibroblasts. *Mol Vis* (2011) 17:2782–8. doi: 10.1006/exer.1997.0353
44. Tsai CC, Kao SC, Cheng CY, Kau HC, Hsu WM, Lee CF, et al. Oxidative stress change by systemic corticosteroid treatment among patients having active graves ophthalmopathy. *Arch Ophthalmol* (2007) 125:1652–6. doi: 10.1001/archopht.125.12.1652
45. Wiersinga WM. Smoking and thyroid. *Clin Endocrinol (Oxf)* (2013) 79:145–51. doi: 10.1111/cen.12222
46. Akarsu E, Buyukhatipoglu H, Aktaran S, Kurtul N. Effects of pulse methylprednisolone and oral methylprednisolone treatments on serum levels of oxidative stress markers in Graves' ophthalmopathy. *Clin Endocrinol (Oxf)* (2011) 74:118–24. doi: 10.1111/j.1365-2265.2010.03904.x
47. Rayman MP. The importance of selenium to human health. *Lancet* (2000) 356:233–41. doi: 10.1016/S0140-6736(00)02490-9
48. Visser TJ. Regulation of thyroid function, synthesis, and function of thyroid hormones. *Thyroid Dis* (2018) 125(12):1652–6. doi: 10.1007/978-3-319-45013-1_1
49. Drutel A, Archambeaud F, Caron P. Selenium and the thyroid gland. *Clin Endocrinol* (2013) 78:155–64. doi: 10.1111/cen.12066

50. Rayman MP. Selenium and human health. *Lancet* (2012) 379:1256–68. doi: 10.1016/S0140-6736(11)61452-9
51. Duntas LH. Selenium and Inflammation: Underlying Anti-inflammatory Mechanisms. *Horm Metab Res* (2009) 41:443–44. doi: 10.1055/s-0029-1220724
52. Duntas LH. Selenium and the thyroid: a close-knit connection. *J Clin Endocrinol Metab* (2010) 95:5180–8. doi: 10.1210/jc.2010-0191
53. Stranges S, Marshall JR, Natarajan R, Donahue RP, Trevisan M, Combs GF, et al. Effects of long term supplementation on the incidence of type 2 diabetes: a randomized trial. *Ann Int Med* (2007) 147:217–22. doi: 10.7326/0003-4819-147-4-200708210-00175
54. Marinò M, Marcocci C, Vitti P, Chiovato L, Bartalena L. Selenium in the treatment of thyroid diseases. *Eur Thyroid J* (2017) 6:113–4. doi: 10.1159/000456660
55. Vrca VB, Mayer L, Skreb F, Rahelić D, Marušić S. Antioxidant supplementation and serum lipids in patients with Graves' disease: effect on LDL-cholesterol. *Acta Pharm* (2012) 62:115–22. doi: 10.2478/v10007-012-0005-2
56. Kahaly GJ, Riedl M, König J, Diana T, Schomburg L. Double-Blind, Placebo-Controlled, Randomized Trial of Selenium in Graves Hyperthyroidism. *J Clin Endocrinol Metab* (2017) 102:4333–41. doi: 10.1210/jc.2017-01736
57. Guerra LN, Ríos de Molina Mdel C, Miler EA, Moiguer S, Karner M, Burdman JA. Antioxidants and methimazole in the treatment of Graves' disease: effect on urinary malondialdehyde levels. *Clin Chim Acta* (2015) 352:115–20. doi: 10.1016/j.cccn.2004.08.020
58. Bartalena L, Baldeschi L, Boboridis K, Eckstein A, Kahaly GJ, Marcocci C, et al. European Group on Graves' Orbitopathy (EUGOGO). The 2016 European Thyroid Association/European Group on Graves' Orbitopathy Guidelines for the Management of Graves' Orbitopathy. *Eur Thyroid J* (2016) 5:9–26. doi: 10.1159/000443828
59. Stan MN, Salvi M. Management of endocrine disease: rituximab therapy for Graves' orbitopathy - lessons from randomized control trials. *Eur J Endocrinol* (2016) 176:R101–9. doi: 10.1530/EJE-16-0552
60. Douglas RS, Kahaly GJ, Patel A, Sile S, Thompson EHZ, Perdok R, et al. Teprotumumab for the Treatment of Active Thyroid Eye Disease. *N Engl J Med* (2020) 382(4):341–52. doi: 10.1056/NEJMoa1910434
61. Smith TJ, Kahaly GJ, Ezra DG, Fleming JC, Dailey RA, Tang RA, et al. Teprotumumab for thyroid-associated ophthalmopathy. *N Engl J Med* (2017) 376:1748–61. doi: 10.1056/NEJMoa1614949
62. Kahaly GJ, Riedl M, König J, Pitz S, Ponto K, Diana T, et al. Combined mycophenolate + prednisolone therapy is more effective than prednisolone in active and moderate-to-severe Graves' Orbitopathy – a randomized, observer blind, multicenter trial. *Lancet Diabetes Endocrinol* (2018) 6:287–98. doi: 10.1530/EJE-16-0552
63. Pérez-Moreiras JV. Treatment of active corticosteroid-resistant Graves' Orbitopathy. *Ophthalmic Plast Reconstr Surg* (2014) 30:162–7. doi: 10.1097/IOP.0000000000000037
64. Sisti E, Coco B, Menconi F, Leo M, Rocchi R, Latrofa F, et al. Intravenous glucocorticoid therapy for Graves' ophthalmopathy and acute liver damage: an epidemiological study. *Eur J Endocrinol* (2015) 172:269–76. doi: 10.1530/EJE-14-0712
65. Sisti E, Coco B, Menconi F, Leo M, Rocchi R, Latrofa F, et al. Age and Dose Are Major Risk Factors for Liver Damage Associated with Intravenous Glucocorticoid Pulse Therapy for Graves; Orbitopathy (2015). *Thyroid* 25:846–50. doi: 10.1089/thy.2015.0061
66. Marcocci C, Watt T, Altea MA, Rasmussen AK, Feldt-Rasmussen Ù, Orgiazzi J, et al. Fatal and non-fatal adverse events of glucocorticoid therapy for Graves' orbitopathy: a questionnaire survey among members of the European Thyroid Association. *Eur J Endocrinol* (2012) 166:247–53. doi: 10.1530/EJE-11-0779
67. Rotondo Dottore G, Chiarini R, De Gregorio M, Leo M, Casini G, Cestari L, et al. Selenium rescues orbital fibroblasts from cell death induced by hydrogen peroxide: another molecular basis for the effects of selenium in Graves' orbitopathy. *Endocrine* (2017) 58:386–9. doi: 10.1007/s12020-016-1226-9
68. Tsai CC, Wu SB, Kao SC, Kau HC, Lee FL, Wei YH. The protective effect of antioxidants on orbital fibroblasts from patients with Graves' ophthalmopathy in response to oxidative stress. *Mol Vis* (2013) 19:927–34. doi: 10.1007/s12020-017-1255-z

21

Rare Co-Occurrence of Ocular Myasthenia Gravis and Thyroid-Associated Orbitopathy (Ophthalmopathy) in an Individual with Hypothyroidism

Ran An[1†]*, Yan Li*[1†]*, Baiyuan Yang*[1,2†]*, Hui Wang*[1] *and Yanming Xu*[1*]

[1] *Department of Neurology, West China Hospital, Sichuan University, Chengdu, China,* [2] *Department of Neurology, Chengdu Seventh People's Hospital, Chengdu, China*

***Correspondence:**
Yanming Xu
neuroxym999@163.com

† *These authors have contributed equally to this work*

Ocular myasthenia gravis (Ocular MG, OMG) shares many clinical features with thyroid-associated orbitopathy or thyroid-associated ophthalmopathy (TAO). In the rare instance of their coexistence, clinicians may fail to diagnose ocular MG when TAO is also present. Here we report the case of a patient with both TAO and ocular MG, whose "hyperthyroidism"—most likely the hashitoxicosis variant of Hashimoto's thyroiditis—rapidly transformed to hypothyroidism after radioactive iodine therapy. This is reminiscent of a previous case of a patient with MG, in whom disease onset coincided with the methimazole-induced transformation from hyper- to hypothyroidism. It is possible that the same transformation from "hyper-" to hypothyroidism, which occurred after radioactive iodine therapy and was accompanied by hypothyroidism-associated orbitopathy (ophthalmopathy), may have induced the development of myasthenia gravis in our patient. The hypothyroidism may have been caused by the radioactive iodine therapy and/or it may simply reflect the natural course of the hashitoxicosis variant of Hashimoto's thyroiditis. The co-occurrence of hypothyroidism, hypothyroidism-associated orbitopathy (ophthalmopathy) and ocular MG has never been reported. Our case highlights the need for clinicians to focus on overlapping symptoms of hyperthyroidism and the hashitoxicosis variant of Hashimoto's thyroiditis, and to carefully differentiate between them, especially when deciding on radioactive iodine therapy. In addition, our case highlights that the possible co-occurrence of TAO should be considered when a patient with thyroid disease displays both ptosis and eye movement dysfunction, and when only the ptosis is dramatically resolved after treatment with pyridostigmine bromide.

Keywords: myasthenia gravis, thyroid-associated orbitopathy, thyroid-associated ophthalmopathy, TAO, hypothyroidism, radioactive iodine therapy, hyperthyroidism, Graves' disease

BACKGROUND

Autoimmune diseases, which result from specific immune responses against self structures, include autoimmune thyroid diseases and myasthenia gravis (MG). In autoimmune thyroid diseases, which include Hashimoto's thyroiditis and Graves's disease (GD), the body mounts immune responses against thyroid antigens (1). In myasthenia gravis, the body usually produces antibodies targeting acetylcholine receptors (AChRs) (1, 2), leading to defective nerve impulse transmissions to muscles and ultimately causing muscle weakness and abnormal susceptibility to fatigue. Autoimmune thyroid diseases and MG show many commonalities.

Ocular myasthenia gravis (Ocular MG, OMG) shares many clinical features with thyroid-associated orbitopathy or thyroid-associated ophthalmopathy (TAO) and is therefore difficult to diagnose when TAO is also present (3, 4). TAO can occur in patients with primary hypothyroidism, though it is more often reported in Graves' thyrotoxicosis. Here we report the case of a patient with TAO and ocular MG who underwent a rapid transformation from "hyper-" to hypothyroidism after radioactive iodine therapy.

CASE REPORT

A 35-year-old Chinese man, employed at a bank, showed the following abnormal thyroid function results during a health examination at our hospital in November 2016: thyroid-stimulating hormone (TSH), < 0.005 mU/L (normal, 0.27–4.2); free triiodothyronine (FT3), 26.11 pmol/L (3.6–7.5); free thyroxine (FT4), 59.16 pmol/L (12.0–22.0); anti-thyroid peroxidase antibodies (TPO-Ab), >600 IU/ml (<34); and anti-thyroglobulin antibodies (TG-Ab), >4,000 IU/ml (<115).

The same man was admitted to a local hospital in March 2017 for further evaluation. He reported palpitations, sweating, heat intolerance, weakness, fatigue, polyphagia, tremors, and increased defecation lasting throughout the previous 6 months. A physical examination revealed no distinctive abnormalities except for a goiter. The results of thyroid function tests were as follows: TSH, < 0.0004 mIU/L (normal, 0.35-4.94); FT3, 17.74 pmol/L (2.63-5.70); FT4, 33.64 pmol/L (9.01-19.05); TPO-Ab, >400 IU/ml (<30); TG-Ab, >2,000 IU/ml (<75); and anti-thyroid-stimulating hormone receptor antibodies (TSHR-Ab), 38.89 IU/L (<1.22). Thyroid ultrasonography revealed an uneven echoic involvement of the parenchyma, with iso-echo nodules of regular shape and a clear boundary in the right lobe and isthmus. The 24-h rate of radioactive iodine uptake increased, with a peak appearing in advance. The patient was diagnosed with "hyperthyroidism" and given the anti-thyroid drug Tapazole orally (10 mg, three times daily). After treatment for 20 days, the patient complained of itchy skin and a red rash. This was interpreted as an allergic reaction, so Tapazole was discontinued, radioactive iodine therapy was then given, and the patient was discharged.

In May 2017, the patient displayed ptosis of the left eye, which grew worse by the end of the day or after exertion, and which improved upon rest. He also exhibited diplopia and limited eye movement in all directions, which at its worst meant that he could not move his eyes at all. In addition, the patient reported generalized muscle ache and weakness. Thyroid function tests at the local hospital gave the following results: TSH, < 47.8642 mIU/L; FT3, <1.54 pmol/L; FT4, <5.15 pmol/L; TPO-Ab, >400 IU/ml; and TG-Ab, >2,000 IU/ml. The patient was diagnosed with hypothyroidism and took levothyroxine (L-T4, 75 mg per day) replacement therapy. Two weeks later, the symptoms of fatigue, muscle weakness and myalgia had completely disappeared. However, after 2 months of L-T4 therapy, ocular symptoms persisted, and the patient was admitted to the neurology department in the same local hospital in July 2017. A physical and neurological examination found no abnormalities except for ptosis of the left eye and the limited movement of both eyes in all directions, without proptosis, periorbital or limb edema. TSH, FT3, and FT4 were normal. TPO-Ab was >400 IU/ml, TG-Ab was 1416.67 IU/ml, and serum lactic acid was 2.4 mmol/L (normal, 0.5–2.2). Complete blood count, tests of liver and kidney function, as well as levels of creatine kinase and serum tumor markers were normal. Magnetic resonance imaging of the brain, cervical vertebra, and the orbital cavity was normal, as were the electrocardiogram and echocardiography. Contrast-enhanced computed tomography of the chest was normal, revealing no obvious thymic hyperplasia or thymoma. Thyroid ultrasonography revealed uneven echoic involvement of the parenchyma, with iso-echo nodules in the right lobe. Low- and high-frequency repetitive nerve stimulation did not reveal abnormal decrease or increase in the amplitude of compound muscle action potential. The Ptosis was apparently alleviated, based on the positive response in the neostigmine test (**Figure 1**) (5, 6), but restricted eye movement and diplopia remained. Conventional enzyme-linked immunosorbent assays (ELISAs) showed normal levels of antibodies against AChRs (0.39 nmol/L; normal, <0.4), muscle-specific kinase (<0.4 U/ml; normal, <0.4), skeletal muscle, myocardium, titin, and SOX1. Ocular MG was suspected, and the patient was prescribed pyridostigmine bromide (60 mg, three times a day) along with the previous L-T4 regimen.

In August 2017, the patient was admitted to our neurology department complaining of restricted eye movements. The following test results were obtained upon admission: serum lactic acid, 2.7 mmol/L (normal, 0.7-2.1); TSH, FT3, and FT4, normal; TPO-Ab, >600 IU/ml; and TG-Ab, >4,000 IU/ml. Normal findings were obtained for complete blood count, erythrocyte sedimentation rate, liver and kidney function, electrolytes, serum glucose, serum lipid, creatine kinase, and serum tumor markers. A thyroid ultrasonography revealed uneven hypoechoic involvement of the parenchyma, with mild hyper-echo nodules in the right lobe. Low- and high-frequency repetitive nerve stimulation did not reveal abnormal changes in the amplitude of compound muscle action potential. Nerve conduction tests and needle electromyography both provided normal findings. Contrast-enhanced magnetic resonance imaging of the orbital cavity revealed thickened extraocular muscles in both eyes, with an obvious uneven enhancement.

Given the possibility of a mitochondrial disease, such as chronic progressive external ophthalmoplegia, a muscle biopsy

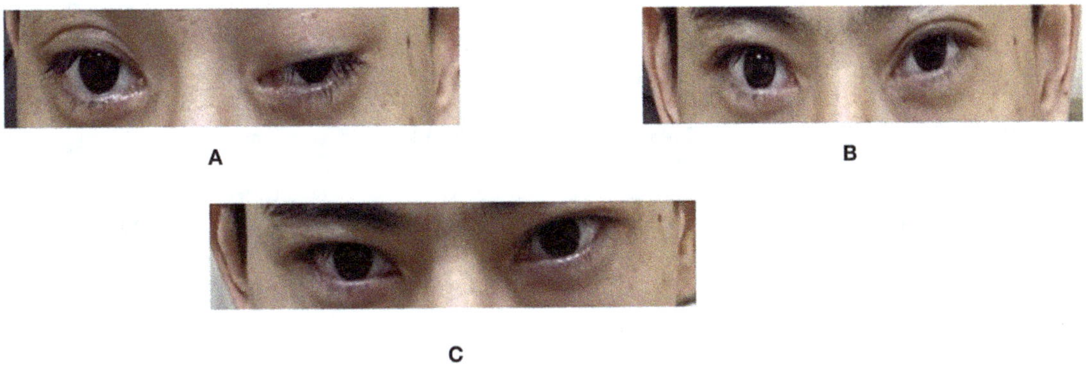

FIGURE 1 | Eyelid symptoms before and after the neostigmine test. **(A)** Before the test. Both eyes, especially the left one, showed ptosis. **(B)** 30 min after the test. Ptosis improved dramatically, to a greater extent in the left eye. **(C)** 60 min after the test. Both eyelids recovered nearly to a normal state. Relative score = 100% (positive). In the neostigmine test, the most severely affected muscle group was chosen, the muscle power at baseline was scored, then neostigmine (1.5 mg) and atropine (0.5 mg) were administered intramuscularly. The patient was then evaluated every 10 min for a total of 60 min. Relative Score = (score at baseline − score when improvement was greatest after injection) / (score at baseline) × 100%. Relative scores ≤ 25% were classified as negative; >25% and <60%, suspected positive; and ≥60%, positive.

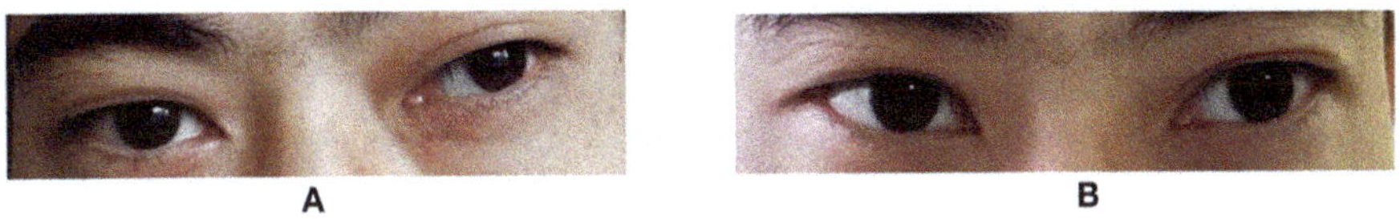

FIGURE 2 | Eyelid symptoms after cessation of pyridostigmine bromide therapy. **(A)** At 1 month after cessation of therapy (Dec. 2017). **(B)** At 3 months after cessation of therapy (Feb. 2018). At both time points, the left eyelid was nearly unaffected, showing only mild abnormality.

was conducted, and findings did not indicate any distinctive abnormalities. The patient was started on combination therapy of L-T4 and pyridostigmine bromide, which led to a stable condition of limited eye movement and mild diplopia. He stopped using pyridostigmine bromide in November 2017 when he began planning for a baby. A follow-up in December 2017 and February 2018 showed only mild abnormality in the left eyelid (**Figure 2**).

Table 1 summarizes the results of the thyroid function tests from the beginning in November 2016 to last follow-up. During the follow-up, radioimmunoprecipitation assays revealed the presence of antibodies against AChRs (7.310 nmol/L; normal, <0.5) and muscle-specific kinase (0.005 nmol/L; normal, <0.05). Later on, titer of anti-AChR antibodies was 0.678 nmol/L (normal, <0.4) based on an ELISA test and 1.864 nmol/L (normal, <0.5) based on a radioimmunoprecipitation assay (**Table 2**).

DISCUSSION

After the patient's first admission to a local hospital in March 2017, he was diagnosed with Graves's disease on the basis of abnormal thyroid function results with hyperthyroidism, increased titers of TPO-Ab, TG-Ab, and TSHR-Ab, and an increased 24-h rate of radioactive iodine uptake. However, a review of the initial ultrasound images of the thyroid gland and repeated ultrasonography which revealed uneven (nodular) hypoechoic areas, raises the possibility of the hashitoxicosis variant of Hashimoto's thyroiditis at the initial presentation rather than Grave's disease, which usually displays on ultrasound images as diffused hypoechogenicity without nodules (4). Unfortunately, because the fine needle puncture of the thyroid was not performed routinely as the first choice for the diagnosis of the thyroid disease, the biopsy and pathological examination of the thyroid gland was not performed, which could have aided in a correct diagnosis at the initial presentation.

The differential diagnosis of hyperthyroidism should include Grave's disease and the hashitoxicosis variant of Hashimoto's thyroiditis. The latter may show a hyperthyroid phase virtually indistinguishable from Graves's disease, including the elevated thyroid uptake of radioactive iodine and the presence of thyroid-stimulating immunoglobulins. However, hyperthyroidism is transient in the hashitoxicosis variant of Hashimoto's thyroiditis, and after 3–24 months evolves into permanent hypothyroidism (7). The hypothyroidism in our patient may have been caused by radioactive iodine therapy and/or the natural progression of the hashitoxicosis variant of Hashimoto's thyroiditis. However, if the suspected diagnosis of the hashitoxicosis variant of Hashimoto's thyroiditis was true in our patient, treatment with radioactive iodine therapy may have been inappropriate, because this can further destroy thyroid tissue and exacerbate the symptoms of hypothyroidism. The present case highlights the need for clinicians to carefully differentiate between the hashitoxicosis variant of Hashimoto's thyroiditis and Graves's hyperthyroidism,

TABLE 1 | Changes in thyroid function results from the beginning to the last follow-up.

No	Date \ Item	TSH	FT3	FT4	TPO-Ab	TG-Ab	TSHR-Ab
1	Nov. 2016	<0.005↓ (0.27–4.2 mU/L)	26.11↑ (3.6–7.5 pmol/L)	59.16↑ (12.0–22.0 pmol/L)	>600↑ (<34 IU/ml)	>4000↑ (<115 IU/ml)	ND
2	Feb. 2017	0.0009↓ (0.35–4.94 mIU/L)	17.96↑ (2.63–5.70 pmol/L)	41.36↑ (9.01–19.05 pmol/L)	>400↑ (<30 IU/ml)	1823.86↑ (<75 IU/ml)	35.11↑ (<1.22 IU/L)
3	Mar. 2017	0.0004↓	17.74↑	33.64↑	>400↑	>2000↑	38.89↑
4	May 2017	47.8642↑	<1.54↓	<5.15↓	>400↑	>2000↑	ND
5	Jun. 2017	2.4451	4.05	13.04	ND	ND	>40↑
6	Jul. 2017	1.8375	3.65	13.63	>400↑	1416.67↑	ND
7	Aug. 2017	0.512	4.28	16.97	>600↑	>4000↑	ND
8	Dec. 2017	0.606	4.55	16.39	>600↑	>4000↑	22.28↑ (<3 IU/L)

FT3, free triiodothyronine; FT4, free thyroxine; ND, not done; TG-Ab, thyroglobulin antibodies; TPO-Ab, thyroid peroxidase antibodies; TSH, Thyroid-stimulating hormone; TSHR-Ab, thyroid-stimulating hormone receptor antibodies. Tests in rows 1, 7, and 8 were performed at our hospital; others were performed at another hospital. In March 2017, radioactive iodine therapy was performed. In May 2017, ocular myasthenia gravis and thyroid-associated orbitopathy occurred, and hypothyroidism was detected.

TABLE 2 | Titers of anti-AChR and anti-MuSK antibodies assayed by ELISA or radioimmunoprecipitation assay.

	ELISA		Radioimmunoprecipitation	
Date	**Anti-AchR (<0.4 nmol/L)**	**Anti-MuSK (<0.4 U/ml)**	**Anti-AchR (<0.5 nmol/L)**	**Anti-MuSK (≤0.05 nmol/L)**
Jul. 2017	0.39	<0.4	ND	ND
10 Dec. 2017	ND	ND	7.310	0.005
20 Dec. 2017	0.678	ND	1.864	ND

ELISA, enzyme-linked immunosorbent assay; AChR, acetylcholine receptor; MuSK, muscle-specific kinase; ND, not done. Normal ranges are indicated below the antibody descriptions.

in light of their overlapping symptoms and the damage that may result from inappropriate application of radioactive iodine therapy. If necessary, the thyroid should be biopsied and analyzed by histopathology in order to ensure accurate, complete diagnosis.

Our patient showed elevated serum concentrations of anti-AChR antibodies (**Table 2**), consistent with previous reports (8). This observation, together with the positive neostigmine test (**Figure 1**) and substantial improvement in ptosis following the first treatment with pyridostigmine bromide, permitted a definite diagnosis of MG. This highlights the usefulness of repeat testing for anti-AChR antibodies if initial results are normal.

In addition to hypothyroidism and ocular symptoms, our patient showed generalized muscle ache and weakness on May 2017, which disappeared after 2 weeks of levothyroxine therapy. Muscle ache and weakness are considered characteristics of hypothyroid myopathy (8). Although most patients with hypothyroidism with MG give a negative result on the edrophonium test (8), while our patient tested positive on a neostigmine test. It is likely that the myopathic signs and symptoms of the patients in that previous study, disappeared with thyroid hormone replacement therapy, in turn suggesting that most myasthenia gravis symptoms in those patients were manifestations of hypothyroid myopathy, and that such symptoms can disappear with thyroid hormone replacement therapy, without the need for anti-myasthenic medication. However, our patient showed ptosis that did not respond to levothyroxin therapy. We concluded that the ptosis was a clinical manifestation of myasthenia gravis and independent of hypothyroid myopathy. Consistent with this idea, the ptosis nearly disappeared after a few months of treatment with pyridostigmine bromide.

Initially, our patient required anti-myasthenic medications to relieve ptosis. Subsequently, even at 1 or 3 months after cessation of pyridostigmine therapy, the left eyelid showed only mild abnormality (**Figure 2**). This leads us to suggest that the thyroid disease and MG were distinct yet interacting conditions in our patient. Controlling the hypothyroidism in our patient may also have alleviated the MG symptoms to some extent. The mild ocular abnormality in our patient, even after withdrawal of pyridostigmine bromide, is consistent with the observation that MG is often milder and more likely to show ocular involvement in patients with autoimmune thyroid disease, than in patients with non-autoimmune thyroid disease or no thyroid disease etc. (3).

Our patient displayed restricted eye movements and thickened extraocular muscles of both eyes, which are typical of TAO. The presence of ptosis in a patient with TAO should alert the clinician to the possible presence of MG, since the clinical features of TAO and ocular MG overlap substantially, and ptosis has been described as a rare feature of TAO (3). Indeed, the ptosis in our patient appears to have been a symptom of MG, further identifying the existence of OMG in the context of TAO. Our case highlights that the possible co-occurrence of TAO should be considered if a patient with thyroid disease displays both ptosis and eye movement dysfunction, and if only the ptosis dramatically resolves after treatment with pyridostigmine bromide. If necessary, magnetic resonance imaging of the orbit can be performed to guide diagnosis and further therapy.

TAO may occur more frequently among Graves' disease patients with ocular MG, than among Graves' disease patients without MG or with generalized MG. Euthyroid ophthalmopathy occurs more frequently among Graves' disease patients when they also have MG, suggesting a preferential association between the ocular manifestations of Graves' disease and MG (9). This previous study suggested that the co-occurrence of ocular MG and TAO may be due to a shared genetic background as well as immunological cross-reactivity against common autoimmune targets in the eye muscle. Our case is consistent with the preferential association between hypothyroidism-associated orbitopathy (ophthalmopathy) and ocular MG. Whole-exome sequencing of our patient and his parents did not identify any obvious gene mutations or polymorphisms in coding regions that may help explain an association between thyroid-associated ophthalmopathy and ocular MG (data not shown). Large genetic studies are needed to examine this potential association in detail.

Previous studies described a patient with MG in whom disease onset coincided with the methimazole-induced transformation from hyper- to hypothyroidism (10). It is possible that the transformation from "hyper-" to hypothyroidism in our patient is analogous, inducing the development of MG, although it occurred after radioactive iodine therapy and was accompanied by hypothyroidism-associated orbitopathy (ophthalmopathy). The hypothyroidism may have been caused by the radioactive iodine therapy and/or it may simply reflect the natural course of the hashitoxicosis variant of Hashimoto's thyroiditis. This appears to be the first report of the triple occurrence of hypothyroidism, hypothyroidism-associated orbitopathy (ophthalmopathy) and ocular MG. This case therefore deserves significant attention because of its implications in research and clinical practice.

CONCLUDING REMARKS

MG is usually reported in hyperthyroidic patients, rarely in patients with hypothyroidism. We present here a rare case of co-occurrence of MG, hypothyroidism and TAO after radioactive iodine therapy for "hyperthyroidism." This case highlights the need for clinicians to be aware of the possible co-occurrence of such comorbidities, which have implications for treatment and management. Clinicians should carefully differentiate between hyperthyroidism and the hashitoxicosis variant of Hashimoto's thyroiditis, especially when considering radioactive iodine therapy. Our case further highlights the need to consider the co-occurrence of TAO if pyridostigmine bromide only partly resolves ocular MG symptoms in patients with thyroid disease. If necessary, magnetic resonance imaging of the orbit can be performed to guide diagnosis and therapy.

ETHICS STATEMENT

The study protocol was approved by the Ethics Committee of Sichuan University and written informed consent was obtained from participants.

AUTHOR CONTRIBUTIONS

RA, YL, BY, and HW collected patient data and wrote the manuscript. YX conducted the study and revised the manuscript.

ACKNOWLEDGMENTS

Written informed consent was obtained from the patient to participating in the study and for publication of this manuscript, including the images in **Figures 1, 2.** We thank the patient and his family for participating in this study.

REFERENCES

1. Lopomo A, Berrih-Aknin S. Autoimmune thyroiditis and myasthenia gravis. *Front Endocrinol.* 8:169. doi: 10.3389/fendo.2017.00169
2. Gilhus NE, Skeie GO, Romi F, Lazaridis K, Zisimopoulou P, Tzartos S. Myasthenia gravis - autoantibody characteristics and their implications for therapy. *Nat Rev Neurol.* (2016) 12:259–68. doi: 10.1038/nrneurol.2016.44
3. Selvan C, Dutta D, Maisnam I, Thukral A, Chakraborthy PP, Roy A, et al. Thyroid associated orbitopathy with ocular myasthenia in primary hypothyroidism: keep those eyes open. *Indian J Endocrinol Metab.* (2013) 17:S657–9. doi: 10.4103/2230-8210.123559
4. De Leo S, Lee SY, Braverman LE. Hyperthyroidism. *Lancet* (2016) 388:906–18. doi: 10.1016/S0140-6736(16)00278-6
5. Li ZY, Xueqiang H. China guidelines for the diagnosis and treatment of myasthenia gravis. *Chin J Neurol.* (2015) 48:11. doi: 10.20517/2347-8659.2015.60
6. Dantao P, Xianhao X, Ziyu S. Study on revive criteria for neostigmine test. *Chin J Neuroimmunol Neurol.* (2007) 14:1. doi: 10.3969/j.issn.1006-2963.2007.01.001
7. Caturegli P, De Remigis A, Rose NR. Hashimoto thyroiditis: clinical and diagnostic criteria. *Autoimmun Rev.* (2014) 13:391–7. doi: 10.1016/j.autrev.2014.01.007
8. Turker H, Bayrak O, Gungor L, Yilmaz A, Terzi M, Turker CM, et al. Hypothyroid myopathy with manifestations of Hoffman's syndrome and myasthenia gravis. *Thyroid* (2008) 18:259–62. doi: 10.1089/thy.2007.0030
9. Marinò M, Barbesino G, Pinchera A, Manetti L, Ricciardi R, Rossi B, et al. Increased frequency of euthyroid ophthalmopathy in patients with Graves' disease associated with myasthenia gravis. *Thyroid* (2000) 10:799–802. doi: 10.1089/thy.2000.10.799
10. Takanami I, Imamuma T, Yamamoto Y, Yamamoto T, Kodaira S. The rapid transformation of hyperthyroidism to hypothyroidism complicated by myasthenia gravis. *J Thorac Cardiovasc Surg.* (1995) 110:852.

22

Not all Orbitopathy is Graves': Discussion of Cases and Review of Literature

Neeraja Boddu[1*], *Maliha Jumani*[1], *Vibhor Wadhwa*[2], *Gitanjali Bajaj*[2] *and Fred Faas*[1†]

[1] *Endocrinology, University of Arkansas for Medical Sciences, Little Rock, AR, United States,* [2] *Radiology, University of Arkansas for Medical Sciences, Little Rock, AR, United States*

Correspondence:
Neeraja Boddu
drneeraja12@gmail.com

†Fred Faas, Deceased (May He Rest in Peace).

Introduction: Graves' orbitopathy is the extra thyroidal manifestation of Graves' disease and the most common cause of exophthalmos. It is also known as thyroid-associated orbitopathy (TAO) as it occasionally occurs in euthyroid or hypothyroid patients with chronic thyroiditis. 5% of patients with Graves' orbitopathy can be euthyroid or hypothyroid as they have low titers of anti-thyrotropin-receptor antibodies, which are difficult to detect in some assays. Orbitopathy has also been seen in a small percentage of patients with Hashimotos thyroiditis. The eye involvement in Graves' is frequently bilateral and symmetric. These patients pose few diagnostic difficulties when the ocular findings occur concomitantly with the thyroid disease. However, when unilateral and asymmetric ocular findings occur with normal or mildly abnormal thyroid function tests, alternate etiologies should also be pursued. We aim to discuss some conditions like sarcoidosis, lymphoma, orbital pseudotumor, and orbital malignancy that mimic TAO.

Cases: Three patients were referred to us with concern for Graves' orbitopathy. After further work-up, we diagnosed the first patient with specific orbital myositis from sarcoidosis. Our second patient had CD10-positive B-cell lymphoma. Our third patient had orbitopathy likely secondary to Hashimotos or orbital pseudotumor.

Conclusion: Our cases and discussion describe some other conditions that clinically mimic TAO and the importance of pursuing further work-up for accurate diagnosis when presentation of orbitopathy is atypical.

Keywords: differential of thyroid-associated orbitopathy, Graves' orbitopathy, orbital lymphoma, sarcoid orbitopathy, orbitopathy

Graves' orbitopathy also referred to as thyroid-associated orbitopathy (TAO) is the extra thyroidal manifestation of Graves' disease and the most common cause of exophthalmos. It is an immune disorder causing inflammation and expansion of orbital fat and muscle. It is seen in 25–50% of patients with Graves' disease and hyperthyroidism. Occasionally, it occurs in those with Graves' disease with no evident clinical symptoms or biochemical thyroid abnormality (1). Few cases have also been reported to occur in patients with Hashimoto's thyroiditis (2). Clinical features of TAO include exophthalmos, lid retraction, periorbital swelling, ophthalmoplegia, and chemosis (3). Diagnosis is based on clinical features and may be supported by abnormal thyroid function tests and positive thyroid antibodies (4). Mostly, eye signs are bilateral but unilateral changes may occur in about 15% of patients and sometimes precede the onset of Graves' (5). Although, this disorder has strong correlation with TSH receptor antibodies, some cases have been reported with antibody negativity (6). When endocrinologists receive referrals for euthyroid patients with negative thyroid antibodies with orbitopathy suspicious for Graves', they need to be aware of other conditions that may mimic Graves' orbitopathy. Some of these disorders are sarcoidosis, lymphoma, orbital pseudotumor, and orbital malignancy. We present three cases of orbitopathy referred to our Endocrine clinic for suspected TAO and a review of literature on the differential diagnosis of the same.

CASE 1

A female aged 40–50 years presented with a 2-month history of intermittent headaches, heat intolerance, fatigue, right facial numbness, double vision, and periorbital swelling. On exam, she had mild thyromegaly with a nodular texture and no palpable cervical adenopathy. Eye exam showed proptosis, periorbital edema, and diplopia. TSH was 5.11 μIU/ml (0.450–4.500 μIU/ml) with a normal free T4 0.88 ng/dl (0.82–1.77 ng/dl). Thyroid peroxidase (TPO) antibodies were elevated at 356 IU/ml (0–34 IU/ml). TSH receptor antibodies (TRAb) were 0.51 IU/L (0.00—1.75 IU/L) and Thyroid stimulating immunoglobulin (TSI) 51% (0–139%). Thyroid ultrasound showed a multinodular goiter with right thyroid lobe enlargement. CT scan of the orbits showed bilateral asymmetric enlargement of extraocular muscles (EOMs) with suspicion for Graves' orbitopathy. MRI of the orbits confirmed EOM enlargement; largest in bilateral lateral rectus, left medial rectus, and left inferior rectus. Closer review of MRI images also showed lacrimal gland enlargement, leptomeningeal enhancement of the surface of the brain and spinal canal, and thickened infundibulum raising concern for sarcoidosis (**Figure 1**). Subsequently, a 1 cm right thyroid nodule was biopsied showing granulomatous changes consistent with sarcoidosis. During the course of her followup, she also developed complete heart block and required pacemaker placement. Patient was started on prednisone 20 mg daily with marked improvement in her visual symptoms. Repeat MRI of the brain after steroids showed marked improvement in size of EOMs, lacrimal glands, and leptomeningeal disease. Repeat thyroid ultrasound showed decrease in the size of the goiter with no discrete nodularity, microcalcifications, or other concerning features. This patient had orbital, neurologic, and cardiac involvement with sarcoidosis. She had no pulmonary nodules or mediastinal findings on further imaging.

CASE 2

A male aged 50–60 years was referred with left eye proptosis progressively getting worse for 2 months. He denied visual changes, headache, eye pain, fatigue, diaphoresis, palpitations, tremor, or weight changes. Visual field testing was normal. Exophthalmos was noted in the left eye with forward displacement of 21 mm compared to 17 mm on the right. MRI of the brain and orbits showed an enhancing circumscribed mass within the superior aspect of the left orbit measuring 4.2 cm in greatest dimension with thickening of the anterior tendinous portion of superior rectus. The globe was displaced inferiorly and laterally. The lacrimal glands showed no enlargement (**Figure 2**). Also noted incidentally was a right sided pituitary macroadenoma measuring 17 mm × 21 mm and extending to the right cavernous sinus with left shift of the pituitary infundibulum but no significant compression of optic chiasm. Differentials for the extraocular muscle involvement were felt to be orbital pseudotumor, unusual asymmetric enlarged muscle in Graves' disease or an infiltrative tumor involving the muscle. Biochemical evaluation for thyroid and pituitary was within normal range. Subsequently, the patient underwent transsphenoidal resection of non-secretory pituitary macroadenoma. He continued to have left eye proptosis and was given empiric steroid taper with temporary resolution of proptosis and decrease in muscle swelling on MRI. However, symptoms recurred when steroids were tapered. Fine needle aspiration (FNA) of left levator palpebrae muscle was performed twice and was negative for malignancy. Due to continued symptoms, patient underwent left lateral orbitotomy with bone removal and biopsy of the lesion. Biopsy showed CD10-positive B-cell lymphoma. This was an indolent follicular/marginal zone lymphoma involving the superior rectus muscle. Patient received radiation therapy with improvement in symptoms.

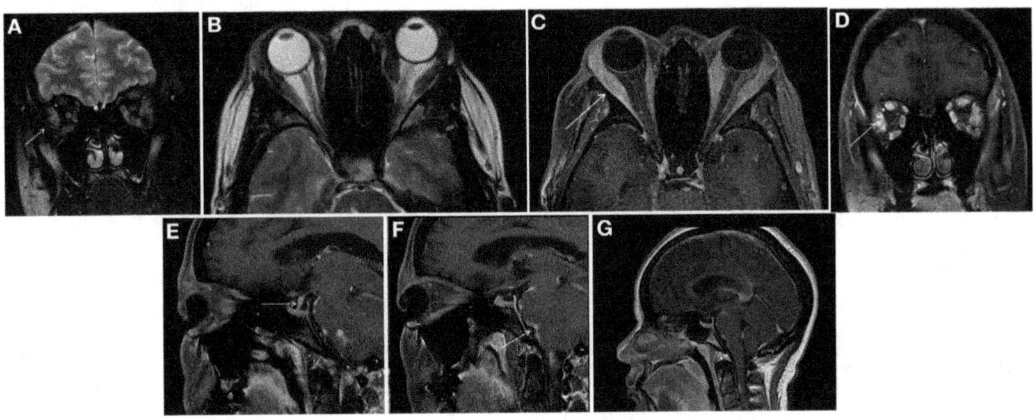

FIGURE 1 | Case 1. Diffuse enlargement and enhancement of muscle bellies and anterior tendinous insertions of bilateral extraocular muscle on coronal and axial T2 **(A,B)** and fat suppressed post contrast T1 **(C,D)** orbital images. Involvement of the tendons and lateral rectus muscle makes Graves' orbitopathy less likely. Additional findings, which favored the diagnosis of sarcoidosis included nodular leptomeningeal enhancement **(F,G)** with thickening of the pituitary stalk **(E)**.

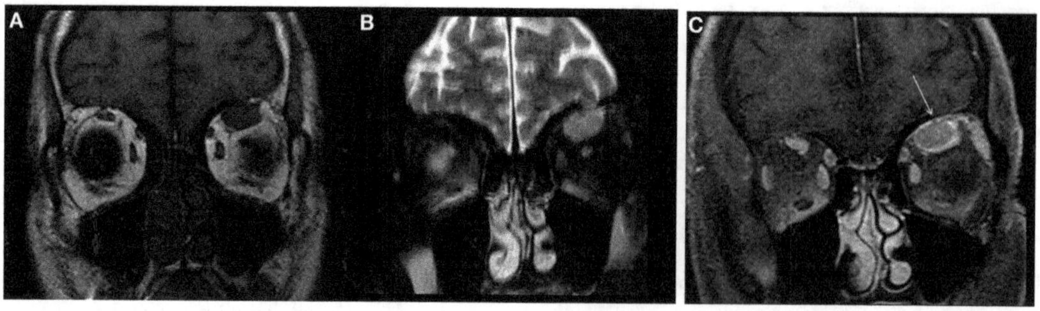

FIGURE 2 | Case 2. T1 hypointense and T2 hyperintense mildly enhancing mass in the left superior rectus muscle seen on coronal T1 **(A)**, fat saturated T2 **(B)**, and post contrast fat saturated T1 **(C)** images of the orbits. Solitary muscle involvement especially of the superior rectus makes thyroid orbitopathy an unlikely etiology.

CASE 3

A male aged 50–60 years was referred with right eye proptosis and double vision of 1-year duration. His only symptom was fatigue. No thyromegaly was noted. He had diplopia on both vertical and horizontal gaze. Exophthalmos was noted, 25 mm on right and 20 mm on left. Biochemical work-up showed a TSH of 149 μIU/ml. TSI and TSH receptor antibodies were negative, but TPO antibodies were positive. Given biochemical confirmation of hypothyroidism, patient was started on levothyroxine. An MRI was obtained for evaluation of orbital disease and it showed mild diffuse mid-belly enlargement and T2 hyperintensity of EOMs bilaterally. There was moderate enlargement of the right inferior rectus muscle (**Figure 3**). His imaging findings were concerning for TAO because of involvement of the right inferior rectus muscle and diffusely hazy orbital fat. Focal sparing of the tendon of the inferior rectus further supported this. He was started on steroid eye drops followed by oral steroids. Orbital swelling improves while on steroids but recurs when the dose is tapered. FNA of inferior rectus was performed while patient was on steroids. The specimen was small and inconclusive and showed mild inflammation only.

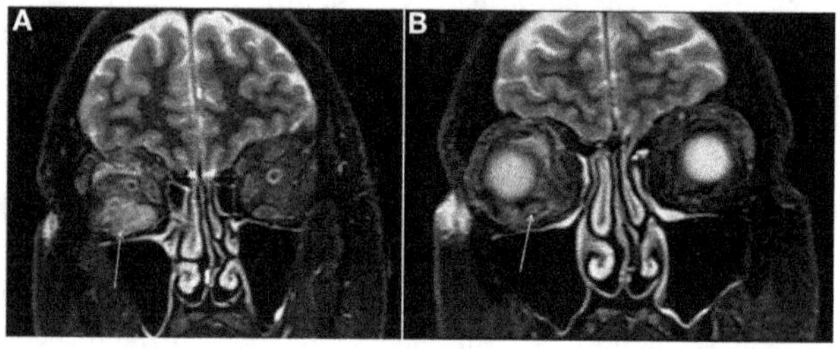

FIGURE 3 | Case 3. Coronal T2W MRI images showing enlargement of the right inferior rectus muscle [arrow in **(A)**] with surrounding fat stranding, features similar to thyroid-associated orbitopathy (TAO). Focal sparing of the anterior tendinous insertion [arrow in **(B)**] is another common finding of TAO.

DISCUSSION

Graves' orbitopathy has an incidence rate of 16 women and 3 men per 100,000 (7). It occasionally occurs in euthyroid or hypothyroid patients with chronic thyroiditis. The 5% of patients with Graves' orbitopathy who are euthyroid or hypothyroid generally have low titers of TRAbs, which are difficult to detect in some assays (3, 7). It may occur in a small percentage of patients with Hashimoto's thyroiditis as well (6, 8). Most speculated mechanism causing Graves' orbitopathy is that autoantibodies are formed against thyrotropin receptors that are found in both the thyroid gland and orbit. This causes activation of T lymphocytes with subsequent release of inflammatory mediators (9). The muscles are infiltrated with inflammatory cells and hyaluron causing enlargement of the EOMs and an increase in the orbital fat volume (10). Ultimately, collagen deposition leads to fibrosis. The involvement is frequently bilateral and symmetric (11). Patients with Graves' Orbitopathy pose few diagnostic difficulties when ocular findings occur concomitantly with the thyroid disease. But unilateral or inconclusive ocular features in the absence of objective evidence of thyroid dysfunction need pursuance of alternate etiologies (12). We aim to discuss some conditions that mimic TAO and our cases provide examples of the potential pitfalls in delineating TAO from these other conditions.

DIAGNOSTIC DIFFICULTIES

Clinically eyelid retraction, proptosis, chemosis, restrictive ophthalmopathy with diplopia, and in worst cases, compressive optic neuropathy are seen with TAO (1). Radiographically extraocular muscle enlargement sparing the tendons is seen (4). Extraocular muscle involvement is frequently bilateral with more than one muscle group involved and with regular borders. However, none of these features are specific. Other etiologies should be considered when the presentation is atypical. These other conditions could be inflammatory, neoplastic, infectious, vascular, or neuromuscular (**Table 1**). Often, autoimmune thyroiditis may also occur in conjunction with other systemic autoimmune conditions like sarcoidosis, Sjogren's disease, systemic sclerosis, systemic lupus erythematosus (SLE), and rheumatoid arthritis, which may further complicate the diagnosis (13). Clinically, time of onset of symptoms and disease progression might provide some clue to alternate diagnosis. Orbital cellulitis is acute and rapidly progressive. Orbital myositis from systemic causes may be subacute in onset over days or weeks and may be associated with pain. Neoplastic involvement may be painless and restrictive

TABLE 1 | Differential diagnosis of Graves' orbitopathy.

Differential diagnosis of Graves' orbitopathy
1. Specific orbital inflammation ~5%
A. Sarcoidosis
B. Systemic lupus erythematosus
C. Crohn's disease
D. Scleroderma
2. Orbital pseudotumor/non-specific orbital inflammation ~40%
3. Neoplasms ~20–40%
A. Lymphomas
B. Benign tumors—hamartomas, primary granulosa cell tumors, rhabdomyomas, liposarcomas
C. Metastases—melanoma, breast, gastrointestinal, and lung carcinomas
4. Others ~10–15%
A. Vascular malformations
B. Infections
C. Neuromuscular dysfunction

and occur more gradually over weeks or months. It also may present as mass effect. Very often orbital biopsy has to be offered to confirm a diagnosis and properly tailor the treatment plan in these cases (12).

Specific Orbital Inflammation and Myositis

This is a less common cause of orbitopathy accounting for ~5% cases compared to non-specific inflammation, which accounts for about 40% cases in a reported study (12). It occurs from systemic inflammatory causes like sarcoidosis, SLE, Crohn's disease, or scleroderma. Our first patient presented with this etiology.

Sarcoidosis is a multisystem granulomatous disease characterized histologically by non-caseating epithelioid-cell granulomas in affected tissue. It presents in the third or fourth decades and more commonly affects blacks. 30–35% of all sarcoidosis patients may have ophthalmic involvement; 7–19% of these patients have systemic disease along with ocular symptoms but others could have isolated orbital disease with lacrimal gland involvement and very rarely extraocular muscle involvement (14, 15). In these cases, incorrect diagnosis of Graves' orbitopathy may be made especially if concomitant thyroid function test abnormality is present. The unilateral or bilateral proptosis in sarcoidosis results from retro-orbital infiltration by sarcoid tissue. The imaging findings are non-specific and include enhancement of EOMs such as in Graves' disease, infiltrative mass identical to orbital pseudotumor or lymphoma and rarely thickening, nodularity of sclera (16, 17). Involvement of other intracranial structures and presence of parenchymal, leptomeningeal, dural, or skull findings may be clue to diagnosis. Sarcoid granuloma in the thyroid is extremely rare, with a prevalence of 4% in autopsied patients with systemic sarcoidosis. Hypothyroidism may occur through extensive infiltration by epithelioid granulomas, which was the case in our patient (18). Also a significantly higher prevalence of clinical hypothyroidism and Graves' disease has been observed in female patients with sarcoidosis than in control subjects. It is important to test thyroid function and thyroid antibodies in these patients (19).

Systemic lupus erythematosus, which is a collagen vascular disease resulting in multisystem involvement and vasculitis may also cause Bilateral orbital involvement and specific myositis in few case reports (20). Other symptoms like rash, photosensitivity, and arthritis may give a clue to diagnosis. This condition also usually responds to high-dose steroids and disease modifying antirheumatic drugs like hydroxychloroquine. Crohn's disease is another granulomatous inflammatory condition of the bowels causing orbital disease in about 13%. It may present as iritis, scleritis, optic neuritis, and retinal involvement. Bilateral involvement of orbital muscles in these patients has been reported. Again excellent response to steroids is seen. The pathogenesis is speculated to be immune complexes, which have affinity for EOMs (21). Scleroderma is another chronic autoimmune condition causing thickening and fibrosis of skin that may also cause inflammation, fibrosis, and extraocular muscle restriction like Graves' (12).

Primary or Secondary Neoplasms

This is a reported cause in about 20–40% of cases with non-thyroid orbitopathy (12). Our second patient had presented with progressively worsening unilateral proptosis. He did not have symptoms of hyperthyroidism on presentation and no prior history of the same. Thyroid antibodies were negative and he had radiologically confirmed unilateral disease. This along with the fact that he only had transient improvement in symptoms with steroids prompted us to look for alternative diagnoses. Indeed, a biopsy revealed lymphoma.

Orbital lymphoma can mimic TAO as it may originate from or infiltrate the EOMs (22). Conjunctival disease is frequent and can be an isolated finding in 20% of cases. A diffuse infiltrative form may occur with intraconal, muscular, or perineural involvement. The involvement is rarely multifocal within the orbit (<5%). Bilateral involvement is seen in 25%, usually with higher grade lesions. The best diagnostic clue on imaging is a solid, homogeneously enhancing orbital tumor that molds to and encases orbital structures. Restricted diffusion within the lesion can be another useful imaging feature to lymphoma as a likely diagnosis. Lymphoma can be primary to the orbit or secondary to systemic disease. Secondary ocular involvement occurs in 2–5% of patients with advanced systemic non-Hodgkin's lymphoma (NHL). However, lymphomas are the most common primary orbital tumors accounting for 55% of malignant orbital tumors in adults 60 years and older. The majority of NHL of the orbit and orbital adnexa are extra nodal marginal-zone B-cell lymphomas of mucosa-associated lymphoid tissue (23). Clinical manifestations of orbital lymphoma include painless proptosis and motility disturbances. Whole body staging is necessary after diagnosis and is most often done with FDG PET CT. Low-grade tumors respond well to radiation therapy while chemotherapy is necessary for high-grade or systemic disease (24).

Other primary orbital tumors involving EOMs simulating TAO are rare. Benign tumors like hamartoma, primary granular cell orbital tumors, rhabdomyomas, and liposarcoma have been described (12, 25, 26). Metastases from distant sites may occur with melanoma, breast cancer, gastrointestinal, and lung carcinoma. They can present as isolated or multiple masses within the EOMs, orbital fat, globe, or bony orbit. Majority of patients have a diagnosis of primary malignancy at presentation (27). Patients may present with diplopia, visual disturbance, proptosis, and movement restriction. All muscles could be involved (28).

Orbital Pseudotumor or Non-Specific Orbital Inflammatory Syndrome

This has been described as the most common differential of TAO occurring in about 40% of cases (12). Our third patient presented with uniocular proptosis and diplopia, hypothyroidism, and right orbital edema with enlargement of inferior rectus muscle on MRI. His orbital biopsy showed mild inflammation only. He had good response to steroids but the swelling did not subside completely. One possibility is orbitopathy related to Hashimoto's thyroiditis. Most euthyroid and hypothyroid patients with orbitopathy are TRAb-positive and they are diagnosed as having euthyroid or hypothyroid Graves' disease. In our patient, TRAb was negative. Cases of orbitopathy have been reported in patients with Hashimoto's thyroiditis with TRAb negativity (6, 29). In these patients, orbitopathy is likely related to the specific production of antibodies to orbital tissue other than TRAb. Alternatively, this patient could also have idiopathic orbital inflammatory syndrome if other secondary systemic disease or metastatic lesion is ruled out.

Idiopathic orbital inflammatory syndrome is an orbital inflammatory process of unknown etiology and is diagnosed by excluding other possible causes of exophthalmos. It was first described by Birch-Hirshfeld to describe an orbital syndrome clinically resembling a neoplasm but surgical pathology showing only inflammation. Over a period of time, many difficult to diagnose systemic inflammatory diseases and lymphomas were falsely classified under this category. With better imaging and diagnostic modalities, this disorder now denotes non-specific benign orbital inflammation without evidence of specific local or systemic cause (29). Good corticosteroid response is seen. It has varied clinical and radiologic presentation. It may present with inflammation and mass effect with symptoms and signs of pain, chemosis, proptosis, and motility restriction. Imaging usually shows a defined or poorly demarcated mass. It occurs in any age or sex group. Single muscle involvement is more common but involvement of bilateral muscles sparing the tendons very similar to Graves' has been noted too (30). Biopsy is required to exclude other diseases. FNA is not helpful as inflammatory cells may be seen even with malignancy and not conclusive for this etiology. Histopathologic material is more informative. It is a self-limiting disorder most of the times. Based on the cellular, stromal, or vascular component, orbital pseudotumor is divided into histopathologic subclasses. These are sclerosing, granulomatous, vasculitic, and eosinophilic varieties. Therapy with steroids is advised during active phase as it rarely has a malignant course with extraocular muscle involvement and optic nerve damage. Steroid therapy classically results in rapid improvement, but cases unresponsive to steroids have been reported. In such cases, low-dose irradiation has been administered with varying success.

OTHER LESS COMMON DIFFERENTIALS

Other conditions, which may resemble TAO are vascular malformations, infections and neuromuscular dysfunction. Some vascular disorders causing myopathy are carotid cavernous fistulas and congenital orbital vascular malformations. In these disorders, arteriovenous shunting into cavernous sinus causes retrograde flow along superior ophthalmic vein causing venous distension and tissue edema with enlargement of muscles. Also, decreased pressure within the microcirculation leads to low tissue perfusion, hypoxia, and ophthalmoplegia (31). Orbital cellulitis from bacterial infections is more common, but uncommon infections like trichinosis, cysticercosis, and Lyme's disease have been described. Neuromuscular disorders like myasthenia gravis cause extraocular muscle weakness, but not enlargement. Chronic progressive external ophthalmoplegia is an extremely rare condition where extraocular muscle size is reduced on imaging (32).

IMAGING

Imaging is very important and may give clues to diagnosis in atypical cases. Observation of muscle shape, size, borders, pattern of involvement, surrounding soft tissues, and bone involvement can help in the differential diagnosis (33, 34). In TAO, enlargement of EOMs and increase in retrobulbar fat volume is noted. The classical criteria is spindle-shaped enlargement of EOMs >4 mm without involvement of the tendon on both MRI and CT. Preferential muscle involvement, starting with rectus inferior followed by the medial rectus, the superior rectus, and finally the lateral is a specific finding, seen best on coronal views (33).

MRI gives better soft-tissue differentiation. T2-weighted images detect edema, inflammation in EOMs, and also help rule out other orbital pathology like infiltrative process. Orbital myositis is the most common etiology mimicking graves. It may involve any extraocular muscle including the tendons, may show medial bowing of the muscle with infiltration of fat. Inflamed muscles show low intensity on T1-weighted images and increased intensity on T2-weighted images. Tumors also have low-signal intensity on T1 and moderate to marked increase on T2 (34).

CT provides good imaging of orbital apex and optic nerve. In Graves' orbitopathy, CT shows fusiform enlargement of the extraocular muscle, smooth borders, and non-involvement of tendons. Orbital fat is normal. Myositis on CT is characterized by contrast enhancement and likely diffuse irregular enlargement of muscles involving tendons in most cases. Orbital fat may be involved suggestive of inflammation. Concomitant periorbital findings may point occasionally to systemic disease. Malignancy may show single nodular muscle enlargement in most cases with sharp borders and occasional bone change. AV malformations may show homogenous enlargement of multiple EOMs with sharply defined borders and distension of superior ophthalmic vein. Infection and orbital cellulitis may show blurred muscle margins, adjacent sinus infiltrate, and orbital fat infiltration (35).

CONCLUSION

Graves' disease is the most common cause of orbitopathy. Hashimotos thyroiditis results in orbitopathy in a small percentage of patients. Alternate etiologies should be considered in the absence of hyperthyroidism and negative thyroid antibodies. Orbital imaging should always be performed. Other rare diagnoses like orbital pseudotumor, orbital lymphoma, orbital sarcoidosis, and orbital neoplasms should be evaluated for in the event of atypical clinical, biochemical, and imaging findings with an orbital biopsy. As vision loss can occur in some of these cases, accurate diagnosis, and treatment are imperative.

ETHICS STATEMENT

Consent: written, informed consent was obtained from all patients mentioned in our manuscript both for the purposes of participating in the research as well as for their personal information to be published.

AUTHOR CONTRIBUTIONS

NB is responsible for coordinating with other authors and writing up the manuscript. MJ was responsible for writing Case 2 and part of the discussion as well as editing of manuscript. VW contributed to editing imaging findings and references. GB provided images and description for the same. FF is the final author who reviewed the manuscript and provided advise.

REFERENCES

1. Bahn RS, Heufelder AE. Pathogenesis of Graves' ophthalmopathy. *N Engl J Med* (1993) 329(20):1468–75. doi:10.1056/NEJM199311113292007
2. Wyse EP, McConahey WM, Woolner LB, Scholz DA, Kearns TP. Ophthalmopathy without hyperthyroidism in patients with histologic Hashimoto's thyroiditis. *J Clin Endocrinol Metab* (1968) 28(11):1623–9. doi:10.1210/jcem-28-11-1623
3. Bahn RS. Graves' ophthalmopathy. *N Engl J Med* (2010) 362(8):726–38. doi:10.1056/NEJMra0905750
4. Dolman PJ. Evaluating Graves' orbitopathy. *Best Pract Res Clin Endocrinol Metab* (2012) 26(3):229–48. doi:10.1016/j.beem.2011.11.007
5. Daumerie C, Duprez T, Boschi A. Long-term multidisciplinary follow-up of unilateral thyroid-associated orbitopathy. *Eur J Intern Med* (2008) 19(7):531–6. doi:10.1016/j.ejim.2008.01.013
6. Yoshihara A, Yoshimura Noh J, Nakachi A, Ohye H, Sato S, Sekiya K, et al. Severe thyroid-associated orbitopathy in Hashimoto's thyroiditis. Report of 2 cases. *Endocr J* (2011) 58(5):343–8. doi:10.1507/endocrj.K11E-019
7. Bartley GB. The epidemiologic characteristics and clinical course of ophthalmopathy associated with autoimmune thyroid disease in Olmsted County, Minnesota. *Trans Am Ophthalmol Soc* (1994) 92:477–588.
8. Verma R, Gupta M, Mehta VK. Thyroid associated orbitopathy. *BMJ Case Rep* (2013) 2013:bcr2013009920. doi:10.1136/bcr-2013-009920
9. Khoo DH, Eng PH, Ho SC, Tai ES, Morgenthaler NG, Seah LL, et al. Graves' ophthalmopathy in the absence of elevated free thyroxine and triiodothyronine levels: prevalence, natural history, and thyrotropin receptor antibody levels. *Thyroid* (2000) 10(12):1093–100. doi:10.1089/thy.2000.10.1093
10. Forbes G, Gorman CA, Brennan MD, Gehring DG, Ilstrup DM, Earnest F IV. Ophthalmopathy of Graves' disease: computerized volume measurements of the orbital fat and muscle. *AJNR Am J Neuroradiol* (1986) 7(4):651–6.
11. Nugent RA, Belkin RI, Neigel JM, Rootman J, Robertson WD, Spinelli J, et al. Graves orbitopathy: correlation of CT and clinical findings. *Radiology* (1990) 177(3):675–82. doi:10.1148/radiology.177.3.2243967
12. Lacey B, Chang W, Rootman J. Nonthyroid causes of extraocular muscle disease. *Surv Ophthalmol* (1999) 44(3):187–213. doi:10.1016/S0039-6257(99)00101-0
13. Fallahi P, Ferrari SM, Ruffilli I, Elia G, Biricotti M, Veta R, et al. The association of other autoimmune diseases in patients with autoimmune thyroiditis: Review of the literature and report of a large series of patients. *Autoimmun Rev* (2016) 15(12):1125–8. doi:10.1016/j.autrev.2016.09.009
14. Baughman RP, Lower EE, Kaufman AH. Ocular sarcoidosis. *Semin Respir Crit Care Med* (2010) 31(4):452–62. doi:10.1055/s-0030-1262213
15. So WL, Hardy TG, McKelvie P. Atypical clinical presentation of isolated extraocular muscle sarcoid. *Case Rep Ophthalmol Med* (2012) 2012:370258. doi:10.1155/2012/370258
16. Heiligenhaus A, Michel D, Koch JM. Nodular scleritis in a patient with sarcoidosis. *Br J Ophthalmol* (2003) 87(4):507–8. doi:10.1136/bjo.87.4.507
17. Imes RK, Reifschneider JS, O'Connor LE. Systemic sarcoidosis presenting initially with bilateral orbital and upper lid masses. *Ann Ophthalmol* (1988) 20(12):466–7.
18. Hoang TD, Mai VQ, Clyde PW, Glister BC, Shakir MK. Multinodular goiter as the initial presentation of systemic sarcoidosis: limitation of fine-needle biopsy. *Respir Care* (2011) 56(7):1029–32. doi:10.4187/respcare.01000
19. Antonelli A, Fazzi P, Fallahi P, Ferrari SM, Ferrannini E. Prevalence of hypothyroidism and Graves disease in sarcoidosis. *Chest* (2006) 130(2):526–32. doi:10.1378/chest.130.2.526
20. Grimson BS, Simons KB. Orbital inflammation, myositis, and systemic lupus erythematosus. *Arch Ophthalmol* (1983) 101(5):736–8. doi:10.1001/archopht.1983.01040010736006
21. Weinstein JM, Koch K, Lane S. Orbital pseudotumor in Crohn's colitis. *Ann Ophthalmol* (1984) 16(3):275–8.
22. Patrinely JR, Osborn AG, Anderson RL, Whiting AS. Computed tomographic features of nonthyroid extraocular muscle enlargement. *Ophthalmology* (1989) 96(7):1038–47. doi:10.1016/S0161-6420(89)32785-0
23. Payne JF, Shields CL, Eagle RC Jr, Shields JA. Orbital lymphoma simulating thyroid orbitopathy. *Ophthal Plast Reconstr Surg* (2006) 22(4):302–4. doi:10.1097/01.iop.0000225422.69538.17
24. Eckardt AM, Lemound J, Rana M, Gellrich NC. Orbital lymphoma: diagnostic approach and treatment outcome. *World J Surg Oncol* (2013) 11:73. doi:10.1186/1477-7819-11-73
25. Purohit BS, Vargas MI, Ailianou A, Merlini L, Poletti PA, Platon A, et al. Orbital tumours and tumour-like lesions: exploring the armamentarium of multiparametric imaging. *Insights Imaging* (2016) 7(1):43–68. doi:10.1007/s13244-015-0443-8
26. Cunniffe G, Fernandez J, Alonso T, Balaguer O, Dinares C, Huguet P, et al. Thyroid orbitopathy obscuring the diagnosis of a rare neuromuscular hamartoma of the superior rectus muscle in an adult. *Orbit* (2010) 29(3):168–70. doi:10.3109/01676830903537146
27. Spraul CW, Lang GE, Lang GK. [Orbital myopathy in metastatic malignant paraganglioma: a paraneoplastic syndrome?]. *K lin Monbl Augenheilkd* (1996) 209(2–3):153–7. doi:10.1055/s-2008-1035296
28. Jaeger MJ, Green WR, Miller NR, Harris GJ. Granular cell tumor of the orbit and ocular adnexae. *Surv Ophthalmol* (1987) 31(6):417–23. doi:10.1016/0039-6257(87)90033-6
29. Grzesiuk W, Szydlarska D, Pragacz A, Bar-Andziak E. Thyroid-associated orbitopathy in patients with Hashimoto's thyroiditis: a case report. *Pol Arch Med Wewn* (2008) 118(5):318–21.
30. Dresner SC, Rothfus WE, Slamovits TL, Kennerdell JS, Curtin HD. Computed tomography of orbital myositis. *AJR Am J Roentgenol* (1984) 143(3):671–4. doi:10.2214/ajr.143.3.671
31. Kirsch E, Hammer B, von Arx G. Graves' orbitopathy: current imaging procedures. *Swiss Med Wkly* (2009) 139(43–44):618–23.
32. Muller-Forell W, Kahaly GJ. Neuroimaging of Graves' orbitopathy. *Best Pract Res Clin Endocrinol Metab* (2012) 26(3):259–71. doi:10.1016/j.beem.2011.11.009
33. Mombaerts I, Goldschmeding R, Schlingemann RO, Koornneef L. What is orbital pseudotumor? *Surv Ophthalmol* (1996) 41(1):66–78. doi:10.1016/S0039-6257(97)81996-0
34. Sanders MD, Hoyt WF. Hypoxic ocular sequelae of carotid-cavernous fistulae. Study of the caues of visual failure before and after neurosurgical treatment in a series of 25 cases. *Br J Ophthalmol* (1969) 53(2):82–97. doi:10.1136/bjo.53.2.82
35. Carlow TJ, Depper MH, Orrison WW Jr. MR of extraocular muscles in chronic progressive external ophthalmoplegia. *AJNR Am J Neuroradiol* (1998) 19(1):95–9.

23

The Role of the Microbiota in Graves' Disease and Graves' Orbitopathy

Jueyu Hou[1,2†], Yunjing Tang[1,2†], Yongjiang Chen[3†] and Danian Chen[1,2]*

[1] The Research Laboratory of Ophthalmology and Vision Sciences, State Key Laboratory of Biotherapy, West China Hospital, Sichuan University, Chengdu, China, [2] The Department of Ophthalmology, West China Hospital, Sichuan University, Chengdu, China, [3] The School of Optometry and Vision Science, University of Waterloo, Waterloo, ON, Canada

***Correspondence:**
Danian Chen
danianchen2006@qq.com
orcid.org/0000-0002-6916-2978

†These authors have contributed equally to this work

Graves' disease (GD) is a clinical syndrome with an enlarged and overactive thyroid gland, an accelerated heart rate, Graves' orbitopathy (GO), and pretibial myxedema (PTM). GO is the most common extrathyroidal complication of GD. GD/GO has a significant negative impact on the quality of life. GD is the most common systemic autoimmune disorder, mediated by autoantibodies to the thyroid-stimulating hormone receptor (TSHR). It is generally accepted that GD/GO results from complex interactions between genetic and environmental factors that lead to the loss of immune tolerance to thyroid antigens. However, the exact mechanism is still elusive. Systematic investigations into GD/GO animal models and clinical patients have provided important new insight into these disorders during the past 4 years. These studies suggested that gut microbiota may play an essential role in the pathogenesis of GD/GO. Antibiotic vancomycin can reduce disease severity, but fecal material transfer (FMT) from GD/GO patients exaggerates the disease in GD/GO mouse models. There are significant differences in microbiota composition between GD/GO patients and healthy controls. *Lactobacillus*, *Prevotella*, and *Veillonella* often increase in GD patients. The commonly used therapeutic agents for GD/GO can also affect the gut microbiota. Antigenic mimicry and the imbalance of T helper 17 cells (Th17)/regulatory T cells (Tregs) are the primary mechanisms proposed for dysbiosis in GD/GO. Interventions including antibiotics, probiotics, and diet modification that modulate the gut microbiota have been actively investigated in preclinical models and, to some extent, in clinical settings, such as probiotics (*Bifidobacterium longum*) and selenium supplements. Future studies will reveal molecular pathways linking gut and thyroid functions and how they impact orbital autoimmunity. Microbiota-targeting therapeutics will likely be an essential strategy in managing GD/GO in the coming years.

Keywords: gut microbiota, Graves' disease, Graves' orbitopathy (GO), TSHR (thyroid-stimulating hormone receptor), Th17 and Treg cells, *Lactobacillus*, *Prevotella*, *Veillonella*

INTRODUCTION

Graves' disease (GD) is an autoimmune disorder characterized by the unique association of an enlarged and overactive thyroid gland, an accelerated heart rate, Graves' orbitopathy (GO), and Graves' dermopathy such as pretibial myxedema (PTM), in its typical presentation. GD is the most common cause of hyperthyroidism. The lifetime risk is about 3% for women and 0.5% for men

(Davies et al., 2020). GD is mediated by autoantibodies to the thyroid-stimulating hormone receptor (TSHR). The TSHR is also expressed in orbital fibroblasts. GO is the most common extrathyroidal complication of GD (Covelli and Ludgate, 2017). About 25%–30% of GD patients have GO, but careful orbital imaging analysis can identify subtle orbital soft tissue abnormalities in 50%–70% of GD patients (Smith and Hegedüs, 2016; Perros et al., 2017; Taylor et al., 2020). The annual GO incidence is about 16 cases per 100,000 Europeans and 10 cases per 100,000 Japanese (Hiromatsu et al., 2014; Perros et al., 2017). GO is characterized by orbital tissue remodeling, retro-orbital inflammation, and glycosaminoglycan accumulation (Hansen et al., 1999). The major clinical features include periorbital edema, eyelid lag, proptosis, limited ocular movement, orbital disfigurement, and diplopia (Ludgate, 2020). Glucocorticoids are the primary treatment for GO at the active stage; smoking cessation, selenium supplements, and ocular lubricants are also helpful. Approximately 2% of GO patients will develop moderate to severe disease. These patients can have a visual loss due to corneal ulcers or GO-related optic neuropathy and eventually need decompression surgery (Davies et al., 2020). Thus, GO has a significant negative impact on the quality of life (Taylor et al., 2020).

GD is a multifactorial disease resulting from complex interactions between genetic and environmental factors that lead to the loss of immune tolerance to thyroid antigens. TSHR, T-cell-mediated immunity, and the mesenchymal stem cell properties of orbital fibroblasts have been implicated in the pathogenesis of GO (Taylor et al., 2020). However, the exact mechanism is still elusive. Some studies support the causative roles of microbiota in the pathogenesis of GD/GO (Kohling et al., 2017; Masetti and Ludgate, 2020).

Trillions of microorganisms exist on the mucosal and epidermal surfaces in the human body, such as skin, mouth, nose, sinuses, gut, respiratory tract, and ocular surface. These microbes are composed of bacteria, viruses, and fungi; usually do not harm; and are beneficial for the human body (Belkaid and Hand, 2014; Khan et al., 2019). The gastrointestinal tract is the primary interface in the human body to host microorganisms. Gut microbiota includes all microorganisms in the gastrointestinal mucosa and has about 10^{14} microbial cells (Szablewski, 2018). Gut microbiota can protect the host from pathogens, accelerate food digestion and mineral uptake (such as selenium, iron, and zinc), and modulate the immune system (Fröhlich and Wahl, 2019; Shivaji, 2019). Dysbiosis is an imbalance of the typical gut microbiota composition (Robles Alonso and Guarner, 2013). Dysbiosis can change the regulatory signaling of the immune system, resulting in pathological conditions of many organs (Gritz and Bhandari, 2015).

Indeed, increasing evidence has revealed that dysbiosis is closely connected to many diseases, including autoimmune diseases [e.g., rheumatoid arthritis (Gianchecchi and Fierabracci, 2019; Alghamdi and Redwan, 2021) and multiple sclerosis (Tsunoda, 2017; Zeng et al., 2019; Wang et al., 2021)], inflammatory diseases [e.g., ankylosing spondylitis (Ciccia et al., 2017; Wen et al., 2017; Berlinberg et al., 2021), infective endocarditis (Del Giudice et al., 2021), and inflammatory bowel disease (Kassam et al., 2018; Gianchecchi and Fierabracci, 2019; Pavel et al., 2021)], and ocular diseases [e.g., age-related macular degeneration (Rowan et al., 2017; Rinninella et al., 2018), diabetic retinopathy (Beli et al., 2018), dry eye (Cavuoto et al., 2019; Trujillo-Vargas et al., 2020), glaucoma (Chen et al., 2018; Doulberis et al., 2019), and uveitis (Fu et al., 2021)].

We will discuss the changes and potential mechanisms of the gut microbiota in the pathogenesis of GD/GO and comment on some possible therapeutic means to treat GD/GO by targeting the gut microbiome in this article.

CHANGES OF THE GUT MICROBIOME IN GD/GO

During the past 20 years, animal model studies have indicated a critical role of the gut microbiota in regulating innate and adaptive immune responses (Virili et al., 2021). Germ-free (GF) mouse models provide the most strong evidence to support that notion, including models of spontaneous ankylosing enteropathy (Rehakova et al., 2000), autoimmune arthritis (Wu et al., 2010), autoimmune encephalomyelitis (Lee et al., 2011), and autoimmune uveitis (Heissigerova et al., 2016; Fu et al., 2021). In these GF animal models, the disease incidence and severity are reduced under the GF environment, indicating the microbiota is crucial for the initiation and progression of these diseases (Vieira et al., 2014; Carding et al., 2015). This conclusion is further confirmed in clinical observations of many patients with ankylosing spondylitis (Ciccia et al., 2017; Wen et al., 2017), rheumatoid arthritis (Gianchecchi and Fierabracci, 2019), uveitis (Huang et al., 2018; Fu et al., 2021), and multiple sclerosis (Tsunoda, 2017; Zeng et al., 2019). GD is an autoimmune thyroid disease (AITD); the role of the gut microbiota in the pathogenesis of GD/GO was only discovered recently, based on both mouse models and clinical investigations (**Table 1**). These results are supported by findings that therapeutic agents of GD/GO (such as antithyroid drugs, glucocorticoids, immunosuppressants, and biologics) can also change the microbiota composition (**Table 2**).

Animal Models of GD/GO

Previously, a GD/GO animal model was established by transferring human TSHR-primed T cells into female BALB/c mice (Many et al., 1999). It was initially established in Brussels, Belgium. Many TSHR-immunized mice developed TSAb (thyroid-stimulating antibody) and GO-like phenotypes. However, this disease model could not be reproduced in Cardiff, UK (Baker et al., 2005). Because both animal facilities in Brussels and Cardiff are not pathogen-free, environmental microbial factors are possible reasons that TSHR-induced GO could not be generated in Cardiff. This result was the first scientific evidence suggesting that gut microbiota may be related to GD/GO pathogenesis (Baker et al., 2005; Masetti and Ludgate, 2020). The commonly used GD/GO mouse models are generally BALB/c female mice, induced by electroporation of DNA

TABLE 1 | Major references connecting the gut microbiome with GD/GO.

Year	Study Type	Subjects	Major Findings	References
2018	Experimental	BALB/c female, two locations	Disease-associated taxonomies explain the GD/GO variations observed	Masetti et al. (2018)
2018	Experimental	BALB/c and C57BL/6J females	Big differences of BALB/c and C57BL/6J gut microbiota composition	Moshkelgosha et al. (2018)
2020	Experimental	BALB/c female, FMT	FMT from GD donor increased the severity of GD	Su et al. (2020)
2021	Experimental	BALB/c female, microbiota modification	Vancomycin reduced, but FMT from GO donor increased the severity of GD/GO	Moshkelgosha et al. (2021)
2018	Clinical-GD	27 GD/12 HC	Diversity reduced, F/B ratio increased	Ishaq et al. (2018)
2019	Clinical-GD	15 GD/15 HC	Diversity reduced, F/B ratio increased	Yang M. et al. (2019)
2020	Clinical-GD	9 GD/11 HC	Diversity reduced	Cornejo-Pareja et al. (2020)
2020	Clinical-GD	58 GD/63 HC	Diversity reduced	Su et al. (2020)
2020	Clinical-GD	39 GD/17 HC	Diversity reduced	Yan et al. (2020)
2021	Clinical-GD	15 GD/14 HC	Diversity reduced	Chen et al. (2021)
2021	Clinical-GD	55 GD/48 HC	Diversity unchanged, F/B ratio decreased	Chang et al. (2021)
2021	Clinical-GD	45 GD/59 HC	Diversity reduced, F/B ratio decreased	Jiang et al. (2021)
2019	Clinical-GO	33 GO/32 HC	Diversity reduced, F/B ratio decreased	Shi et al. (2019b)
2019	Clinical-GO	31 GO	Links between the gut microbiota and GO-related traits are identified	Shi et al. (2019a)
2021	Clinical-GD/GO	30 GD/33 GO/32 HC	Random forest algorithm can identify the three groups with 70–80% accuracy	Shi et al. (2021)

GD, Graves' disease; GO, Graves' orbitopathy; F/B ratio, Firmicutes/Bacteroidetes ratio; HC, healthy controls.

plasmids expressing human TSHR A-subunit (Moshkelgosha et al., 2013) or injection of adenovirus expressing human TSHR A-subunit (Ad-TSHR289) (Chen et al., 2006). Both electroporation and Ad-TSHR289 can successfully induce GO-like phenotypes (Zhao et al., 2011).

GD/GO Mouse Models in Two Locations (Essen and London)

A recent study investigated the TSHR plasmid-immunized mice in two locations (Essen in Germany and London in the UK) by 16S rRNA gene sequencing and routine microbiological tests (Berchner-Pfannschmidt et al., 2016; Masetti et al., 2018). These female BALB/c mice showed different gut microbiota compositions between these two SPF (specific pathogen-free) facilities. Essen mice had more abundant *Lactobacillaceae*, *Ruminococcaceae*, and *Porphyromonadaceae*, but did not have *Bifidobacteria*. The *Firmicutes : Bacteroidetes* (F/B) ratio changed in TSHR mice of both locations. Orbital adipogenesis in Essen mice was correlated positively with *Firmicutes* OTUs (operational taxonomic units) and negatively with *Bacteroidetes* phyla. Disease-associated taxonomies have been identified and explained the clinical differences observed between Essen and London (**Figure 1A**). These findings suggest that gut microbiota may modulate the clinical heterogeneity of GD/GO in TSHR-immunized mice (Masetti et al., 2018).

GD/GO Models in Two Mouse Strains (C57BL/6 and BALB/c)

After being immunized with TSHR plasmids, female C57BL/6 mice had produced both TSAb and TSBAb (TSH stimulating blocking antibody). However, none of these mice had GD or any

TABLE 2 | Major references connecting the gut microbiome with therapeutic agents for GD/GO.

Year	Study Type	Therapeutic Agent	Subjects	References
2020	Experimental	PTU	Adult male SD rat	Shin et al. (2020)
2020	Experimental	PTU/MMI	Adult female SD rat	Sun et al. (2020)
2020	Clinical	PTU/MMI	GD patient	Sun et al. (2020)
2021	Clinical	MMI	GD patient	Chen et al. (2021)
2021	Clinical	MMI	GD patient	Huo et al. (2021)
2011	Experimental	Stress (increased steroid)	Mouse	Bailey et al. (2011)
2018	Experimental	GCs	Bird	Noguera et al. (2018)
2019	Clinical	GCs	Patient with GC-induced obesity	Qiu et al. (2019)
2020	Experimental	GCs (short term)	Mouse	Zhao et al. (2020)
2020	Experimental	GCs (long term)	Mouse	Schepper et al. (2020)
2021	Clinical	AZA	Crohn's disease patient	Effenberger et al. (2021)
2018	Experimental	MMF	Mouse	Flannigan et al. (2018)
2021	Experimental	MMF	Spontaneously hypertensive rat (SHR)	Robles-Vera et al. (2021)
2019	Clinical	Anti-TNF-α antibody	Crohn's disease patient	Yilmaz et al. (2019)
2021	Clinical	Anti-TNF-α antibody	Enteropathic arthritis patient	Ditto et al. (2021)
2021	Clinical	Anti-TNF-α antibody	Crohn's disease patient	Effenberger et al. (2021)

AZA, azathioprine; GD, Graves' disease; GCs, glucocorticoids; GO, Graves' orbitopathy; MMI, methimazole; MMF, mycophenolate mofetil; PTU, propylthiouracil; TNF-α, antitumor necrosis factor-α.

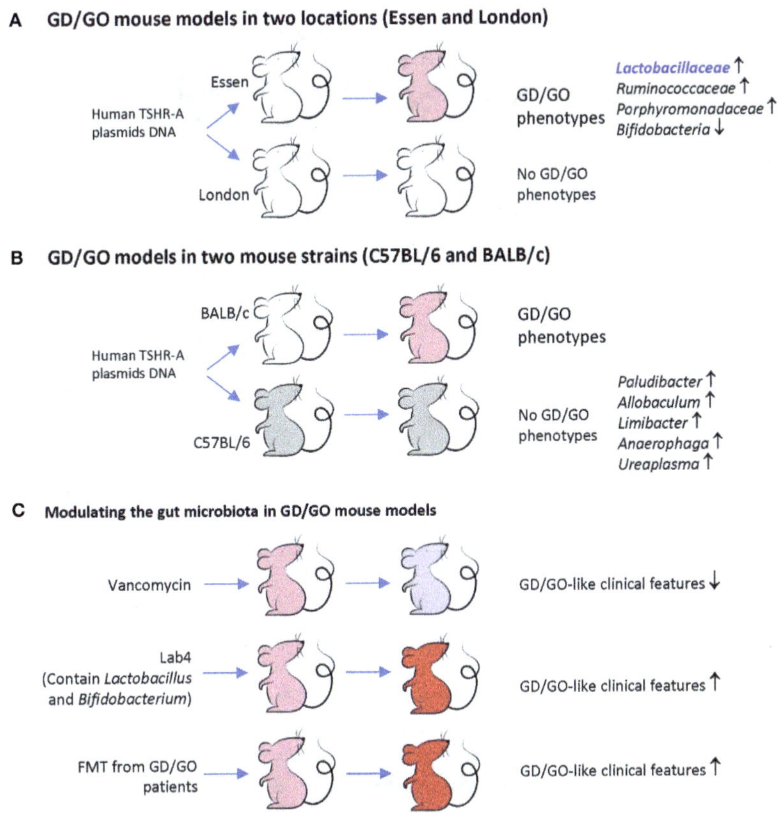

FIGURE 1 | Animal model of Graves' disease (GD)/Graves' orbitopathy (GO) and gut microbiota. **(A)** BALB/c female mice were immunized with human TSHR-A plasmid DNA. The mice in Essen but not in London developed GD/GO phenotypes (pink). These mice have different gut microbiome profiles. Note, Essen mice have more *Lactobacillaceae*, which is also increased in GD patients and a component in Lab4. **(B)** BALB/c and C57BL/6 female mice were immunized with human TSHR-A plasmid DNA. Only BALB/c but not C57BL/6 female mice developed GD/GO phenotypes (pink). These mice have different gut microbiome profiles. **(C)** Modify the gut microbiota of TSHR immunized mice (pink) by antibiotic vancomycin, probiotic Lab4, and fecal material transfer (FMT) from GD/GO patients, resulting in changed GD/GO-like clinical features (light purple or red). Derived from Berchner-Pfannschmidt et al. (2016); Masetti et al. (2018); Moshkelgosha et al. (2018); Su et al. (2020), and Moshkelgosha et al. (2021).

orbital soft tissue changes, while BALB/c female animals showed GD and GO-like phenotypes. Splenic T cells isolated from C57BL/6 mice did not grow upon TSHR stimulation and mainly produced IL-10, but not proinflammatory cytokines such as IFN-γ (Moshkelgosha et al., 2018). 16S rRNA sequencing revealed increased beta-diversity between BALB/c and C57BL/6J gut microbiome and differential abundance of five genera (*Paludibacter*, *Allobaculum*, *Limibacter*, *Anaerophaga*, and *Ureaplasma*). These two mice strains had different correlations between gut microbiota and clinical manifestations; for instance, TSAb in C57BL/6J mice was correlated negatively with increased *Limibacter*. These results indicate that gut microbiota can modulate the immune activity, which explains different thyroid/orbit changes in different inbred mouse strains receiving TSHR immunization (**Figure 1B**).

Modulating the Gut Microbiota in GD/GO Mouse Models

To investigate whether the above-observed correlation indicates causation, the same research team altered the microbiota composition before the TSHR immunization by antibiotic vancomycin, probiotic Lab4, and fecal material transfer (FMT) from GO patients (Moshkelgosha et al., 2021). The antibiotic vancomycin was administered through drinking water, and probiotic Lab4 and FMT powder were administered through gavage. Vancomycin reduced the richness and diversity of gut microbiota. It depleted *Firmicutes* genera but increased *Bacteroides*, thus reducing the F/B ratio. It also significantly reduced $CD4^{+}CD25^{+}$ regulatory T cells (Tregs) in orbital lymph nodes and GD/GO-like clinical features. TSHR mice receiving FMT from GO patients had a similar microbiota composition with their donors at the early stage after the transfer. GD-like features and orbital brown adipose tissue (BAT) volumes increased after FMT.

Lab4 are lactic acid bacteria that have been isolated from the gut flora of healthy humans. It combines four strains of lactic acid bacteria, including two strains of *Lactobacillus acidophilus*, one *Bifidobacterium animalis* subsp. *lactis*, and a *Bifidobacterium bifidum*. Despite Lab4 containing two *Bifidobacteria* species, none of them can be detected in any mice fed with Lab4, and the reason was unknown. Lab4 increased Tregs in orbital lymph nodes only in mice without TSHR immunization but not in mice receiving TSHR immunization. Lab4 exacerbated TSHR-induced autoimmune GD and GO-like phenotypes. Thus, although Lab4 increases orbital Tregs in normal mice, it cannot prevent TSHR-induced tolerance breakdown (Moshkelgosha et al., 2021).

In another BALB/c mouse model injected with Ad-TSHR289, FMT from GD patients before TSHR immunization also increased total T4, thyrotropin receptor antibody (TRAb), and IL-17A and doubled the GD incidence (Su et al., 2020). These findings suggest that the gut microbiota is involved in the development of GD/GO-like phenotypes (**Figure 1C**).

In summary (**Table 1** and **Figure 1**), experimental GD/GO models of the same mouse strain but housed in two different animal facilities (Masetti et al., 2018), or different mouse strains from the same animal facility (Moshkelgosha et al., 2018), revealed significant differences in gut microbiota composition which explain variations in clinical manifestations. Modulating gut microbiota can change the incidence and severity of GD/GO (Su et al., 2020; Moshkelgosha et al., 2021). These results uncovered a crucial role of gut microbiota in initiating and developing GD/GO mouse models (Masetti and Ludgate, 2020).

Changes of the Gut Microbiome in GD/GO Patients

There have been more than 10 clinical observational studies since 2018 comparing the gut microbiota of GD/GO patients to healthy controls (HCs). In total, fecal samples from 293 GD patients, 33 GO patients, and 271 healthy controls have been analyzed by 16S rRNA gene sequencing (**Table 1**).

Gut Microbiota in GD Patients

Until July 2021, there are eight papers, including 263 GD/239 HC samples, studying the gut microbiome of GD patients (**Table 1**). Overall, about 29 taxa are reported as differentially represented in GDs compared with HCs (**Figure 2**), and the gut microbial diversity decreased in most studies (Ishaq et al., 2018; Yang M. et al., 2019; Cornejo-Pareja et al., 2020; Su et al., 2020; Yan et al., 2020;

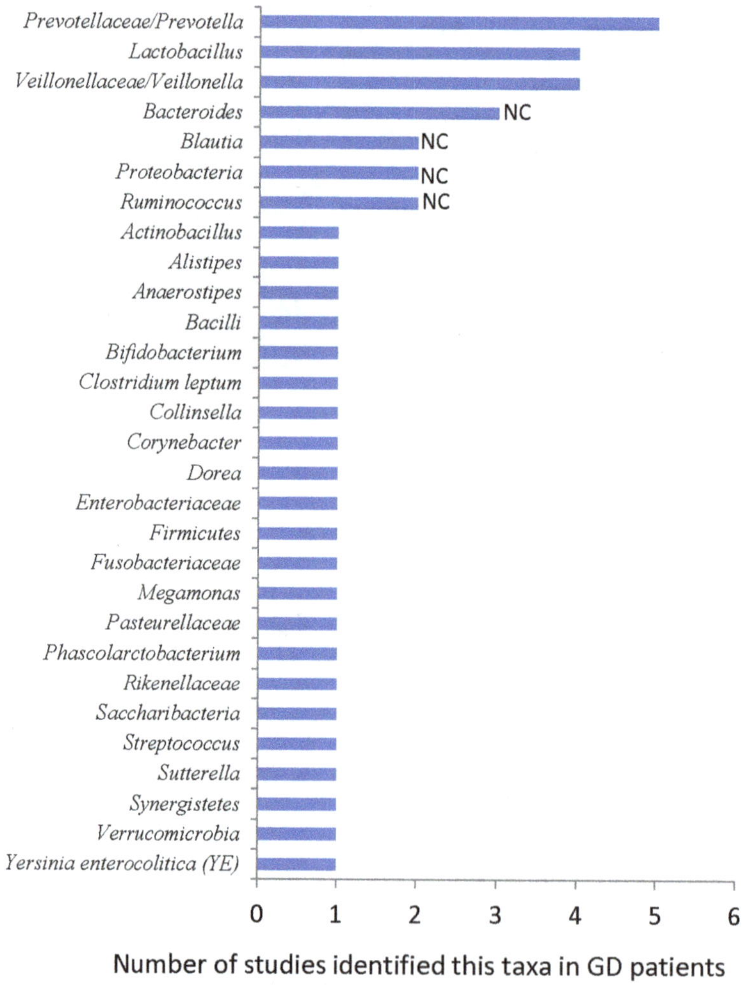

FIGURE 2 | Reported gut microbiota taxa changed in GD patients. NC: results are not consistent between studies.

Changet al., 2021; Chen et al., 2021; Jiang et al., 2021). However, other results across these studies lack consistency. Differences in sample size, subject heterogeneity, study design, geographical location, and sequencing platform may contribute to the lack of reproducibility. Despite these limitations, several taxa were identified in three or more studies, including *Prevotellaceae* and *Veillonellaceae* at the family level and *Bacteroides, Lactobacillus, Prevotella*, and *Veillonella* at the genus level (**Figure 2**).

In a study comparing 27 GD patients and 11 HCs, *Prevotellaceae* increased in GD patients (Ishaq et al., 2018). In another study with 58 GD patients and 63 HCs, the random forest analysis showed that GD patients could be distinguished from HCs with 85% accuracy by three bacteria species, including *Prevotella* (Su et al., 2020). *Prevotella* also increased in GD patients in another study (Yan et al., 2020). Furthermore, *Prevotellaceae* and *Prevotella* were identified as the core microbiome of the GD group (Cornejo-Pareja et al., 2020). Moreover, they were found to be closely associated with GD patients (Chang et al., 2021). *Prevotella* has been linked with rheumatoid arthritis (RA), as specific antigens of *Prevotella* can shape or amplify immune responses in RA joints (Scher et al., 2013; Pianta et al., 2017; Pianta et al., 2021).

At the genus level, *Bacteroides* of GD patients decreased in two studies (Ishaq et al., 2018; Su et al., 2020) but increased in another one (Jiang et al., 2021). The *Firmicutes* and *Bacteroidetes* phyla are the major components of the human and mouse microbiota. The F/B ratio of their abundance is often used as a dysbiosis marker. The F/B ratio increased in GD patients in two studies (Ishaq et al., 2018; Yang M. et al., 2019) but decreased in another two (Chang et al., 2021; Jiang et al., 2021), suggesting that this index may not be related to the pathogenesis of GD.

In three studies, *Lactobacillus* increased in GD patients (Yan et al., 2020; Chen et al., 2021; Jiang et al., 2021). Interestingly, the TRAb level was correlated positively with *Lactobacillus*, and the abundance of *Lactobacillus* decreased after oral methimazole (MMI) treatment (Chen et al., 2021). The TSHR plasmid-immunized GD/GO mice in Essen also had more abundant *Lactobacillaceae* (**Figure 1**) (Berchner-Pfannschmidt et al., 2016; Masetti et al., 2018). *Lactobacillus* is generally not pathogenic in the human body, and it is a recognized element in some probiotics such as Lab4 (Moshkelgosha et al., 2021). However, some studies also suggested that *Lactobacillus* can induce macrophages to secrete proinflammation cytokines, such as IL-6 and TNF-α (Rocha-Ramírez et al., 2017), and the abundance of *Lactobacillus* increased in autoimmune hepatitis (Wei et al., 2020) and Crohn's disease (Wang et al., 2014; Effenberger et al., 2021). These results are consistent with the observed effects of Lab4 on mice. Lab4 increases orbital Tregs in normal mice but exacerbates TSHR-induced autoimmune GD and GO-like phenotypes (**Figure 1**) (Moshkelgosha et al., 2021).

The abundance of the family *Veillonellaceae* or the genus *Veillonella* increased in GD patients (Yan et al., 2020; Chang et al., 2021; Chen et al., 2021). *Veillonella* is a symbiotic bacterium in humans and can become a conditional pathogenic bacterium. For instance, *Veillonella* acts as a pathogen in various inflammatory diseases such as pneumonia (Shah et al., 2008). *Veillonella* is also associated with the disease activity of autoimmune hepatitis (Wei et al., 2020) and recurrent Crohn's disease (De Cruz et al., 2015). The role of *Prevotella, Lactobacillus*, and *Veillonella* in the pathogenesis of GD needs further investigation.

Gut Microbiota in GO Patients

There are fewer studies regarding the gut microbiota of GO patients. Until July 2021, there are only three reports from a single institute, including 30 GD, 33 GO, and 30 HC samples (**Table 1**). In one study, 33 active GO patients and 32 HCs were compared (Shi et al., 2019b). Community diversity decreased in GO patients, consistent with most observations of GD patients (Ishaq et al., 2018; Yang M. et al., 2019; Cornejo-Pareja et al., 2020; Su et al., 2020; Chen et al., 2021; Jiang et al., 2021). The F/B ratio decreased in the GO group, consistent with some recent findings in GD patients (Su et al., 2020; Chang et al., 2021; Jiang et al., 2021). Metabolic-network-driven analysis of 31 hyperthyroid GO patients indicated that TRAb was associated with *Prevotellaceae* OTUs, CAS (clinical activity score) was associated with *Bacteroides* OTUs, and thyroglobulin autoantibodies were associated with OTUs from the *Bacteroides stercoris* species (Shi et al., 2019a). They also compared the original GO cohort (33 GO/32 HCs) with 30 GD patients taking antithyroid drugs. They identified bacterial phyla with different abundances between GD and GO patients, including *Deinococcus-Thermus, Cyanobacteria, Chloroflexi*, and *Actinobacteria*. At the genus level, *Blautia, Anaerostipes, Dorea*, and *Butyricicoccus* were more abundant in the GD group, while *Subdoligranulum* and *Bilophila* were more abundant in the GO group. Random forest analysis could differentiate GO patients, GD patients, and HCs with 70%–80% accuracy. *Deinococcus-Thermus, Cyanobacteria*, and *Chloroflexi* were the major taxa determining the classification accuracy (Shi et al., 2021). These results need to be confirmed with more studies on larger groups of patients.

In summary, clinical studies concluded that GD/GO patients and healthy controls have a much different gut microbiota composition. Whether these gut microbiota alterations in GD/GO patients could contribute to disease pathogenesis or are just a consequence remains unknown. However, FMT from GD/GO patients significantly increased GD/GO incidence in the GD/GO mouse model, suggesting a fundamental pathogenic role of gut microbiota in the development of GD/GO (Su et al., 2020; Moshkelgosha et al., 2021).

THE EFFECTS ON THE GUT MICROBIOTA OF THERAPEUTIC AGENTS FOR GD/GO

The primary goal in the treatment of GD is restoring normal thyroid hormone levels. To reach this goal, antithyroid drugs (such as thionamides), radioiodine, and thyroidectomy are commonly used. The treatment of GO is stage-dependent. The anti-inflammatory agent is recommended for active progressive disease, and rehabilitative surgery is performed only in the stable inactive stage (Davies et al., 2020). Glucocorticoids (GCs) are the first-line treatment; if an insufficient response is observed after 6 weeks, second-line therapy, including immunosuppressants (such as mycophenolate mofetil and azathioprine) and biologic agents (such as rituximab, infliximab tocilizumab, and teprotumumab) should be considered (Davies et al., 2020; Taylor et al., 2020). Recent studies indicated that some of these therapeutic agents (including antithyroid drugs, glucocorticoids, immunosuppressants, and biologics) could also affect the gut microbiota (**Table 2**).

Antithyroid Drugs and Gut Microbiota

Methimazole (MMI) and propylthiouracil (PTU) are the commonly used antithyroid drugs (ATDs). ATD can change the gut microbiota structure in wild-type adult rats (Shin et al., 2020; Sun et al., 2020) and GD patients (Sun et al., 2020; Chen et al., 2021; Huo et al., 2021).

The effects of PTU on microbiota were studied in adult male SD rats (Shin et al., 2020). After treatment for 4 weeks, the alpha-diversity did not change. However, *Christensenellaceae*, *Tenericutes*, and *Mollicutes* increased, while *Ruminococcaceae*, *Prevotella*, *Mogibacteriaceae*, *Alcaligenaceae*, *Betaproteobacteria*, *Burkholderiales*, *Sutterella*, and *Ruminococcus* decreased (Shin et al., 2020). The effects of MMI/PTU on microbiota were also measured in female adult SD rats (Sun et al., 2020). ATDs increased the alpha-diversity, different from the results in female rats (Shin et al., 2020). The ATD group had more *Bacteroidetes*, *Proteobacteria*, and *Spirochaetae*, but fewer *Firmicutes* at the phylum level and more *Prevotellaceae* and *Ruminococcaceae* but fewer *Lactobacillaceae* and *Peptostreptococcaceae* at the family level. Compared with the MMI group, the PTU group had more *Spirochaetae* at the phylum level and more *Spirochaetaceae* and *Clostridiaceae_1* but less *Lachnospiraceae* and *Rikenellaceae* at the family level. The microbial dysbiosis index (MDI) increased after ATD treatment, indicating that the gut microbiota structure was disturbed in the treatment group. The MDI of the MMI group was higher than that of the PTU group (Sun et al., 2020).

ATDs can also affect the gut microbiota composition of GD patients. The fecal samples from 20 MMI-treated GD patients, 20 PTU-treated GD patients, and 50 healthy controls were analyzed by 16S rRNA sequencing. The MMI group had a higher Ace index than the PTU group. The community diversity was different between the two drug treatment groups. The MMI group had more *Firmicutes* at the phylum level, while the PTU group had more *Bacteroidetes.* The MMI group had more *Blautia* and *Escherichia–Shigella* at the genus level, while the PTU group had more *Bacteroides* and *Lachnoclostridium.* The MDI and the F/B ratio suggested that dysbiosis occurred in both drug-treated groups. Interestingly, ATD treatment reduced short-chain fatty acid (SCFA)-producing bacteria, including *Faecalibacterium*, *Ruminococcaceae*, *Lactobacillus*, and *Blautia* (Sun et al., 2020).

In a recent study with 15 GD patients, MMI treatment reduced the abundance of *Blautia*, *Lactobacillus*, and *Streptococcus* but increased *Proteobacteria* (Chen et al., 2021). In another study with 8 GD patients, MMI treatment for 6 months also reduced the microbial Shannon index and *Faecalibacterium prausnitzii*, *Ligilactobacillus salivarius*, *Lactococcus lactis*, and some species of the genera *Porphyromonas* and *Prevotella* (Huo et al., 2021).

Glucocorticoids and Gut Microbiota

GCs are the first-line treatments for moderate to severe active GO. GCs are potent immune-modulating drugs with a number of side effects, such as GC-induced obesity or osteoporosis, but little is known about the effect of steroid treatment on gut microbiota in GO patients. In patients with GC-induced obesity, gut microbial diversity decreased, *Firmicutes* (e.g., genus *Streptococcus*) increased, and *Bacteroidetes* were depleted. Concomitantly, the SCFA level decreased in gut microbial metabolites of these patients (Qiu et al., 2019).

In animal models, GCs can change the composition of gut microbiota. In mice, dexamethasone increased the abundance of *Actinobacteria*, *Bifidobacterium*, and *Lactobacillus* compared with controls (Huang et al., 2015). A recent study found different results regarding *Lactobacillus* (Zhao et al., 2020). At the phyla level, short-term dexamethasone treatment increased the abundance of *Firmicutes.* At the genus level, dexamethasone increased the abundance of *Lachnospiraceae*, *Oscillibacter*, *Ruminococcaceae*, *Ruminiclostridium*, *Anaerotruncus*, and *Butyricicoccus* but reduced the abundance of *Lactobacillus*, *Enterorhabdus*, and *Pseudomonas* (Zhao et al., 2020).

It is also proven in mice that subcutaneous prednisolone implants for 8 weeks can promote dysbiosis, cause intestinal barrier leaks, and raise serum endotoxin levels. GCs reduced *Verrucomicobiales* and *Bacteriodales* and increased *Clostridiales.* These effects mediated the GC-induced osteoporosis (Schepper et al., 2020). In birds (yellow-legged gull *Larus michahellis*), corticosterone implants reduced *Mycoplasma* and *Microvirga*, which were potentially pathogenic avian bacteria, and increased *Firmicutes*, which was beneficial for birds (Noguera et al., 2018).

GCs can also alter the gut microbiota through changes in brain function. Stress can increase serum corticosteroid levels; stress also changes the mouse microbiome, and it reduces intestinal *Bacteroides* while increasing the relative abundance of bacteria in the genus *Clostridium* (Bailey et al., 2011). This effect is similar to the results of long-term subcutaneous prednisolone implants (Schepper et al., 2020).

Immunosuppressant Drugs Have a Direct Effect on Microbiota

Recent clinical trials concluded that combining steroids with immunosuppressant drugs (azathioprine and mycophenolate mofetil) has beneficial effects for GO patients (Kahaly et al., 2018; Rajendram et al., 2018). While these effects are generally attributed to their immunosuppressive activity, azathioprine (AZA) and mycophenolate mofetil (MMF) directly affect the microbiota. In liver cells, AZA is metabolized to 6-mercaptopurine (MP), which can inhibit the maturation of B and T lymphocytes and the synthesis of DNA/RNA and proteins in immune cells. AZA can inhibit the growth of *Campylobacter concisus*, *Bacteroides fragilis*, *Bacteroides vulgatus*, *Escherichia coli*, and *Mycobacterium Avium paratuberculosis* (Shin and Collins, 2008; Antoniani et al., 2013; Liu et al., 2017). AZA is commonly used to treat inflammatory bowel disease (IBD). AZA can restore intestinal microbial diversity in patients with Crohn's disease by decreasing *Proteobacteria* but increasing *Bacteroidetes* (Effenberger et al., 2021).

MMF is an inhibitor of inosine-5′-monophosphate dehydrogenase (IMPDH). MMF inhibits both T-cell and B-cell activities by blocking purine synthesis and is widely used in organ transplant recipients to reduce immune rejection (Ritter and Pirofski, 2009). MMF has some antibacterial (such as *Staphylococcus epidermidis*), antifungal (such as *Cryptococcus*, *Aspergillus*, *Pneumocystis jirovekii*, and *Candida albicans*), and antiviral (such as *Camelpox virus*, *Cowpox virus*, *Monkeypox virus*, and *Vaccinia virus*) activities, as it inhibits the synthesis of microbial DNA/RNA (Jones, 2020).

MMF treatment can cause gastrointestinal (GI) toxicity in organ transplant recipients. In mice, MMF reduced the overall gut microbial diversity and increased *Proteobacteria*. MMF-induced GI toxicity could be reversed or prevented using broad-spectrum antibiotics and was absent in germ-free animals (Flannigan et al., 2018; Taylor et al., 2019). Spontaneously hypertensive rats (SHR) are commonly used hypertension animal models. They have decreased gut microbial richness and acetate- and butyrate-producing bacteria and increased F/B ratio and lactate-producing bacteria (Yang T. et al., 2019). MMF can reduce blood pressure in SHR (Rodríguez-Iturbe et al., 2002). MMF triggered substantial changes in the SHR microbiota taxa and reduced gut dysbiosis by reducing the F/B ratio and lactate-producing bacteria and increasing acetate- and butyrate-producing bacteria (Robles-Vera et al., 2021).

Biological Agents and Gut Microbiota

Several biological agents that can be used as a novel therapy for GO patients. Even though there were very few studies regarding the effects of these agents on gut microbiota, their underlying pathways can interact with gut microbiota. For example, rituximab (RTX), a chimeric human-murine anti-CD20 monoclonal antibody, has been used to treat active moderate–severe GO for more than 15 years (Vannucchi et al., 2021). RTX eliminates orbital and peripheral B cells, therefore, reducing the production of antibodies. B-cell-produced IgA is the most abundant antibody in the mucosa; secretory IgA (SIgA) is secreted into the lumen of the gut. IgA can bind to multiple distinct taxonomic groups of the microbiota and is involved in the elimination, neutralization, and colonization of gut microbiota. IgA can also regulate bacterial gene expression (Weis and Round, 2021). Thus, RTX should have some effects on gut microbiota, but this has not been specifically addressed.

Tocilizumab, a humanized recombinant IL-6R monoclonal antibody, can improve disease activity and severity in corticosteroid-resistant GO patients (Perez-Moreiras et al., 2018; Sánchez-Bilbao et al., 2020). Infliximab, an antitumor necrosis factor (TNF)-α antibody, has been successfully used to treat sight-threatening GO (Durrani et al., 2005; Komorowski et al., 2007; Fallahi et al., 2021). Both IL-6 and TNF-α are monocyte-derived key proinflammation cytokines. Gut microbiota can modulate the production of these cytokines through their metabolites. The microbial tryptophan metabolite tryptophol potently influences cytokine production, which has strong inhibitory effects on the TNF-α response. On the other hand, palmitoleic acid can affect the production of monocyte-derived cytokines (TNF-α, IL-1β, IL-6) but not lymphocyte-derived cytokines (IFN-γ, IL-17, IL-22) (Schirmer et al., 2016). *Lachnospiraceae* and *Ruminococcaceae* families, typically producing SCFAs, define the frequently relapsing disease and poor treatment response to anti-TNF-α in Crohn's disease (Yilmaz et al., 2019). Like AZA, the anti-TNF-α antibody can restore intestinal microbial diversity in patients with Crohn's disease by decreasing *Proteobacteria* but increasing *Bacteroidetes* (Effenberger et al., 2021). In 20 enteropathic arthritis patients who followed a Mediterranean diet, anti-TNF-α antibody treatment for 6 months could increase *Lachnospiraceae* family and *Coprococcus* genus and also induce a decreasing trend in *Proteobacteria* and *Gammaproteobacteria* and an increasing trend in *Clostridia* (Ditto et al., 2021).

Teprotumumab, an insulin-like growth factor-1 receptor (IGFR-1) inhibiting monoclonal antibody, was approved in the USA to treat GO (Kahaly et al., 2021). Gut microbiota can modulate circulating IGF-1 in the host. Microbiota-derived metabolites such as SCFAs are sufficient to induce IGF-1 (Yan and Charles, 2018). How teprotumumab affects gut microbiota has not yet been explored.

In summary, the fact that ATDs, GCs, AZA, and MMF can change the microbiota composition is consistent with the notion that modifying the gut microbiota may reduce the severity of GD/GO, thus strengthening the concept that GD/GO and dysbiosis are tightly connected. The relationship between biological agents and gut microbiota needs further study in the future.

HOW GUT MICROBIOTA AFFECT GD/GO DEVELOPMENT

Two major mechanisms are proposed, namely, molecular/antigenic mimicry and imbalance of proinflammation T helper 17 cells (Th17) and Treg cells (**Figure 3**).

Antigenic Mimicry

Yersinia enterocolitica (YE) and *Helicobacter pylori* (HP) were thought to be possible environmental risk factors for GD for a long time (Wolf et al., 1991). The structural or conformational similarity between different antigens can lead to cross-reactivity, also known as molecular or antigenic mimicry. Cross-reactivity between gut microbial peptides and self-antigens can produce autoreactive T cells and induce autoimmunity (Avni and Koren, 2018; Rojas et al., 2018; Wildner and Diedrichs-Möhring, 2020). If microbes have similar protein structures in their host, they will escape immune detection (**Figure 3A**).

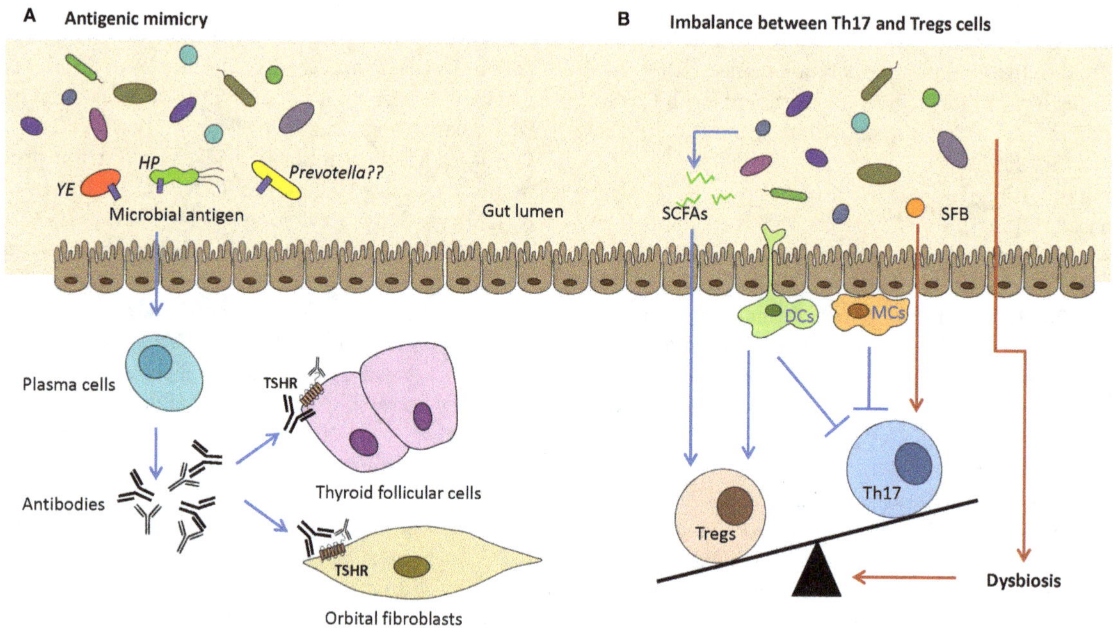

FIGURE 3 | Two potential proposed mechanisms of GD/GO are caused by dysbiosis of the gut microbiome. **(A)** Antigenic mimicry. Antigenic mimics in the gut microbiome, which have a highly similar structure or sequence with the autoantigens (e.g., TSHR), could activate plasma cells to produce antibodies that can bind TSHR on the thyroid follicular cells and orbital fibroblasts. Possible pathogenic microbes include *Yersinia enterocolitica* (YE), *Helicobacter pylori* (HP), and *Prevotella*. **(B)** Imbalance between Th17 and Tregs cells. Intestinal dysbiosis may cause the absence of beneficial microbiota and the reduction in beneficial anti-inflammatory metabolites such as SCFAs, which can increase the production of Tregs. SFB can promote the differentiation and maturation of Th17 cells. The imbalance between Th17 and Tregs cells can indirectly promote the progression of GD/GO. TSHR, thyroid-stimulating hormone receptor; SCFA, short-chain fatty acids; SFB, segmented filamentous bacteria.

Such similarities can be shared by amino acid and nucleotide sequence or protein 3D structures (Miraglia and Colla, 2019). YE porin proteins have sequence similarity with TSHR and can stimulate B cells to produce autoantibodies to TSHR (Wang et al., 2010; Hargreaves et al., 2013). The IgG from YE-infected patients can induce GD-like changes in human thyroid structures, and GD patients have a higher YE infection rate than the healthy controls (Wolf et al., 1991). Although YE is considered involved in the development of GD, 16S rRNA gene sequencing did not detect it in GD patients. However, PCR analysis could easily detect YE in GD patients with diarrhea (Su et al., 2020).

HP in the human gastric mucosa can also affect the development of GD/GO (Bassi et al., 2010). Human TSHR is partly aligned with nine HP proteins such as NADH dehydrogenase subunit L, ABC transporter, and radical SAM protein (Figura et al., 2019). The most virulent HP strains express the cytotoxin-associated gene A antigens (CagA). GD patients have a much higher prevalence of CagA$^+$ HP than healthy controls (Bassi et al., 2010). While these clinical observations support that antigenic mimicry may trigger GD/GO, it has not been proven in any animal model yet.

Several recent studies revealed that *Prevotellaceae* and *Prevotella* consistently increase in GD patients (Ishaq et al., 2018; Cornejo-Pareja et al., 2020; Su et al., 2020; Yan et al., 2020; Chang et al., 2021). *Prevotella* has been linked with rheumatoid arthritis (RA), as specific antigens of *Prevotella*, such as Pc-27 and *N*-acetylglucosamine-6-sulfatase (GNS), can trigger antigenic mimicry with RA joints (Scher et al., 2013; Pianta et al., 2017; Pianta et al., 2021). If these *Prevotella*-related antigens have similarities with human TSHR, they need further investigation.

Imbalance Between Th17 and Treg Cells

The gut-associated lymphoid tissue has many T-cell populations, including proinflammation helper T (Th) cells and anti-inflammation Tregs. T helper cells include Th1, Th2, and Th17 cells. Th17 cells are the most important autoimmunity-related cells. Autoimmune diseases are closely related to abnormal Th17 cells (Bettelli et al., 2007; Pandiyan et al., 2019). Usually, Th17 and Tregs cells are in a dynamic balance to maintain the immune homeostasis of the gut mucosa. Gut microbiota can keep the balance between Th17/Tregs (Omenetti and Pizarro, 2015) (**Figure 3B**).

For instance, some gut microorganisms, such as *Intestinimonas* and *Roseburia*, can produce SCFAs, including primarily acetic acid, propionic acid, and butyric acid. SCFAs can increase Tregs in the gut mucosa (Smith et al., 2013). *Segmented filamentous bacteria* (SFB) promote the differentiation and maturation of Th17 cells (Ivanov et al., 2008; Hedblom et al., 2018). Gut microbiota can affect gut dendritic cells and macrophage cells. Gut dendritic cells can secrete transforming growth factor-beta (TGF-β), promoting the differentiation of

Th17 and Treg cells. Dendritic cells also produce retinoic acid, which can promote Treg development but suppress Th17 cells. Gut macrophages can inhibit Th17 development by producing IL-2 and IL-10 (Masetti and Ludgate, 2020). Thus, dysbiosis may increase Th17 cells and suppress Treg production, which can cause many intestine inflammatory conditions and some extraintestinal diseases such as autoimmune uveitis (Zhuang et al., 2017).

As expected, GD patients have much less circulating $CD4^+Foxp3^+$ Tregs but more $CD4^+IL\text{-}17^+$ Th17 cells (Qin et al., 2017; Su et al., 2020). Gas chromatography–mass spectrometry (GC–MS) analysis generated metabolic profiles of gut microbiota in GD patients and indicated that two important SCFAs (propionic acid and butyric acid) were significantly decreased in GD patients (Su et al., 2020). SCFA-producing *Bacteroides fragilis* YCH46 strain (B.f.S) was significantly reduced in GD patients. The culturing medium of B.f.S increased Tregs and IL-10 levels but reduced Th17 cells and IL-17A levels in peripheral blood mononuclear cells (PBMCs) from healthy individuals. B.f.S also exacerbated the imbalance of Treg/Th17 cells in GD patients (Su et al., 2020). GO patients also have much more Th17 cells and higher IL-17A expression than normal controls (Fang et al., 2016). These results are further confirmed by single-cell sequencing of retrobulbar tissues from GO patients (Fang et al., 2019). Single-cell sequencing identified six major cell clusters in retrobulbar tissues, including orbital fibroblasts and lymphocytes. In the $CD4^+CD8^-$ T-cell subset, both IFN-γ–producing and IL-17A–producing T cells increased, but $FoxP3^+$ Tregs decreased in GO orbits (Fang et al., 2019). Thus, increased Th17 and impaired Treg responses may be involved in GD/GO pathogenesis.

Removing $CD4^+CD25^+$ Tregs afforded some GD-resistant C57BL/6 mice susceptible to Ad-TSHR289 immunization and increased the GD severity in susceptible BALB/c mice. Removing $CD4^+CD25^+$ Tregs also promoted TSAB production but suppressed thyroid-blocking antibody synthesis. These results indicate that Tregs are essential for Ad-TSHR289–induced GD phenotypes (Saitoh and Nagayama, 2006). However, the importance of Th17 cells in the immune response of the GD mouse model varies among different genetic backgrounds (Horie et al., 2011). BALB/c and NOD-H2(h4) mouse strains with wild-type (WT) or knockout (KO) IL-17 genes were immunized with Ad-TSHR289. BALB/c mice developed GD with WT or KO IL17 gene, but NOD-H2(h4) mice developed GD only in some animals with WT IL17 gene. This result suggested that IL-17 is essential for the GD development only in NOD-H2(h4) but not in BALB/c background (Horie et al., 2011).

These findings suggest that Th17/Treg imbalance is involved in developing GD/GO in some genetic backgrounds or ethnic groups (for instance, all these abovementioned clinical observations are from the Asian population).

TARGETING THE GUT MICROBIOTA TO TREAT GD/GO

Dysbiosis is closely related to the development of GD/GO; therapeutic approaches targeting the gut microbiota may provide potential benefits to GD/GO patients. Currently, antibiotics, probiotics, diet modifications, and fecal microbial transplantation are the four major strategies proposed.

Antibiotics

Antibiotics can change the gut microbiome. It was shown that oral antibiotic vancomycin could reduce the GD/GO severity in mouse models by reducing gut microbiota richness and diversity (**Figure 1C**). The reduced orbital pathology was correlated positively with *Akkermansia* (Moshkelgosha et al., 2021). As HP infection of the gastric mucosa is associated with GD through an increased inflammatory status and molecular mimicry, anti-HP therapy may also benefit GD/GO patients (Figura et al., 2019).

Probiotics

Probiotics are live microorganisms with health benefits, which improve or restore the gut microbiota. Probiotics can promote the differentiation of Tregs, thus modifying the intestine immune homeostasis (Lin, 2019). Probiotics have been tested in GD/GO mouse models (Moshkelgosha et al., 2021) and GD patients (Huo et al., 2021).

The probiotic Lab4 is a consortium comprising of *Lactobacillus* and *Bifidobacterium*. Lab4 elevated the orbital $CD25^+$ Treg cells but promoted the GD/GO phenotypes of TSHR-immunized mice (Moshkelgosha et al., 2021). One possible reason is that *Lactobacillus* in Lab4 may be pathogenic to GD as it frequently increases in fecal samples from GD patients (Yan et al., 2020; Chen et al., 2021; Jiang et al., 2021). These results also suggest that probiotics alone are not enough to suppress GD/GO development. Treatment with MMI and probiotic *Bifidobacterium longum* (2×10^7 CFU per day) for 6 months improved thyroid function and significantly reduced the TRAb concentration of nine GD patients (Huo et al., 2021). This treatment increased *Bifidobacterium adolescentis*, *Bifidobacterium angulatum*, *Bifidobacterium breve*, *B. longum*, and *Faecalibacterium prausnitzii* and reduced *Blautia hansenii*, *Clostridium esterthеticum*, and *Klebsiella pneumoniae.* Several microbial metabolic pathways were enriched in subjects receiving the probiotic *B. longum* treatment, including fatty acid biosynthesis, toluene degradation, phenylacetate degradation, and flavin biosynthesis. SCFAs also increased in these patients (Huo et al., 2021). The above results from animal models and GD patients support the idea that *Lactobacillus* may not benefit GD patients.

Future studies need to optimize the beneficial microbe stains in the probiotics formula; for instance, the formula should not include *Lactobacillus*, *Prevotella*, and *Veillonella*, as their abundance often increases in GD patients (Ishaq et al., 2018; Yang M. et al., 2019; Cornejo-Pareja et al., 2020; Su et al., 2020; Yan et al., 2020; Chang et al., 2021; Chen et al., 2021; Jiang et al., 2021).

Diet Modifications and Selenium Supplements

The diet can shape the microbiome composition. Culture and geographic-related diet differences can cause microbiome composition changes, for instance, *Firmicutes* enriched in the USA and Russia, *Bacteroides* spp. enriched in France and China, and *Prevotella* spp. enriched in Germany and India (Fröhlich and Wahl, 2019). Most GD patients have a reduced microbial diversity, which can be helped by a fiber-rich, low-calorie diet (Meijnikman et al., 2018). Diet with more vegetables increases SCFAs and *Bifidobacteria*, but animal fat increases the production of secondary bile acids (Ercolini and Fogliano, 2018). Diet with eicosapentaenoic acid (EPA) can inhibit IFN-γ and IL-17 productions, thus attenuating experimental autoimmune encephalomyelitis (EAE) (Unoda et al., 2013).

The Mediterranean diet (MD) is consumed in countries bordering the Mediterranean sea and is characterized by a high intake of vegetables and fruits, legumes, and whole grains combined with a moderate amount of red wine and olive oil. It is well known that MD plays a protective role in preventing cardiovascular diseases, type 2 diabetes mellitus, obesity, Alzheimer's or Parkinson's disease, and cancer. MD was associated with a higher abundance of *Bacteroidetes*, *Prevotellacea*, and *Prevotella* and a lower concentration of *Firmicutes* and *Lachnospiraceae*. MD can also induce fecal propionate and butyrate (De Filippis et al., 2016; Gutiérrez-Díaz et al., 2016). As discussed above, *Prevotellacea* and *Prevotella* often increase in GD patients (Yan et al., 2020; Chang et al., 2021; Chen et al., 2021), and MD may not be a good choice for GD/GO patients. However, these results are mainly from research in Asia; if MD has any beneficial effects on GD/GO patients in the other geographic locations needs further study.

In the 2021 European Group on Graves' orbitopathy (EUGOGO) clinical practice guidelines for the medical management of GO, oral selenium supplementation is recommended for patients with mild GO (Bartalena et al., 2021). Mild GO patients from selenium-deficient areas can benefit from oral selenium supplementation. A double-blind, randomized clinical trial confirmed that sodium selenite could improve both the quality of life and overall ocular outcome and slow the progression in mild GO patients (Marcocci et al., 2011). These effects may be partially related to the role of selenium on gut microbiota. In adult C57BL/6 male mice, selenium in the diet can increase the microbiota diversity (Kasaikina et al., 2011), increase *Turicibacter* and *Akkermansia*, but reduce *Mucispirillum* (Qixiao Zhai et al., 2018). *Turicibacter* has been reported to display potential anti-inflammatory activities in the gut, and *Akkermansia* plays an essential role in the gut barrier protection, immune modulation, and metabolic regulation of the host (Qixiao Zhai et al., 2018). *Akkermansia* is also correlated positively with reduced orbital pathology in vancomycin-treated GO mouse models (**Figure 1C**) (Moshkelgosha et al., 2021). Thus, selenium supplementation increased the gut microbial diversity and positively modulated health beneficial microbes and negatively modulated the deleterious microbes in mice models. However, the effects of selenium supplementation on human gut microbiota are still unknown (Ferreira et al., 2021).

Fecal Microbiota Transplantation

Fecal microbiota transplantation (FMT) transfers fecal bacteria and other microbes from a healthy donor into the patient to replace their dysbiotic microbiota. FMT has been successfully used to treat *Clostridium difficile* infection in colitis by increasing the diversity of the host microbiota (Cheng et al., 2019). FMT has also been used to treat rheumatoid arthritis (Zeng et al., 2021). FMT from GD/GO patients can increase the severity of induced GD/GO-like features in TSHR immunization mouse models (Su et al., 2020; Moshkelgosha et al., 2021), but if FMT from healthy donors can suppress established GD/GO manifestation has not been tested yet.

CONCLUSIONS AND FUTURE DIRECTIONS

The relationship between gut microbiota and GD/GO has been uncovered during the past 4 years. Oral antibiotic vancomycin reduces disease severity in GD/GO mouse models, but FMT from GD/GO patients exaggerates the disease. There are significant differences in microbiota composition between GD/GO patients and healthy controls. *Lactobacillus*, *Prevotella*, and *Veillonella* often increase in GD patients. GCs are the first-line treatment for GO and can also change the composition of the microbiota. Two immunosuppression drugs (AZA and MMF) for GO have some antimicrobial properties; two AIDs (MMI and PTU) can change microbiota composition. Antigenic mimicry and imbalance of Th17/Tregs are likely the mechanisms for the effects of dysbiosis on GD/GO phenotypes.

Interventions including antibiotics, probiotics, and diet modification that modulate the gut microbiota have been actively investigated in preclinical models and clinical settings. However, only limited data exist on their effects on GD/GO patients. More research is needed to reveal molecular pathways linking gut and thyroid functions and how they impact orbital autoimmunity. For instance, the gut microbial features of GO patients need to be determined in more geographic locations; the effects of different probiotic formulas on GD/GO mouse model and patients need to be investigated; and how *Lactobacillus*, *Prevotella*, and *Veillonella* affect GD/GO phenotypes is still unknown. We believe microbiota-targeting therapeutics will be an important strategy in the management of GD/GO. This conclusion requires not only a thorough understanding of the distinct gut microbial composition and function of GD/GO patients but also carefully designed clinical trials.

AUTHOR CONTRIBUTIONS

JH, YT, YC, and DC conceived and designed the manuscript, and all authors wrote, edited, and approved the manuscript.

REFERENCES

1. Alghamdi, M. A., and Redwan, E. M. (2021). Interplay of Microbiota and Citrullination in the Immunopathogenesis of Rheumatoid Arthritis. *Probiotics Antimicrob. Proteins*. doi: 10.1007/s12602-021-09802-7
2. Antoniani, D., Rossi, E., Rinaldo, S., Bocci, P., Lolicato, M., Paiardini, A., et al. (2013). The Immunosuppressive Drug Azathioprine Inhibits Biosynthesis of the Bacterial Signal Molecule Cyclic-Di-GMP by Interfering With Intracellular Nucleotide Pool Availability. *Appl. Microbiol. Biotechnol.* 97, 7325–7336. doi: 10.1007/s00253-013-4875-0
3. Avni, O., and Koren, O. (2018). Molecular (Me)micry? *Cell Host Microbe* 23, 576– 578. doi: 10.1016/j.chom.2018.04.012
4. Bailey, M. T., Dowd, S. E., Galley, J. D., Hufnagle, A. R., Allen, R. G., and Lyte, M. (2011). Exposure to a Social Stressor Alters the Structure of the Intestinal Microbiota: Implications for Stressor-Induced Immunomodulation. *Brain Behav. Immun.* 25, 397–407. doi: 10.1016/j.bbi.2010.10.023
5. Baker, G., Mazziotti, G., Von Ruhland, C., and Ludgate, M. (2005). Reevaluating Thyrotropin Receptor-Induced Mouse Models of Graves' Disease and Ophthalmopathy. *Endocrinology* 146, 835–844. doi: 10.1210/en.2004-1015
6. Bartalena, L., Kahaly, G. J., Baldeschi, L., Dayan, C. M., Eckstein, A., Marcocci, C., et al. (2021). The 2021 European Group on Graves' Orbitopathy (EUGOGO) Clinical Practice Guidelines for the Medical Management of Graves' Orbitopathy. *Eur. J. Endocrinol.* 185, G43–g67. doi: 10.1530/EJE-21-0479
7. Bassi, V., Santinelli, C., Iengo, A., and Romano, C. (2010). Identification of a Correlation Between Helicobacter Pylori Infection and Graves' Disease. *Helicobacter* 15, 558–562. doi: 10.1111/j.1523-5378.2010.00802.x
8. Beli, E., Yan, Y., Moldovan, L., Vieira, C. P., Gao, R., Duan, Y., et al. (2018). Restructuring of the Gut Microbiome by Intermittent Fasting Prevents Retinopathy and Prolongs Survival in Db/Db Mice. *Diabetes* 67, 1867–1879. doi: 10.2337/db18-0158
9. Belkaid, Y., and Hand, T. W. (2014). Role of the Microbiota in Immunity and Inflammation. *Cell* 157, 121–141. doi: 10.1016/j.cell.2014.03.011
10. Berchner-Pfannschmidt, U., Moshkelgosha, S., Diaz-Cano, S., Edelmann, B., Görtz, G. E., Horstmann, M., et al. (2016). Comparative Assessment of Female Mouse Model of Graves' Orbitopathy Under Different Environments, Accompanied by Proinflammatory Cytokine and T-Cell Responses to Thyrotropin Hormone Receptor Antigen. *Endocrinology* 157, 1673–1682. doi: 10.1210/en.2015-1829
11. Berlinberg, A. J., Regner, E. H., Stahly, A., Brar, A., Reisz, J. A., Gerich, M. E., et al. (2021). Multi 'Omics Analysis of Intestinal Tissue in Ankylosing Spondylitis Identifies Alterations in the Tryptophan Metabolism Pathway. *Front. Immunol.* 12, 587119. doi: 10.3389/fimmu.2021.587119
12. Bettelli, E., Oukka, M., and Kuchroo, V. K. (2007). T(H)-17 Cells in the Circle of Immunity and Autoimmunity. *Nat. Immunol.* 8, 345–350. doi: 10.1038/ ni0407-345
13. Carding, S., Verbeke, K., Vipond, D. T., Corfe, B. M., and Owen, L. J. (2015). Dysbiosis of the Gut Microbiota in Disease. *Microb. Ecol. Health Dis.* 26, 26191. doi: 10.3402/mehd.v26.26191
14. Cavuoto, K. M., Banerjee, S., and Galor, A. (2019). Relationship Between the Microbiome and Ocular Health. *Ocul. Surf.* 17, 384–392. doi: 10.1016/j.jtos.2019.05.006
15. Chang, S. C., Lin, S. F., Chen, S. T., Chang, P. Y., Yeh, Y. M., Lo, F. S., et al. (2021). Alterations of Gut Microbiota in Patients With Graves' Disease. *Front. Cell Infect. Microbiol.* 11, 663131. doi: 10.3389/fcimb.2021.663131
16. Chen, C. R., Aliesky, H. A., Guo, J., Rapoport, B., and Mclachlan, S. M. (2006). Blockade of Costimulation Between T Cells and Antigen-Presenting Cells: An Approach to Suppress Murine Graves' Disease Induced Using Thyrotropin Receptor-Expressing Adenovirus. *Thyroid* 16, 427–434. doi: 10.1089/ thy.2006.16.427
17. Chen, H., Cho, K.-S., Vu, T. H. K., Shen, C.-H., Kaur, M., Chen, G., et al. (2018). Commensal Microflora-Induced T Cell Responses Mediate Progressive Neurodegeneration in Glaucoma. *Nat. Commun.* 9, 3209. doi: 10.1038/ s41467-018-05681-9
18. Cheng, Y. W., Phelps, E., Ganapini, V., Khan, N., Ouyang, F., Xu, H., et al. (2019). Fecal Microbiota Transplantation for the Treatment of Recurrent and Severe Clostridium Difficile Infection in Solid Organ Transplant Recipients: A Multicenter Experience. *Am. J. Transplant.* 19, 501–511. doi: 10.1111/ajt.15058
19. Chen, J., Wang, W., Guo, Z., Huang, S., Lei, H., Zang, P., et al. (2021). Associations Between Gut Microbiota and Thyroidal Function Status in Chinese Patients With Graves' Disease. *J. Endocrinol. Invest.* 44 (9), 1913–1926. doi: 10.1007/ s40618-021-01507-6
20. Ciccia, F., Guggino, G., Rizzo, A., Alessandro, R., Luchetti, M. M., Milling, S., et al. (2017). Dysbiosis and Zonulin Upregulation Alter Gut Epithelial and Vascular Barriers in Patients With Ankylosing Spondylitis. *Ann. Rheum. Dis.* 76, 1123– 1132. doi: 10.1136/annrheumdis-2016-210000
21. Cornejo-Pareja, I., Ruiz-Limón, P., Gómez-Pérez, A. M., Molina-Vega, M., Moreno-Indias, I., and Tinahones, F. J. (2020). Differential Microbial Pattern Description in Subjects With Autoimmune-Based Thyroid Diseases: A Pilot Study. *J. Pers. Med.* 10. doi: 10.3390/jpm10040192
22. Covelli, D., and Ludgate, M. (2017). The Thyroid, the Eyes and the Gut: A Possible Connection. *J. Endocrinol. Invest.* 40, 567–576. doi: 10.1007/s40618-016-0594-6 Davies, T. F., Andersen, S., Latif, R., Nagayama, Y., Barbesino, G., Brito, M., et al. (2020). Graves' Disease. *Nat. Rev. Dis. Primers* 6, 52. doi: 10.1038/s41572-020-0184-y
23. De Cruz, P., Kang, S., Wagner, J., Buckley, M., Sim, W. H., Prideaux, L., et al. (2015). Association Between Specific Mucosa-Associated Microbiota in Crohn's Disease at the Time of Resection and Subsequent Disease Recurrence: A Pilot Study. *J. Gastroenterol. Hepatol.* 30, 268–278. doi: 10.1111/jgh.12694
24. De Filippis, F., Pellegrini, N., Vannini, L., Jeffery, I. B., La Storia, A., Laghi, L., et al. (2016). High-Level Adherence to a Mediterranean Diet Beneficially Impacts the Gut Microbiota and Associated Metabolome. *Gut* 65, 1812–1821. doi: 10.1136/gutjnl-2015-309957
25. Del Giudice, C., Vaia, E., Liccardo, D., Marzano, F., Valletta, A., Spagnuolo, G., et al. (2021). Infective Endocarditis: A Focus on Oral Microbiota. *Microorganisms* 9. doi: 10.3390/microorganisms9061218
26. Ditto, M. C., Parisi, S., Landolfi, G., Borrelli, R., Realmuto, C., Finucci, A., et al. (2021). Intestinal Microbiota Changes Induced by TNF-Inhibitors in IBD- Related Spondyloarthritis. *RMD Open* 7. doi: 10.1136/rmdopen-2021-001755
27. Doulberis, M., Polyzos, S. A., Papaefthymiou, A., Katsinelos, P., and Kountouras, J. (2019). Comments to the Editor Concerning the Paper Entitled "The Microbiome and Ophthalmic Disease" by Baim Et Al. *Exp. Biol. Med.* 244, 430–432. doi: 10.1177/1535370218824340
28. Durrani, O. M., Reuser, T. Q., and Murray, P. I. (2005). Infliximab: A Novel Treatment for Sight-Threatening Thyroid Associated Ophthalmopathy. *Orbit* 24, 117–119. doi: 10.1080/01676830590912562
29. Effenberger, M., Reider, S., Waschina, S., Bronowski, C., Enrich, B., Adolph, T. E., et al. (2021). Microbial Butyrate Synthesis Indicates Therapeutic Efficacy of Azathioprine in IBD Patients. *J. Crohns Colitis* 15, 88–98. doi: 10.1093/ecco- jcc/jjaa152
30. Ercolini, D., and Fogliano, V. (2018). Food Design To Feed the Human Gut Microbiota. *J. Agric. Food Chem.* 66, 3754–3758. doi: 10.1021/acs.jafc.8b00456 Fallahi, P., Ferrari, S. M., Elia, G., Ragusa, F., Paparo, S. R., Patrizio, A., et al. (2021). Cytokines as Targets of Novel Therapies for Graves' Ophthalmopathy. *Front. Endocrinol. (Lausanne)* 12, 654473. doi: 10.3389/fendo.2021.654473
31. Fang, S., Huang, Y., Wang, S., Zhang, Y., Luo, X., Liu, L., et al. (2016). IL-17a Exacerbates Fibrosis by Promoting the Proinflammatory and Profibrotic Function of Orbital Fibroblasts in TAO. *J. Clin. Endocrinol. Metab.* 101, 2955–2965. doi: 10.1210/jc.2016-1882
32. Fang, S., Huang, Y., Wang, N., Zhang, S., Zhong, S., Li, Y., et al. (2019). Insights Into Local Orbital Immunity: Evidence for the Involvement of the Th17 Cell Pathway in Thyroid-Associated Ophthalmopathy. *J. Clin. Endocrinol. Metab.* 104, 1697–1711. doi: 10.1210/jc.2018-01626
33. Ferreira, R. L. U., Sena-Evangelista, K. C. M., De Azevedo, E. P., Pinheiro, F. I., Cobucci, R. N., and Pedrosa, L. F. C. (2021). Selenium in Human Health and Gut Microflora: Bioavailability of Selenocompounds and Relationship With Diseases. *Front. Nutr.* 8, 685317. doi: 10.3389/fnut.2021.685317
34. Figura, N., Di Cairano, G., Moretti, E., Iacoponi, F., Santucci, A., Bernardini, G., et al. (2019). Helicobacter Pylori Infection and Autoimmune Thyroid Diseases: The Role of Virulent Strains. *Antibiot. (Basel)* 9. doi: 10.3390/antibiotics9010012
35. Flannigan, K. L., Taylor, M. R., Pereira, S. K., Rodriguez-Arguello, J., Moffat, A. W., Alston, L., et al. (2018). An Intact Microbiota is Required for the

Gastrointestinal Toxicity of the Immunosuppressant Mycophenolate Mofetil. *J. Heart Lung Transplant.* 37, 1047–1059. doi: 10.1016/j.healun.2018.05.002

36. Fröhlich, E., and Wahl, R. (2019). Microbiota and Thyroid Interaction in Health and Disease. *Trends Endocrinol. Metab.* 30, 479–490. doi: 10.1016/j.tem.2019.05.008
37. Fu, X., Chen, Y., and Chen, D. (2021). The Role of Gut Microbiome in Autoimmune Uveitis. *Ophthalmic Res.* 64, 168–177. doi: 10.1159/000510212
38. Gianchecchi, E., and Fierabracci, A. (2019). Recent Advances on Microbiota Involvement in the Pathogenesis of Autoimmunity. *Int. J. Mol. Sci.* 20, 283. doi: 10.3390/ijms20020283
39. Gritz, E. C., and Bhandari, V. (2015). The Human Neonatal Gut Microbiome: A Brief Review. *Front. Pediatr.* 3, 17. doi: 10.3389/fped.2015.00017
40. Gutiérrez-Dıaz, I., Fernández-Navarro, T., Sánchez, B., Margolles, A., and González, S. (2016). Mediterranean Diet and Faecal Microbiota: A Transversal Study. *Food Funct.* 7, 2347–2356. doi: 10.1039/C6FO00105J
41. Hansen, C., Rouhi, R., Förster, G., and Kahaly, G. J. (1999). Increased Sulfatation of Orbital Glycosaminoglycans in Graves' Ophthalmopathy. *J. Clin. Endocrinol. Metab.* 84, 1409–1413. doi: 10.1210/jc.84.4.1409
42. Hargreaves, C. E., Grasso, M., Hampe, C. S., Stenkova, A., Atkinson, S., Joshua, G. W., et al. (2013). Yersinia Enterocolitica Provides the Link Between Thyroid- Stimulating Antibodies and Their Germline Counterparts in Graves' Disease. *J. Immunol.* 190, 5373–5381. doi: 10.4049/jimmunol.1203412
43. Hedblom, G. A., Reiland, H. A., Sylte, M. J., Johnson, T. J., and Baumler, D. J. (2018). Segmented Filamentous Bacteria - Metabolism Meets Immunity. *Front. Microbiol.* 9, 1991. doi: 10.3389/fmicb.2018.01991
44. Heissigerova, J., Seidler Stangova, P., Klimova, A., Svozilkova, P., Hrncir, T., Stepankova, R., et al. (2016). The Microbiota Determines Susceptibility to Experimental Autoimmune Uveoretinitis. *J. Immunol. Res.*, 2016, 5065703. doi: 10.1155/2016/5065703
45. Hiromatsu, Y., Eguchi, H., Tani, J., Kasaoka, M., and Teshima, Y. (2014). Graves' Ophthalmopathy: Epidemiology and Natural History. *Intern. Med.* 53, 353– 360. doi: 10.2169/internalmedicine.53.1518
46. Horie, I., Abiru, N., Saitoh, O., Ichikawa, T., Iwakura, Y., Eguchi, K., et al. (2011). Distinct Role of T Helper Type 17 Immune Response for Graves' Hyperthyroidism in Mice With Different Genetic Backgrounds. *Autoimmunity* 44, 159–165. doi: 10.3109/08916931003777247
47. Huang, E. Y., Inoue, T., Leone, V. A., Dalal, S., Touw, K., Wang, Y., et al. (2015). Using Corticosteroids to Reshape the Gut Microbiome: Implications for Inflammatory Bowel Diseases. *Inflamm Bowel Dis.* 21, 963–972. doi: 10.1097/MIB.0000000000000332
48. Huang, X., Ye, Z., Cao, Q., Su, G., Wang, Q., Deng, J., et al. (2018). Gut Microbiota Composition and Fecal Metabolic Phenotype in Patients With Acute Anterior Uveitis. *Invest. Ophthalmol. Vis. Sci.* 59, 1523–1531. doi: 10.1167/iovs.17-22677
49. Huo, D., Cen, C., Chang, H., Ou, Q., Jiang, S., Pan, Y., et al. (2021). Probiotic Bifidobacterium Longum Supplied With Methimazole Improved the Thyroid Function of Graves' Disease Patients Through the Gut-Thyroid Axis. *Commun. Biol.* 4, 1046. doi: 10.1038/s42003-021-02587-z
50. Ishaq, H. M., Mohammad, I. S., Shahzad, M., Ma, C., Raza, M. A., Wu, X., et al. (2018). Molecular Alteration Analysis of Human Gut Microbial Composition in Graves' Disease Patients. *Int. J. Biol. Sci.* 14, 1558–1570. doi: 10.7150/ijbs.24151
51. Ivanov, Ii, Frutos, R. D. E., Manel, N., Yoshinaga, K., Rifkin, D. B., Sartor, R. B., et al. (2008). Specific Microbiota Direct the Differentiation of IL-17-Producing T-Helper Cells in the Mucosa of the Small Intestine. *Cell Host Microbe* 4, 337– 349. doi: 10.1016/j.chom.2008.09.009
52. Jiang, W., Yu, X., Kosik, R. O., Song, Y., Qiao, T., Tong, J., et al. (2021). Gut Microbiota May Play a Significant Role in the Pathogenesis of Graves' Disease. *Thyroid* 31, 810–820. doi: 10.1089/thy.2020.0193
53. Jones, N. P. (2020). Immunosuppression in the Management of Presumed Non-Infective Uveitis; Are We Sure What We are Treating? Notes on the Antimicrobial Properties of the Systemic Immunosuppressants. *Ocul. Immunol. Inflamm.* 28 (6), 994–1003. doi: 10.1080/09273948.2019.1643030
54. Kahaly, G. J., Douglas, R. S., Holt, R. J., Sile, S., and Smith, T. J. (2021). Teprotumumab for Patients With Active Thyroid Eye Disease: A Pooled Data Analysis, Subgroup Analyses, and Off-Treatment Follow-Up Results From Two Randomised, Double-Masked, Placebo-Controlled, Multicentre Trials. *Lancet Diabetes Endocrinol.* 9, 360–372. doi: 10.1016/S2213-8587(21)00056-5
55. Kahaly, G. J., Riedl, M., König, J., Pitz, S., Ponto, K., Diana, T., et al. (2018). Mycophenolate Plus Methylprednisolone Versus Methylprednisolone Alone in Active, Moderate-to-Severe Graves' Orbitopathy (MINGO): A Randomised, Observer-Masked, Multicentre Trial. *Lancet Diabetes Endocrinol.* 6, 287–298. doi: 10.1016/S2213-8587(18)30020-2
56. Kasaikina, M. V., Kravtsova, M. A., Lee, B. C., Seravalli, J., Peterson, D. A., Walter, J., et al. (2011). Dietary Selenium Affects Host Selenoproteome Expression by Influencing the Gut Microbiota. *FASEB J.* 25, 2492–2499. doi: 10.1096/fj.11- 181990
57. Kassam, F., Gurry, T., Aldarmaki, A., Nguyen, T., Kassam, Z., Beck, P. L., et al. (2018). The Impact of the Gut Microbiome in Developing Uveitis Among Inflammatory Bowel Disease Patients: A Case-Control Study. *Gastroenterology* 154, S-415. doi: 10.1016/S0016-5085(18)31664-0
58. Khan, R., Petersen, F. C., and Shekhar, S. (2019). Commensal Bacteria: An Emerging Player in Defense Against Respiratory Pathogens. *Front. Immunol.* 10, 1203. doi: 10.3389/fimmu.2019.01203
59. Kohling, H. L., Plummer, S. F., Marchesi, J. R., Davidge, K. S., and Ludgate, M. (2017). The Microbiota and Autoimmunity: Their Role in Thyroid Autoimmune Diseases. *Clin. Immunol.* 183, 63–74. doi: 10.1016/j.clim.2017.07.001
60. Komorowski, J., Jankiewicz-Wika, J., Siejka, A., Lawnicka, H., Kłysik, A., Goś, R., et al. (2007). Monoclonal Anti-TNFalpha Antibody (Infliximab) in the Treatment of Patient With Thyroid Associated Ophthalmopathy. *Klin. Oczna.* 109, 457–460.
61. Lee, Y. K., Menezes, J. S., Umesaki, Y., and Mazmanian, S. K. (2011). Proinflammatory T-Cell Responses to Gut Microbiota Promote Experimental Autoimmune Encephalomyelitis. *Proc. Natl. Acad. Sci. U. S. A.* 108 (Suppl 1), 4615–4622. doi: 10.1073/pnas.1000082107
62. Lin, P. (2019). Importance of the Intestinal Microbiota in Ocular Inflammatory Diseases: A Review. *Clin. Exp. Ophthalmol.* 47, 418–422. doi: 10.1111/ ceo.13493
63. Liu, F., Ma, R., Riordan, S. M., Grimm, M. C., Liu, L., Wang, Y., et al. (2017). Azathioprine, Mercaptopurine, and 5-Aminosalicylic Acid Affect the Growth of IBD-Associated Campylobacter Species and Other Enteric Microbes. *Front. Microbiol.* 8, 527. doi: 10.3389/fmicb.2017.00527
64. Ludgate, M. (2020). Fibrosis in Dysthyroid Eye Disease. *Eye (Lond)* 34, 279–284. doi: 10.1038/s41433-019-0731-5
65. Many, M. C., Costagliola, S., Detrait, M., Denef, F., Vassart, G., and Ludgate, M. C. (1999). Development of an Animal Model of Autoimmune Thyroid Eye Disease. *J. Immunol.* 162, 4966–4974.
66. Marcocci, C., Kahaly, G. J., Krassas, G. E., Bartalena, L., Prummel, M., Stahl, M., et al. (2011). Selenium and the Course of Mild Graves' Orbitopathy. *N. Engl. J. Med.* 364, 1920–1931. doi: 10.1056/NEJMoa1012985
67. Masetti, G., and Ludgate, M. (2020). Microbiome and Graves' Orbitopathy. *Eur. Thyroid J.* 9, 78–85. doi: 10.1159/000512255
68. Masetti, G., Moshkelgosha, S., Köhling, H. L., Covelli, D., Banga, J. P., Berchner- Pfannschmidt, U., et al. (2018). Gut Microbiota in Experimental Murine Model of Graves' Orbitopathy Established in Different Environments may Modulate Clinical Presentation of Disease. *Microbiome* 6, 97. doi: 10.1186/s40168-018- 0478-4
69. Meijnikman, A. S., Gerdes, V. E., Nieuwdorp, M., and Herrema, H. (2018). Evaluating Causality of Gut Microbiota in Obesity and Diabetes in Humans. *Endocr. Rev.* 39, 133–153. doi: 10.1210/er.2017-00192
70. Miraglia, F., and Colla, E. (2019). Microbiome, Parkinson's Disease and Molecular Mimicry. *Cells* 8. doi: 10.3390/cells8030222
71. Moshkelgosha, S., Masetti, G., Berchner-Pfannschmidt, U., Verhasselt, H. L., Horstmann, M., Diaz-Cano, S., et al. (2018). Gut Microbiome in BALB/c and C57BL/6J Mice Undergoing Experimental Thyroid Autoimmunity Associate With Differences in Immunological Responses and Thyroid Function. *Horm. Metab. Res.* 50, 932–941. doi: 10.1055/a-0653-3766
72. Moshkelgosha, S., So, P. W., Deasy, N., Diaz-Cano, S., and Banga, J. P. (2013). Cutting Edge: Retrobulbar Inflammation, Adipogenesis, and Acute Orbital Congestion in a Preclinical Female Mouse Model of Graves' Orbitopathy Induced by Thyrotropin Receptor Plasmid-*In Vivo* Electroporation. *Endocrinology* 154, 3008–3015. doi: 10.1210/en.2013-1576
73. Moshkelgosha, S., Verhasselt, H. L., Masetti, G., Covelli, D., Biscarini, F., Horstmann, M., et al. (2021). Modulating Gut Microbiota in a Mouse Model of Graves' Orbitopathy and its Impact on Induced Disease. *Microbiome* 9, 45. doi: 10.1186/s40168-020-00952-4

74. Noguera, J. C., Aira, M., Pérez-Losada, M., Domınguez, J., and Velando, A. (2018). Glucocorticoids Modulate Gastrointestinal Microbiome in a Wild Bird. *R. Soc. Open Sci.* 5, 171743. doi: 10.1098/rsos.171743

75. Omenetti, S., and Pizarro, T. T. (2015). The Treg/Th17 Axis: A Dynamic Balance Regulated by the Gut Microbiome. *Front. Immunol.* 6, 639. doi: 10.3389/ fimmu.2015.00639

76. Pandiyan, P., Bhaskaran, N., Zou, M., Schneider, E., Jayaraman, S., and Huehn, J. (2019). Microbiome Dependent Regulation of T(regs) and Th17 Cells in Mucosa. *Front. Immunol.* 10, 426. doi: 10.3389/fimmu.2019.00426

77. Pavel, F. M., Vesa, C. M., Gheorghe, G., Diaconu, C. C., Stoicescu, M., Munteanu, M. A., et al. (2021). Highlighting the Relevance of Gut Microbiota Manipulation in Inflammatory Bowel Disease. *Diagn. (Basel)* 11. doi: 10.3390/diagnostics11061090

78. Perez-Moreiras, J. V., Gomez-Reino, J. J., Maneiro, J. R., Perez-Pampin, E., Romo Lopez, A., Rodrıguez Alvarez, F. M., et al. (2018). Efficacy of Tocilizumab in Patients With Moderate-To-Severe Corticosteroid-Resistant Graves Orbitopathy: A Randomized Clinical Trial. *Am. J. Ophthalmol.* 195, 181- 190. doi: 10.1016/j.ajo.2018.07.038

79. Perros, P., Hegedüs, L., Bartalena, L., Marcocci, C., Kahaly, G. J., Baldeschi, L., et al. (2017). Graves' Orbitopathy as a Rare Disease in Europe: A European Group on Graves' Orbitopathy (EUGOGO) Position Statement. *Orphanet J. Rare Dis.* 12, 72. doi: 10.1186/s13023-017-0625-1

80. Pianta, A., Arvikar, S., Strle, K., Drouin, E. E., Wang, Q., Costello, C. E., et al. (2017). Evidence of the Immune Relevance of Prevotella Copri, a Gut Microbe, in Patients With Rheumatoid Arthritis. *Arthritis Rheumatol.* 69, 964–975. doi: 10.1002/art.40003

81. Pianta, A., Chiumento, G., Ramsden, K., Wang, Q., Strle, K., Arvikar, S., et al. (2021). Identification of Novel, Immunogenic HLA-DR-Presented Prevotella Copri Peptides in Patients With Rheumatoid Arthritis: Patients With Rheumatoid Arthritis. *Arthritis Rheumatol.* 73 (12), 2200–2205. doi: 10. 1002/art.41807

82. Qin, J., Zhou, J., Fan, C., Zhao, N., Liu, Y., Wang, S., et al. (2017). Increased Circulating Th17 But Decreased CD4(+)Foxp3(+) Treg and CD19(+) CD1d(hi) CD5(+) Breg Subsets in New-Onset Graves' Disease. *BioMed. Res. Int.*, 2017, 8431838. doi: 10.1155/2017/8431838

83. Qiu, D., Xia, Z., Deng, J., Jiao, X., Liu, L., and Li, J. (2019). Glucorticoid-Induced Obesity Individuals Have Distinct Signatures of the Gut Microbiome. *Biofactors* 45, 892–901. doi: 10.1002/biof.1565

84. Qixiao Zhai, S. C., Peng, L, Fengwei, T., Jianxin, Z., Hao, Z., and Wei, C. (2018). Effects of Dietary Selenium Supplementation on Intestinal Barrier and Immune Responses Associated With Its Modulation of Gut Microbiota. *Environ. Sci. Technol. Lett.* 5 (2), 724–730. doi: 10.1021/acs.estlett.8b00563

85. Rajendram, R., Taylor, P. N., Wilson, V. J., Harris, N., Morris, O. C., Tomlinson,

86. M., et al. (2018). Combined Immunosuppression and Radiotherapy in Thyroid Eye Disease (CIRTED): A Multicentre, 2 × 2 Factorial, Double-Blind, Randomised Controlled Trial. *Lancet Diabetes Endocrinol.* 6, 299–309. doi: 10.1016/S2213-8587(18)30021-4

87. Rehakova, Z., Capkova, J., Stepankova, R., Sinkora, J., Louzecka, A., Ivanyi, P., et al. (2000). Germ-Free Mice do Not Develop Ankylosing Enthesopathy, a Spontaneous Joint Disease. *Hum. Immunol.* 61, 555–558. doi: 10.1016/S0198- 8859(00)00122-1

88. Rinninella, E., Mele, M. C., Merendino, N., Cintoni, M., Anselmi, G., Caporossi, A., et al. (2018). The Role of Diet, Micronutrients and the Gut Microbiota in Age-Related Macular Degeneration: New Perspectives From the Gut(-)Retina Axis. *Nutrients* 10. doi: 10.3390/nu10111677

89. Ritter, M. L., and Pirofski, L. (2009). Mycophenolate Mofetil: Effects on Cellular Immune Subsets, Infectious Complications, and Antimicrobial Activity. *Transpl. Infect. Dis.* 11, 290–297. doi: 10.1111/j.1399-3062.2009.00407.x

90. Robles Alonso, V., and Guarner, F. (2013). Linking the Gut Microbiota to Human Health. *Br. J. Nutr.* 109 Suppl 2, S21–S26. doi: 10.1017/ S0007114512005235

91. Robles-Vera, I., de la Visitación, N., Toral, M., Sánchez, M., Gómez-Guzmán, M., Jiménez, R., et al. (2021). Mycophenolate Mediated Remodeling of Gut Microbiota and Improvement of Gut-Brain Axis in Spontaneously Hypertensive Rats. *BioMed. Pharmacother.* 135, 111189. doi: 10.1016/ j.biopha.2020.111189

92. Rocha-Ramırez, L. M., Pérez-Solano, R. A., Castañón-Alonso, S. L., Moreno Guerrero, S. S., Ramırez Pacheco, A., Garcıá Garibay, M., et al. (2017). Probiotic Lactobacillus Strains Stimulate the Inflammatory Response and Activate Human Macrophages. *J. Immunol. Res.*, 2017, 4607491. doi: 10.1155/2017/4607491

93. Rodrıguez-Iturbe, B., Quiroz, Y., Nava, M., Bonet, L., Chávez, M., Herrera-Acosta, J., et al. (2002). Reduction of Renal Immune Cell Infiltration Results in Blood Pressure Control in Genetically Hypertensive Rats. *Am. J. Physiol. Renal Physiol.* 282, F191–F201. doi: 10.1152/ajprenal.0197.2001

94. Rojas, M., Restrepo-Jimenez, P., Monsalve, D. M., Pacheco, Y., Acosta-Ampudia, Y., Ramirez-Santana, C., et al. (2018). Molecular Mimicry and Autoimmunity. *J. Autoimmun.* 95, 100–123. doi: 10.1016/j.jaut.2018.10.012

95. Rowan, S., Jiang, S., Korem, T., Szymanski, J., Chang, M. L., Szelog, J., et al. (2017). Involvement of a Gut-Retina Axis in Protection Against Dietary Glycemia- Induced Age-Related Macular Degeneration. *Proc. Natl. Acad. Sci. U. S. A.* 114, E4472–E4481. doi: 10.1073/pnas.1702302114

96. Saitoh, O., and Nagayama, Y. (2006). Regulation of Graves' Hyperthyroidism With Naturally Occurring CD4+CD25+ Regulatory T Cells in a Mouse Model. *Endocrinology* 147, 2417–2422. doi: 10.1210/ en.2005-1024

97. Sánchez-Bilbao, L., Martınez-López, D., Revenga, M., López-Vázquez,, Valls-

98. Pascual, E., Atienza-Mateo, B., et al. (2020). Anti-IL-6 Receptor Tocilizumab in Refractory Graves' Orbitopathy: National Multicenter Observational Study of 48 Patients. *J. Clin. Med.* 9 (9), 2816. doi: 10.3390/jcm9092816

99. Schepper, J. D., Collins, F., Rios-Arce, N. D., Kang, H. J., Schaefer, L., Gardinier, J. D., et al. (2020). Involvement of the Gut Microbiota and Barrier Function in Glucocorticoid-Induced Osteoporosis. *J. Bone Miner Res.* 35, 801–820. doi: 10.1002/jbmr.3947

100. Scher, J. U., Sczesnak, A., Longman, R. S., Segata, N., Ubeda, C., Bielski, C., et al. (2013). Expansion of Intestinal Prevotella Copri Correlates With Enhanced Susceptibility to Arthritis. *Elife* 2, e01202. doi: 10.7554/eLife.01202

101. Schirmer, M., Smeekens, S. P., Vlamakis, H., Jaeger, M., Oosting, M., Franzosa, E. A., et al. (2016). Linking the Human Gut Microbiome to Inflammatory Cytokine Production Capacity. *Cell* 167, 1125–1136.e1128. doi: 10.1016/ j.cell.2016.10.020

102. Shah, A., Panjabi, C., Nair, V., Chaudhry, R., and Thukral, S. S. (2008). Veillonella as a Cause of Chronic Anaerobic Pneumonitis. *Int. J. Infect. Dis.* 12, e115–e117. doi: 10.1016/j.ijid.2008.03.018

103. Shi, T. T., Hua, L., Wang, H., and Xin, Z. (2019a). The Potential Link Between Gut Microbiota and Serum TRAb in Chinese Patients With Severe and Active Graves' Orbitopathy. *Int. J. Endocrinol.*, 2019, 9736968. doi: 10.1155/2019/9736968

104. Shin, N. R., Bose, S., Wang, J. H., Nam, Y. D., Song, E. J., Lim, D. W., et al. (2020). Chemically or Surgically Induced Thyroid Dysfunction Altered Gut Microbiota in Rat Models. *FASEB J.* 34, 8686–8701. doi: 10.1096/ fj.201903091RR

105. Shin, S. J., and Collins, M. T. (2008). Thiopurine Drugs Azathioprine and 6-Mercaptopurine Inhibit Mycobacterium Paratuberculosis Growth *In Vitro*. *Antimicrob. Agents Chemother.* 52, 418–426. doi: 10.1128/AAC.00678-07

106. Shivaji, S. (2019). Connect Between Gut Microbiome and Diseases of the Human Eye. *J. Biosci.* 44, 110. doi: 10.1007/s12038-019-9931-1

107. Shi, T. T., Xin, Z., Hua, L., Wang, H., Zhao, R. X., Yang, Y. L., et al. (2021). Comparative Assessment of Gut Microbial Composition and Function in Patients With Graves' Disease and Graves' Orbitopathy. *J. Endocrinol. Invest.* 44, 297–310. doi: 10.1007/s40618-020-01298-2

108. Shi, T. T., Xin, Z., Hua, L., Zhao, R. X., Yang, Y. L., Wang, H., et al. (2019b). Alterations in the Intestinal Microbiota of Patients With Severe and Active Graves' Orbitopathy: A Cross-Sectional Study. *J. Endocrinol. Invest.* 42, 967–978. doi: 10.1007/s40618-019-1010-9

109. Smith, T. J., and Hegedüs, L. (2016). Graves' Disease. *N Engl. J. Med.* 375, 1552- 1565. doi: 10.1056/NEJMra1510030

110. Smith, P. M., Howitt, M. R., Panikov, N., Michaud, M., Gallini, C. A., Bohlooly, Y. M., et al. (2013). The Microbial Metabolites, Short-Chain Fatty Acids, Regulate Colonic Treg Cell Homeostasis. *Science* 341, 569–573. doi: 10.1126/ science.1241165

111. Sun, J., Zhao, F., Lin, B., Feng, J., Wu, X., Liu, Y., et al. (2020). Gut Microbiota Participates in Antithyroid Drug Induced Liver Injury Through the Lipopolysaccharide Related Signaling Pathway. *Front. Pharmacol.* 11, 598170. doi: 10.3389/fphar.2020.598170

112. Su, X., Yin, X., Liu, Y., Yan, X., Zhang, S., Wang, X., et al. (2020). Gut Dysbiosis Contributes to the Imbalance of Treg and Th17 Cells in Graves' Disease Patients by Propionic Acid. *J. Clin. Endocrinol. Metab.* 105 (11), 3526–3547. doi: 10.1210/clinem/dgaa511
113. Szablewski, L. (2018). Human Gut Microbiota in Health and Alzheimer's Disease. *J. Alzheimers Dis.* 62, 549–560. doi: 10.3233/JAD-170908
114. Taylor, M. R., Flannigan, K. L., Rahim, H., Mohamud, A., Lewis, I. A., Hirota, S. A., et al. (2019). Vancomycin Relieves Mycophenolate Mofetil-Induced Gastrointestinal Toxicity by Eliminating Gut Bacterial b-Glucuronidase Activity. *Sci. Adv.* 5, eaax2358. doi: 10.1126/sciadv.aax2358
115. Taylor, P. N., Zhang, L., Lee, R. W. J., Muller, I., Ezra, D. G., Dayan, C. M., et al. (2020). New Insights Into the Pathogenesis and Nonsurgical Management of Graves Orbitopathy. *Nat. Rev. Endocrinol.* 16, 104–116. doi: 10.1038/s41574- 019-0305-4
116. Trujillo-Vargas, C. M., Schaefer, L., Alam, J., Pflugfelder, S. C., Britton, R. A., and De Paiva, C. S. (2020). The Gut-Eye-Lacrimal Gland-Microbiome Axis in Sjogren Syndrome. *Ocul. Surf.* 18 (2), 335–344. doi: 10.1016/j.jtos.2019.10.006
117. Tsunoda, I. (2017). Lymphatic System and Gut Microbiota Affect Immunopathology of Neuroinflammatory Diseases, Including Multiple Sclerosis, Neuromyelitis Optica and Alzheimer's Disease. *Clin. Exp. Neuroimmunol.* 8, 177–179. doi: 10.1111/cen3.12405
118. Unoda, K., Doi, Y., Nakajima, H., Yamane, K., Hosokawa, T., Ishida, S., et al. (2013). Eicosapentaenoic Acid (EPA) Induces Peroxisome Proliferator-Activated Receptors and Ameliorates Experimental Autoimmune Encephalomyelitis. *J. Neuroimmunol.* 256, 7–12. doi: 10.1016/j.jneuroim.2012.12.003
119. Vannucchi, G., Campi, I., Covelli, D., Currò, N., Lazzaroni, E., Palomba, A., et al. (2021). Efficacy Profile and Safety of Very Low-Dose Rituximab in Patients With Graves' Orbitopathy. *Thyroid* 31, 821–828. doi: 10.1089/thy.2020.0269
120. Vieira, S. M., Pagovich, O. E., and Kriegel, M. A. (2014). Diet, Microbiota and Autoimmune Diseases. *Lupus* 23, 518–526. doi: 10.1177/0961203313501401
121. Virili, C., Stramazzo, I., and Centanni, M. (2021). Gut Microbiome and Thyroid Autoimmunity. *Best Pract. Res. Clin. Endocrinol. Metab.* 35, 101506. doi: 10.1016/j.beem.2021.101506
122. Wang, W., Chen, L., Zhou, R., Wang, X., Song, L., Huang, S., et al. (2014). Increased Proportions of Bifidobacterium and the Lactobacillus Group and Loss of Butyrate-Producing Bacteria in Inflammatory Bowel Disease. *J. Clin. Microbiol.* 52, 398–406. doi: 10.1128/JCM.01500-13
123. Wang, X., Liang, Z., Wang, S., Ma, D., Zhu, M., and Feng, J. (2021). Role of Gut Microbiota in Multiple Sclerosis and Potential Therapeutic Implications. *Curr. Neuropharmacol.* doi: 10.2174/1570159X19666210629145351
124. Wang, Z., Zhang, Q., Lu, J., Jiang, F., Zhang, H., Gao, L., et al. (2010). Identification of Outer Membrane Porin F Protein of Yersinia Enterocolitica Recognized by Antithyrotopin Receptor Antibodies in Graves' Disease and Determination of its Epitope Using Mass Spectrometry and Bioinformatics Tools. *J. Clin. Endocrinol. Metab.* 95, 4012–4020. doi: 10.1210/jc.2009-2184
125. Wei, Y., Li, Y., Yan, L., Sun, C., Miao, Q., Wang, Q., et al. (2020). Alterations of Gut Microbiome in Autoimmune Hepatitis. *Gut* 69, 569–577. doi: 10.1136/ gutjnl-2018-317836
126. Weis, A. M., and Round, J. L. (2021). Microbiota-Antibody Interactions That Regulate Gut Homeostasis. *Cell Host Microbe* 29, 334–346. doi: 10.1016/ j.chom.2021.02.009
127. Wen, C., Zheng, Z., Shao, T., Liu, L., Xie, Z., Le Chatelier, E., et al. (2017). Quantitative Metagenomics Reveals Unique Gut Microbiome Biomarkers in Ankylosing Spondylitis. *Genome Biol.* 18, 142. doi: 10.1186/s13059-017-1271-6 Wildner, G., and Diedrichs-Möhring, M. (2020). Molecular Mimicry and Uveitis. *Front. Immunol.* 11, 580636. doi: 10.3389/fimmu.2020.580636
128. Wolf, M. W., Misaki, T., Bech, K., Tvede, M., Silva, J. E., and Ingbar, S. H. (1991). Immunoglobulins of Patients Recovering From Yersinia Enterocolitica Infections Exhibit Graves' Disease-Like Activity in Human Thyroid Membranes. *Thyroid* 1, 315–320. doi: 10.1089/thy.1991.1.315
129. Wu, H. J., Ivanov, Ii., Darce, J., Hattori, K., Shima, T., Umesaki, Y., et al. (2010). Gut-Residing Segmented Filamentous Bacteria Drive Autoimmune Arthritis *via* T Helper 17 Cells. *Immunity* 32, 815–827. doi: 10.1016/j.immuni.2010.06.001
130. Yan, H. X., An, W. C., Chen, F., An, B., Pan, Y., Jin, J., et al. (2020). Intestinal Microbiota Changes in Graves' Disease: A Prospective Clinical Study. *Biosci. Rep.* 40. doi: 10.1042/BSR20191242
131. Yan, J., and Charles, J. F. (2018). Gut Microbiota and IGF-1. *Calcif. Tissue Int.* 102, 406–414. doi: 10.1007/s00223-018-0395-3
132. Yang, T., Aquino, V., Lobaton, G. O., Li, H., Colon-Perez, L., Goel, R., et al. (2019). Sustained Captopril-Induced Reduction in Blood Pressure Is Associated With Alterations in Gut-Brain Axis in the Spontaneously Hypertensive Rat. *J. Am. Heart Assoc.* 8, e010721. doi: 10.1161/JAHA.118.010721
133. Yang, M., Sun, B., Li, J., Yang, B., Xu, J., Zhou, X., et al. (2019). Alteration of the Intestinal Flora may Participate in the Development of Graves' Disease: A Study Conducted Among the Han Population in Southwest China. *Endocr. Connect* 8, 822–828. doi: 10.1530/EC-19-0001
134. Yilmaz, B., Juillerat, P., yås, O., Ramon, C., Bravo, F. D., Franc, Y., et al. (2019). Microbial Network Disturbances in Relapsing Refractory Crohn's Disease. *Nat. Med.* 25, 323–336. doi: 10.1038/s41591-018-0308-z
135. Zeng, Q., Junli, G., Liu, X., Chen, C., Sun, X., Li, H., et al. (2019). Gut Dysbiosis and Lack of Short Chain Fatty Acids in a Chinese Cohort of Patients With Multiple Sclerosis. *Neurochem. Int.* 129, 104468. doi: 10.1016/j.neuint.2019.104468
136. Zeng, J., Peng, L., Zheng, W., Huang, F., Zhang, N., Wu, D., et al. (2021). Fecal Microbiota Transplantation for Rheumatoid Arthritis: A Case Report. *Clin. Case Rep.* 9, 906–909. doi: 10.1002/ccr3.3677
137. Zhao, H., Jiang, X., and Chu, W. (2020). Shifts in the Gut Microbiota of Mice in Response to Dexamethasone Administration. *Int. Microbiol.* 23, 565–573. doi: 10.1007/s10123-020-00129-x
138. Zhao, S. X., Tsui, S., Cheung, A., Douglas, R. S., Smith, T. J., and Banga, J. P. (2011). Orbital Fibrosis in a Mouse Model of Graves' Disease Induced by Genetic Immunization of Thyrotropin Receptor cDNA. *J. Endocrinol.* 210, 369–377. doi: 10.1530/JOE-11-0162
139. Zhuang, Z., Wang, Y., Zhu, G., Gu, Y., Mao, L., Hong, M., et al. (2017). Imbalance of Th17/Treg Cells in Pathogenesis of Patients With Human Leukocyte Antigen B27 Associated Acute Anterior Uveitis. *Sci. Rep.* 7, 40414. doi: 10.1038/srep40414

24

Corticosteroid Pulse Therapy for Graves' Ophthalmopathy Reduces the Relapse Rate of Graves' Hyperthyroidism

Rosario Le Moli [1†‡], Pasqualino Malandrino [1†], Marco Russo [1], Fabrizio Lo Giudice [1], Francesco Frasca [1], Antonino Belfiore [1] and Riccardo Vigneri [1,2]*

[1] *Endocrinology, Department of Clinical and Experimental Medicine, Garibaldi-Nesima Medical Center, University of Catania, Catania, Italy,* [2] *Institute of Crystallography, Structural Chemistry and Biosystems, CNR-ICCSB, Catania, Italy*

Correspondence:
Rosario Le Moli
lemoli.rosario@tiscali.it

† These authors have contributed equally to this work

Background: A course of anti-thyroid drugs (ATD) is the most common first line treatment for Graves' hyperthyroidism. However, hyperthyroidism relapse is frequent (30–70%). Due to the autoimmune nature of Graves' disease, the immunosuppressive treatment used for active Graves' orbitopathy (GO) may reduce the relapses after ATD discontinuation.

Objective: To evaluate the recurrence rate in Graves' patients who, in addition to standard ATD, were treated or not treated with parenteral methylprednisolone (MPDS) for GO.

Methods: Single-center retrospective study in a continuous series of 162 newly diagnosed Graves' patients, with or without GO, all gone into remission and followed-up until hyperthyroidism recurrence or at least 4 years after ATD discontinuation. Patients with moderate-severe active GO underwent middle dose MPDS treatment according to the EuGoGo guidelines. Cox proportional-hazard model was used to comparatively evaluate the risk of recurrence and the predictive factors in patients treated or not treated with MPDS pulse therapy.

Results: MPDS treatment was the most significant factor that independently correlated with a reduced risk of hyperthyroidism relapse (HR = 0.53, 95% C.I. = 0.31–0.89). FT3 and female sex were also independent protective factors, while age almost reached the significance level, $p = 0.062$. The efficacy of MPDS was very high in patients aged <40 years (42.1% decrease in relapses, $p < 0.01$) but it was not significant in older patients.

Discussion: Our study found that after ATD discontinuation the frequency of Graves' hyperthyroidism relapse was reduced in patients treated with MPDS pulse therapy for GO. This effect was more marked in young patients.

Keywords: Graves' hyperthyroidism, corticosteroid pulse therapy, Graves' ophthalmopathy, relapse of Graves' hyperthyroidism, anti-thyroid drugs

INTRODUCTION

Graves' disease (GD) is an autoimmune disorder characterized by the excess production of thyroid hormones due to the overstimulation of the thyroid gland by thyrotropin (TSH)-receptor autoantibodies (TRAbs). GD is the most frequent cause of hyperthyroidism, with a prevalence of ~0.5% in the general population, with a female-to-male ratio of ~3:1. (1–3). The treatment options for GD are antithyroid drugs (ATD), radioiodine administration (RAI) or thyroidectomy (Tx). The most frequent long-term unfavorable consequences of these treatments are life-long hypothyroidism for Tx and RAI (4), radiation exposure for RAI (5) and hyperthyroidism recurrence for ATD (6, 7). Since a course of ATD (minimum 12–18 months) is now the most common first line treatment of GD, the risk of relapse is a relevant clinical problem. The overall relapse rate after a single course of ATD is ~50% although it may greatly vary from 30 to 70% in different studies, also depending from the length of the patient follow-up (7). Although several risk factors are believed to influence the relapse rate of GD after ATD treatment, the contribution of each risk factor is controversial and varies among studies (8–10). Recently, a predictive model based on simple clinical data detected at presentation of GD (patient age, goiter size, free thyroxine levels and TRAbs serum levels) and called GREAT (Graves' Recurrent Events After Therapy) has been proposed and validated (11–13).

Attempts to enhance the remission rate and to reduce hyperthyroidism recurrence after ATD treatment have been limited and have met little success. The autoimmune nature of GD and the curative effect of ATD are well established (14, 15).

Few studies have tested the effect of adding immunosuppressive agents to the standard ATD treatment on hyperthyroidism outcome. In this regard, a recent meta-analysis evaluated seven studies in which immunosuppressive drugs were added to the ATD treatment and concluded that the combined treatment reduced the relapse risk (16). However, the examined studies had a moderate/high risk of bias because of small effect and poor design (16).

More specifically, corticosteroids were used in four studies. In one study (17) the number of relapses was reduced in patients treated with the combined therapy; however, in the other study, methylprednisolone (MPDS) pulse therapy had only a temporary effect on the TBII decrease in Japanese patients, with no significant difference at 12 months after ATD discontinuation (18). The other two studies evaluated the effect of local thyroid treatment with corticosteroid and methimazole (MMI) in Chinese patients. In both series (19, 20) the relapse rate of hyperthyroidism was reduced.

Considering the clinical relevance of this issue, that the available data are mainly from patients of Asian ethnicity and the peculiar route of steroid administration, and considering also that high dose corticosteroid (pulse therapy) is the first line treatment for medium/severe active Graves' orbitopathy (GO), we retrospectively evaluated the effect of immunosuppressive corticosteroid therapy on the risk of hyperthyroidism recurrence rate in a continuous series of Graves' patients treated either with ATD alone or with corticosteroid pulse therapy for GO in addition to the standard ATD treatment.

METHODS

Study Design

In this retrospective, observational, single-center study, 162 consecutive patients with newly diagnosed Graves' hyperthyroidism from 2004 to 2013 were selected from 1,162 Graves' hyperthyroidism patients referred to our thyroid tertiary center (Endocrinology, University of Catania, Sicily). The selection criteria are summarized in **Figure 1**. All 162 patients received ATD continuously for almost 18 months in most cases and underwent clinical and biochemical hyperthyroidism remission after ATD treatment (MMI in all cases). Additionally, as an inclusion criterion to enter the study, all patients were continuously followed-up in our Center until hyperthyroidism recurrence or until at least 4 years after ATD discontinuation.

Among the 162 selected patients, 43 (26.5%) who had moderate to severe active Graves' orbitopathy also received a course of treatment with parenteral MPDS.

Graves' Hyperthyroidism

GD was diagnosed based on typical clinical signs and symptoms of hyperthyroidism confirmed by laboratory tests: TSH < 0.4 mU/L, free thyroxine (FT4) > 23.0 pmol/L and/or free triiodothyronine (FT3) > 2.7 pmol/L and diffuse homogeneous uptake on thyroid scintigraphy (99mTc-pertechnetate).

Anti-thyroid Treatment

As ATD treatment we employed a block and replace (B/R) regimen to better standardize the time intervals between one clinical examination and another (15–30 mg methimazole and L-thyroxine in a dose to maintain constantly normal thyroid function) in 122 cases while only titrated MMI administration was used in 40 patients in whom the combined regimen was not accepted. The treatment lasted a minimum period of 18 months or longer, until the normalization of clinical signs and laboratory data.

Graves' Orbitopathy

GO severity and clinical activity stage were evaluated at presentation by trained investigators. GO severity was evaluated according to the EuGoGo guidelines (21). The lid fissure width was evaluated in millimeters by a router, and proptosis was evaluated with a Hertel exophthalmometer. Diplopia

Abbreviations: GH, Graves' hyperthyroidism; GO, Graves' ophthalmopahty; ATD, anti thyroid drugs; B/R, block and replace therapy, MPDS, metilprednisolone; EuGoGo, The European Group on Graves' Orbitopathy; RAI, radioiodine administration; Tx, thyroidectomy; GREAT, Graves' Recurrent Events After Therapy; FT3, triiodothyronine; FT, thyroxine or tetraiodothyronine; TSH, thyroid stimulating hormone; TRAB, thyrotropin (TSH)-receptor autoantibodies; TBII, TSH binding inhibitor immunoglobulins; MMI, methimazole; ROC, receiver operator characteristics; POM, potential outcome mean; ATE, average treatment effect; RR, relative risk; IPWRA, inverse probability weight regression adjustment analysis.

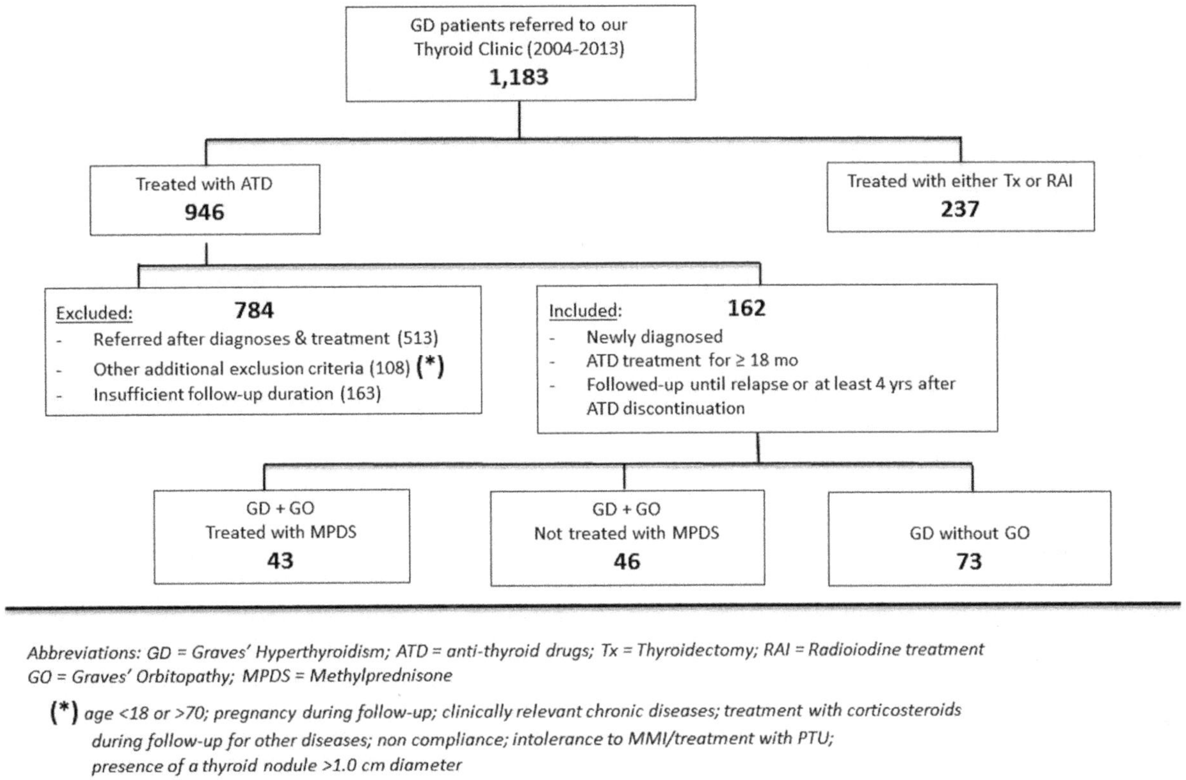

FIGURE 1 | Flow chart of Graves' patients selection.

was classified according to the Gorman score. A complete ophthalmological evaluation was carried out by an expert ophthalmologist. The GO was defined as moderate to severe when eye disease had a sufficient impact on daily life with one or more of the following: lid retraction 2 mm or more, moderate or severe soft tissue involvement, exophthalmos three or more mm above 21, and inconstant or constant diplopia. GO was considered active when the clinical activity score (CAS) was ≥3 (22). Corticosteroid treatment for GO was administered to patients with moderate to severe active GO (21) and consisted of intravenous MPDS (Solumedrol; Pfizer, Karlsruhe, Germany) injections with a cumulative dose of 4.5 g subdivided in 12 weekly infusions (500 mg each week for 6 weeks followed by 250 mg week for 6 weeks); this treatment was initiated in all patients within 8 months after starting ATD and following the EuGoGo protocol (23, 24).

Graves' Hyperthyroidism Remission

GD remission was defined as the condition of normal thyroid function after ATD discontinuation, documented both clinically and biochemically. Follow-up consisted of the control of clinical and laboratory parameters according to our well-established protocol which includes the first control visit 45 days after MMI discontinuation and then at 3, 6, and 12 months and every 6 months thereafter.

Graves' Hyperthyroidism Relapse

GD relapse was defined as overt hyperthyroidism, occurring after documented remission lasting at last 3 months and confirmed by the clinical signs and symptoms of hyperthyroidism and by the laboratory values of serum TSH <0.4 mU/L in combination with elevated FT4 (>23.0 pmol/L) and/or elevated serum FT3 (>2.7 pmol/L) and diffuse homogeneous uptake on thyroid scintigraphy (99mTc-pertechnetate). In all the patients the following clinical parameters were recorded at baseline as they could potentially influence the risk of Graves' hyperthyroidism relapse: age, sex, BMI (body mass index), goiter size as assessed by ultrasound imaging (18), presence of GO and smoking behavior. Moreover, the GREAT class of each patient was also calculated as an overall indicator of the risk of hyperthyroidism recurrence after discontinuation of ATD treatment (11).

Laboratory Measurements

Serum hormones were measured by microparticle enzyme immunoassay (Abbot AxSYM-MEIA) with inter-assay coefficients of variation of <10% over the analytical ranges of 1.7–46.0 pmol/L for FT3, 5.15–77.0 pmol/L for FT4 and 0.03–10.0 mU/L for TSH. The within-run and between-run precisions for FT3, FT4 and TSH assays showed coefficients of variation <5%. The TSH receptor antibodies (TRAbs) were measured by a radio-receptor assay (RADIM, Italy). Positivity was >9 UI/L.

Statistical Analysis

The Mann Whitney U test was used to analyze the variables without normal distribution, and the chi-square test was used to study the categorical variables. Cut-off values for putative predictor variables were obtained by receiver operating characteristic (ROC) curve analysis. We carried out uni- and multivariate Cox regression analysis to identify the independent factors predictive of GD relapse and to determine the specific relevance of each factor. Independent predictors were identified by a p-value <0.05. We included in the multivariate statistical model all variables that were significantly different by univariate analysis between the relapsed and not relapsed patients, and also smoke, FT4 and TRAb values that are known predictive factors for GD relapse. Additionally, to minimize the effects of selection bias from non-randomized treatment assignment, the potential outcome mean (POM), average treatment effect (ATE) and relative risk (RR) were calculated by combining the outcome and treatment models through an inverse probability weight regression adjustment (IPWRA) analysis.

The outcome was modeled as a function of sex, age at methylprednisolone administration, TRAbs positivity, cigarette smoke and FT3 values. The treatment was modeled as a function of sex, age at MPDS administration, B/R therapy and cigarette smoke. Thereafter, we assessed the standardized differences and considered a value $<10\%$ to be indicative of negligible imbalance in the baseline covariates between treated and untreated subjects (25). Statistical analyses were carried out using the STATA 15.1 statistical package (StataCorp LP, College Station, Texas, USA).

RESULTS

The clinical and biochemical characteristics of the 162 Graves' hyperthyroidism patients at presentation are shown in **Table 1**. The mean duration of ATD therapy was 26.4 ± 9.3 months. GO was present in 89/162 (54.9%) patients; however, according to the EuGoGo criteria, active GO of moderate to severe grade was diagnosed in only 43 patients who received early (within 4.1 ± 3.0 months from diagnosis) MPDS treatment. The most frequent side effect of this treatment was skin flushing after the i.v. MPDS (14 cases); of more relevance, hyperglycemia requiring 2–6 weeks treatment occurred in three patients (metformin was used in all cases), and development or worsening of hypertension occurred in six cases. After the ATD was withdrawn, the patients were followed-up for an average of 55.1 ± 27.1 months (range 19-124). Hyperthyroidism relapsed in 97/162 patients (59.9%) after a median disease-free interval of 24 months (range 3–103) after ADT discontinuation, while 65 patients (40.1%) remained euthyroid during the observation period (in no case shorter than 48 months after ADT withdrawal). The clinical

TABLE 1 | Clinical and laboratory characteristics of the studied patients at presentation subdivided according to Graves' ophthalmopathy presence and therapy with methylprednisolone.

	GD without GO	GD + GO without MPDS therapy	GD + GO + MPDS therapy	P
Patients	73	46	43	
Age (years, m ± SD)	38.9±13.6	41.4 ± 11.1	45.5 ± 11.1	0.021
Sex (m/f)	17/56	16/30	11/32	0.38
BMI (Kg/m^2, m ± SD)	22.1 ± 2.6	23.5 ± 3.6	29.6 ± 5.0	<0.001
Smoking	25 (34.2)	17 (37.0)	22 (51.2)	0.18
TSH (μU/ml, m ± SD)	0.03 ± 0.11	0.01 ± 0.03	0.02 ± 0.03	0.35
FT3 (pmol/L, m ± SD)	13.8 (7.2)	14.6 (10.3)	12.5 (6.6)	0.45
FT4 (pmol/L, m ± SD)	47.7 (20.7)	42.5 (21.4)	41.8 (21.0)	0.24
TRAB (IU/L, median, IQR)	37.1 (13.5–80.3)	27.3 (6.3–87.3)	25.4 (12.6–65.9)	0.55
Thyroid volume (ml, m ± SD)	21.8 ± 10.9	19.4 ± 11.4	22.2 ± 14.0	0.46
GREAT SCORE				
Class 0	18 (24.7%)	18 (39.1%)	16 (37.2%)	0.20
Class 1	39 (53.4%)	23 (50.0%)	23 (53.5%)	
Class 2	16 (21.9%)	5 (10.9%)	4 (9.3%)	
ATD duration (months, m ± SD)	28.6 ± 10.5	24.2 ± 8.2	25.1 ± 7.5	0.024
B/R therapy	41 (56.2%)	42 (91.3%)	39 (90.7%)	<0.001
GD relapse	51 (69.9%)	28 (60.9%)	18 (41.9%)	0.012
Disease free interval (months, m ± SD)	26.5 ± 25.7	24.7 ± 20.6	37.0 ± 28.9	0.045

GD, Graves' Disease; GO, Graves' Ophthalmopathy; MPDS, methylprednisolone.

TABLE 2 | Clinical and laboratory characteristics of untreated and MPDS- treated Graves' disease patients.

	MPDS untreated	MPDS treated	p
N. cases	119	43	
Female gender	86 (72.3%)	32 (74.4%)	0.79
Age (years, m ± SD)	39.8 ±12.7	45.5 ± 11.1	0.011
BMI (Kg/m^2, m ± SD)	23.0 ± 3.3	29.6 ± 5.0	<0.001
Smoking	42 (35.3%)	22 (51.2%)	0.06
TSH (μU/ml, m ± SD)	0.03 ± 0.09	0.02 ± 0.03	0.65
FT3 (pmol/L, m ± SD)	14.1 ± 8.5	12.5 ± 6.6	0.25
FT4 (pmol/L, m ± SD)	45.7 ± 21	41.8 ± 21	0.3
TRAb (IU/L, median, IQR)	25.4 (12.6–65.9)	32.9 (12.6–80.3)	0.64
Thyroid volume (ml, m ± SD)	20.9 ± 11.1	22.2 ± 14	0.54
GREAT SCORE			
Class 0	36 (30.3%)	16 (37.2%)	0.38
Class 1	62 (52.1%)	23 (53.5%)	
Class 2	21 (17.6%)	4 (9.3%)	
ATD duration (months, m ± SD)	26.9 ± 9.9	25.1 ± 7.5	0.28
B/R treatment	83 (69.7%)	39 (90.7%)	0.006
Follow-up after ATD discontinuation (months, m ± SD)	52.7 ± 26.2	62 ± 28.5	0.051
GD relapse	79 (66.4%)	18 (41.9%)	0.005
Disease free interval (months, m ± SD)	25.8 ± 23.8	37 ± 28.9	0.014

TABLE 3 | Variables associated with the Graves' disease relapse in the study population (uni- and multivariate Cox regression analysis).

	Univariate analysis		Multivariate analysis	
	Hazard ratio (95% CI)	*P*	Hazard ratio (95% CI)	*P*
Age <40 yrs	1.57 (1.05–2.34)	0.029	1.48 (0.98–2.22)	0.062
Male sex	1.58 (1.02–2.43)	0.038	1.56 (1.00–2.43)	0.048
BMI	0.95 (0.87–1.03)	0.18		
Smoking	1.23 (0.82–1.85)	0.31	1.27 (0.84–1.93)	0.26
GO	0.67 (0.45–1.00)	0.048		
FT3	1.03 (1.00–1.06)	0.02	1.04 (1.00–1.07)	0.036
FT4	1.00 (0.99–1.01)	0.63	0.99 (0.98–1.01)	0.24
TRAb	1.00 (0.99–1.00)	0.22	1.00 (0.99–1.00)	0.27
Thyroid volume	1.00 (0.99–1.02)	0.58		
GREAT SCORE				
1	1.04 (0.67–1.63)	0.86		
2	1.40 (0.76–2.56)	0.28		
ATD duration	1.12 (0.75–1.67)	0.58		
B/R pulse therapy	1.14 (0.71–1.84)	0.58		
MPDS therapy	0.52 (0.31–0.88)	0.014	0.53 (0.31–0.89)	0.017

BMI, body mass index; GO, Graves' ophthalmopathy; TRAb, thyrotropin receptor antibody; ATD, anti thyroid drug; B/R, block and replace; MPDS, methylprednisolone.

and biochemical characteristics of the patients with or without Graves' hyperthyroidism relapse are shown in **Table 1** and indicate that significant differences were observed for age (more frequent relapse in younger patients; $p < 0.01$) and for MPDS treatment (less frequent relapse in MPDS-treated patients, $p < 0.005$). The data indicate that the presence of GO was similar between relapsed and not relapsed patients ($p = 0.5$, **Table 1**). To further confirm this observation, we compared the 46 patients that had minimal or non-active GO and who were, therefore, not treated with MPDS ($n = 46$) with patients without GO ($n = 73$). No significant difference was observed between the two groups in terms of the clinical and biochemical parameters, except that the B/R scheme of ATD treatment was more frequent in the patients having GO who also had a shorter ATD treatment period (24.2 ± 8.2 vs. 28.6 ± 10.5 months). Additionally, the GREAT classes did not differ between these two groups ($p = 0.14$), indicating a similar risk of relapse at presentation. Therefore, these 119 patients were considered to be a single group (control group) to be compared with the 43 patients that had both Graves'

TABLE 4 | Inverse probability weight regression analysis (IPWRA) for Graves' disease relapse according to MPDS pulse therapy and patient age.

	All patients ($n = 162$)		Age < 40 y ($n = 67$)		Age ≥ 40 y ($n = 95$)	
	MPDS −	MPDS +	MPDS −	MPDS +	MPDS −	MPDS +
POM	65.5% (56.8–74.3)	40.5% (27.3–53.6)	78.9% (68.1–89.6)	53.5% (36.5–70.5)	56.4% (44.1–68.7)	38.0% (22.9–53.1)
ATE	−25.1% (−40.6 to −9.6)		−25.4% (−45.0 to −5.8)		−18.4% (−37.6 to 0.8)	
RR	1.62* (1.15–2.29)		1.47* (1.05–2.07)		1.48^ns (0.95–2.33)	

POM, potential outcome mean (i.e., the percentage of Graves' disease relapse); ATE, average treatment effect (i.e., the difference of relapse between MPDS-treated and untreated patients); RR, relative risk (i.e., the risk ratio of MPDS-treated to untreated patients).
Values between brackets indicate 95% confidential intervals.
**P < 0.05.*
ns, not significant.

hyperthyroidism and moderate to severe active GO and who received MPDS pulse therapy. When the control and the MPDS-treated groups were compared, most of the clinical and all the biochemical parameters at diagnosis were similar. Significant differences were observed only for age (higher in the group treated with MPDS, $p = 0.011$) and BMI (higher in the MPDS group). These patients were also more frequently treated with the B/R scheme (**Table 2**). The GREAT classes were not significantly different ($p = 0.38$) between the groups, confirming that the risk of hyperthyroidism relapse evaluated at presentation was similar. Remarkably, the prevalence of hyperthyroidism relapse after ATD withdrawn was significantly lower in the patients who received MPDS ($p = 0.005$). In addition, in these patients the disease-free interval was significantly longer ($p = 0.014$) than that in the control group. Hazard ratios indicated that MPDS treatment, sex and FT3 were the only significant factors predicting the risk of relapse, while age almost reached the significance level ($p = 0.062$) (**Table 3**). The role of MPDS therapy in reducing the risk of relapse was further confirmed by the IPWRA method. Indeed, we observed that the POM (i.e., the percentage of relapse) was 65.5% (95% CI = 56.8–74.3%) and 40.5% (95% CI = 27.3–53.6%) for patients who were untreated or treated with MPDs, respectively. Thus, if no patient was treated with MPDS the risk of relapse would have been 1.62 times higher (95% CI = 1.15–2.29, $p = 0.006$) than if all the patients had received the MPDS treatment. As shown in **Table 4** and **Figure 2** the beneficial effect of pulse MPDS treatment on reducing relapse was more marked in young patients (<40 years), effectively counteracting the higher propensity toward relapse among patients in this age group (10). In contrast, MPDS pulse therapy did not significantly reduce the risk of relapse in patients older than 40 years ($p = 0.084$) (**Table 4** and **Figure 2**).

DISCUSSION

Hyperthyroidism due to Graves' disease is a common disorder that is currently treated with ATD in most cases. However, recurrence of hyperthyroidism after ATD discontinuation is

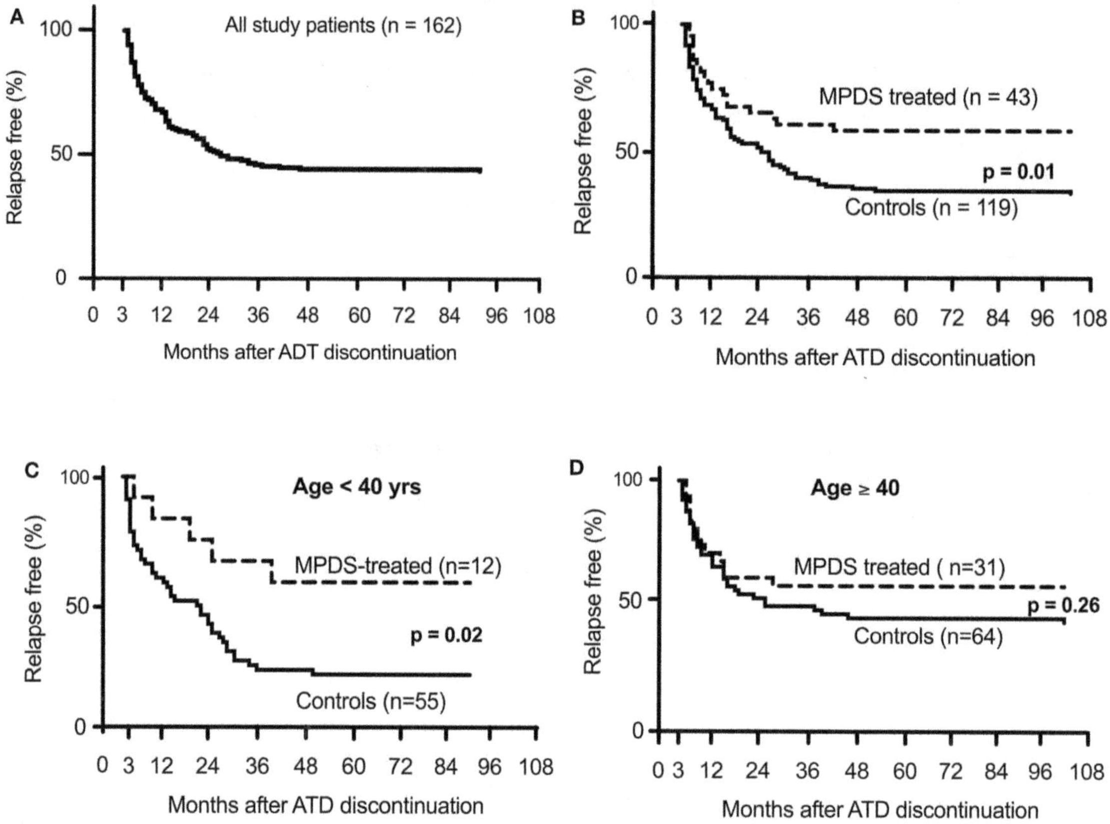

FIGURE 2 | Percentage of relapse-free Graves' patients after discontinuation of anti-thyroid drug therapy. **(A)** shows all patients included in the study. **(B)** shown the difference between MPDS-treated and untreated patients. **(C,D)** show the different relapse rate according to patient age.

frequent, with cumulative occurrence being time-dependent even if most cases relapse within 2 years after therapy withdrawal. Due to the autoimmune nature of the disease, immunosuppressive drugs in combination with ATD treatment seem to be a rationale treatment from an etiopathogenetic approach. This approach, however, has not been adequately studied because of the potentially severe adverse events associated with chronic immunosuppression. Corticosteroids, which represent the standard treatment for many autoimmune diseases, can cause serious side effects, including metabolic disturbances, osteoporosis and hypertension. In this study we observed no major side effect in the patients treated with MPDS pulse therapy, although severe adverse events have been reported (26, 27). However, the risks inherent to chronic corticosteroid administration are acceptable for treating severe orbitopathy, which is a frequent complication of Graves' disease. MPDS pulse therapy is, in fact, the first line treatment for patients with moderate to severe active GO.

The present study, although with limitations, shows that immunosuppression with MPDS for active GO significantly reduces the risk of hyperthyroidism relapse. This effect was already nearly significant at 1 year after MMI withdrawal ($p = 0.07$), and further increased up to 4 years, when it reached a plateau with a >42% decrease in the relapse rate relative to patients not treated with MPDS ($p = 0.01$) (**Figure 2**). Although late recurrence may occur, the prognosis is excellent after 4 years without relapse (28). Moreover, even in cases of relapse, MPDS-treated patients benefit from a longer disease-free interval ($p = 0.014$) (**Table 2**).

The multivariate analysis indicated that MPDS pulse therapy most effectively predicts reduced risk of GD recurrence and is a more effective predictor than patient sex, age or FT3 which are well-known risk factors for relapse (**Table 3**) (10, 12, 29).

In our series, other risk factors for GD relapse such as high TRAbs concentrations, large goiter size were not significantly different between relapsed and not relapsed patients and were not included in multivariate analysis. In contrast to other studies (30) we found no association between GO and an increased risk of hyperthyroidism recurrence. In any case, we found that in young GO patients, that in some studies are considered at higher risk of recurrent hyperthyroidism, MPDS treatment reduced the relapse rate to levels lower than those in patients without GO.

A remarkable observation of our study is that MPDS pulse treatment showed different effects at different patient ages. It is well known that the remission rate is lower and the relapse rate is higher in young age patients with Graves' disease (31). The Cox regression and the IPWRA analyses (**Table 4**) as well as the Kaplan-Meier curves (**Figure 2**) indicated that MPDS treatment was highly effective in reducing the relapse rate in younger patients (<40 years) but not in older Graves' disease patients. The reason for the different age-related responses to corticosteroids is unclear, as is the reason why disease outcome tends to be worse in younger patients. Higher levels of TRAbs and circulating thyroid hormones and larger thyroid volume in younger patients have been previously discussed as possible causative factors for worse Graves' disease outcome among younger patients (29). We did not observe similar differences in our series (TRAbs difference $p = 0.99$; FT4 $p = 0.93$ and thyroid volume $p = 0.81$ between patients younger or older than 40 years). Corticosteroid absorption, distribution and efficacy on immunocompetent cells are possible reasons for greater efficacy in younger patients.

These potential differences include the effects of glucocorticoid receptor activation on a series of regulators. Both non-genomic effects such as cytokine and growth factors cross-talk (32–34) and epigenetic modifications in many target tissues may determine a different individual responses across patient's lifespan (35). There is no evidence that a longer treatment with ATD is associated with a reduced relapse rate (24), but when combined with steroids ATD treatment may contribute to a higher remission rate. However, in our study ATD treatment length was no longer in patients treated with MPDS.

From a clinical point of view, among young patients for whom surgery or radioiodine is usually indicated due to the patient's higher likelihood of failure to respond to ATD treatment, MPDS pulse therapy, required for the presence of GO, may reverse the therapeutic advice in favor of ATD.

Our study has some limitations inherent to retrospective studies and lacks familial and genetic characteristics of the studied patients (11, 16, 30).

In addition, repeated TRAbs analysis during follow-up might have provided useful information. On the other hand the long 4-year follow-up during remission, the standardized protocol with complete data from all patients and the robust statistical analyses of the results are strengths of this study.

CONCLUSIONS

In conclusion we observed that Graves' patients treated with MPDS pulse therapy for GO have a significantly reduced risk of hyperthyroidism relapse, confirming the important role of immunosuppression in the clinical outcomes of Graves' patients. This steroid effect is more relevant in younger patients who more frequently undergo hyperthyroidism relapse. When GO is present, in these patients the combined medical treatment reduces the relapse risk and should be considered as an alternative to more definitive treatments such as surgery or radioiodine. However, a prospective study is necessary to confirm these statements.

ETHICS STATEMENT

The studies involving human participants were reviewed and approved by Ethics Committee Garibaldi Nesima Hospital - Catania. Written informed consent for participation was not required for this study in accordance with the national legislation and the institutional requirements.

AUTHOR CONTRIBUTIONS

RL and RV: conception and design of the study. RL, PM, MR, and FL: data collection. RL and PM: statistical analysis. RL, FL, PM, and MR: figures. RL, RV, AB, FF, PM, and MR: writing and revision of the manuscript. All authors read and approved the final manuscript.

ACKNOWLEDGMENTS

The authors gratefully acknowledge the clinical support of the day-hospital staff coordinator (Dr. M. Arpi) who managed patients' care and the secretarial support of Ms Rita Pennisi.

REFERENCES

1. Cooper DS. Treatment of thyrotoxicosis. In: *Werner and Ingbar's The Thyroid: A Fundamental and Clinical Text.* 10th ed. Philadelphia, PA: LippincottWilliams and Wilkins (2013). p. 492–516.
2. Wemeau JL, Klein M, Sadoul JL, Briet C, Velayoudom-Cephise FL. Graves' disease: introduction, epidemiology, endogenous and environmental pathogenic factors. *Ann Endocrinol.* (2018) 79:599–607. doi: 10.1016/j.ando.2018.09.002
3. Tanda ML, Piantanida E, Liparulo L, Veronesi G, Lai A, Sassi L, et al. Prevalence and natural history of Graves' orbitopathy in a large series of patients with newly diagnosed Graves' hyperthyroidism seen at a single center. *J Clin Endocrinol Metab.* (2013) 98:1443–9. doi: 10.1210/jc.2012-3873
4. Burch HB, Burman KD, Cooper DS. A 2011 survey of clinical practice patterns in the management of Graves' Disease. *J Clin Endocrinol Metab.* (2012) 97:4549–58. doi: 10.1210/jc.2012-2802
5. Metso S, Auvinen A, Huhtala H, Salmi J, Oksala H, Jaatinen P. Increased cancer incidence after radioiodine treatment for hyperthyroidism. *Cancer.* (2007) 109:1972–9. doi: 10.1002/cncr.22635
6. Laurberg P, Berman DC, Andersen S, Pedersen IB. Sustained control of Graves' hyperthyroidism during long-term low-dose antithyroid drug therapy of patients with severe Graves' orbitopathy. *Thyroid.* (2011) 21:951–6. doi: 10.1089/thy.2011.0039
7. Elbers L, Mourits M, Wiersinga WM. Outcome of very long-term treatment with antithyroid drugs in Graves' hyperthyroidism associated with Graves' orbitopathy. *Thyroid.* (2011) 21:279–8. doi: 10.1089/thy.2010.0181

8. Katagiry Y, Kobayashi S, Sasaki S. Effect of excess iodine intake on thyroid diseases in different populations: a systematic review and meta-analyses including observational studies. *PLoS ONE.* (2017) 12:e0173722. doi: 10.1371/journal.pone.0173722
9. Strieder TG, Prummel MF, Tijssen JG, Endert E, Wiersinga WM. Risk factors for and prevalence of thyroid disorders in a cross-sectional study among healthy female relatives of patients with autoimmune thyroid disease. *Clin Endocrinol.* (2003) 59:396–401. doi: 10.1046/j.1365-2265.2003.01862.x
10. Allahabadia A, Daykin J, Holder RL, Sheppard MC, Gough SC, Franklyn JA. Age and gender predict the outcome of treatment for Graves' hyperthyroidism. *J Clin Endocrinol Metab.* (2000) 85:1038–42. doi: 10.1210/jc.85.3.1038
11. Vos G, Endert E, Zwinderman K, Tijssen J, Wiersinga WM. Predicting the risk of recurrence before the start of antithyroid drug therapy in patients with Graves' hyperthyroidism. *J Clin Endocrinol Metab.* (2016) 101:1381–9. doi: 10.1210/jc.2015-3644
12. Struja T, Kaeslin M, Boesiger F, Jutzi R, Imahorn N, Kutz A, Bernasconi L, et al. External validation of the GREAT score to predict relapse risk in Graves' disease: results from a multicenter, retrospective study with 741 patients. *Eur J Endocrinol.* (2017) 176:413–9. doi: 10.1530/EJE-16-0986
13. Masiello E, Veronesi G, Gallo D, Premoli P, Bianconi E, Rosetti S, et al. Antithyroid drug treatment for Graves'disease: baseline predictive models of relapse after treatment for a patient-tailored management. *J Endocrinol Invest.* (2018) 41:1425–32. doi: 10.1007/s40618-018-0918-9
14. Laurberg P, Andersen S, Karmisholt J. Antithyroid drug therapy of Graves' hyperthyroidism: realistic goals and focus on evidence. *Expert Rev Endocrinol Metab.* (2006) 1:91–102. doi: 10.1586/17446651.1.1.91
15. Cooper DS. Antithyroid drugs. *N Engl J Med.* (2005) 352:905–17. doi: 10.1056/NEJMra042972
16. Struja T, Guebelin L, Kutz A, Fehlberg H, Mueller B, Schuetz P. Does immunosuppressive therapy improve outcomes in Graves' disease? A systematic review and meta-analysis. *Thyroid.* (2016) 26:634–40 doi: 10.1089/thy.2015.0647
17. Olbios G, Mesa J, Simo R, Garcia L, Garcia C, Tresànces JM. Effect of carbimazole and dexamethasone on TSH bond (TBII) inhibiting immunoglobulins in Graves-Basedow disease. *Rev Clin Esp.* (1988) 183:401–4.
18. Kubota S, Ohye H, Nishihara E, Kudo T, Ito M, Fukata S, et al. Effect of high dose methylprednisolone pulse therapy followed by oral prednisolone administration on the production of anti - TSH receptor antibodies and clinical outcome in Graves' disease. *Endocr J.* (2005) 52:735–41. doi: 10.1507/endocrj.52.735
19. Chen L, Wang HQ, Gao YY, Liang J, Wang M, Bay J, et al. Comparison of methimazole/idrocortisone ointment with oral methimazole in patients with Graves' disease: a prospective, randomized, open label, parallel group, 18-month study. *Curr Ther Res Clin Exp.* (2008) 69:305–17. doi: 10.1016/j.curtheres.2008.08.004
20. Mao XM, Li HQ, Li Q, Li DM, Xie XJ, Yin GP, et al. Prevention of relapse of Graves' disease by treatment with an intrathyroid injection of dexamethasone. *J Clin Endocrinol Metab.* (2009) 94:4984–91. doi: 10.1210/jc.2009-1252
21. Bartalena L, Baldeschi L, Boboridis K, Eckstein A, Kahaly GJ, Marcocci C, et al. The 2016 European Thyroid Association/ European Group on Graves' Orbitopathy Guidelines for the management of Graves' Orbitopathy. *Eur Thyroid J.* (2016) 5:9–26 doi: 10.1159/0004 43828
22. Mourits MP, Prummel MF, Wiersinga WM, Koornneef L. Clinical activity score as a guide in the management of patients with Graves' ophthalmopathy. *Clin Endocrinol.* (1997) 47:9–14. doi: 10.1046/j.1365-2265.1997.2331047.x
23. Bartalena L, Krassas GE, Wiersinga WM, Marcocci C, Salvi M, Daumerie C, et al. Efficacy and safety of three different cumulative doses of intravenous methylprednisolone for moderate to severe and active Graves' Orbitopathy. *J Clin Endocrinol Metab.* (2012) 97:4454–63. doi: 10.1210/jc.2012-2389
24. Kahaly GJ, Bartalena L, Hegedüs L, Leenhardt L, Poppe L, Pearce SH. European Thyroid Association guideline for the management of Graves' hyperthyroidism. *Eur Thyroid J.* (2018) 7:167–86. doi: 10.1159/000490384
25. Stuart EA. Matching methods for causal inference: a review and a look forward. *Stat Sci.* (2010) 25:1–21. doi: 10.1214/09-STS313
26. Le Moli R, Baldeschi L, Saeed P, Regensburg N, Mourits MP, Wiersinga W. Determinants of liver damage associated with intravenous methylprednisolone pulse therapy in Graves' ophthalmopathy. *Thyroid.* (2007) 17:357–62. doi: 10.1089/thy.2006.0267
27. Marinó M, Morabito E, Brunetto MR, Bartalena L, Pinchera A, Marocci C. Acute and severe liver damage associated with intravenous glucocorticoids pulse therapy in patients with Graves' ophthalmopathy. *Thyroid.* (2004) 14:403–6. doi: 10.1089/1050725047741 93276
28. Mohlin E, Filipsson HN, Eliasson M. Long-term prognosis after medical treatment of Graves' disease in a northern Swedish population 2000–2010. *Eur J Endocrinol.* (2014) 170:419–27. doi: 10.1530/EJE-13-0811
29. Bano A, Gan E, Addison C, Narayanan K, Weaver JU, Tsatlidis V, et al. Age may influence the impact of TRAbs on thyroid function and relapse-risk in patients with Graves disease. *J Clin Endocrinol Metab.* (2019) 104:1378–85. doi: 10.1210/jc.2018-01738
30. García-Mayor RV, Álvarez-Vázquez P, Fluiters E, Valverde D, Andrade A. Long-term remission following antithyroid drug withdrawal in patients with Graves' hyperthyroidism: parameters with prognostic value. *Endocrine.* (2019) 63:316–22. doi: 10.1007/s12020-018-1785-z
31. Wiersinga WM. Graves' Disease: can it be cured? *Endocrinol Metab.* (2019) 34:29–38. doi: 10.3803/EnM.2019.34.1.29
32. Enuka Y, Feldman ME, Chowdhury A, Srivastava S, Lindzen M, Sas-Chen A, et al. Epigenetic mechanisms underlie the crosstalk between growth factors and a steroid hormone. *Nucleic Acids Res.* (2017) 45:12681–99. doi: 10.1093/nar/gkx865
33. Newton R, Shah S, Altonsy MO, Gerber AN. Glucocorticoid and cytokine crosstalk: feedback, feedforward, and co-regulatory interactions determine repression or resistance. *J Biol Chem.* (2017) 292:7163–717. doi: 10.1074/jbc.R117.777318
34. Panettieri RA, Schaafsma D, Amrani Y, Koziol-White C, Ostrom R, Tliba O. Non-genomic effects of glucocorticoids: an updated view. *Trends Pharmacol Sci.* (2019) 40:38–49. doi: 10.1016/j.tips.2018.11.002
35. Zannas AS, Chrousos GP. Epigenetic programming by stress and glucocorticoids along the human lifespan. *Mol Psychiatry.* (2017) 22:640–6. doi: 10.1038/mp.2017.35

25

Antithymocyte Globulin as Second-Line Therapy in Graves Orbitopathy

Monika Sarnat-Kucharczyk[1†], Maria Świerkot[2†], Gabriela Handzlik[2], Grażyna Kulawik[2], Krystyna Jagoda[3], Iga Grochoła-Małecka[2], Joanna Fryżewska[2], Ewa Mrukwa-Kominek[1] and Jerzy Chudek[2]*

[1] Department of Ophthalmology, Faculty of Medical Sciences in Katowice, Medical University of Silesia, Katowice, Poland, [2] Department of Internal Medicine and Oncological Chemotherapy, Faculty of Medical Sciences in Katowice, Medical University of Silesia, Katowice, Poland, [3] Department of Hematology and Bone Marrow Transplantation, Faculty of Medical Sciences in Katowice, Medical University of Silesia, Katowice, Poland

***Correspondence:**
Gabriela Handzlik
ghandzlik@sum.edu.pl

[†]These authors have contributed equally to this work

Objective: Management of Graves' orbitopathy remains a challenge. Our previous case report has shown promising results for rabbit antithymocyte globulin (rATG) in the treatment of Graves' orbitopathy.

Design: We present the response of 7 individuals with active moderate-to-severe steroid-resistant Graves' orbitopathy to rATG, representing preliminary results from a prospective single-center study.

Methods: rATG was administered intravenously at a dose of 0.8–1.0 mg/kg daily (cumulative dose of 150–200 mg). The primary outcome measures at weeks 24 and 48 were ≥2-point reduction in Clinical Activity Score from baseline, a proptosis response, a diplopia response, and improvement of distant best-corrected visual acuity and mean retinal sensitivity. Key secondary outcomes included stabilization of ganglion cell complex thickness, a decrease of retinal nerve fiber layer in OCT, and a reduction in CD4/CD8 ratio and TRAb at 48 weeks.

Results: An improvement in clinical activity score was observed in all patients, with disease inactivation in 3 cases. Proptosis reduction equal to or greater than 2 mm was noted for 8 of 10 eyes. Diplopia improved in three of 6 patients. There was an improvement in best-corrected visual acuity (from 0.69 to 0.78) and mean retinal sensitivity (from 20.8 to 23.5 dB). In addition, there was a long-lasting improvement in CD4/CD8 ratio in 6 patients. Two patients experienced adverse events (influenza and serum sickness).

Conclusion: rATG therapy offers a long-lasting improvement in moderate-to-severe steroid-resistant Graves' orbitopathy with improvement in functional vision (reduction of diplopia, improvement of visual acuity, retinal sensitivity, and VEP pattern). The therapy is well-tolerated.

Clinical Trial Registration: ClinicalTrials.gov, identifier NCT05199103.

Keywords: Graves' orbitopathy, Graves' disease, antithymocyte globulin, proptosis, thyroid eye disease

1 INTRODUCTION

Graves' orbitopathy (GO), also known as thyroid eye disease, is the most common extrathyroidal manifestation of Graves' disease, affecting 25% of patients with this complex autoimmune disorder (1). Graves' disease is more prevalent in women than in men; however, if present in men, it takes a more severe form. Smoking and radioiodine therapy are strong risk factors for the development of sight-threatening orbitopathy (2).

Most cases of GO are benign, but 5%–6% of patients are classified as an active moderate-to-severe disease, in whom corticosteroid systemic administration is a mainstay of treatment recommended by EUGOGO (3). However, 20%–30% of patients refractory to standard steroid therapy require second-line treatment with repeated and high courses of corticosteroids, orbital radiotherapy, cyclosporin A, or rituximab. Over the past 5 years, novel hypotheses in the pathogenesis of GO created potential new therapeutic targets affecting immunological and inflammatory reactions, survival and proliferation of fibroblasts and adipocytes, and extracellular matrix production (4, 5). Among emerging agents are monoclonal antibodies against the interleukin-6 receptor (tocilizumab) and the insulin-like growth factor 1 receptor (teprotumumab) (5).

The mechanisms underlying the development of GO are complex and still not entirely elucidated, with key pathogenetic processes applying to autoimmune-induced extraocular muscle enlargement, orbital fat expansion, fibroblasts proliferation followed by their differentiation into myofibroblasts and adipocytes (6). Early orbital T-cell infiltration and local release of proinflammatory cytokines emerge as a triggering mechanism and become a basis for further therapeutic research. Infiltration of CD4+ cells to orbital tissues plays an essential role in the molecular pathways leading to the proliferation and differentiation of orbital fibroblasts. T regulatory (Treg) cells are considered substantial for suppression of immunological responses in autoimmune disorders. The activity of Treg cells may be influenced by the abnormal CD4 to CD8 ratio observed in GO (7).

Rabbit antithymocyte globulin (rATG, Thymoglobulin) is an anti-T-cell agent widely used in the management of acute cellular rejection after organ transplantation. rATG induces T-cell depletion and affects the cell surface and adhesion molecules regulating T-cell function. It has also anti-B-cell activity *via* induction of naïve plasma B-cell apoptosis (8). *In vitro*, incubation of peripheral blood mononuclear cells from GO patients with rATG resulted in restored CD4 to CD8 ratio and significantly increased the number of T CD3+ lymphocytes with the phenotype of Treg cells: FOXP3+ CD4+ CD25+ $CD127^{low}$ (7). Of note, Lee et al. described the resolution of GO shortly after induction therapy with ATG (1.5 mg/kg/dose for five doses) with a triple immunosuppressive regimen (including glucocorticoids) in the kidney transplantation recipient previously untreated for GO. The clinical improvement, in this case, was followed by the disappearance of TSHR antibody titters that remained undetectable 12 months after the procedure (9).

Compressive optic neuropathy in the course of GO causes damage to the retinal ganglion cell axons of the optic nerve by mechanical damage. It usually results in a progressive and structural and functional deterioration of the optic nerve (10). The evaluation of both structure and function in optic neuropathies at the time of presentation provides crucial information about the status of the disease and is useful for monitoring the clinical progression and recovery after treatment (11).

It was shown that the peripapillary retinal nerve fiber layer (RNFL) is altered in compressive optic neuropathies of different causes depending on the stage of the disease (12).

In this paper, we report preliminary analyses of the ongoing single-center academic-driven research on the efficacy and safety of rATG in patients with steroid-resistant moderate-to-severe Graves' orbitopathy.

2 PATIENTS AND METHODS

This prospective interventional, single-center study enrolled adult patients with active moderate-to-severe GO after ineffective treatment with moderate-to-high doses of glucocorticoids. The study protocol was approved by the local bioethics committee of the Medical University of Silesia (KNW-1-075/N/8/K). All patients gave their written informed consent.

Euthyroid adult patients (>18 years of age) with active moderate-to-severe GO, with clinical activity score (CAS) of ≥3/7, and who were previously ineffectively treated (partial response, recurrence, or progression of symptoms) with moderate-to-high doses of glucocorticoids (at least 4.5 g of methylprednisolone) were considered eligible for enrollment.

The exclusion criteria were as follows: hypersensitivity to rabbit proteins or any product excipients, active acute or chronic infections, latent tuberculosis, leucopenia below 3,000/μl, lymphopenia below 400/μl, thrombocytopenia below 75,000/μl, coagulation disorders, active malignancy, and pregnancy.

Presented results describe effectiveness in seven patients who met all the inclusion criteria. Each eligible patient received 0.8–1.0 mg/kg of rATG (cumulative dose of 150–200 mg given intravenously in two or three divided doses, 24 h apart) after premedication with 1 mg of clemastine—and an antihistaminic agent orally, methylprednisolone (in the total dose of 375 mg), and 1,000 mg paracetamol given intravenously. Subsequent doses were preceded by complete blood count assessment (CBC) and dose postponement in case of lymphocyte count <100/μl (required in a single case).

To assess the efficacy and safety of rATG therapy, patients were evaluated at baseline and 6, 12, 24, and 48 weeks. Baseline evaluation involved medical history, physical examination, including eye examination, laboratory assessment thyroid-stimulating hormone (TSH), flow cytometry, TSH-receptor antibody (TRAb) titer, CBC), and orbital magnetic resonance imaging (MRI). Physical re-evaluations were conducted by the same endocrinologist and ophthalmologist.

Eye examinations were performed using:

- Hertl's ophthalmometry,
- seven-point CAS assessment (spontaneous retrobulbar pain, pain on attempted eye movements, conjunctival hyperemia, eyelid redness, chemosis, swelling of the caruncle, swelling of the eyelids),

- classification of Graves' orbitopathy: NOSPECS (0, no signs or symptoms; 1, only signs no symptoms; 2, soft-tissue involvement; 3, proptosis [amount of protrusion of the eye from the orbital rim]; 4, extraocular muscle involvement; 5, corneal involvement; 6, sight loss),
- diplopia Gorman's scale: a score of 0 indicates no diplopia; 1, intermittent diplopia; 2, inconstant diplopia, and 3, constant diplopia,
- Ishihara color plates,
- distant uncorrected/best-corrected visual acuity (DUCVA/DBCVA),
- static visual field—mean sensitivity (MS)
- pattern visual evoked potentials (PVEP),
- posterior segment optical coherent tomography (OCT) of ganglion cell complex (GCC) in the macula and the retinal nerve fiber layer (RNFL) around the optic nerve.

2.1 Visual Evoked Potential Measurement

Visual evoked potential (VEP) measurements were performed using the Reti-Port electrophysiological apparatus from Roland Consult (Brandenburg a.d. Havel, Germany), following the standards of the International Society for Clinical Electrophysiology of Vision (ISCEV) (13). A black and white checkerboard pattern with alternating phase change (pattern reversal VEP, PVEP) was used to elicit a visual cortical response. The reversal rate was 2 reversals/s. Each VEP test was preceded by checking the visual acuity of the distance in the patient's correction with glasses using Snellen charts, an intraocular pressure test using a Goldmann applanation tonometer. Before the fundus examination, short-acting (4–6 h) mydriatics were given: parasympatholytic (1% Tropicamidum, Polfa, Warsaw, Poland) or sympathomimetic (10% Neosynephrin-POS, Ursapharm, Saarbrücken, Germany) drops. The amplitude and the latency of the P100 (PVEP) waves were analyzed.

2.2 Flow Cytometry

Flow cytometry was performed on the lymphocyte subpopulation extracted from peripheral blood samples collected by venipuncture to EDTA tubes. The cells were stained using a reagent kit with six-color fluorochrome-labeled monoclonal antibodies (BD Multitest 6-color TBNK, Becton Dickinson Biosciences): CD3-FITC, CD16-PE + CD56-PE, CD45-PerCP-Cy5.5, CD4-PE-Cy7, CD19-APC, and CD8-APC-Cy7. The staining procedure was performed according to the manufacturer's recommendations. Briefly, 50 µl of anticoagulated whole blood was added to 20 µl of reagent and incubated for 15 min in the dark at room temperature. Erythrocytes were briefly lysed, and samples were immediately acquired in an 8-color flow cytometer (FACSCanto II, Becton Dickinson Biosciences). In addition, the WBC count and the percentage of lymphocytes among leucocytes were counted on the Sysmex XN-10 cell counter. The acquisition process was followed by analysis according to the manufacturer's instructions. The results were expressed as the percentage of T, T helper, T suppressor, B, and NK cell subpopulations among the lymphocytes and as the absolute number of these cells per 1 µl of blood. For further analysis, CD4/CD8 ratio was calculated.

2.3 Measurement of Clinical Outcomes

The primary outcome measures at weeks 24 and 48 were as follows: ≥2-point reduction in CAS from baseline, a proptosis response (defined as ≥2 mm reduction in proptosis), a diplopia response (defined as a reduction in diplopia of ≥1 grade from baseline using Gorman's subjective diplopia score), and improvement of distant best-corrected visual acuity (considered significant if improved by ≥1 row in Snellen visual acuity chart) and mean retinal sensitivity (considered significant if increased by ≥2 dB).

Key secondary outcomes included: stabilization of ganglion cell complex thickness (defined as a change of less than ±2 µm), a decrease of retinal nerve fiber layer in OCT ≥2 µm, increase in 1° amplitude in Pattern VEP by 1 µV, changes in CD4/CD8 ratio (considered significant if reduced by at least 50%), and changes in TRAb.

2.4 Statistical Analysis

Data are presented as median values with interquartile ranges (1-3Q). Mean values were calculated to show changes in quantitative data with time. ANOVA for repeated measurements with Dunnett's test as *post hoc* test and Student's *t*-test for dependent data were conducted, as appropriate. Statistical significance was set at a *p*-value below 0.05.

3 RESULTS

3.1 Study Group Characteristics

Seven patients (5 women and 2 men) with steroid-resistant and active Graves' orbitopathy (CAS ≥4 pts) have completed the study protocol and were included in the intention-to-treat analysis. There were no dropouts, and all patients were examined after 6, 12, 24, and 48 weeks after the administration of rATG. Demographic data are presented in **Table 1**. Ophthalmologic examination and analysis included fourteen eyes.

Severe violations of the study protocol took place in two patients (both men) and were related to the unscheduled use of glucocorticoids related to severe optic neuropathy followed by orbital radiotherapy.

3.2 Primary Outcomes

3.2.1 Changes in Clinical Activity Score

In all patients with baseline CAS 4 and more, CAS has reduced at the end of the observational period, with a median improvement of 4 points at 48 weeks. Disease inactivation (CAS = 0) at the end of the observational period occurred in three patients. Two of them received unscheduled doses of glucocorticoids with orbital radiotherapy.

3.2.2 Proptosis and Diplopia Response

Proptosis was initially observed in 10 eyes. Mean proptosis before treatment was 23.8 mm (max 30 mm), and after the treatment was 21.4 mm. In eight eyes, the reduction of proptosis was equal to or more than 2 mm.

According to Gorman's score at the initial examination, constant diplopia was present in primary position in four

TABLE 1 | Baseline patients' clinical data.

Sex [*N* (%)]	
Men	2 (29)
Women	5 (71)
Age (years)	59 (49–71)
Duration of Graves' disease (years)	6 (4–15)
Duration of Graves' orbitopathy (months)	11 (6–18)
Smokers (*n*) (%)	5 (71%)
Therapy of Graves' disease [*N* (%)]	
Thiamazole	2 (29)
Thyroxine	5 (71)
Thyroidectomy	1 (14)
Radioactive iodine therapy	4 (57)
Patients with diplopia [*N* (%)]	6 (86)
CAS (pts)	4 (4–5)
TSH (uIU/ml)	0.54 (0.42–1.33)
FT4 (ng/dl)	1.01 (0.91–1.18)
Anti-TSH receptor (TRAb) (IU/ml)	2.08 (1.26–38.3)

Data are shown as medians with interquartile range.

patients, inconstant in one patient, intermittent in one patient, and was absent in one patient. After the treatment with rATG, an improvement of 1 point in Gorman's score was noticed in three of 6 patients (**Table 2**).

3.2.3 Best-Corrected Visual Acuity and Mean Retinal Sensitivity

Visual acuity was impaired in 11 eyes. After rATG therapy, the improvement in best-corrected visual acuity (BCVA) was observed in seven eyes (64%) while remaining stable in six eyes. The mean BCVA increased from 0.69 to 0.78 (**Figure 1**). A more significant improvement was noted for eyes with initially worse BCVA in comparison with those with better BCVA before starting rATG treatment.

In one patient with severe optic neuropathy and unscheduled doses of glucocorticoid followed by orbital radiotherapy, the initial BCVA examination showed no light perception in the left eye in the initial period, but, at the end of the study, BCVA has improved to 1.0.

Mean retinal sensitivity (MRS) in the static visual field has improved from 20.8 to 23.5 dB before and at the end of the treatment, respectively (**Figure 1**). The improvement reaches statistical significance at 6-week and all subsequent measurements ($p < 0.05$).

3.3 Secondary Outcomes

3.3.1 Optical Coherent Tomography and Retinal Nerve Fiber Layer

In OCT, GCC values remained at a similar level after the treatment, suggesting no further progression of optic neuropathy and further reduction of GCC due to GO.

RNFL thickness slightly decreased in comparison with the initial values after the treatment from 91 to 88 μm (**Figure 1**). In three patients, RNFL decreased ≥2 μm.

3.3.2 Visual Evoked Potentials

The amplitude in 1° tended to increase from 5.86 ± 3.26 to 6.52 ± 1.98 μV, and latencies have elongated in 1°, after the treatment with rATG (**Table 3**).

3.3.3 Color Vision

There was a single patient with severe optic neuropathy manifested by severe deterioration of color vision (Ishihara Color Plates RE 11/16, LE 10/16) with full recovery (Ishihara Color Plates RE and LE 16/16) after 24 weeks since the rATG infusion. The patient did not receive unscheduled doses of glucocorticoids/orbital radiotherapy.

3.3.4 Immune Parameters

Five of 7 patients had initially detectable TRAb. One patient became seronegative at the end of the follow-up. One patient obtained about a 40% reduction of TRAb titter after 48 weeks. In the remaining 4 patients, a transient decrease in TRAb values, most prominent at 6 weeks was observed. GO inactivation (assessed by CAS) at the end of follow-up was observed in two subjects with a 40% decline in TRAb titter. In the third patient with the disease inactivation, there was no decline in TRAb titter.

Notwithstanding, a long-lasting improvement in the CD4/CD8 ratio was found in 6 of 7 studied patients. Six of the 7 subjects achieved a 50% reduction of the CD4/CD8 ratio at 6 weeks, which persisted at 48 weeks in 3 of them.

3.3.5 Safety and Adverse Events

No anaphylaxis and local reactions during and after the administration of rATG were noted. There was, however, one case of mild influenza infection (H1N1) within 1 week after rATG administration. In addition, one patient developed serum

TABLE 2 | Diplopia according to the Gorman's score in patients with active moderate-to-severe GO at baseline and after therapy in patients treated with rATG.

Diplopia	*N* (%)	
Present at baseline	6 (86%)	
Improved at 48 weeks	3 (43%)	
Gorman's score (patient's No.)	At baseline	At 48 weeks
1	Constant	Inconstant
2	Constant	Constant
3	Intermittent	Absent
4	Constant	Constant
5	Absent	Absent
6	Constant	Inconstant
7	Inconstant	Inconstant

sickness with fever, rash, myalgia, and pruritus 14 days after treatment. Both patients made a complete recovery.

4 DISCUSSION

According to the literature, our study is the first of its kind to assess the usefulness of rATG treatment in steroid-resistant GO in a group of seven patients. Until now, two cases of the patient treated with rATG showing its usefulness in GO were reported (9). The case of GO published by Lee et al. was not previously treated with steroids and received rATG as a part of induction therapy after kidney transplantation. The second one was a part of this study (14). In our series of cases, improvement in the CAS scale was followed by beneficial changes in functional and structural parameters, regardless

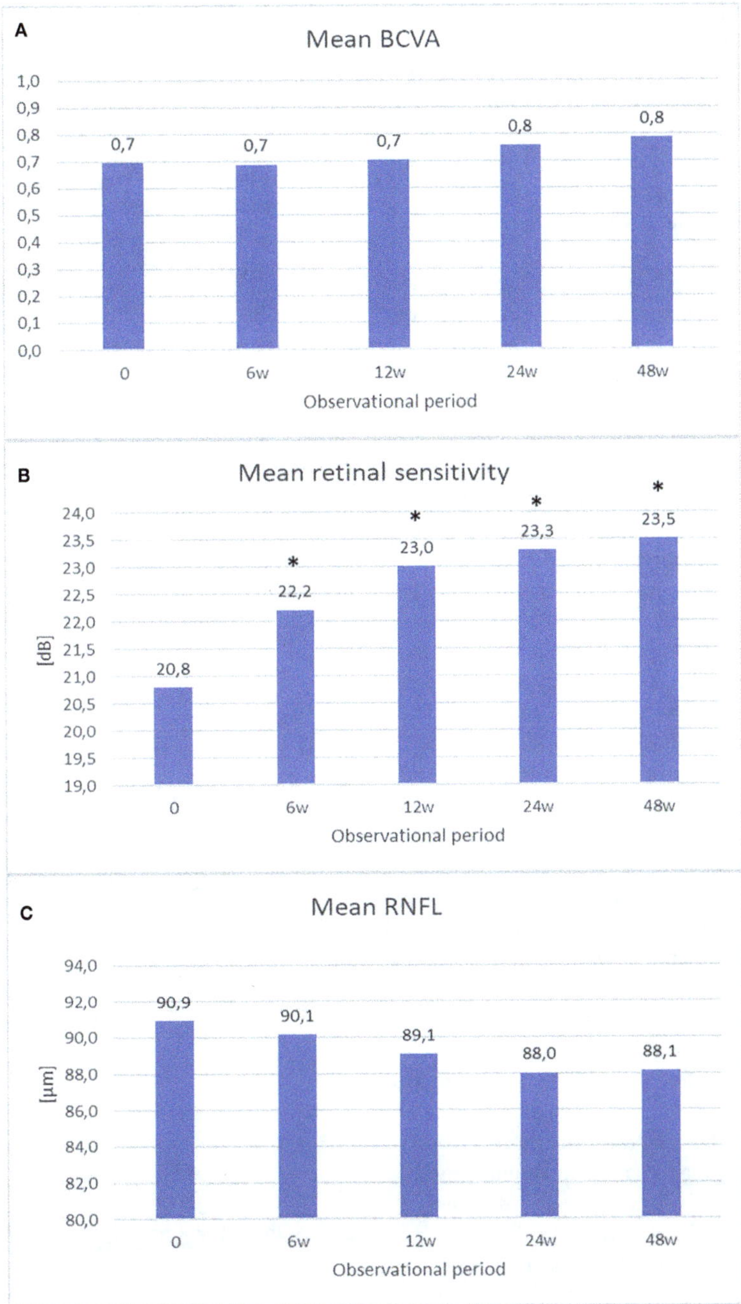

FIGURE 1 | The graphs show **(A)** mean best-corrected visual acuity (BCVA), **(B)** mean retinal sensitivity, **(C)** mean retinal nerve fiber layer (RNFL) – at baseline and at 6, 12, 24, 48 weeks after treatment. *$P < 0.05$ vs. baseline measurement.

TABLE 3 | Visual evoked potentials.

	Initially	After 48 weeks	*p*-value
1°			
Latency (ms)	117 ± 15	119 ± 11	0.78
Amplitude (μV)	5.9 ± 3.3	6.5 ± 2.0	0.37
15 min			
Latency (ms)	128 ± 11	137 ± 11	0.05
Amplitude (μV)	8.0 ± 5.5	7.5 ± 4.2	0.52

p-values were calculated with Student's t-test.

of the long-lasting activity of moderate-to-severe GO refractory to intravenously administered glucocorticoids.

We have observed long-lasting improvement in CAS and even inactivation of the disease in 3 of 7 patients (43%), reduction of proptosis in 8 eyes (57%), and diplopia in 3 of 6 patients (50%) with the advanced stage of the disease. Of note, an absence of the change in diplopia score in two patients with persistent disease activity may be related to advanced irreversible fibrosis of the extraocular muscles.

In addition, we observed improvement in optic nerve dysfunction probably related to some extent to the reversion of compressive neuropathy after rATG treatment. Advanced damage to the optic nerve and severe fibrosis of extraocular muscles and other intraorbital structures during long-lasting GO caused to a certain degree their irreversible dysfunction.

Visual acuity improved in seven out of 11 eyes, including a spectacular sight recovery in one patient with no light perception to full visual acuity at the end of the study. This proves that visual recovery is possible even in such severely affected patients when optic nerve compression does not cause irreversible damage to the optic nerve fibers.

Mean retinal sensitivity is an important indicator for the evaluation of visual capacity and is frequently used in the measurement of the outcome of as well as pharmacological treatment (15) and surgical decompression for GO (16). In the presented study, increased retinal mean sensitivity at 6-week and all subsequent measurements suggests an improvement of visual function due to rATG treatment.

Dave et al. have shown increased RNFL thickness in the active stage of GO in comparison with the inactive phase (10). Initial increased RNFL thickness in some patients could have been caused by axonal swelling and then resolved with time. As a consequence, the resultant ischemia would have caused a loss of integrity and, therefore, RNFL thinning. These results suggest that patients with more severe Graves' orbitopathy may have thicker RNFL than patients with a less severe form of the disease in the active phase.

PVEP is a useful method in assessing the function of the optic nerve in GO (17, 18). In our study, an increase in amplitude in 1° PVEP after the treatment with rATG may indicate a decrease of optic nerve compression in GO. Patients included in the study had prolonged optic nerve compression due to steroid-resistant disease, so to some extent, irreversible damage to the optic nerve fibers has occurred. This could be the reason why other parameters, such as latency in 1° PVEP and both latency and amplitude in 15-min PVEP have not improved after rATG treatment. Therefore, PVEP can be used to assess the severity of nerve damage and to monitor dysthyroid optic neuropathy before and after the treatment with rATG.

We have to acknowledge the use of unscheduled doses of glucocorticoids and orbital radiotherapy in two cases, both men, that obtained inactivation of the disease at the end of the study. This observation indicates the potential usefulness of combined therapies in the management of moderate-to-severe GO refractory to intravenously administered glucocorticoids.

The limitation of our study is the small number of participants. Due to the outbreak of the COVID-19 pandemic, we encountered problems associated with low patient attendance, as well as our and the patients' fear of undergoing immunosuppressive treatment, which could potentially endanger their lives. Despite severe influenza in one patient, no other serious infectious adverse events were present in other patients. Furthermore, viral infection was present in typical winter to early springtime, so to prevent this complication, if possible, rATG should be administered in the summer to early autumn period.

5 CONCLUSIONS

rATG therapy offers long-lasting improvement in moderate-to-severe steroid-resistant Graves' orbitopathy with improvement in functional vision (reduction of diplopia, improvement of visual acuity, retinal sensitivity, and VEP pattern). The therapy is well tolerated. However, further research in this field is needed to confirm the usefulness of rATG in the clinical setting in patients with GO.

ETHICS STATEMENT

The studies involving human participants were reviewed and approved by the ethics committee of the Medical University of Silesia. The patients/participants provided their written informed consent to participate in this study.

AUTHOR CONTRIBUTIONS

JC and MŚ conceived the concept of the study and designed the study. MŚ, GK, IG-M I, JF, and GH managed the patients. MS-K performed all ophthalmology assessments. KJ performed flow cytometry assessments. MS-K, MŚ, and GH drafted the manuscript. All authors contributed to data interpretation and the writing and editing of the manuscript. JC and EM-K approved the final version of the manuscript. All authors listed have made a substantial, direct, and intellectual contribution to the work and approved it for publication.

REFERENCES

1. Tanda ML, Piantanida E, Liparulo L, Veronesi G, Lai A, Sassi L, et al. Prevalence and Natural History of Graves' Orbitopathy in a Large Series of Patients With Newly Diagnosed Graves' Hyperthyroidism Seen at a Single Center. *J Clin Endocrinol Metab* (2013) 98(4):1443–9. doi: 10.1210/jc.2012-3873
2. Ehlers M, Schott M, Allelein S, Endocrinology S, Faculty M. Graves ' Disease in Clinical Perspective. *Front Biosci* (2019) 24:35–47. doi: 10.2741/4708
3. Bartalena L, Kahaly J, Baldeschi L, Dayan C, Eckstein A, Marcocci C, et al. The 2021 European Group on Graves' Orbitopathy (EUGOGO) Clinical Practice Guidelines for the Medical Management of Graves' Orbitopathy. *Eur J Endocrinol* (2021) 185(4):G43–67. doi: 10.1530/EJE-21-0479
4. Smith TJ, Bartalena L. Will Biological Agents Supplant Systemic Glucocorticoids as the First-Line Treatment for Thyroid-Associated Ophthalmopathy? *Eur J Endocrinol* (2020) 181(5):1–28. doi: 10.1530/EJE-19-0389
5. Taylor PN, Zhang L, Lee RWJ, Muller I, Ezra DG, Dayan CM, et al. New Insights Into the Pathogenesis and Nonsurgical Management of Graves Orbitopathy. *Nat Rev Endocrinol* (2020) 16(2):104–16. doi: 10.1038/s41574-019-0305-4
6. Khong JJ, McNab AA, Ebeling PR, Craig JE, Selva D. Pathogenesis of Thyroid Eye Disease: Review and Update on Molecular Mechanisms. *Br J Ophthalmol* (2016) 100(1):142–50. doi: 10.1136/bjophthalmol-2015-307399
7. Kahaly GJ, Shimony O, Gellman YN, Lytton SD, Eshkar-Sebban L, Rosenblum N, et al. Regulatory T-Cells in Graves' Orbitopathy: Baseline Findings and Immunomodulation by Anti-T Lymphocyte Globulin. *J Clin Endocrinol Metab* (2011) 96(2):422–9. doi: 10.1210/jc.2010-1424
8. Zand MS, Vo T, Huggins J, Felgar R, Liesveld J, Pellegrin T, et al. Polyclonal Rabbit Antithymocyte Globulin Triggers B-Cell and Plasma Cell Apoptosis by Multiple Pathways. *Transplantation* (2005) 79(11):1507–15. doi: 10.1097/01.tp.0000164159.20075.16
9. Lee Y, Butani L, Glaser N, Nguyen S. Resolution of Graves' Disease After Renal Transplantation. *Pediatr Transplant* (2016) 20(4):590–3. doi: 10.1111/petr.12709
10. Dave TV, Laghmisetty S, Krishnamurthy G, Bejjanki K, Ganguly A, Jonnadula GB, et al. Retinal Vascularity, Nerve Fiber, and Ganglion Cell Layer Thickness in Thyroid Eye Disease on Optical Coherence Tomography Angiography. *Orbit* (2022) 41(2):170–7. doi: 10.1080/01676830.2020.1846761
11. Laowanapiban P, Chirapapaisan N, Kemahayung S, Srikong M. Variable Structure and Function Relationship of Compressive Optic Neuropathy at the Time of Diagnosis. *Clin Ophthalmol* (2019) 13:1599–608. doi: 10.2147/OPTH.S215115
12. Rajabi MT, Ojani M, Riazi Esfahani H, Tabatabaei SZ, Rajabi MB, Hosseini SS. Correlation of Peripapillary Nerve Fiber Layer Thickness With Visual Outcomes After Decompression Surgery in Subclinical and Clinical Thyroid-Related Compressive Optic Neuropathy. *J Curr Ophthalmol* (2019) 31(1):86–91. doi: 10.1016/j.joco.2018.11.003
13. Odom JV, Bach M, Brigell M, Holder GE, McCulloch DL, Mizota A, et al. ISCEV Standard for Clinical Visual Evoked Potentials: (2016 Update). *Doc Ophthalmol* (2016) 133(1):1–9. doi: 10.1007/s10633-016-9553-y
14. Świerkot M, Kulawik G, Sarnat-Kucharczyk M, Jagoda K, Mrukwa-Kominek E, Chudek J. Long-Term Remission of Steroid-Resistant Graves' Orbitopathy After Administration of Anti-Thymocyte Globulin. *Endokrynol Pol* (2020) 71 (2):198–9. doi: 10.5603/EP.a2019.0067
15. Freitag SK, Tanking T. A Nomenclature to Describe the Sequence of Visual Field Defects in Progressive Thyroid Eye Disease–Compressive Optic Neuropathy (An American Ophthalmological Society Thesis). *Am J Ophthalmol* (2020) 213:293–305. doi: 10.1016/j.ajo.2019.12.005
16. Gulati S, Ueland HO, Haugen OH, Danielsen A, Rødahl E. Long-Term Follow-Up of Patients With Thyroid Eye Disease Treated With Endoscopic Orbital Decompression. *Acta Ophthalmol* (2015) 93(2):178–83. doi: 10.1111/aos.12469
17. Iao TWU, Rong SS, Ling AN, Brelén ME, Young AL, Chong KKL. Electrophysiological Studies in Thyroid Associated Orbitopathy: A Systematic Review. *Sci Rep* (2017) 7(1):1–10. doi: 10.1038/s41598-017-11998-0
18. Labonia AF, Carnovale-Scalzo G, Paola A, De'Morelli G, Scorcia V, Bruzzichessi D, et al. Subclinical Visual Field Alterations are Commonly Present in Patients With Graves' Orbitopathy and are Mainly Related to the Clinical Activity of the Disease. *Exp Clin Endocrinol Diabetes* (2008) 116 (6):347–51. doi: 10.1055/s-2008-1042401

Permissions

All chapters in this book were first published by Frontiers; hereby published with permission under the Creative Commons Attribution License or equivalent. Every chapter published in this book has been scrutinized by our experts. Their significance has been extensively debated. The topics covered herein carry significant findings which will fuel the growth of the discipline. They may even be implemented as practical applications or may be referred to as a beginning point for another development.

The contributors of this book come from diverse backgrounds, making this book a truly international effort. This book will bring forth new frontiers with its revolutionizing research information and detailed analysis of the nascent developments around the world.

We would like to thank all the contributing authors for lending their expertise to make the book truly unique. They have played a crucial role in the development of this book. Without their invaluable contributions this book wouldn't have been possible. They have made vital efforts to compile up to date information on the varied aspects of this subject to make this book a valuable addition to the collection of many professionals and students.

This book was conceptualized with the vision of imparting up-to-date information and advanced data in this field. To ensure the same, a matchless editorial board was set up. Every individual on the board went through rigorous rounds of assessment to prove their worth. After which they invested a large part of their time researching and compiling the most relevant data for our readers.

The editorial board has been involved in producing this book since its inception. They have spent rigorous hours researching and exploring the diverse topics which have resulted in the successful publishing of this book. They have passed on their knowledge of decades through this book. To expedite this challenging task, the publisher supported the team at every step. A small team of assistant editors was also appointed to further simplify the editing procedure and attain best results for the readers.

Apart from the editorial board, the designing team has also invested a significant amount of their time in understanding the subject and creating the most relevant covers. They scrutinized every image to scout for the most suitable representation of the subject and create an appropriate cover for the book.

The publishing team has been an ardent support to the editorial, designing and production team. Their endless efforts to recruit the best for this project, has resulted in the accomplishment of this book. They are a veteran in the field of academics and their pool of knowledge is as vast as their experience in printing. Their expertise and guidance has proved useful at every step. Their uncompromising quality standards have made this book an exceptional effort. Their encouragement from time to time has been an inspiration for everyone.

The publisher and the editorial board hope that this book will prove to be a valuable piece of knowledge for researchers, students, practitioners and scholars across the globe.

List of Contributors

Terry J. Smith
Department of Ophthalmology and Visual Sciences, Kellogg Eye Center, Ann Arbor, MI, United States
Division of Metabolism, Endocrinology, and Diabetes, Department of Internal Medicine, University of Michigan Medical School, Ann Arbor, MI, United States

Zhanjun Mei, Xue Jiang and Yuhong Shi
Department of Nuclear Medicine, The Second Affiliated Hospital of Chengdu Medical College, China National Nuclear Corporation 416 Hospital, Chengdu, China

Wenling Tu
School of Bioscience and Technology, Chengdu Medical College, Chengdu, China
Department of Nuclear Medicine, The Second Affiliated Hospital of Chengdu Medical College, China National Nuclear Corporation 416 Hospital, Chengdu, China

Jia Yao
Research and Development Center, Chengdu SuAn Technology Co., Ltd, Chengdu, China

Xianqun Fan
Department of Ophthalmology, Shanghai Ninth People's Hospital, Shanghai JiaoTong University School of Medicine, Shanghai, China
Shanghai Key Laboratory of Orbital Diseases and Ocular Oncology, Shanghai Ninth People's Hospital, Shanghai JiaoTong University School of Medicine, Shanghai, China

Sijie Fang, Yi Lu and Yazhuo Huang
Department of Ophthalmology, Shanghai Ninth People's Hospital, Shanghai JiaoTong University School of Medicine, Shanghai, China
Shanghai Key Laboratory of Orbital Diseases and Ocular Oncology, Shanghai Ninth People's Hospital, Shanghai JiaoTong University School of Medicine, Shanghai, China
Shanghai Institute of Immunology, Shanghai JiaoTong University School of Medicine, Shanghai, China
Department of Immunology and Microbiology, Shanghai JiaoTong University School of Medicine, Shanghai, China

Irene Campi and Guia Vannucchi
Department of Endocrine and Metabolic Diseases, Istituto Auxologico Italiano IRCCS, Milan, Italy

Elisa Lazzaroni, Martina Dainese, Benedetta Montacchini, Danila Covelli and Mario Salvi
Graves' Orbitopathy Center, Endocrinology, Fondazione IRCCS Cà Granda, Ospedale Maggiore Policlinico Milan, Milan, Italy

Maura Arosio
Graves' Orbitopathy Center, Endocrinology, Fondazione IRCCS Cà Granda, Ospedale Maggiore Policlinico Milan, Milan, Italy
Department of Clinical Sciences and Community Health, University of Milan, Milan, Italy

Ilaria Muller
Graves' Orbitopathy Center, Endocrinology, Fondazione IRCCS Cà Granda, Ospedale Maggiore Policlinico Milan, Milan, Italy
Department of Clinical Sciences and Community Health, University of Milan, Milan, Italy
Division of Infection and Immunity, School of Medicine, Cardiff University, Cardiff, United Kingdom

Nicola Currò
Ophthalmology, Fondazione IRCCS Cà Granda, Ospedale Maggiore Policlinico Milan, Milan, Italy

Claudio Guastella and Lorenzo Pignataro
Otolaryngology, University of Milan and Fondazione IRCCS Cà Granda, Milan, Italy

Laura Fugazzola
Department of Endocrine and Metabolic Diseases, Istituto Auxologico Italiano IRCCS, Milan, Italy
Department of Pathophysiology and Transplantation, University of Milan, Milan, Italy

Luigi Bartalena, Eliana Piantanida, Daniela Gallo, Adriana Lai and Maria Laura Tanda
Endocrine Unit, Department of Medicine and Surgery, University of Insubria, ASST dei Sette Laghi, Varese, Italy

Sen-Hsu Wang and Chia-Chun Wang
Department of Ophthalmology, National Taiwan University Hospital, Taipei, Taiwan

Yi-Hsuan Wei
Department of Ophthalmology, National Taiwan University Hospital, Taipei, Taiwan
Graduate Institute of Clinical Medicine, College of Medicine, National Taiwan University, Taipei, Taiwan

Shu-Lang Liao and Chang-Hao Yang
Department of Ophthalmology, National Taiwan University Hospital, Taipei, Taiwan
Department of Ophthalmology, College of Medicine, National Taiwan University, Taipei, Taiwan

Sita Virakul and Tanapat Palaga
Department of Microbiology, Faculty of Science, Chulalongkorn University, Bangkok, Thailand

Trairak Pisitkun
Center of Excellence in Systems Biology, Research affairs, Faculty of Medicine, Chulalongkorn University, Bangkok, Thailand

Poorichaya Somparn
Center of Excellence in Systems Biology, Research affairs, Faculty of Medicine, Chulalongkorn University, Bangkok, Thailand
Translational Research in Inflammation and Immunology Research Unit (TRIRU), Department of Microbiology, Faculty of Medicine, Chulalongkorn University, Bangkok, Thailand

Peter J. van der Spek
Department of Bioinformatics, Erasmus University Medical Center, Rotterdam, Netherlands

Willem A. Dik
Department of Immunology, Laboratory Medical Immunology, Erasmus University Medical Center, Rotterdam, Netherlands

Virgil A. S. H. Dalm
Department of Immunology, Laboratory Medical Immunology, Erasmus University Medical Center, Rotterdam, Netherlands
Department of Internal Medicine, Division of Clinical Immunology, Erasmus University Medical Center, Rotterdam, Netherlands

P. Martin van Hagen
Department of Immunology, Laboratory Medical Immunology, Erasmus University Medical Center, Rotterdam, Netherlands
Department of Internal Medicine, Division of Clinical Immunology, Erasmus University Medical Center, Rotterdam, Netherlands
Rotterdam Eye Hospital, Rotterdam, Netherlands

Dion Paridaens
Rotterdam Eye Hospital, Rotterdam, Netherlands
Department of Ophthalmology, Erasmus Medical Center, Rotterdam, Netherlands

Nattiya Hirankarn
Center of Excellence in Immunology and Immune Mediated Diseases, Department of Microbiology, Faculty of Medicine, Chulalongkorn University, Bangkok, Thailand

Soma Farag and Karim Meeran
Imperial College School of Medicine, Imperial College London, London, United Kingdom
Department of Metabolism, Digestion and Reproduction, Imperial College London, London, United Kingdom

Claire Feeney
Department of Metabolism, Digestion and Reproduction, Imperial College London, London, United Kingdom
Department of Ophthalmology, The Western Eye Hospital, Imperial College Healthcare National Health Service (NHS) Trust, London, United Kingdom

Sonali Nagendran
Department of Ophthalmology, Central Middlesex Hospital, London North West Healthcare NHS Trust, London, United Kingdom

Rajni Jain and Rashmi Akishar
Department of Ophthalmology, The Western Eye Hospital, Imperial College Healthcare National Health Service (NHS) Trust, London, United Kingdom

Ahmad Aziz
Department of Ophthalmology, The Western Eye Hospital, Imperial College Healthcare National Health Service (NHS) Trust, London, United Kingdom
Department of Ophthalmology, Central Middlesex Hospital, London North West Healthcare NHS Trust, London, United Kingdom
The Western Eye Hospital, Imperial College Healthcare NHS Trust, London, United Kingdom

Grigorios Panagiotou
Department of Acute and Intensive Care Medicine, Northwick Park Hospital, London North West University Healthcare NHS Trust, Harrow, United Kingdom

Petros Perros
Department of Endocrinology, Royal Victoria Infirmary, Newcastle-upon-Tyne, United Kingdom

Mary Kelada
Imperial College School of Medicine, Imperial College London, London, United Kingdom
Department of Metabolism, Digestion and Reproduction, Imperial College London, London, United Kingdom

Parizad Avari and Vassiliki Bravis
Department of Metabolism, Digestion and Reproduction, Imperial College London, London, United Kingdom

Vickie Lee
The Western Eye Hospital, Imperial College Healthcare NHS Trust, London, United Kingdom Department of Ophthalmology, Central Middlesex Hospital, London North West Healthcare NHS Trust, London, United Kingdom Department of Ophthalmology, The Western Eye Hospital, Imperial College Healthcare National Health Service (NHS) Trust, London, United Kingdom

Yan Wang, Xiao-Min Ma and Hong-Song Yu
Department of Immunology, Special Key Laboratory of Ocular Diseases of Guizhou Province, Zunyi Medical University, Zunyi, China

Xin Wang, Xin Sun, Ling-Jun Wang, Xin-Qi Li and Xiao-Yan Liu
School of Basic Medical Sciences, Special Key Laboratory of Gene Detection and Therapy of Guizhou Province, Zunyi Medical University, Zunyi, China

Adriano Naselli, Diletta Moretti, Concetto Regalbuto, Maria Luisa Arpi, Fabrizio Lo Giudice, Francesco Frasca, Antonino Belfiore and Rosario Le Moli
Endocrinology, Department of Clinical and Experimental Medicine, University of Catania, Garibaldi Nesima Medical Center, Catania, Italy

Augustine George, Tanja Diana, Jan Längericht and George J. Kahaly
Molecular Thyroid Research Laboratory, Department of Medicine I, Johannes Gutenberg University (JGU) Medical Center, Mainz, Germany

Poupak Fallahi and Gabriella Cavallini
Department of Translational Research of New Technologies in Medicine and Surgery, University of Pisa, Pisa, Italy

Silvia Martina Ferrari, Giusy Elia, Francesca Ragusa, Sabrina Rosaria Paparo, Armando Patrizio, Stefania Camastra and Mario Miccoli
Department of Clinical and Experimental Medicine, University of Pisa, Pisa, Italy

Salvatore Benvenga
Section of Endocrinology, Department of Clinical and Experimental Medicine, University of Messina, Messina, Italy
Master Program on Childhood, Adolescent and Women's Endocrine Health, University of Messina, Messina, Italy
Interdepartmental Program of Molecular & Clinical Endocrinology, and Women's Endocrine Health, University Hospital, A.O.U. Policlinico Gaetano Martino, Messina, Italy

Alessandro Antonelli
Department of Surgical, Medical and Molecular Pathology and Critical Care, University of Pisa, Pisa, Italy

Giulia Lanzolla, Claudio Marcocci and Michele Marinò
Department of Clinical and Experimental Medicine, Endocrinology Unit II, University of Pisa and University Hospital of Pisa, Pisa, Italy

Yu Wu, Yinwei Li, Jing Sun and Huifang Zhou
Department of Ophthalmology, Shanghai Ninth People's Hospital, Shanghai JiaoTong University School of Medicine, Shanghai, China
Shanghai Key Laboratory of Orbital Diseases and Ocular Oncology, Shanghai Ninth People's Hospital, Shanghai, China

Lei Zhang, Colin Dayan and Marian Ludgate
Thyroid Research Group, Cardiff University School of Medicine, Cardiff, United Kingdom

Mohd Shazli Draman
Thyroid Research Group, Cardiff University School of Medicine, Cardiff, United Kingdom
KPJ Healthcare University College, Nilai, Malaysia

Ga Eun Lee
Yonsei University College of Medicine, Seoul, South Korea

Jinjoo Kim, Jihei Sara Lee, Jae Sang Ko and Jin Sook Yoon
Department of Ophthalmology, Severance Hospital, Institute of Vision Research, Yonsei University College of Medicine, Seoul, South Korea

Eun Jig Lee
Department of Endocrinology, Severance Hospital, Yonsei University College of Medicine, Seoul, South Korea

Benping Zhang, Weijie Xu and Gang Yuan
Department of Endocrinology, Tongji Hospital, Tongji Medical College, Huazhong University of Science and Technology, Wuhan, China

Yaling Li
Department of Critical Care Medicine, Wuhan No.1 Hospital, Wuhan, China

Bei Peng
Department of Endocrinology, Taikang Tongji (Wuhan) Hospital, Wuhan, China

Ran An, Yan Li, Hui Wang and Yanming Xu
Department of Neurology, West China Hospital, Sichuan University, Chengdu, China

Baiyuan Yang
Department of Neurology, West China Hospital, Sichuan University, Chengdu, China
Department of Neurology, Chengdu Seventh People's Hospital, Chengdu, China

Neeraja Boddu, Maliha Jumani and Fred Faas
Endocrinology, University of Arkansas for Medical Sciences, Little Rock, AR, United States

Vibhor Wadhwa and Gitanjali Bajaj
Radiology, University of Arkansas for Medical Sciences, Little Rock, AR, United States

Jueyu Hou, Yunjing Tang and Danian Chen
The Research Laboratory of Ophthalmology and Vision Sciences, State Key Laboratory of Biotherapy, West China Hospital, Sichuan University, Chengdu, China
The Department of Ophthalmology, West China Hospital, Sichuan University, Chengdu, China

Yongjiang Chen
The School of Optometry and Vision Science, University of Waterloo, Waterloo, ON, Canada

Pasqualino Malandrino and Marco Russo
Endocrinology, Department of Clinical and Experimental Medicine, Garibaldi-Nesima Medical Center, University of Catania, Catania, Italy

Riccardo Vigneri
Endocrinology, Department of Clinical and Experimental Medicine, Garibaldi-Nesima Medical Center, University of Catania, Catania, Italy
Institute of Crystallography, Structural Chemistry and Biosystems, CNR-ICCSB, Catania, Italy

Monika Sarnat-Kucharczyk and Ewa Mrukwa-Kominek
Department of Ophthalmology, Faculty of Medical Sciences in Katowice, Medical University of Silesia, Katowice, Poland

Maria Świerkot, Gabriela Handzlik, Grażyna Kulawik, Iga Grochoła-Małecka, Joanna Fryżewska and Jerzy Chudek
Department of Internal Medicine and Oncological Chemotherapy, Faculty of Medical Sciences in Katowice, Medical University of Silesia, Katowice, Poland

Krystyna Jagoda
Department of Hematology and Bone Marrow Transplantation, Faculty of Medical Sciences in Katowice, Medical University of Silesia, Katowice, Poland

Index

O

P

Q

R

S

T

V

www.ingramcontent.com/pod-product-compliance
Lightning Source LLC
LaVergne TN
LVHW081022210926
848485LV00004B/926